A╌╌╌╌ ╌╌╌╌╌╌╌╌╌ MURDOCK'S

THE NEW ART OF DYING

"Like never before, we have the opportunity to create a most personal end-of-life journey. This thoughtful, practical book can help each of us chart the course by which we live and ultimately, die."

—DIANNE GRAY, CEO, HOSPICE AND
HEALTHCARE COMMUNICATIONS, AND PRESIDENT,
ELISABETH KÜBLER-ROSS FOUNDATION

"This down-to-earth book cuts through the rhetoric and hysteria often surrounding issues of dying; it should significantly benefit many families with its sensible, straightforward advice."

—BRUCE C. VLADECK, SENIOR ADVISOR, NEXERA, INC.,
AND FORMER ADMINISTRATOR OF HCFA, NOW CMS

"Without pretense or presumption, this book teaches that amidst medical advancements and legal restrictions there is truly an art to planning a life's end that complements our life journey. Murdock also codeveloped a mHealth app, revolutionizing the communication of our end-of-life wishes."

—CHARLES R. HOFHEIMER, ATTORNEY
AND DIANE HOFHEIMER, MOTHER, DAUGHTER,
GRANDMOTHER, CAREGIVER

The
New Art
of Dying

HOW TO PERSONALIZE

THE MOST IMPORTANT DECISIONS

FOR YOURSELF

AND YOUR LOVED ONES

DIANE BURNSIDE MURDOCK

Developmental editing by Alan Rinzler
Copy editing by Doreen Major-Ryan
Cover and interior design by Ingrid Paulson

Care has been taken to confirm the accuracy of the information
presented. The author and publisher are not responsible
for errors or omissions or for any consequences from application
of the information in this book and make no warranty, expressed or
implied, with respect to the contents of the publication.

The contents provided herein are informational only. Professionals
who are familiar with the medical history or condition of you
or your loved one should confirm any application of principles or
information contained in this manuscript.

The names of individuals have been altered to preserve confidentiality.
Other names are fictional characters created to bring this book to life.
The names of institutions have been changed or otherwise obscured.

The Vermont Ethics Network's Patient Values Questionnaire has been
adapted with permission. Vermont Ethics Network, 61 Elm Street,
Montpelier, VT 05602 802-828-6558, www.vtethicsnetwork.org.

Published 2014 in the United States by
The Murdocks, LLC
Virginia Beach, Virginia
www.dianemurdock.com

Printed in the United States of America.

To Weez, Elwood, Chris, Steve

It is necessary to meditate early, and often,
on the art of dying to succeed later in doing it
properly just once.
—*Umberto Eco*, The Island of the Day Before

CONTENTS

FOREWORD

How we die is significantly affected by many changes in medicine, its practice, and our new longevity. Manuals for the art of dying appeared as early as the fifteenth century, informing the dying about what to expect and prescribing prayers, actions, and attitudes leading to a "good death." With today's many possibilities and choices, a new art of dying is needed. This book is that new guidebook for how to make your dying deeply personal and all about you.

As a physician who worked in hematology and oncology for many years, I had the privilege of working with patients and families as they struggled to make decisions regarding treatments and interventions that might prolong life with little chance of curing. *The New Art of Dying* helps us see the importance of having a plan well in advance of serious illness and not waiting until you are facing death to figure out how you wish to die. This practical book helps you know the ways to communicate your desires for end-of-life care. It makes it possible for you to have those much-needed conversations with family, caregivers, and physicians about how you wish to die and to put these wishes in writing.

There's no "right way" to die, but most people will tell you they'd like to go quickly, peacefully, and with dignity. Some of us know clearly what we want done and what we don't want done when faced with decisions related to dying care. Some can say, in the event of a terminal illness, "I do not want any intervention that will prolong life." Others may say, "I would like everything done to prolong my life for as long as humanly possible." But we don't know what we don't know. *The New Art of Dying* explores those things. It's meticulous and comprehensive in helping you figure out your unique way of dying.

For the rest of us who need to think about it a bit, you will find *The New Art of Dying* is powerful in its description of what we face on a personal and societal level. It gives you an honest look at the medical terrain of dying, allowing you to create an advance care plan that's about you. With a menu of questions, you're guided to take a look at the many aspects of your life and background that affect your approach to death. *The Art of Dying* clearly defines the procedures, treatments, and interventions that are frequently a part of the process of dying and that must be understood if reasoned decisions are to be made about what interventions are desired and for how long.

An important creation that came about in writing this book is a new mobile health app, My Health Care Wishes, that stores and retrieves your advance directives for instant availability on your smartphone whenever and wherever needed. This solves one of the major issues surrounding advance directives, that of having them immediately available in the emergency room or health care setting to convey in writing and in the proper format your wishes for care.

This book presents a down-to-earth, clear, and complete look at the problems you potentially face as you near the end of your time that can get in the way of your dying plan. Through text, examples, and facts, *The New Art of Dying* gives us a new tool that will prove useful to all, and one that promises the development of a unique ever changing plan for dying.

—Elwood Headley, M.D.

PREFACE

In 2008, my good friend Louise Wilson and I became impassioned on the subject of dying and how we die these days. I talked about my Mom, who died of cancer at 64, and the powerful last things a person remembers. How could Mom's dying have been different—better for her and better for us? How is it that when a loved one dies, so many of my friends say, "I don't want that to happen to me?"

Weez, in her 80s, had moved to an independent living place that offered continuing care. To her annoyance, she noticed no one talked about dying. She talked about its inevitability. "Everyone's doing it. Why not know about it?"

I developed this habit of writing about ways of dying on slips of paper and reading them to her. Weez finally turned to me and said, "Where's the book?"

Then my father died. I was flooded with the same questioning that surrounded my Mom's passing. Hadn't I learned anything about dying? I know Dad wouldn't have wanted my brothers and me to feel the way we did about his death—the overwhelming guilt and ruminations. We never did sit with him and talk about his wishes, and I don't think he gave them much thought either. He had a boilerplate advance medical directive that included the words "no extraordinary measures." But what does extraordinary measures mean, and what did it mean to him? Alzheimer's made it too late to have a conversation.

The book began as a catharsis and then was becoming the most incredible advance directive form in the world. But what really nagged me was this central question: If you have a plan and had the talk, what if you aren't getting what you want? What if you're getting unwanted care that equates to wrongful care?

And there are also these facts: Too many of us believe advance directives are for people who are very sick or old. Many of us want to die at home, but few actually do. Only one-third of patients in the ICU have some kind of advance directive. Different people have different ideas about what's best for them.

These facts led me to examine common dying practices in America. I believe there is an art to dying, one where you can feel protected, where your wishes for care are intact. The book grew into and is a study of everything that can go wrong, what you can control and what you can't, and how to get at your attitudes about health care and rethink what you think to get to an advance care plan that's about you and about dying how you wish.

The *ars moriendi*, the art of dying, relates to Latin texts from the early 15th to 18th century offering advice on how to die well. Practical guides informed the dying and family about what to expect, prescribing prayers, actions, and attitudes leading to a good death and salvation. Final hours were made sacred, and last words came to hold a particular place of reverence.

Medicine has made it possible to postpone dying, and families struggle with how and when to accept that the battle is lost. We often panic and insist everything be done, forgetting that dying is all about you, not your illness or treatment.

Some may feel this book displays a bias against expensive, heroic interventions even when the patient wants them. I believe this tension is inherent in discussions of how we die today—how we don't talk about dying, have a plan, or take control of our destiny.

I wrote *The New Art of Dying* as a handbook for our time.

INTRODUCTION

Everyone is doing it. Why not know about it?
—My friend Louise Wilson, b 1921

How would you like to die? How can you help your family and other loved ones to have a death that gives them comfort and support?

Only you can answer this. Each of us has our own feelings, hopes, fears, and desires around this universal issue. These days, dying can happen in many different ways because of high-intensity therapies that prolong life and postpone death. The proliferation of choices, possibilities, and alternatives can be overwhelming. There is no one answer for dying correctly. Each of us wants to get it right and do it our own way.

It's not easy to think about death, whether that of a loved one or ourselves. We instinctively avoid it, don't want to think or talk about it. That's normal human behavior. But we've all heard or experienced painful stories of terror, confusion, useless and expensive extension of hopeless bad health, huge financial losses that lead only to inevitable conclusions. The fact is, these chaotic, passive, and dysfunctional experiences can be eliminated. Yes, we all are going to die, but it doesn't have to be a passive, helpless, out-of-control nightmare. If we prepare and make plans, we can make it more like what we want. Facing the inevitability and figuring out how we want to do it can be a tremendous help for when it happens, for us and those we care for.

That's why I wrote *The New Art of Dying*. It's a constructive and thorough guide to empower you to make your own choices. It is progressive about patient rights, making you the central figure and enabling you to experience dying the way you have experienced life— by being in charge of your own destiny. It's for you only, a continuing reference and source of inspiration.

Your changing attitudes about life influence how you wish to die. How you feel about death and dying at forty may not be the same as when you're seventy-five. I hope this book helps you find consistency with who you are, what you are about, and how to live life to its end. I hope you'll find this a book that you can put down and pick up again over the years as you grow and age and refashion your dying wishes.

—*Diane Murdock, Virginia Beach 2012*

Part 1
Who Are
You?

Who am I? And how, I wonder, will this story end?
—The Notebook, *Nicholas Sparks*

The most important time in your life is not the moment of your death, but the time as it approaches.
—Elisabeth Kübler-Ross, M.D., psychiatrist, hospice pioneer, author of *On Death and Dying*

1

HOW WE DIE

There's no doubt that how we die lives on in those who survive us. We're gone, but those who live on carry our last days with them forever.

It's heartbreaking that so many of us aren't happy or at peace with what happened to a loved one who died recently or even a long time ago. Frequently we hear people express guilt that they couldn't prevent someone's death or help them get through it with less pain and suffering. Others say they feel remorse because they couldn't let a loved one go, and that led to unnecessary suffering and pain. Often those who've lost a loved one are devastated because they decided to "pull the plug" and felt they were on what amounted to their loved one's "death panel."

Such feelings are common. How can we help our loved ones die more peacefully? And how can we plan a better death for ourselves? We can stop such ruminations by knowing who we are and what we believe constitutes a good death. We can have our dying reflect our core values and who we've been all of our lives.

Questions about dying elicit different responses simply because we are different people. For example:

1. Who should take care of you when you approach death? Do you believe that caring for a dying person is the responsibility of those who are closest and most loving, or a difficult burden that should be passed along to a professional caregiver?

2. Do you believe that life should be preserved as long as possible? Do you believe there is always a chance for a miracle, for recovery with a decent quality of existence remaining?

3. How do your own experiences with illness and death impact how you wish to die? Have you lived through difficult end-of-life situations as either a child or adult?

4. What are the specific medical issues you or your loved ones are facing now or may face in the future?

We even give different answers to what family means. Its definition is evolving to include the traditional and nontraditional, extended families, blended families, partners, and close friends. These days, family captures whoever is significant and part of an entourage of special people touching our lives. When you see the word "family" as you read through this book, interpret it as you define it.

Our personal histories make it possible for us to answer these questions. And the answers are uniquely our own. If we ask the right questions and take the time to answer them honestly and thoughtfully, we can get past our apprehensions, blocks, and dreads. Then we can become masters in creating our own peaceful exit.

Most of us are overwhelmed when we face end-of-life choices. It's that tumultuous feeling that it's impossible to know what to do because there are so many facts and so much to know. How can you hope to make the right choices?

It is natural to feel this way. The medical facts are important, but they are only part of the whole. It isn't only about your illness, your treatment, or a procedure, it is about you. It is knowing what you are about that allows you to say, "I am a person with a whole life history behind me who is dying, not just the fragment of myself you see lying here now."

The practice of medicine has changed dramatically in the last century, largely due to technology, and changes in medicine continue to expand at an alarming rate. We find that medical, legal, and moral decisions are intertwined with how we die. We hear of ugly disputes between medical staff and a patient's family on what is or is not to be done for a person. It's as if medical technology is in a face-off with patients' rights.

The fact remains that you do have rights. You can request to be cared for the way you want. You can say what you don't want and decline treatments. You can also ask for everything to be done, but the treatment team may decline treatments it does not consider medically appropriate.

Inevitably, an ill person reaches a point when medical interventions can do little to stave off death and may even prolong the process of dying and cause suffering. If we don't think about dying now, we force those who love and care for us into deliberating and guessing what is best, negotiating about limiting or discontinuing therapies, and deciding whether or not to resuscitate us. These situations are distressing because when death happens, we may believe that it was a direct result of our decision rather than the inevitable outcome of the illness. A wise old woman recently said, "It is my first time growing old and so I haven't had much practice." We are not taught or told how to age. We have to learn the connection between aging and deciding how we wish to die.

Most of us don't talk about dying or plan for serious illness and death until someone dear to us or we ourselves become seriously ill. Morrie Schwartz, the old professor and humanist in Mitch Albom's book *Tuesdays with Morrie,* said: "There's a better approach. To know you're going to die, and to be prepared for it at any time. That's better."

2

....

EXPERIENCES
AND EXPECTATIONS

One thing is certain. There is a range of individual expectations and experiences about dying. We often find ourselves saying, "When death comes, the lucky among us will go out peacefully with dignity." But is it really about luck? Many of us have heard of end-of-life situations involving family members, neighbors, or people in the news. They evoke powerful images and lessons for handling difficult aspects of the end of our journey. Some deaths escalate from merely bad to ugly. Others are more peaceful.

It's true different people want different care. But the stories we hear tell us that we often don't know what outlooks we have about health care and how these attitudes have everything to do with how we die. We don't know how to take stock of ourselves to make better end-of-life decisions.

Because we are built from our experiences, the following questions are designed to help you explore who you are and how this applies to dying. To get started you can select from the menu, picking and choosing among the various topics.

There is no set order; this allows you to construct a personalized tool for determining what was ingrained in you by family, friends, religion, community, and experiences. It requires reflecting on your concerns, distresses, beliefs, fears, tolerances, limits, and spiritual needs. It gets at what's behind your choices you may have considered so far, such as your feelings about living wills and do-not-resuscitate (DNR) orders.

Clearly, you are not born knowing yourself, and you don't get to know yourself simply by getting older. However, answering these questions can help. This customized tool can guide your thinking and help you look at areas where you might want to change your opinions or tailor health care wishes to be in line with who you are now.

Not knowing yourself becomes problematic sooner or later. Some of the stories on dying we've heard about or experienced show this. But sad endings aren't just about ignoring dying. They are about ignoring yourself.

What's more, your needs, values, and understanding of these things change, as does your appreciation of quality of life, as you grow older. Keep coming back then to these questions, because your wishes for care change as you age and change.

Give yourself time to rethink what you think. You are building your own profile and over time, your profile will change.

Think of these questions as ones to look over while at your kitchen table with a cup of coffee, sitting with someone you are close to, and talking about the sorts of issues that surround health care and dying. Get a sense of why you feel the way you do, what's behind your attitudes toward health care, how these views are shaped, and how they apply to dying and creating an advance care plan.

FAMILY BACKGROUND AND ETHNICITY

▸ Do your family background, ethnicity, and inter-relationships affect how you see illness, health care, and dying?

▸ Does anything in your background influence whom you believe should care for you when you approach death?

▸ Do your views on end-of-life care and death and dying also pertain to a religion? Particular customs? Rituals? Family traditions?

▸ Did you grow up feeling restrained or uncomfortable asking questions about health and illness with your doctor or other physicians and health care professionals?

▸ Were you raised to believe that it's best to keep personal issues to yourself? Were you taught to withhold or hide your emotions?

RELIGIOUS BELIEFS AND SPIRITUALITY

▸ What role does religion, spirituality, and philosophy play when seriously ill or dying?

▸ Do you believe life should always be preserved as long as possible?

▸ For you, is it permissible to use life support to save and extend life?

▸ Do you believe that at some point, aggressive medical intervention to maintain life can interfere with the will of God or some higher power? The natural course of life and death?

PAST EXPERIENCES

▸ Do you feel that life history lessons, what is instilled in you and your actions or reactions to them, carry over in deciding what care you want at end of life?

▸ Have your views of dying care been shaped by your experiences with aging and illness?

▸ How does your attitude toward past medical experiences carry over to decision making regarding end-of-life care?

- Did past experiences with death and dying affect your thoughts about your own mortality?

VALUES

- What beliefs or values should those making medical decisions for you consider if you are unable to speak for yourself?

- What is important in your life? Walking? Eating? Thinking clearly? Traveling? Communicating with others? Living independently?

- Would you feel that life would still be worth living if you were unable to enjoy some or most of these things? Why or why not?

- How much are you willing to compromise on who you are to postpone dying?

CURRENT SITUATION

- Do you feel responsible for the welfare of your family? Financially? Emotionally? Do you feel that your family would fall apart without you?

- Do you feel that your education and areas of study impact your decisions about what care you want when dying? How easy it is for you to communicate with health care professionals? To understand what they are saying?

- Does your career and what you do influence your thinking about how to die? About whether you can die the way you want?

FAMILY

- What was your family like? Was it close? Estranged? A blended family? Biracial?

- What is your family like now?

- Are you concerned you can't get good care because you can't speak English? Because of your ethnicity? Because you're gay?

- Are you without family? Have you outlived your family?

- Who can help you talk through these concerns? Who is it safe to talk to about these issues?

- Have you thought about the implications of close relationships and strong support systems for the kind of care you envision when dying?

- Does your immediate family live nearby? How does this affect the potential for family support?

COST OF CARE

- Do you worry about the cost of health care when very sick or near the end of life?

► Should financial considerations influence decisions about your medical care? Should cost be a factor in the care wanted or given?

► Do you feel that having money gives you opportunities for better health care at end of life?

► Do you feel entitled to all the care you want, even at end of life?

► Would you want to be asked, "Can you afford this?"

CURRENT ATTITUDES ON DYING

► What care do you feel you deserve when dying? How would you define the best care possible?

► Do you want to concentrate on comfort and peace, or on efforts to extend life?

► Do you feel you would keep fighting as death nears? That your family should do the same for you?

► How important is "allowing nature to take its course"? Is it acceptable? Is allowing nature to take its course giving up?

ATTITUDES ON LIFE-SUSTAINING TREATMENT

► Do you believe it's a personal choice to fight all the way to the end with the most aggressive possible care?

► Is there a limit to what you feel should be done medically to save a life?

- Would you be hesitant to forgo treatments? Do you equate this with giving up?

- Once a person is on life support, it is wrong to withdraw it? When is it permissible to withdraw care?

- Do you believe withholding treatment is the same as withdrawing treatment? Do you perceive withdrawing treatment as more problematic than withholding?

- Would your approach to accepting or rejecting care depend on how old you were at the time of treatment?

ATTITUDES ON MEDICAL AID IN DYING

- Do you think it's right for a terminally ill person to take control of their own destiny and ingest medications that end their life?

- Is physician-assisted suicide or assisted dying something you would consider? What if you were suffering a painful dying experience? Is it allowed or prohibited by the religion you follow?

- Have you ever known someone who hastened his or her own death?

- Do you approve of mercy killing (active euthanasia) or suicide if terminally ill? Diagnosed with Alzheimer's? Is it prohibited by your beliefs?

ATTITUDES ON WHERE TO DIE

► Where do you wish to be as you approach the end of life? Does this matter to you as long as your loved ones are with you?

► Do you feel that the best place to die depends on your care needs and available support, costs, and admission criteria?

► Would you do everything possible to fight your disease, even if it meant spending more time in the hospital? Would you consider hospice?

► Would you like to die at home? If so, is there any way you could?

Part 2
What Are Your Choices?

Before the light in my mind faded and the shadows lengthened too much for me to see anymore, I chose at least, at last, to be master of my farewell.
—*Eugene O'Kelly*, Chasing Daylight

Every day thousands of people across the country are experiencing the wrong kind of final chapter— needlessly painful, fruitlessly prolonged, dehumanizing and undignified.
—*Stephen Kiernan*, Last Rights

All of us deal with dying in our own unique way. Our decisions for end-of-life care are certainly our own. But the choices we make about death and dying are complicated and bring into play life-sustaining treatments and procedures, palliative care, and legal documents on advance care planning. You can think about your life and what it means in the context of its end, but how do you make decisions for approaching death if you don't know your choices?

The next sections describe high-intensity therapies for life support, palliative care for managing pain and suffering, and legal documents available for stating health care wishes. Getting to know these therapies and treatments and how they may affect your exit is key to protecting your rights as a patient. This knowledge will ultimately help you express wishes that are consistent with who you are and define your specific advance medical directive.

In an ideal world your wishes would be known, understood, and honored, and you would die surrounded by your loved ones. But imagining a peaceful death won't just make it happen. You have to tell your family what you want and put it in writing.

3

MEDICAL CHOICES

The treatments and techniques we can either select or decline fall into two basic categories: life supporting and life sustaining. It's important to know the difference.

Life-supporting interventions literally keep us alive when we are in critical condition by supporting basic life functions, such as providing blood, food, and oxygen. They stop bleeding, fight infection, remove toxins, provide antidotes to poison, remove ruptured or infected organs, and relieve pain. Life-supporting interventions comprise these treatments when applied in an emergency situation in which recovery is expected.

Life-sustaining interventions comprise these same treatments when used to support life in a situation in which recovery is unlikely. It is often said that in this circumstance, the interventions prolong dying rather than sustain life.

These terms are generally used interchangeably, regardless of the clinical situation. But it's important to make a distinction at times when it may not be desirable to begin life-supporting treatments in patients with terminal illnesses like cancer, chronic pulmonary disease, dementia, or congestive heart failure in the end stages.

Beginning these interventions requires careful thought if you have a serious, perhaps terminal illness, because while effective in keeping you alive, they are not intended to treat the underlying illness. They don't fix what's seriously wrong. This emphasizes the need to know what life-supporting treatments are about, what they do and don't do, when they are required, and when they are beneficial or detrimental.

Life-supporting care is designed to keep you alive. It includes treatments, devices, and medications to keep your heart pumping (cardiopulmonary resuscitation [CPR], defibrillation), help you breathe (mechanical ventilation, intubation), give you food and water (intravenous [IV] hydration, IV nutrition, feeding tube), get rid of bacterial infections (antibiotics), and clean your body of toxins (renal dialysis). Usually, life-support treatments take place initially in the ICU and sometimes in the ER, and they then can be shifted to other settings.

These procedures are aggressive, and the outcome can be uncertain. They stabilize a critical situation. They may be painful physically and emotionally, and they often expose a patient to risks of additional medical complications. Life-supporting treatments:

1. Sustain vital signs by keeping your heart beating, keeping your lungs moving to bring in and exhale air, and maintaining blood pressure in a normal range
2. Provide treatment for any life-threatening condition that may be present or arise
3. Provide comfort from pain
4. Allow time for a cure, if it is possible

Deciding to forgo a particular treatment is generally based on the belief that the burdens of the treatment outweigh the potential benefits, but an individual's hopes, values, and history are a big part of the decision process, if not the biggest part.

Who is more apt to face these choices? There's the frail elderly, for whom there is really no single thing that is seriously wrong; they simply are failing, and their medical needs are more demanding. There are patients burdened by accumulated pains and disabilities from illnesses and the side effects of treatments. And there are those with end-stage medical conditions, advanced illness, or chronic conditions that can't be cured or reversed.

What follows are descriptions of life-support therapies to help make sense of what our choices are.

WHAT IF MY HEART STOPS?

Cardiopulmonary resuscitation (CPR) is a treatment for cardiac arrest (cardiopulmonary arrest or circulatory arrest) when the normal circulation of blood stops because the heart failed to contract effectively. Cardiac arrest is different from a heart attack, in which blood flow to the muscle of the heart is impaired, but it may be caused by a heart attack.

With cardiac arrest, the lack of a beating heart to provide blood circulation prevents delivery of oxygen to the body, and the lack of oxygen to the brain causes loss of consciousness and abnormal or absent breathing. This is serious because brain injury is likely if cardiac arrest isn't reversed within five minutes. Immediate and decisive treatment—CPR—is imperative for the best chance of survival and neurological recovery.

Most of us know CPR is the process of blowing air into a patient's mouth and pressing on a patient's chest, called basic life support. But CPR involves more than cardiac compression and mouth-to-mouth resuscitation. It can require insertion of a breathing tube (endotracheal intubation), use of IV medications (advanced cardiac life support), and electric shock (defibrillation). If the heartbeat is restored but the patient is still not breathing, a ventilator may be used.

CPR can save lives, but because it is aggressive and can cause painful injuries such as fractured ribs and punctured lungs, CPR sometimes offers more risks or harm than benefits, especially to those seriously ill and not expected to recover.

WHAT IF I STOP BREATHING?

Mechanical ventilation is a method to assist or replace spontaneous normal breathing. This involves a breathing machine called a ventilator (respirator) that performs one of the most complex functions of the body, the inhaling of oxygen and exhaling of carbon dioxide. A ventilator helps people breathe when breathing is difficult or they can't breathe on their own.

The ventilator provides air to the lungs using a tube inserted through the mouth (endotracheal intubation), the nose, or a hole in the throat (tracheostomy or trach). There are several methods of ventilation ranging from noninvasive to long-term invasive with a trach. Many patients can be taken off a ventilator, but some have little or no chance of breathing without its assistance and must continue to use one for the rest of their life.

Whether or not to start mechanical ventilation is one of the most controversial areas of life support, because once started, it's complicated to stop. Generally it's easier to decide to use ventilation in situations that appear reversible, with problems that may be expected to correct with treatment over time. Used appropriately, ventilation is a godsend. In other situations, its use is viewed as a "crossing the Rubicon" event, passing a point of no return.

Mechanical ventilation is what the medical world calls an *invasive procedure*. Invasive procedures enter the body by cutting or puncturing the skin or inserting instruments into a body orifice for diagnosis or treatment. We don't think of such routine procedures as colonoscopy or Pap smears as invasive, but they are. Life-supporting treatments such as intubation, IVs, and tracheostomy are also invasive. And major surgical procedures dealing with an acute, serious complication are invasive too.

What's necessary and actually required before any invasive procedure is a discussion between you or your family and the doctor about why it's being recommended, what's the expected outcome and benefit, and whether the proposed procedure improves your chance of survival and/or quality of life. It's your choice whether to have an invasive procedure, but either way, you or your proxy must sign an informed consent.

IV lines are the most effective way to deliver fluids (hydration and nutrition) and medications for infections (antibiotics) and pain. IV devices can be used for drawing blood for testing (phlebotomy), and the only way to give blood transfusions is intravenously. Intravenous means "within a vein."

Some terms you may hear referring to IVs are:

1. A *drip*, which is just another way of saying IV therapy or IV administration of liquid substances directly into a vein.

2. *Lining them up,* which is the placement of multiple tubes either into a vein in the hand, arm, foot, or scalp (peripheral IV line) or into a vein in the neck, chest, or groin that feeds to the heart (central IV line).

3. A *peripherally inserted central catheter (PICC), port,* or *tunneled catheter/IV,* which refers to types of central IV lines in which a catheter is inserted directly into one of the major large veins of the body.

4. *Arterial catheterization lines* (art-lines or a-lines) which can only be used in the ICU. A catheter is inserted into an artery at the wrist (or possibly the forearm near the elbow, the groin, or the foot) to monitor blood pressure.

If you intend to say no to IV lines, catheters, or IV needles no matter what's administered, consider not being transported to a hospital from home or a nursing facility. This is a big decision and deeply personal, one only you can make.

WHAT IF I NEED FLUIDS OR NUTRITION?

Administration of artificial hydration (IV hydration) is about delivering fluids when a person is unable to drink enough liquid, take water by mouth, or swallow properly. An IV can be used for as little as a few hours to provide fluids to a patient during a short surgical procedure or to rehydrate a patient who is dehydrated from any cause. It may provide fluid when a person can no longer drink, but it cannot supply the nutrition needed to stay alive.

Keep in mind that dehydration is a normal part of the dying process in patients confronting terminal illness. This dehydration is a result of decreased intake of liquids combined with the disease itself. While dehydration is common at the end of life, thirst and hunger are not. Using IV hydration can prolong dying. But even if IV fluids improve hydration, the sensation of thirst and dry mouth might persist, possibly as a side effect from medications for pain, blood pressure, and nausea. Some comforting things to relieve these symptoms are moistening the lips and swabbing the inside of the mouth.

Administration of artificial nutrition or IV nutrition is "feeding" a person intravenously, bypassing the usual process of eating and digesting. Typically, IV nutrition is a short-term measure given to patients who can't consume enough nutrients or who can't eat due to an illness, surgery, or accident. But many at the end of life may refuse to eat because they no longer have the urge or desire. There are two types of IV nutrition:

- *Partial parenteral nutrition (PPN)*, given temporarily and short term, replaces some daily required nutrients and supplements oral intake. PPN is administered via a small tube (a catheter) inserted into a vein in the lower part of the arm.
- *Total parenteral nutrition (TPN)*, given for an extended period, is for a patient who cannot eat and must receive all required nutrients daily. TPN is adminis-

tered through a PICC inserted into a central vein closer to the heart, under the collarbone. TPN is definitely more invasive than PPN and should call attention to an escalation in the level of care.

Complications resulting from IV nutrition include bacterial infections, which require administration of antibiotics, and liver dysfunction associated with prolonged TPN.

Is IV nutrition always a good thing? And can't this question be asked about any life-sustaining treatments? Maybe Morrie Schwartz, the professor in *Tuesdays with Morrie,* can help to answer this: "Don't let go too soon, but don't hang on too long." We can die our own way, but our experience rests on decisions such as whether to start, stop, or continue IV nutrition. There are some like Dr. Stanley A. Terman, author of *The Best Way to Say Goodbye*, whose advice to those who wish to avoid prolonged, unnecessary end-of-life suffering is to exercise the legal peaceful choice of voluntary refusal of food and fluids.

Consoling words shared by Ira Byock, a physician specializing in palliative care and the author of *Dying Well*, are also worth repeating: "Dying of a progressive inability to eat is probably one of the most natural and physiologically gentle ways to expire. In the context of advanced illness, hunger is rarely, if ever, a source of discomfort. The same is true with thirst."

WHAT IF I CAN'T SWALLOW?

A *feeding tube* is a life-sustaining intervention in which a tube is placed in the gastrointestinal tract to provide nutrition and/or fluids for those who no longer can take food or water by mouth. Tube feeding may be temporary for the treatment of acute conditions or lifelong in the case of chronic disabilities. There are a variety of feeding tubes. For short-term feeding and nutrition, a tube (nasogastric or NG-tube) is passed through the nostrils down the esophagus and into the stomach. For the long term, a tube can be inserted directly into the stomach (a gastric feeding tube, G-tube, or button) or the intestines (percutaneous endoscopic gastrostomy or PEG tube).

But when do you need a feeding tube? Only when you either have difficulty swallowing (dysphagia) or just can't swallow at all. A PEG doesn't fix this, but it can provide the time needed for someone to heal and swallow properly again. For patients with multiple conditions, especially those with advanced dementia, recovering the ability to swallow is unlikely, and a PEG provides them the nourishment they need to live.

Tube feeding provides needed nutrition and allows nutrients to enter the stomach when there's difficulty swallowing, and it prevents aspiration, the inhalation of food or fluids into the lungs related to impaired swallowing. But it doesn't prevent saliva and stomach contents from coming back up into the esophagus (reflux), and patients may still develop aspiration pneumonia. A feeding tube can be a good thing, but it can't fix all problems.

WHAT IF I HAVE A
LIFE-THREATENING INFECTION?

Antibiotics are a life-sustaining treatment for an infection such as pneumonia or urinary tract infection. They are powerful medicines that fight bacterial infections and, used properly, can save lives. Penicillin and streptomycin are examples of antibiotics.

Seriously ill individuals often develop life-threatening infections requiring antibiotics, which commonly cause side effects such as diarrhea, fever, nausea, and rash. With frequent use of antibiotics comes the effect of overuse. In the process of continually fighting infections in a patient, different and more serious strains of bacteria may surface, resistant to one antibiotic after another. Many patients in hospitals or nursing homes develop methicillin-resistant Staphylococcus aureus (MRSA), which is difficult to treat. There are times when no antibiotic can combat the infection and death occurs.

While antibiotics treat an infection, they do not necessarily improve a patient's underlying condition or quality of life. For example, patients with advanced Alzheimer's are at risk of pneumonia because food swallowed goes down the wrong pipe and into the lungs (aspiration pneumonia). Antibiotics help with the pneumonia, but they don't cure the Alzheimer's or the swallowing problem that led to the pneumonia in the first place.

If care is futile you can stop antibiotics, permit a natural death, and switch to palliative sedation. If you don't want antibiotics, you may want to consider not going to see a doctor or transferring to a hospital, because either implies you want something done, and that's a mixed message.

WHAT IF MY KIDNEYS STOP WORKING?

Renal dialysis is a life-sustaining treatment for people whose kidneys stop working. Renal dialysis removes toxins and excess fluid from your blood, a function normally performed by the kidneys. A majority of dialysis patients are given hemodialysis, where a line is made into an artery and a vein (a shunt) and connected to the dialysis machine. This machine becomes an artificial kidney through which the patient's blood is pumped and impurities removed, a process that typically takes several hours and is done several times a week. Patients can be maintained on chronic hemodialysis for years or for life.

Dialysis can be a temporary measure for someone recovering from an illness or waiting for a kidney transplant, or a permanent one if a transplant is not an option. Kidney failure is a relatively common complication in seriously ill individuals and can be fatal. When kidney failure is only a small part of a patient's declining health, dialysis fails to alter the big picture. Here again, you have to ask, what's accomplished? Why undergo dialysis when it's fixing only one of many grave problems and illnesses?

In the presence of such serious conditions, David Feldman and Andrew Lasher (*The End of Life Handbook*) tell us, "Passing away from kidney failure is peaceful. Patients usually become sleepier and lapse into a coma...."

WHAT IF I HAVE CANCER AND TIME GROWS SHORT?

Chemotherapy and *radiation therapy* can cause cancer to go into remission or deter its progress. These therapies may slow down the progression of the cancer and give pain relief to a dying patient who is terminally ill, even in the end stages of cancer, when treatments have become ineffective. There are some health care professionals who object to high-dose chemotherapy for cancer patients who have failed one or more protocols when an expected death is thought to be within hours or days, considering such treatment as too aggressive.

When deciding whether or not to have such treatments near the end of life, weigh the anticipated benefits versus the side effects, or simply whether it will make you feel better rather than make you better. Ask the question "Is this right for me?" And if necessary, be assertive with an oncologist to stop treatment.

4

PALLIATIVE CARE CHOICES

WHAT IS PALLIATIVE CARE?

Palliative care centers on treating symptoms of an illness rather than on the underlying disease. Palliative care doesn't mean do not treat, but rather treat all symptoms as aggressively as possible so that the patient and family are relieved of stress and discomfort, either during the course of an illness or in the final stages.

As Dr. Diane Meier, a leader in the field of palliative care and the recipient of a MacArthur Foundation "genius award," asserts, "The single most important message is that palliative care is a concurrent care mode, delivered at the same time as all other appropriate therapies whether the goal is cure, life prolongation, or achieving a peaceful death." Palliative care can be appropriate at any stage of an illness and at any age if a serious illness is present.

Many believe palliative care is an alternative to life-sustaining therapies, a way to avoid multiple admissions to the hospital, lengthy stays in the ICU, and daily regimens of vitals taken, fingers poked, catheters inserted, and IVs administered. They see palliative care as a way to avoid burdensome transitions, transfers, or multiple hospitalizations in the last few days of life.

These impressions are partially true, but palliative care is absolutely not a replacement for medical care. Think of palliative care as a blanket term covering the care associated with relieving suffering, managing and alleviating pain and stress, and addressing other debilitating symptoms that result from an illness. Hospice and comfort care are pieces of this blanket. This section clarifies what palliative care is about so you can fully understand and appreciate palliative care choices.

All good clinicians provide elements of palliative care, but a formal palliative care specialist or team is most often utilized in chronic or incurable illnesses with intractable symptoms. Palliative care providers work with specialists treating the underlying disease.

The palliative care team consists of physicians, nurses, nurse practitioners, social workers, psychologists, chaplains, and therapists, all of whom are specialists, not in attempting to cure disease, but rather in attempting to alleviate symptoms both in the patient and their loved ones. Symptoms may be physical, such as pain or shortness of breath, or they may be emotional, spiritual, or financial.

One of the most important aspects of palliative care is relief of pain. In this day and age, there's virtually no reason why a person in the advanced stage of any illness should suffer from pain. The Joint Commission, an organization that accredits health care organizations, places great emphasis on adequate pain management in the care of patients. It has identified pain as one of the vital signs, measurements of the body's most basic functions, along with body temperature, pulse rate, rate of breathing, and blood pressure.

There are effective medications for pain relief called opioids, ranging from oral medications like Percocet or Vicodin to IV administration of drugs like Demerol and morphine. There are also drugs with excellent sedative properties that, when administered with analgesics, can enhance the relief of pain and control nausea, a side effect of narcotic administration.

One of the most recent advances in management of pain is self-administered IV pain medication. The patient pushes a button to deliver medication by a programmable pump when experiencing discomfort but can't take an overdose. When considering advanced stages of illness, there's no real concern regarding addiction or abuse, and adequate analgesia (pain medication) should be provided. This is true for all patients, whether in a formal palliative care program, receiving active medical care for any illness with pain as a significant component, or in comfort care.

For now, palliative care programs are not universally available, but accessibility is improving. You can find out if they are available in your area by contacting your local hospital. Palliative care is a force for shifting care for those with serious illnesses away from hospitalization and medicalization to the home and community, coordinating across care settings and giving support in coping with curative treatments or the final stages of a terminal illness.

WHAT'S THE DIFFERENCE BETWEEN PALLIATIVE AND HOSPICE CARE?

Hospice care is end-of-life palliative care for those diagnosed with a terminal illness and expected to live for six months or less. The underlying illness is not treated and vital signs are usually not taken. Hospice care can be provided for patients with a variety of terminal conditions including cancer, renal disease, end-stage dementias, and degenerative diseases such as ALS (amyotrophic lateral sclerosis or Lou Gehrig's disease), congestive heart failure, and chronic obstructive pulmonary disease.

Eligibility and acceptance for hospice must be determined before a patient can be admitted to the program. If time is short or the patient and family are undecided about hospice, a "bridge" program or comfort care may be the answer. Some home health agencies, with or without hospital affiliation, have established prehospice bridge programs staffed by hospice nurses, and some hospice agencies are considering such programs.

Hospice care can be provided in the home, in freestanding hospice care facilities, in skilled nursing facilities, or in dedicated units in inpatient hospitals. Hospice services provide everything necessary for patient comfort and family support including medications to control pain, nausea, and constipation; skin care; medical supplies and equipment; medical and social services; and bereavement counseling for family members.

Some patients and family members believe that the use of medications in palliative care hastens death. They feel that in the effort to manage a terminally ill patient's pain, the necessary dosage may unintentionally shorten the patient's life. In bioethics, this is an example of the principle of double effect. There is little evidence validating this view, but such thinking can lead to undertreatment of pain in the dying patient.

There are obviously different feelings toward qualifying for hospice services. I found some people are skittish about taking the legal steps necessary to admit a loved one or themselves to hospice, believing it signals that you or your family is giving up. They don't want these services, even with pain and life growing short. They want to continue with medical interventions with the hope for a cure or a miracle. Others believe that hospice care is best if there is no hope of recovery. Think about what hospice means to you. Think about the kind of dying you believe fits your care wishes.

Here's a story my friend Charlie shared with me about how hospice care allowed his Mom to die at home and without pain.

The situation with my Mom was pretty amazing. Her mother lived to be ninety-five and her father, eighty-five. She always thought she'd live longer. Mom's philosophical orientation to life and dying basically was framed around not fighting reality. She said, "This is what's happening and this is what we will do." She said she had had a wonderful life and no one was to be sad for her.

At eighty-six she felt she wanted to move to an independent/continuous care facility while she was still healthy enough to build a social network. She found a perfect place near where she grew up and where her brother and her daughter, my sister Cynthia, lived. She was on a waiting list for one year. She made the final payment in December 2009 and was to greet the New Year by moving in.

But then everything changed. Mom had been diagnosed with breast cancer in 2005 but it had been in remission for the past four years. Now, right before the big move she had planned and paid for, the cancer was back and had traveled from her breast to her liver. The drugs did not control it anymore; they weren't effective. She said yes when more drug cocktails were proposed to hold things at bay even though she was told she only had three to six months to live.

She didn't fight the process. She accepted it.

She decided to stay in her home in Alabama. She had enough money to hire staff to come and be with her during the day until early evening and then she'd go to bed. She stopped driving and let the caregivers take her wherever she needed to go. Our family took turns coming into town.

It was now the end of July, and her doctor said she was not responding to the latest treatment. Hospice was requested. She called her children together and all came to spend precious time with her, including her great granddaughter.

Cynthia and I were with her the last week of her life. During that week she said, "I'm ready to die."

I said, "They don't teach us how to do that, do they?"

Cynthia said, "Mom, maybe you're not ready to go. Are you hungry?"

She said, "Yes."

"Do you want some ice cream?"

"Why yes, I do."

She was sharp and totally cognizant close to the end; she really had no pain until the last couple of days. Morphine was given. She slept a lot. Mom passed away on August 17, 2010. She gave us so much peace with what she said and how she died.

WHAT DOES COMFORT CARE MEAN?

Comfort care was a popular term before palliative care was introduced and is still a commonly used term in health care to indicate palliative care that is aimed not at treating the underlying condition but rather at alleviating symptoms and making the patient comfortable. It's generally known to mean dying care for patients who are not yet ready or eligible for hospice, or who are referred too late. Comfort care changes the focus from curing illness to caring for the dying, and the patient most likely returns home or goes to a nursing facility. Because the term is used loosely, comfort care is also seen as the intention of hospice care.

Comfort care may refer to a more narrowly defined life expectancy than hospice care. Some health care professionals use "comfort care" to refer to care provided to patients when they are expected to die within hours to days; it alerts medical staff that efforts should be made to bring as much symptomatic care as possible to the patient and avoid activities that may bring discomfort such as blood drawing, frequent vital signs, or other tests or procedures.

Another interpretation held by physicians is that comfort care means the health care team places the patient's comfort above everything else; treatment can still continue if the patient or family wishes, as long as the patient is comfortable. It's probably a good idea to ask the medical staff for clarification on how they are using the term.

I include Minnie's story as an example of comfort care, honoring your loved one's wishes, strength of family, and dying naturally at home.

I'm the oldest of six raised by Granma. When Granma became gravely ill, she asked to be taken care of at home surrounded by all of us. The family didn't want that. We didn't like the idea of hospice because to us, it meant giving up. It didn't feel right. It wasn't right.

But dying at home is what she grew up expecting and you didn't argue with Granma. We all rallied around her and her wishes including the congregation and neighbors to make her comfortable. We chose not to go and seek out hospice care.

We told her that we never wanted her to go and she didn't want to leave us either. She was our rock. She was what grew us into family and held us together.

One day I could tell she was ready. I found myself leaning over and whispering, "We will be okay, Granma, you can go now." It was the words she needed to hear. I saw her die in peace; I saw her go to heaven.

I understand now why Granma wanted to die at home. It was our place of love. It's where we belong. I sometimes go into her room and lie down in her bed and think: Granma taught me how to live. She has taught me how to die.

5

....

LEGAL CHOICES

What forms should you complete to let family and health care professionals know how you want to live the end of your life? What are the legal choices available to state your medical choices, your advance care plans?

WHAT IS ALL THIS PAPERWORK?

There are a number of forms you'll come across dealing with your health care when you can't speak for yourself, and these forms cover basically three things:

1. Telling people who gets to make medical decisions for you
2. Telling people what to do for you
3. Having a physician order the care you want

These three things refer to advance medical directives that tell your loved ones and health care professionals what you want for care. If you do these forms right, you don't have to worry about anything else. That's a big statement, I know, but I believe it is true. But it requires knowing yourself and your medical and legal choices, and it requires your loved ones knowing and understanding your choices.

You may already know about legal forms covering life-sustaining treatments and end-of-life decisions. Living wills and DNRs have been around since the 1970s, and health care power of attorney (HCPOA) or health care proxy documents since the 1980s. But you may not be acquainted with a form created in 1991, the physician orders for life-sustaining treatment (POLST), a comprehensive end-of-life medical order. *Advance care planning* is the catchall term for facilitating the idea of expressing your care wishes in advance about medical situations or emergencies in writing and in discussions with those you love. Advance medical directives are the forms and documents.

Charles Sabatino, Director of the American Bar Association's Commission on Law and Aging, said, "The document is only worth the discussion it's based on." Yes, you need to know yourself, what you hold dear, and how your beliefs tie to your wishes about how you die. And you certainly should know about life-sustaining treatments and palliative care. But knowing all this doesn't count for much if you don't talk with loved ones about it all and put it down on paper.

Why the urgency to use these forms and resort to such methods for communicating wishes? They exist so individuals like you and me can record our wishes for care when seriously ill and at the end of life, when we're unable to speak for ourselves.

The stories of Karen Ann Quinlan and Terri Schiavo, important figures in the right to die controversy in the United States, tell us more. Their stories are disturbing, but they show how something so private and personal became so loudly and publicly debated.

Karen Quinlan was left in a coma after ingesting drugs and alcohol in 1975 at twenty-one years of age. Shortly afterwards, she was removed from a ventilator and lived nine more years with artificial nutrition and hydration before infection and pneumonia killed her in 1985. In 1990, Terri Schiavo entered into a persistent vegetative state after having a cardiac arrest at twenty-six, and a fifteen-year saga of disputes began. She required no ventilator, dialysis, or other life-sustaining equipment except a PEG for seven years starting in 1998. She died in 2005 when the PEG was removed.

Neither woman had an advance directive, and that's still true for many of us. That fact alone prompted legal battles among family members, medical professionals, and even elected officials over what these women's wishes were, what their values were, and what really was the right thing to do for them. Personal choices about dying became furious public debate about human rights and limiting medical treatment.

If you don't have a plan, it's not likely your end of life will be publicized nationally or spark a legal case with such public scrutiny, but your care is more likely to be questioned by family members and medical staff, and family discord and confusion are conceivable. We should have end-of-life conversations—open, honest discussions with family—because how can you expect your wishes to be followed otherwise? It's not easy, but talking about dying and writing your wishes down is how you avoid the disquieting repercussions evident in the stories of Karen Quinlan and Terri Schiavo.

A tough concept to grasp about advance care planning is that your wishes for care are projected into the future but are based on who you are now. How in the world can you make these documents relevant? It helps to think of advance care planning as something legal and organic (living), changing as you change and evolving as you grow older, expressing something different from what was stated in its original form.

That's why an ongoing conversation with family is important. That's why your stated or written care decisions need to be turned over in your mind regularly and renewed. Decisions most likely would change as you change with every decade that goes by, with a serious diagnosis, a divorce, a death of a loved one, or a physical or psychological decline. Advance care planning forms can be amended or replaced at any time and should be. What care you'd want at thirty is different from what you'd want at sixty or eighty. And if your plans are so broad in scope that the need to update them seems immaterial, you may want to open up and talk about what you are or are not communicating.

WHAT ABOUT ACCESSIBILITY?

If you haven't created an advance care plan, then it's not available during an emergency because it doesn't exist! But even if you have, there's no guarantee that it will be available and respected. Availability at the time of an emergency and in the ER is rare. This is a critical barrier to your plan for dying as you wish. The information isn't there when you need it. It's not there for your proxy or health care providers.

Let's look at why this happens. You have a plan and you made copies of the documents. You either put them in a safety deposit box or in the top drawer of your desk. You give a copy to your doctor to put in your medical records and a copy to your proxy.

But these documents don't belong tucked away in a safety deposit box. They are personal but not confidential, like a last will and testament, which is only brought out for review after your death. They belong in a designated place somewhere safe in your house that is known to your proxy and others. Maybe you carry an advance care plan wallet card indicating the location of the documents and how to contact your proxy. But the documents are still not there when you most need them, reinforcing the sustained criticism that your plan for dying is only as good as its known existence and accessibility.

Your advance care information may be registered with a state or private national registry, a central repository for storing advance directive documents and information for a proxy or health care provider to access. But does a registry improve access? The focus of registries is registering, not information sharing with providers and proxies. Registries merely seem to protect against misplacement of documents by the recipient. Some registries limit access to those who have the patient's identification access code. This is an inherent flaw, because your documents aren't necessarily available when you need them. Accessibility is definitely improved with electronic registries that allow providers access independent of a registrant's code.

Hospitals' medical records and electronic health records systems are possible resources for physicians to access a patient's AMD using a direct search feature. In effect, the electronic health records system is a registry. But your plan isn't readily available unless you're admitted at hospitals within that system, and the system doesn't allow instant availability of documents to a patient or proxy wherever they are.

So what about accessibility? Where could you keep your advance directive secure and easily accessible just in case? You can store PDF versions of your plan on your smartphone. Many of us have one and it's with us almost

24/7. You could also import and store those of your spouse, parent(s), children, or anyone you care for deeply. Loved ones can carry yours and you can carry theirs. An mHealth app that does this is described in the back of the book.

The following descriptions help you know the available legal instruments for health care planning so you can think about which ones fit who you are now, work with your beliefs, and can be fashioned to express personal wishes.

DECIDING WHO MAKES MEDICAL DECISIONS
FOR YOU WHEN YOU CAN'T

Durable health care power of attorney (HCPOA) goes by many names: health care proxy, durable power of attorney for health care, agent, or surrogate. But all mean the same thing and refer to appointing someone to make health care decisions for you if and when you are not able to make them for yourself. HCPOA is not the same as durable power of attorney (POA) and is not the same as your agent designated in the Health Insurance Portability and Accountability Act of 1996 (HIPAA) form.

To sign the HCPOA, you must be mentally competent and understand what you are signing. It's also customary to appoint someone as a backup, an alternate proxy, just in case your first choice is unavailable in a crisis.

When is HCPOA activated? Your proxy steps in at any point in time when you require medical care or are hospitalized, even briefly, and are unable to speak for yourself and a decision needs to be made. Your proxy will make medical decisions for you anytime you aren't capable, so even if the situation is not life threatening—for example, if you're knocked unconscious in an accident and can't be easily revived—your proxy is still your spokesperson.

Whom you choose as your proxy is important because doctors will only talk with the proxy. Choose someone who knows you well, can be easily reached, stays calm under stressful situations, is a good listener, and is capable of grasping the big picture. You need a take-charge person who can separate his or her own wishes from your own.

Your proxy should be outspoken and strong enough to speak for you and not question themselves while representing your wishes. Situations can get awkward and intense for the proxy. It's not easy facing physicians and disagreeing with what they are suggesting. It's really difficult not to question yourself as proxy when another family member adamantly opposes decisions the proxy made believing they were consistent with the patient's stated wishes.

Logic tells you if you are married, you choose your spouse; if you are widowed or divorced, you choose your adult child. If you have no children, choose a close friend or relative. There's no legal requirement for an individual to choose a proxy, and if someone is not chosen, the law often states that a person's closest family member has the right to make decisions for him or her.

This kind of logic may not always work. Many medical professionals and lawyers say a spouse may be the worst person to choose as your proxy. While your spouse is a natural first choice, think about who truly can be there for you, calm, discerning, unflinching in the midst of a medical crisis, ready to say what you want or don't want for prolonging life or postponing dying.

What about choosing a family member who's a doctor as proxy? That seems to be the best choice because they know all about things clinical. But here also, consider the situation carefully. Here's what a bioethicist said to a doctor who was proxy for his father: "You are not a doctor here, you are the son. You can't say to yourself, 'I'm a doctor, I can fix this.' Your dad needs you as his son."

Choosing the best person as your health care proxy is a great chance for you to take charge of your health care, avoid the possibility of family resistance to your wishes for dying care, and avoid quarreling among your family. Think about a person who can separate his or her wishes from yours. Choose someone who could handle situations in which other family members or loved ones want to make decisions that differ from what you wanted and requested. This person should be easily reachable if needed, live close by, or be willing to travel to be with you. Talk with your family about the kind of care you would want and who you are choosing as your spokesperson and why.

BRINGING THE RIGHT FORM
TO THE HOSPITAL

In a medical crisis, clearly that's not the time to discover you brought the wrong form or a family member never completed the correct one in the first place. Critical time can be lost in the care of a loved one because one form is confused with another. There's good reason to know about three acronyms—HCPOA, POA, and HIPAA—that refer to important documents protecting the rights of a person and a patient.

It's true that both HCPOA and POA designate some-one to speak for you when you are incapacitated, but they are not the same. HCPOA is specific to health care decision making, appointing someone you trust as your health care proxy. POA is not. POA is a document autho-rizing a designated person as your agent to act on your behalf in business and legal matters. That's why, with only a POA document, you cannot speak for a person in a medical emergency.

But what does durable mean anyway? It's indicating the document is designed to take effect when a loved one can no longer make decisions for themselves. For example, you as HCPOA can step in at any point in time when someone you love is hospitalized, even briefly, and unable to speak for themselves, and a health care decision needs to be made. An HCPOA document ought to include language alluding to durability.

Let's say your mother appointed you as health care proxy and you are both her POA and HCPOA. If you show up at the ER with only the POA document, the medical staff won't talk to you about what is happening to your mother. You will not be able to make critical health care decisions on her behalf without presenting the proper form, the advance medical directive (AMD) stating her care wishes and appointing you as her HCPOA or proxy.

There's another area of confusion, HCPOA and HIPAA agent. We're all familiar with the HIPAA form at a doctor's office because we're asked to complete one. The Health Insurance Portability and Accountability Act of 1996 (HIPAA) is a federal law that protects patients' health care privacy and restricts health care providers' disclosure of protected information. By completing the HIPAA form and designating a person (or persons) as your agent or personal representative, health care providers can talk with them about what's happening regarding either an office visit or hospital care.

It may seem odd that the HIPAA form is not the "correct" one for you to bring to the ER. The HCPOA or health care proxy speaks for people when they cannot speak for themselves; the HIPAA representative can't do that. Health care providers will only talk with a proxy about the current situation and life-sustaining treatment choices. What can help a proxy is having an AMD that includes some clause within the HCPOA section that authorizes all health care providers to release to the proxy any protected health care information as set forth in HIPAA standards.

With the right document in hand in the ER or hospital inpatient setting, you won't have to face this predicament, and you can be there the way you want.

IS VAGUENESS THE PERFECT CURSE?

Instructions are often vague and don't always protect us from unwanted medical interventions in the future or at the end of life. Then again, the more specific an advance care plan, the more restraining and possibly irrelevant. A patient's wishes may not be clear because the real limitations or consequences of saying "I do" or "I do not" want a particular treatment are not understood. Also, a healthy person may believe that he would never want a certain treatment, and yet under certain circumstances, he would choose to have this very treatment performed if his life could be saved. This could apply to any life-sustaining therapy, from administration of IV hydration to ventilators.

How then can the proxy possibly take vague instructions and carry out what you really wanted? Is having the last word, as Susan P. Shapiro of the American Bar Foundation says, an elusive goal? It's a good thing your agent has the power to interpret what is written, because it may not perfectly match the situation.

Yes, your choice of proxy is so critical! Obviously you can't craft a perfect document, but you can entrust your final moments to that special discerning someone who happens to be your proxy who attends to the outcomes rather than the processes. But being discerning isn't easy when the "best" outcome isn't necessarily what the dying person expressed they wanted.

WHAT IS A LIVING WILL?

A *living will* is a commonly used written advance directive giving instructions in advance for health care at a time when you are incapacitated and cannot speak for yourself. I should point out that it's an older term for AMD that's still used but is becoming obsolete. "Incapacity" means the inability to give, withdraw, or withhold informed consent regarding health care, typically if the person is terminally ill with no chance of recovery.

Each state has its own requirements for a living will and related forms. You don't have to use your state's form, and many states accept other forms. You can customize the living will, adding instructions about care other than medical such as personal, spiritual, and emotional wishes. If you choose to write your own living will or customize a standard form, make sure, in addition to your signature, you obtain the signature of two witnesses, unrelated by marriage or blood; otherwise it will not be legitimate. The living will must also be notarized. It's interesting that most treating facilities will honor written wishes even if they are not in the approved format. Theoretically you can use a napkin, write your wishes on it, sign it, and have two witnesses unrelated to you also sign it. It will hold up as representing your wishes.

Living wills are often vague and limited in scope. But you can give broad or precise instructions for care, state that you want your life prolonged as long as possible, and be specific about what you want in the event of trauma or a prolonged state of unconsciousness or coma. Some health care professionals contend that you should not specify time frames for treatments in a living will. They feel it's better simply to have your proxy know what you want and apply it to the situation.

You may find conventional living wills use words such as terminal, extraordinary, or heroic. These clearly can have more than one meaning depending on age, stage of disease, and most importantly your background, beliefs, and values. For some, extraordinary is irrelevant. They want everything done, because that's what they believe should happen. For others, extraordinary means just that, and care should be taken not to cross a line where treatments are given that aren't wanted because they compromise what is held dear about life.

This is why it's so important to understand what you're reading, know what you want to say, and express what you mean. Signing anything that you don't understand and can't interpret is definitely something to watch for and avoid.

WHAT IS AN ADVANCE MEDICAL DIRECTIVE?

An *advance medical directive (AMD)* is an instructional directive intended to compensate for limitations of the traditional living will, with its vagueness and focus on dying. With an advance directive, you are asked to decide in advance which life-supporting or life-sustaining treatments you would want in scenarios such as coma with a small or virtually no chance of recovery, or advanced dementia with or without a terminal illness. Advance directives usually include designation of a health care proxy.

Even detailed advance directives may fail to distinguish between short-term use of an intervention for a potentially reversible illness and long-term treatment for a chronic condition. The instructions don't take into account the most common situation in the final years of life, physical decline, in which limiting treatment may be appropriate, especially in light of your values. You can customize an advance directive to account for these factors, but a proxy can also interpret your wishes in light of the situation.

Too many of us believe advance directives are for people who are very sick or old. This isn't so. Advance directives are a good idea for anyone over eighteen. At the very least, all adults should have a health care proxy to prevent ambiguity or disputes over treatments or legal consequences over who has the right to make decisions for them.

It's true an AMD is a legal instrument, but a lawyer is not required to create or assist in completing one, and neither is a physician. Usually when you sit with an attorney to review your estate plan, you're asked about whether you have a living will and proxy designation. The lawyer is making you aware of your rights as a patient regarding future health care and the need for you to take action. But that doesn't mean you have to complete an AMD with legal assistance.

It's not necessary to talk with your doctor when completing an AMD, although you can seek clarification about life-sustaining therapies. Health care professionals and lawyers may guide you in making educated choices, but they can't make choices for you. It's you who must decide what care you want in a medical crisis.

There are requirements for completing an AMD properly. Signing and dating it in the presence of a notary public and obtaining the signatures of two witnesses are usually required. Make copies to give to your physician and health care proxy. Sometimes a wallet-sized card accompanies an AMD, summarizing key contacts and indicating where the AMD is stored. Keep this in your wallet.

An AMD is not about ending your life but about what interventions you do or do not want if you become seriously ill and have a life-threatening condition. It doesn't mean, "Do not treat."

While an AMD is a legal document recounting your treatment wishes, a physician is not legally obligated to honor them. Physicians can refuse to comply with care wishes if they consider them medically inappropriate.

Most patients' wishes, however, are honored. If a physician is uncomfortable complying with a patient's wishes, there's a procedure for turning the patient's care over to another physician who will comply. Most hospitals have an ethics committee that will become involved in such situations.

EXAMPLES OF ADVANCE MEDICAL DIRECTIVES

The following are four excerpts from actual AMDs, sections of living wills, or proxy designations. They are examples of how these forms are written and what they cover. Implications of certain phrasings are also provided.

EXCERPT 1: DOROTHY

My agent is aware of my wishes with respect to artificial nutrition and hydration and I give him full authorization to make decisions with respect to the same.

Dorothy is an eighty-five-year-old woman. She used a form provided by her lawyer. She appointed her husband, Tom, as proxy. These instructions are simple and only about two procedures. These are broad guidelines.

I don't know whether Dorothy and Tom discussed other life-sustaining procedures and specifics on administration (whether, when, and for what duration). Dorothy's instructions are vague and she may not be protected from unwanted medical interventions. But it is also not known whether these broad guidelines are intentional. Dorothy may simply trust Tom to make decisions with her best interest in mind. She may believe Tom will intervene appropriately on her behalf when life-sustaining procedures are being proposed.

EXCERPT 2: ALBERT

I, Albert, the author of this document, request that, if my condition is deemed terminal or if I am determined to be permanently unconscious, I be allowed to die and not be kept alive through life support systems. By terminal condition, I mean that I have an incurable or irreversible medical condition which, without the administration of life support systems, will, in the opinion of my attending physician, result in death within a relatively short time.

By permanently unconscious I mean that I am in a permanent coma or persistent vegetative state that is an irreversible condition in which I am neither aware of myself nor of the environment and show no behavioral response to the environment.

The life support systems that I do not want include, but are not limited to artificial respiration, cardiopulmonary resuscitation and artificial means of providing nutrition and hydration. I do want sufficient pain medication to maintain my physical comfort. I do not intend any direct taking of my life, but only that my dying not be unreasonably prolonged. I ask that drugs be mercifully administered to me for terminal suffering even if they hasten the moment of my death.

I hope you who care for me will feel morally bound to follow my request. I recognize it places a heavy burden of responsibility upon you, and it is with the intention of sharing that responsibility and of mitigating any feelings of guilt that this statement is made.

Albert, a ninety-three-year-old man, wrote his own AMD. His directive is clearly more detailed than Dorothy's. It consists of health care instructions and appointment of a heath care proxy—his daughter, Becky. She is authorized to

1. *Convey to my [Albert's] physician my wishes concerning the withholding or removal of life support systems;*
2. *Take whatever actions are necessary to ensure that my wishes are given effect;*
3. *Consent, refuse or withdraw consent to any medical treatment as long as such action is consistent with my wishes concerning the withholding or removal of life support systems; and*
4. *Consent to any medical treatment designed solely for the purpose of maintaining physical comfort.*

Albert's words are carefully chosen and precise. But if, in the attending physician's opinion, the medical condition is curable, life-support systems may be deemed advantageous to save Albert's life rather than prolong his dying. Becky, his daughter, is aware of this possibility and knows she can disagree with the physician's opinion in knowingly acting on her father's true wishes.

EXCERPT 3: ETTA

I, Etta, declare:

If at any time my attending physician should determine that I have a terminal condition where the application of life-prolonging procedures would serve only to artificially prolong the dying process, I direct that such procedures be withheld or withdrawn, and that I be permitted to die naturally with only the administration of medication or the performance of any medical procedure deemed necessary to provide me with comfort care or to alleviate pain.

The power of my agent shall include the following:

To consent to or refuse or withdraw consent to any type of medical care, treatment, surgical procedure, diagnostic procedure, medication and the use of mechanical or other procedures that affect any bodily function, including, but not limited to, artificial respiration, artificially administered nutrition and hydration, and cardiopulmonary resuscitation.

Etta used a state's AMD form. She is an active healthy woman of seventy-two years. Etta chose her two children, Harold and Charlie, as primary proxies. They both live near Etta. Either one can make health care choices for Etta when she is no longer able to make these choices for herself. Like Albert's directive, decisions are based on the determination of the attending physician. This is customary wording in many directives.

Etta selected Harold and Charlie as proxy with equal power of decisions, but they are very different people. Harold, a professor of applied math, is analytical. He wants to find out what the problem is and how to treat it. His reasoning lends itself to pursuing treatment aggressively if a cure possibly exists. Charlie, a salesman at a department store, is a vegetarian and fitness fanatic. He avoids prescription drugs and looks for natural herbal cures. Charlie's experience and observations lead to a different stance with regard to his mom's end of life.

Etta was good about updating her advance directive over the years, but she didn't put any thought into it. She didn't know what she wanted, didn't talk about it with Charlie and Harold, and didn't see the potential conflict looming in the future for her two children as they faced decisions about her care when she was unable to speak for herself.

EXCERPT 4: PAUL

Paul is a sixty-year-old corporate executive, married for twenty years with two adult children. He was considering two AMD forms but noticed they had very different wording in designating a health care agent or proxy. And he realized the words in one versus the other could lead to very different situations for his family if and when he was unable to make health care choices for himself.

Form A reads:

I, Paul, hereby appoint my wife, Debra, and my children, Sarah and Richard; any one of my wife and my children may act alone without the others, as my agents to make health care decisions on my behalf as authorized in this document.

Form B reads:

The person I choose as my health care agent is:

First Choice Name: Debra
[Contact Information]

If this person is not able or willing to make these choices for me, OR is divorced or legally separated from me, OR this person has died, then these people are my next choices:

Second Choice Name: Richard
[Contact Information]

Third Choice Name: Sarah
[Contact Information]

With Form A, Paul is appointing three proxies, each with the same powers of decision making about Paul's care. This clearly gives flexibility to his family. If one person cannot be there in a medical emergency, another can step in. Yes, each is able to decide separately, but this leaves them open to potential conflict between each other and with the physician if all three proxies don't agree on what should be done. Paul chose Form B because his family was more likely to avoid such circumstances, especially if Paul talked with them about dying.

At 87, Paul revised and revalidated Form B. His wife Debra had passed away five years before, so he designated Richard his first choice as proxy and Sarah, his second choice. Both children are well aware of what is important to their dad because he's been good about telling them what he wants at end of life and what tranquility means to him.

In Paul's final days, Richard made decisions about withdrawal of certain life-sustaining treatments guided by his dad's conversations and shared these decisions with Sarah. Sarah agreed these were hard choices but consistent with what their dad wanted. Their dad's open dialogues guided Sarah and Richard.

Paul passed away with his children by his bedside.

The take-away message is: You should have a plan. Create your art of dying, communicate your wishes to your loved ones, and put them in writing.

MAKING YOUR CARE WISHES AN ORDER

There comes a time when making your care wishes into an order may make sense. That's when there's a very serious and terminal illness, or you are very old or frail and quality of life as you define it is greatly affected.

A physician order is an AMD requiring a physician's signature. These forms list options with a yes or no answer. A DNR order is very specific and narrowly defined, while physician orders for life-sustaining treatment (POLST) is a DNR order plus other orders specifying things you do or don't want such as antibiotics, IV nutrition, and IV hydration.

WHAT A DNR IS AND IS NOT

A *DNR* order is a special category of advance directive that applies only to resuscitation in the event of cardiac arrest. You may have also heard *do-not-attempt resuscitation (DNAR)*. The DNR does not apply to any other medical interventions and should never be interpreted to mean do not treat. It doesn't mean discontinue all prescribed treatments such as fluids, antibiotics, or pain medications.

There's another way to explain this. The DNR document isn't worth much, at least in protecting you from unwanted and intrusive tests or procedures, because the DNR is only for a specific, narrowly defined episode: cardiac arrest. In the absence of an appointed proxy and any other AMD beyond a DNR, the doctor is obligated to do everything possible to save a life.

It's such a significant directive that a physician's signature is required in all states. Other signature requirements vary by state and type of DNR form and may include the signature of the patient or proxy or even witnesses and another physician.

Who should consider a DNR? While anyone may consider initiating a DNR order, individuals with end-stage terminal illness are most likely to consider electing not to have resuscitation in the event of cardiac arrest. The choice whether to have a DNR can be affected by your age, general health, and progression of illness, but it depends mostly on who you are and whether a DNR is consistent with your beliefs.

Ideally a DNR order is black and white: you don't want to be resuscitated in the event of cardiac arrest or you do. But in some cases patients are allowed to pick and choose which CPR procedures they do or don't want. For example, you might desire cardiac compression and limited short-term ventilation but not to be shocked by a defibrillator or put on a ventilator for life. The reality is this makes things much more complicated for the treatment team and can lead to unwanted CPR measures being taken.

DNR forms don't only apply to hospital inpatient and emergency departments. In some states, DNRs can be portable and apply across all health care settings—home, hospital, or other health care facility. Some states offer DNRs for nonhospital settings such as a prehospital DNR; if you prefer not to be resuscitated and want that known and honored in hospital and nonhospital settings, you would need two DNR forms. Another example of a non-hospital DNR is the comfort care DNR, where emergency medical technicians (EMTs) honor a patient's request for no resuscitation and provide palliative care, even if the person has a pulse and/or is breathing. Here again two DNRs are needed: one for the in-hospital and one for the nonhospital setting.

How does this play out when a 911 call is made? Normally, if the patient is not breathing and the heart is not beating, EMTs will immediately start CPR and then take the person to the hospital. If you have a prehospital DNR or portable DNR, post it in a prominent place in your home and wear a bracelet or necklace that communicates your DNR wishes. In the absence of the DNR form, EMTs must do CPR. If you have a prehospital DNR, some maintain that you should not call 911. However, in states where the comfort care DNR is available, EMTs can provide comfort measures and support short of resuscitation in the event of cardiac arrest.

If you want to execute a DNR, it makes sense to know what your state requires as you develop your advance care plan. How many forms you actually need to state your preference on resuscitation depends on where you live.

DNR status is almost universally honored, but there are rare instances where a physician overrides a DNR. Physicians consider the situation and whether a DNR is appropriate. A doctor may resuscitate when it's clear an arrest has occurred or is imminent because the physician sees the situation as easily reversible and feels it would be medically inappropriate not to treat. An example of this might be a drug reaction or a patient choking on food.

A DNR never supplants medical judgment made in context of the situation. Clearly, clinical situations are often not clear-cut, and room must be made for interpretation of the patient's wishes in light of the clinical setting. For example, it may be necessary to resuscitate a nonterminal patient during surgery. In this case, the patient would be asked to revoke the DNR temporarily before surgery.

A proxy might override a DNR too if they believe the situation is not terminal, they do not want to give up, or they believe the circumstances conflict with the patient's own expressed wishes and beliefs. This is why it's so important to appoint someone you feel is discerning and will weigh your wishes in the context of any situation.

What are your feelings toward DNR? What do you believe influences your choice to have or not have a DNR? Answering these questions requires you to know whether you see a DNR as a way to bring about the end of your life or feel resuscitation interferes with a natural death, whether attempting or not attempting resuscitation is against your beliefs, and whether you think your loved ones would object to your decision.

WHAT ARE PHYSICIAN ORDERS FOR LIFE-SUSTAINING TREATMENT?

Physician orders for life-sustaining treatment (POLST) is a voluntary form that can also be part of advance care planning. The POLST is a portable set of medical orders designed to follow a patient across care settings including hospital, home, long-term care, hospice, and emergency medical settings. These medical orders are specific to a patient's end-of-life treatment preferences based on wishes expressed in the AMD and on the person's recent medical conditions. A POLST complements rather than replaces an AMD.

POLST is intended for persons who have terminal, advanced, debilitating, or chronic progressive illnesses, and the prognosis is death within a year. There's no doubt a POLST improves on the relevance of an AMD, because the need to focus on end-of-life care is more immediate and urgent.

POLST medical orders include a portable DNR order applying to in-hospital treatment and nonhospital settings. But POLSTs are about more than whether or not to resuscitate. They provide crucial information about specific types and levels of treatment you wish to receive, depending on your medical history and current status. The medical orders reflected in a POLST apply to the most common life-supporting techniques, including CPR, artificially administered nutrition and hydration, painkillers, antibiotics, and other treatments.

The POLST form would accompany an AMD, but an AMD is not required for the orders to be valid. A POLST may override any conflicting directives in a patient's AMD. Appointing a proxy still applies. An AMD, living will, and HCPOA are legal instruments executed by individuals. A DNR and POLST are medical orders issued by a physician.

Completing a POLST requires an in-depth conversation between the seriously ill person and a health care professional (a physician or, if permitted where you live, a nurse practitioner or physician assistant). Treatment wishes are then turned into medical orders familiar to physicians and emergency medical staff.

Without a physician's signature the POLST is not valid. Your signature is also required, providing evidence of informed consent. The POLST usually comes in a uniformly bright color for easy recognition within a patient's records.

Currently a POLST program has been adopted in nearly twenty states. The names, policies, and forms vary, but the orders are basically the same. Another twenty-seven states are developing a program. If a POLST program does not exist in your state, then you can't use a POLST form. To find out if your state or region has a POLST program, go to www.polst.org.

As with any advance care plan forms, a POLST should be reviewed periodically. If your treatment preferences change, your condition worsens, or your care level or health care setting changes, a new form must be completed. What's important is knowing about high-intensity therapies before expressing your preferences. Clearly, you'd want to know about them long before your health deteriorates and reaches the point that a POLST is recommended.

Here are two examples of POLST forms from North Carolina and California. You will see that the forms have slight differences.

HIPAA PERMITS DISCLOSURE OF MOST TO OTHER HEALTH CARE PROFESSIONALS AS NECESSARY

Medical Orders for Scope of Treatment (MOST)

This is a Physician Order Sheet based on the person's medical condition and wishes. Any section not completed indicates full treatment for that section. When the need occurs, **first** follow these orders, **then** contact physician.

Patient's Last Name:	Effective Date of Form:
	Form must be reviewed at least annually.
Patient's First Name, Middle Initial:	Patient's Date of Birth:

Section A — Check One Box Only	**CARDIOPULMONARY RESUSCITATION (CPR): Person has no pulse and is not breathing.**
	☐ Attempt **R**esuscitation (CPR) ☐ **D**o **N**ot Attempt **R**esuscitation (DNR/no CPR)
	When not in cardiopulmonary arrest, follow orders in B, C, and D.

Section B — Check One Box Only	**MEDICAL INTERVENTIONS: Person has pulse and/or is breathing.**
	☐ **Full Scope of Treatment:** Use intubation, advanced airway interventions, mechanical ventilation, cardioversion as indicated, medical treatment, IV fluids, etc.; also provide comfort measures. **Transfer to hospital if indicated.**
	☐ **Limited Additional Interventions:** Use medical treatment, IV fluids and cardiac monitoring as indicated. Do not use intubation or mechanical ventilation; also provide comfort measures. **Transfer to hospital if indicated. Avoid intensive care.**
	☐ **Comfort Measures:** Keep clean, warm and dry. Use medication by any route, positioning, wound care and other measures to relieve pain and suffering. Use oxygen, suction and manual treatment of airway obstruction as needed for comfort. **Do not transfer to hospital** unless comfort needs cannot be met in current location.
	Other Instructions _____

Section C — Check One Box Only	**ANTIBIOTICS**
	☐ Antibiotics if life can be prolonged.
	☐ Determine use or limitation of antibiotics when infection occurs.
	☐ No Antibiotics (use other measures to relieve symptoms).
	Other Instructions _____

Section D — Check One Box Only in Each Column	**MEDICALLY ADMINISTERED FLUIDS AND NUTRITION: Offer oral fluids and nutrition if physically feasible.**
	☐ IV fluids long-term if indicated ☐ Feeding tube long-term if indicated
	☐ IV fluids for a defined trial period ☐ Feeding tube for a defined trial period
	☐ No IV fluids (provide other measures to ensure comfort) ☐ No feeding tube
	Other Instructions _____

Section E — Check The Appropriate Box	**DISCUSSED WITH AND AGREED TO BY:** *Basis for order must be documented in medical record.*	☐ Patient ☐ Parent or guardian if patient is a minor ☐ Health care agent ☐ Legal guardian of the person ☐ Attorney-in-fact with power to make health care decisions ☐ Spouse	☐ Majority of patient's reasonably available parents and adult children ☐ Majority of patient's reasonably available adult siblings ☐ An individual with an established relationship with the patient who is acting in good faith and can reliably convey the wishes of the patient

MD/DO, PA, or NP Name (Print):	MD/DO, PA, or NP Signature (Required):	Phone #:

Signature of Person, Parent of Minor, Guardian, Health Care Agent, Spouse, or Other Personal Representative (Signature is required and must either be on this form or on file)

I agree that adequate information has been provided and significant thought has been given to life-prolonging measures. Treatment preferences have been expressed to the physician (MD/DO), physician assistant, or nurse practitioner. This document reflects those treatment preferences and indicates informed consent.

If signed by a patient representative, preferences expressed must reflect patient's wishes as best understood by that representative. Contact information for personal representative should be provided on the back of this form.
You are not required to sign this form to receive treatment.

Patient or Representative Name (print)	Patient or Representative Signature	Relationship (write "self" if patient)

SEND FORM WITH PATIENT/RESIDENT WHEN TRANSFERRED OR DISCHARGED

North Carolina's MOST (page 1 of 2)
Reprinted with permission.

HIPAA PERMITS DISCLOSURE OF MOST TO OTHER HEALTH CARE PROFESSIONALS AS NECESSARY

Contact Information

Patient Representative:		Relationship:	Phone #:	
			Cell Phone #:	
Health Care Professional Preparing Form:		Preparer Title:	Preferred Phone #:	Date Prepared:

Directions for Completing Form

Completing MOST

- MOST must be reviewed and prepared by a health care professional in consultation with the patient or patient representative.
- MOST is a medical order and must be reviewed and signed by a licensed physician (MD/DO), physician assistant, or nurse practitioner to be valid. **Be sure to document the basis for the order in the progress notes of the medical record.** Mode of communication (e.g., in person, by telephone, etc.) also should be documented.
- The signature of the patient or their representative is required; however, if the patient's representative is not reasonably available to sign the original form, a copy of the completed form with the signature of the patient's representative must be placed in the medical record and "on file" must be written in the appropriate signature field on the front of this form or in the review section below.
- Use of original form is required. **Be sure to send the original form with the patient.**
- MOST is part of advance care planning, which also may include a living will and health care power of attorney (HCPOA). If there is a HCPOA, living will, or other advance directive, a copy should be attached if available. **MOST may suspend any conflicting directions in a patient's previously executed HCPOA, living will, or other advance directive.**
- **There is no requirement that a patient have a MOST.**
- MOST is recognized under N.C. Gen. Stat. 90-21.17.

Reviewing MOST

This MOST must be reviewed at least annually or earlier if:

- The patient is admitted and/or discharged from a health care facility;
- There is a substantial change in the patient's health status; or
- The patient's treatment preferences change.

If MOST is revised or becomes invalid, draw a line through Sections A – E and write "VOID" in large letters.

Revocation of MOST

This MOST may be revoked by the patient or the patient's representative.

		Review of MOST		
Review Date	Reviewer and Location of Review	MD/DO, PA, or NP Signature (Required)	Signature of Patient or Representative (Required)	Outcome of Review
				☐No Change ☐FORM VOIDED, new form completed
				☐No Change ☐FORM VOIDED, new form completed ☐FORM VOIDED, no new form
				☐No Change ☐FORM VOIDED, new form completed ☐FORM VOIDED, no new form
				☐No Change ☐FORM VOIDED, new form completed ☐FORM VOIDED, no new form
				☐No Change ☐FORM VOIDED, new form completed ☐FORM VOIDED, no new form

SEND FORM WITH PATIENT/RESIDENT WHEN TRANSFERRED OR DISCHARGED

DO NOT ALTER THIS FORM!

NCDHHS/DHSR/DHSR/EMS   1112   Rev. 10/07   North Carolina Department of Health and Human Services

North Carolina's MOST (page 2 of 2)
Reprinted with permission.

HIPAA PERMITS DISCLOSURE OF POLST TO OTHER HEALTH CARE PROFESSIONALS AS NECESSARY

Physician Orders for Life-Sustaining Treatment (POLST)

EMSA #111 B
(Effective 1/1/2009)

First follow these orders, then contact physician. This is a Physician Order Sheet based on the person's current medical condition and wishes. Any section not completed implies full treatment for that section. Everyone shall be treated with dignity and respect.

Last Name

First /Middle Name

Date of Birth   Date Form Prepared

A
Check
One

CARDIOPULMONARY RESUSCITATION (CPR): *Person has no pulse and is not breathing.*

☐ Attempt Resuscitation/CPR   ☐ Do Not Attempt Resuscitation/DNR (Allow Natural Death)
(Section B: Full Treatment required)

When not in cardiopulmonary arrest, follow orders in **B** and **C**.

B
Check
One

MEDICAL INTERVENTIONS: *Person has pulse and/or is breathing.*

☐ **Comfort Measures Only** Use medication by any route, positioning, wound care and other measures to relieve pain and suffering. Use oxygen, suction and manual treatment of airway obstruction as needed for comfort. Antibiotics only to promote comfort. *Transfer if comfort needs cannot be met in current location.*

☐ **Limited Additional Interventions** Includes care described above. Use medical treatment, antibiotics, and IV fluids as indicated. Do not intubate. May use non-invasive positive airway pressure. Generally avoid intensive care.

☐ *Do Not Transfer to hospital for medical interventions. Transfer if comfort needs cannot be met in current location.*

☐ **Full Treatment** Includes care described above. Use intubation, advanced airway interventions, mechanical ventilation, and defibrillation/cardioversion as indicated. *Transfer to hospital if indicated. Includes intensive care.*

Additional Orders: _____

C
Check
One

ARTIFICIALLY ADMINISTERED NUTRITION: *Offer food by mouth if feasible and desired.*

☐ No artificial nutrition by tube.   ☐ Defined trial period of artificial nutrition by tube.

☐ Long-term artificial nutrition by tube.

Additional Orders: _____

D

SIGNATURES AND SUMMARY OF MEDICAL CONDITION:
Discussed with:
☐ Patient ☐ Health Care Decisionmaker ☐ Parent of Minor ☐ Court Appointed Conservator ☐ Other:

Signature of Physician
My signature below indicates to the best of my knowledge that these orders are consistent with the person's medical condition and preferences.

Print Physician Name | Physician Phone Number | Date

Physician Signature (required) | Physician License #

Signature of Patient, Decisionmaker, Parent of Minor or Conservator
By signing this form, the legally recognized decisionmaker acknowledges that this request regarding resuscitative measures is consistent with the known desires of, and with the best interest of, the individual who is the subject of the form.

Signature (required) | Name (print) | Relationship (write self if patient)

Summary of Medical Condition | Office Use Only

SEND FORM WITH PERSON WHENEVER TRANSFERRED OR DISCHARGED

California's POLST (page 1 of 2)
Reprinted with permission.

HIPAA PERMITS DISCLOSURE OF POLST TO OTHER HEALTH CARE PROFESSIONALS AS NECESSARY			
Patient Name (last, first, middle)		Date of Birth	Gender: M F
Patient Address			

Contact Information			
Health Care Decisionmaker	Address		Phone Number
Health Care Professional Preparing Form	Preparer Title	Phone Number	Date Prepared

Directions for Health Care Professional

Completing POLST

- Must be completed by health care professional based on patient preferences and medical indications.
- POLST must be signed by a physician and the patient/decisionmaker to be valid. Verbal orders are acceptable with follow-up signature by physician in accordance with facility/community policy.
- Certain medical conditions or medical treatments may prohibit a person from residing in a residential care facility for the elderly.
- Use of original form is strongly encouraged. Photocopies and FAXes of signed POLST forms are legal and valid.

Using POLST

- Any incomplete section of POLST implies full treatment for that section.

Section A:

- No defibrillator (including automated external defibrillators) should be used on a person who has chosen "Do Not Attempt Resuscitation."

Section B:

- When comfort cannot be achieved in the current setting, the person, including someone with "Comfort Measures Only," should be transferred to a setting able to provide comfort (e.g., treatment of a hip fracture).
- IV medication to enhance comfort may be appropriate for a person who has chosen "Comfort Measures Only."
- Non-invasive positive airway pressure includes continuous positive airway pressure (CPAP), bi-level positive airway pressure (BiPAP), and bag valve mask (BVM) assisted respirations.
- Treatment of dehydration prolongs life. A person who desires IV fluids should indicate "Limited Interventions" or "Full Treatment."

Reviewing POLST

It is recommended that POLST be reviewed periodically. Review is recommended when:

- The person is transferred from one care setting or care level to another, or
- There is a substantial change in the person's health status, or
- The person's treatment preferences change.

Modifying and Voiding POLST

- A person with capacity can, at any time, void the POLST form or change his/her mind about his/her treatment preferences by executing a verbal or written advance directive or a new POLST form.
- To void POLST, draw a line through Sections A through D and write "VOID" in large letters. Sign and date this line.
- A health care decisionmaker may request to modify the orders based on the known desires of the individual or, if unknown, the individual's best interests.

This form is approved by the California Emergency Medical Services Authority in cooperation with the statewide POLST Task Force.

For more information or a copy of the form, visit **www.capolst.org**.

SEND FORM WITH PERSON WHENEVER TRANSFERRED OR DISCHARGED

California's POLST (page 2 of 2)
Reprinted with permission.

CONSIDERING ORGAN DONATION

Organ donation is the process of giving an organ or a part of an organ for the purpose of transplantation into another person. For a person to become an organ donor, blood and oxygen must flow through the organs until the time of organ recovery to ensure viability. Donation is possible only after all efforts to save the patient's life have been exhausted, tests performed to confirm the absence of brain or brain stem activity, and brain death declared.

If the potential donor is not found on the registry, a legally authorized representative (usually a spouse, relative, or close friend) is offered the opportunity to authorize the donation.

Tissue donation includes skin, bone, and heart valves. Donated tissues must be initiated within 24 hours of death. Unlike organs, tissue can be processed and stored for an extended period of time for use in such situations as burn cases, ligament repair, and bone replacement.

Cornea donation has to do with the cornea, the clear dome-like window covering the front of the eye that allows light to pass through to the retina, enabling us to see. Most deceased individuals are potential donors. This kind of donation usually happens within 12 hours of death, and corneas are transplantable for up to 14 days after recovery.

Every adult (18 years or older) can designate himself or herself as a donor by taking one of three actions:

- ► Registering with his or her state's donor registry
- ► Signing and carrying a Uniform Donor Card
- ► Indicating willingness to donate on his or her driver's license application

People younger than 18 years old can designate themselves as donors with parental or guardian consent.

Even if you expressed wishes to be a donor, a designated family member (possibly your proxy) will be asked to sign an organ donation consent form at the time of your death. Family members may refuse permission because they were unaware of your preference to donate and because certain organs need to be removed while you are still on life support.

Here's where you can help your family through yet another part of your dying. It means deciding whether donating your organs or tissues for someone else's benefit or donating your whole body for medical research or education is important to you, and that it is not problematic or against your beliefs. If you are already registered as a donor, tell your loved ones about your decisions. Make sure that some medical instructions, such as a DNR, do not conflict with your desire to donate organs. And if you feel it is inappropriate for the hospital staff to ask you or your family about organ donation, then say it up front.

Part 3
What Are the Problems?

I don't mind my disease killing me,
but it's killing my family, too.
—*2009 film adaptation of the book*
My Sister's Keeper, *Jodi Picoult*

There are problems that can get in the way of your well-crafted plan, things you probably haven't thought about much, especially if you've never experienced a medical crisis or serious illness. These things can unsettle you and your family enough so that your wishes for care are hindered or derailed. Most of these problems didn't even exist just a short time ago. No one had to confront them before medicine and the delivery of health care got so complicated. They weren't around before, but now they are—and you have to face them.

So you've created your plan for dying that's true to who you are. Your family knows your wishes, and you picked a health care proxy you can trust to honor them. But how can you keep unpredictable problems from upsetting what you want?

I have a new approach to this that has proven helpful. First, consider that the potential problems fall into two basic categories: internal, in which control is often within your reach, and external, where the problem is out of your control and something you have to accept. For both, it's crucial to remember that the nature of dying is experiential and not medical. You and your family are experiencing this event, and not the doctors, nurses, or insurance companies.

You may not agree completely with the categorization. Some internal problems may strike you as external and vice versa, and in fact, some are a little of both. You may feel some problems depicted as inside your control are not, and some depicted as outside your control can be modified and controlled. But no matter, you need to be aware of them and know what can go awry.

6

INTERNAL PROBLEMS

Internal problems are about you and your family. They are personal and subjective and can usually be solved. Such things as whether or not to act on a physician's opinions, giving informed consent, and which member of the family is actually in charge—just the proxy or the proxy with the advice of other individuals. These are important decisions you and your loved ones must make. Family dynamics can disrupt what's already going on during a medical crisis, and family dysfunction can affect how you die.

KNOWING WHEN YOU'RE REALLY DYING

One of the biggest internal problems during the approach to anyone's death, yours or a loved one's, is determining exactly when it is time to let go, to say this

is it. No more struggling to stay alive. No more unnecessary painful procedures. No more fruitless expense.

It's not always clear when dying is occurring. People
often cling to hope and want to believe they or their
loved one isn't done with life yet. This can be heartrend-
ing when someone actually is dying, because their
family may feel they would let the person down if they
didn't beg the medical staff to keep trying.

You may ask, isn't it enough to have put it in writing? Yes, that's very important, but if there's no
acknowledgement it's the end by a physician or your
family is in denial, it may become impossible to prevent interventions you specifically said you didn't
want. Your health care wishes can be unintentionally
ignored. That's an unpredictable internal problem: the
perception that your condition, even if you're unconscious or so medicated as to be dysfunctional, is not
necessarily incurable or irreversible, and therefore
treatment may continue even if your written directions
say otherwise.

Dying is not always a dramatic scene where a patient
is in a critical care unit with tubes and needles lined up.
In the powerful words of Ira Byock, the director of palliative medicine at Dartmouth–Hitchcock Medical
Center in Lebanon, New Hampshire: "End-of-life care
is unlike elective surgery, fracture management, treatment of the flu, surgery for acute appendicitis, or even
something as serious as a heart attack from which one
can be expected to survive. One of the key features that

distinguish end-of-life care from other aspects of medicine is that, for the terminally ill patient, life cannot simply be put on hold while treatment is endured."

Observe the care given and ask yourself some questions. What life support is being performed? Is it the least invasive? Is it a lot of invasive little things? Are they happening more and more frequently? How many tests are being done and how often? Are there repeat hospital admissions over a short time? Was it IV hydration and now a central IV line? Are multiple organs failing? Are highly invasive procedures being proposed, including dialysis and ventilation with a trach?

All of the above reflect elevation in complexity and care, and it's difficult to know when you're crossing an invisible threshold that you may not wish to cross in efforts to prolong life. Renowned surgeon, writer, and researcher Atul Gawande notes: "It isn't always possible to know who is dying and who isn't." There is some point where dying care is not about curing and medicine.

Dying isn't just about solving physical problems. There's also your spiritual needs, the impact on your loved ones, and of course financial considerations. It is about you deciding how you want to live your last days, and your family allowing itself to experience these moments with you.

I do know this: Recognizing that dying is happening is not obvious when dealing with aging, frailty, and illness burdens, as Barbara's experiences demonstrate.

It was October 2008, and my dad of dads had just turned ninety. I called him TOM *(the old man) even though his name was Bob. He lived at the Good Shepherd, an assisted living center in Lexington, Massachusetts.*

My dad had broken his hip in early September. Because of the type of break, he needed a titanium rod. Dad had an Alzheimer's-type dementia but always found the perfect words to bring a radiant smile to any woman's face. He had high blood pressure, type II diabetes, and prostate cancer. He was on twenty-four medications a day.

He returned to Good Shepherd from the hospital almost two weeks after his fall and was provided physical therapy. His cronies who sat with him for meals had kept his seat open—regardless of their memory loss, all knew Bob's seat was reserved for Bob. Mr. B. (as the staff called him) was back!

Only two weeks later, Dad was gagging on food and drinks and choking. He was eating little and drinking rarely.

A nurse at Good Shepherd mentioned that Dad could stay and receive comfort care if we chose not to have him transported back to the hospital. While Dad was reluctant to go, not taking him for medical care didn't seem right. So an ambulance was called.

If this next part makes you uncomfortable, it made me uncomfortable too. What follows are the terms that were thrown at us. We didn't understand any of it and felt totally inadequate. We were dealing with a crisis and felt helpless.

He had aspiration pneumonia and was administered IV antibiotics. He was severely dehydrated and begun on IV hydration. He was placed on total parenteral nutrition (TPN), since he was malnourished. Over a three-week period in the ICU, he was found to have MRSA and was given a different antibiotic via a port. The antibiotic was administered along with TPN via a subcutaneous port because Dad was yanking at the IVs and pulling them out. He grew tired of being poked and prodded, which was a part of his daily regimen.

He then acquired C. difficile or C. diff. He had edema in his legs. And then Dad was diagnosed with congestive heart failure.

Needless to say, Dad was a very sick man, but he rarely spoke about it. It could have been the Alzheimer's. I feel it was just as much about being the John Wayne type he was, the World War II vet with Purple Hearts, a Bronze Star, and a Silver Star. He was a real honest-to-God, bigger-than-life hero.

We understood that he couldn't tell us what he truly wanted to happen. By now, many specialists were involved in his care. Each one focused on a certain function or specific medical problem.

Dad didn't know any of these health care professionals. They were caring strangers but strangers all the same. They knew Dad only as a sick man with medical problems. His general practitioner of several years made rounds, usually daily, around 7 a.m. While these doctors probably talked together, it was unclear how frequently. I began feeling that we were all clustered on a bus heading somewhere with no driver and no map.

In the midst of these activities, Dad kept up an affable jokester demeanor. This behavior, I was convinced, was a façade. Occasionally this mask of affability would slip and Dad would turn to my brother or me and proclaim, "I can't stand this, boy" or "Honey, I can't stand this." He didn't want to eat, he didn't want to drink, and he didn't want meds. He wanted to be left alone. He wanted to go home to Good Shepherd and sit outside on the seat of his walker, shirt off, basking in the afternoon sun.

It was now mid-October. It was cold and dark, about 6 a.m. I was driving to be with Dad at a hospital in Middlesex County. I kept saying, over and over to myself, "I wish someone could take me by the hand and tell me what I should do for my dad."

He had a living will. In it he had expressed that if he was dying he did not want extraordinary measures to sustain life. He had a DNR. He had selected a proxy—three of us to be precise. This was part of the problem. There was no one in charge. We didn't know if he was dying, the doctors were giving no indication that his time was near, and we couldn't agree on what to do. We anguished over decisions and because we could not agree on what to do, Dad kept getting treated.

We wished Dad had been more specific in his living will and that he had talked to us, his proxies, and clearly expressed his wishes.

I stopped at Starbucks on Bedford Street for a cup of coffee. I ran in as they opened and right behind me was another woman in as much hurry as I was.

"Why are you up so early on a Sunday morning?" she asked.

I told her I was going to the hospital to be with my dad who was very sick. I treated her to coffee and asked "What about you?"

"I work at a hospital on the south side of town. I'm a doctor. I'm a doctor for seriously ill children. Do you want to talk?"

We sat and I shared my story. She listened and then said, "Give your dad the dignity you feel he deserves. His body is telling you that he wants to go."

She was my someone. And if she reads this, I hope she will know and recognize herself. I want to thank her for her words and the peace she gave me.

That same morning after meeting my someone at Starbucks, I spoke with Dad's general practitioner, who was making his 7 A.M. rounds. I asked, "Is my Dad's time short? Is he indicating to us that it is time?" The doctor said, "No, we will get him back." He then asked me, "Is he suffering? Are there visible signs?" I did not know how to respond!

Our family decided to go the distance. There were three proxies for Dad—my two brothers and me. We all had different views on what was happening and consequently what should happen next. No one of us was willing to overrule the other. We had to find consensus otherwise bedlam would ensue. We knew we would have to agree on everything.

I convinced myself that making different decisions about Dad's care was not possible simply because of family dynamics. I could have been more vocal with my views. But the point is to what end except to aggravate an already very tense situation?

A friend said to me during the crisis: "Stay with the living." In other words, don't burn bridges; let those who are passing, pass in peace. Stay with the living. I grow still with these words and see more clearly. Mom, Dad; weren't they the ONLY ones who could have changed these dynamics?

What did Dad's advance medical directive (his wishes for treatment at end of life) mean? Since each of us had our own opinions on whether he was at the "end of life," our interpretation of his wishes were different.

If he were not seen as dying, the advance directive words "the application of life-prolonging procedures would serve only to artificially prolong the dying process" were rendered meaningless. And if he was not dying, who among us wanted to bring on his death unnecessarily? Who wants the anxiety from the belief that you let him down and "let him die," rather than that he died as a result of an illness?

Since he was defined by his heroics in WWII, who among us wanted to say that he would want to stop the life-sustaining treatments? Decisions were based on avoiding guilt and pursuing any chance, no matter how slim, for his continued survival.

His doctor suggested a PEG. The doctor said that if this were his Dad, he would want this procedure done for him. Give him time to get back to his old self. We all agreed to say no.

Dad developed sepsis and a systemic yeast infection in his bloodstream.

Five weeks after readmission and two weeks after the encounter with my someone, my Dad was discharged from the hospital to go "home" to die. His face and very being expressed relief.

He died one day later at his home away from home, surrounded by family and the caring staff at Good Shepherd. The song playing on the satellite radio '40s music station was "Bugle Boy Blues." His designated seat for meals had remained empty for nearly seven weeks, his buddies awaiting his return.

THE IMPORTANCE OF INFORMED CONSENT

Informed consent is something most of us are familiar with. Any time a physician needs to perform a treatment or procedure, you're asked first to sign a form indicating your informed consent, whether for a mammogram, blood work, surgery, or life support.

Before you sign an informed consent form, physicians are required to disclose the risks, benefits, and alternatives to a proposed treatment, nontreatment, or procedure. The physician should go over the risk of dying (mortality) versus the probability of living (survival), as well as complications and possible adverse outcomes, or the outcomes of not having the procedure done. Only then do you sign, indicating you're informed and giving consent.

Consent is voluntary and can only be given when you're mentally competent and understand what is being signed. And if you're seriously ill or legally declared mentally incapable, your proxy steps in, and his or her consent must also be voluntary. But you and your family can avoid the problem of last minute decision making by choosing not to wait until you're seriously ill or incapacitated.

Physicians may or may not give their personal opinions on what decision ought to be made. Not all doctors will say, "If this were my parent, I would do such and such" or "If this were me, I would want this done or that done."

Some physicians fear sounding authoritarian and steer away from giving you their opinion. They don't want to feel they are leading you to select what they suggest. Others believe that you and your family are paying for their expertise and training and feel they should give their opinion. Still others are prompted to propose a treatment because they believe it is unfair to place the entire decision on the family, as that may leave the patient and family not knowing what to do.

You and your family ultimately are the ones deciding what course to take. Your family or proxy is not obligated to follow whatever the doctor says, but our backgrounds affect decisions we make as patients and family members. For some of us, discussions about advance directive planning are a sign of disrespect, and the family actually prefers the health care provider to initiate the discussions and make all the decisions about life-sustaining treatment. That's fine, there's nothing wrong with this point of view. You do have the option to turn the decision making over to the medical staff and let them take the lead. But consider how this affects your wishes about how you would like to die.

What's often missing is an honest discussion about dying care. Who should sit down with you and your family to talk about how you want to die: your primary care physician, the hospitalist, or a specialist? Who knows you best? Sometimes such experts are helpful, but many of us these days elect to sort this out by ourselves.

Dying is all about you and requires more than discussing your illness or treatments with medical care givers.

There are more than a few lessons to learn from this story about Aunt Nell. One of them is that conveying and understanding choices isn't easy and can lead to unwanted wrongful care.

My Aunt Nell was ninety years old. She lived in an adult apartment complex. Aunt Nell never had children of her own, and Uncle Bob passed away three years before. She was very sick. She had a lung disease and diabetes, and her heart was failing. We were her niece and nephew and the only family she had left.

We took her to the ER because she was acting confused. At the ER they found a sore on her toe from all the time spent lying in bed that wouldn't heal. It was a terrible infection and the hospital said she was septic. She had to be admitted and given antibiotics.

Her heart was failing and her circulation was bad. Because of all this she was put on a breathing machine. Then her leg got worse and gangrene set in because her circulation was so bad. My brother and I couldn't believe all this was happening. I mean from a toe sore to all these huge problems. We didn't see Aunt Nell wanting all this, being hooked up and all. We're sure we heard the hospital tell us that she wouldn't live if she was taken off the ventilator. She wouldn't want to be like this. We told the hospital to take her off the breathing machine. Don't give her any more medical stuff. Just make her comfortable.

She kept breathing after the machine was stopped! We freaked out. So we decided to change what we had said to do for Aunt Nell. It just made sense to do everything to save her now that she was breathing on her own.

But there seemed to be no end to things we were supposed to say yes or no to. We were asked to decide whether to have her leg cut off or not. We told the doctors to do everything to save Aunt Nell but don't cut off her leg. She wouldn't want to have just one leg.

The gangrene in her leg kept getting worse and they told us that her kidneys were failing. We were asked if we wanted Aunt Nell to receive dialysis. We said no. She wouldn't want that.

This was horrible. And the hospital was getting really mad at us. We believed that for Aunt Nell to get better she needed to eat and drink. She needed to fight the infections. We couldn't stop giving her IV fluids and nutrition. We couldn't stop the antibiotics. We didn't think she'd want her leg amputated and couldn't imagine that she'd want all these machines like the ventilator or dialysis.

The hospital and doctors kept at us, talking to us, telling us we didn't understand, that we were confused. That what we were asking for was incompatible with standard medical practice. They said that we should consent to amputation and dialysis because without that she would die or we should take her off everything and go back to comfort care. That didn't make sense to us. What's really amazing to us is that we got the feeling that they believed she was suffering because of what care we wanted for her. We did agree on giving her pain pills.

Finally, she died because her kidneys stopped working right.

Why did the hospital have to make all of this so ugly? All we were trying to do was think about what was best for Aunt Nell and save her life.

REDUCING PAIN AND SUFFERING

Many of us believe that end of life, pain, and suffering are inseparable, and this can lead to problems for you and your family. End of life and pain don't, in fact, always go hand-in-hand. There's almost no reason why anyone with a terminal illness should endure pain. Pain can be controlled, and it can be controlled the way you want.

Tell your proxy, and put in writing, how much pain you would be willing to accept if your chances of recovery from an illness or injury were good (fifty-fifty or better) or poor (less than one in ten). Tell them what life support you wouldn't want any longer if you were in severe pain or discomfort. Be clear about whether you would want adequate medication to relieve pain or just enough to ease the pain but also be aware of your surroundings and what's going on.

There are some patients who fear addiction or being overly sedated, and they prefer traditional healing practices. Personal history with drugs and addiction can be a factor in resisting medication, especially painkillers like Vicodin, morphine, and Demerol. Culture can influence a patient's response to the meaning and expression of pain. Pain may be perceived as a sign of the body fighting towards recovery. It can be seen as a test of faith, a means of achieving higher religious status, or a punishment for a sin. Asking for pain medication can be considered a sign of weakness. If these beliefs are held, patients may not ask for pain medication or expect pain relief.

In some cultures, not wanting to complain or be a burden to family may lead to unnecessary pain and suffering. In a culture that relies on an indirect communication style, the patient may wait to be asked if medication is needed to avoid a public display of emotion and confrontation. Some patients create barriers through stoicism and fatalism.

Not acknowledging pain and suffering or their intensities makes it difficult to effectively manage pain. Providers can't assume that if a patient is not expressing pain, then pain doesn't exist. That could lead to undertreatment. But overtreatment could result for an openly expressive patient without further confirmation of suffering. Pain management must be culturally sensitive and within the context of an individual's perception and response to pain, whether or not the patient asks for it or whether traditional healing practices take precedence over Western medical treatment.

Suffering is actually a broader concept than pain. Suffering can be physical, emotional, spiritual, existential, and social. Pain is physical suffering. The actions of doctors, nurses, and others can unintentionally but too frequently contribute to a patient's suffering. In the effort to save a patient's life, unwanted treatments may be initiated that prolong life and cause suffering. This is also true for families that can't let a loved one go and whose care decisions lead to a patient's unnecessary suffering and pain.

You can help your family recognize the big part they may play in controlling pain and suffering by having conversations and easing each other's minds, freeing your family and other loved ones to let you go as you wish.

FAMILY DYSFUNCTION

There may be disagreements about what a loved one needs even in the most harmonious of families. But too many stories about dying are a result of longstanding family dissonance, conflict, and dysfunction.

A hospital ethicist I know shared how much he'd like to admonish families who stand over a parent in the ICU and argue. "The disagreement isn't over what care should be provided to their parent but about who gets what. It's unimaginable what a patient must be thinking, having to lie there and hear these last words."

A chaplain told me, "Let's say there's a daughter or son from out of town and wanting to take over and show how involved they want to be, but in reality, they've been removed or cut off from the family for years. But these are the same children who make unrealistic demands for curing their parent. It's to erase their guilt. The needs of their parent are not addressed." He asks that this kind of agenda be left at the door, but his requests routinely fall on deaf ears.

There are many examples of an adult child living at a parent's home who wants to keep the Social Security check and the roof over their heads. Or a family doesn't want to spend down the patient's money to qualify for

Medicaid because they're worried about losing their inheritance or home.

It's extremely difficult for dysfunctional family members to deal with each other and for physicians to deal with dysfunctional families. A family member can ignore recommendations by a physician while looking only for personal gain, and clashes between medical staff and family can escalate. It may get to the level where staff believe they can deal with such situations, but it eventually hits bottom, and the ethics committee must try to get the situation back under control.

A vast majority of these problems can be resolved if a strong and reliable proxy is appointed who will honor your wishes for dying care. But that can be a problem too. Some families have such dysfunction and behavioral issues it's impossible to find a relative to appoint, or the proxy may be ignored and rendered ineffective.

If you are the proxy and this kind of dysfunction emerges, make sure you know the wishes of the person you are to speak for. Honor your loved one and tune out the others. Remember this: Don't do what you think you would want and don't guess at what your loved one would want. Do only what you know was requested and apply it to the situation.

The powerful, debilitating effect family dysfunction has on dying is evident in Leonard's story.

My sister Etta and I never got along. When Mom was very sick with all sorts of illnesses, we couldn't even stay in the same hospital room at the same time. But Mom had not chosen a proxy.

Since we were her closest relatives, we were to decide together what care we felt was best for her or choose between ourselves who should be the decision maker for her care. Etta felt she should be proxy because she had been Mom's caregiver for some time. I felt that I needed to be proxy because I wanted to be involved and have a say in the final care decisions. So we sued each other over guardianship because we didn't agree on what was to be done for her. Meanwhile, Mom was hooked up to everything until a court decision could be made.

Now I know why my sister wanted to keep Mom alive. I just couldn't say it out loud. Etta is what I call a "placenta mate." She is living with Mom and she is living off Mom. I've known about the Social Security check that is in the joint account. I know Etta's never left home since coming back after college. She hasn't had a job in many years. She has no other place to go. She says Mom needs her, but it's the other way around.

Then Etta used the smoke screen of religion to cover her own ass. She said she was waiting for a message from God; she was waiting for the miracle cure. She said, "Only God has priority over living. Only God can heal you." Now it's okay if she believed this, but she didn't, and that really disturbed me.

All efforts to save Mom continued as Etta took us to a point of no return. The hospital didn't have a clue

how to get involved and head this off. How do you
challenge that kind of reasoning—a belief?

I watched as Mom's health deteriorated. Mom did
not wait around for this lawsuit thing to get resolved.
She died in agony and there was nothing I could do
to stop that. I still don't talk with my sister and never
plan to speak to her again.

RACE, DISCRIMINATION, AND EQUAL RIGHTS

Racial discrimination and prejudice often have a negative impact on access to care, quality of care, and
outcomes among diverse ethnic, racial, and cultural
groups. African Americans, Hispanics, Chinese, Japanese,
Filipinos, Vietnamese, Cambodians, Thais, Laotians,
Indians, Native Americans, and other people of color
are all familiar with such bias, whether it's blatant and
explicit, or subtle and devious. It's important to understand the impact of prejudice and ethnic discrimination
on health care if our nation is serious about achieving
a more just and equitable society. This becomes even
more urgent as our population shifts to include a greater
percentage of minorities, and this increasing majority of
Americans faces the issues of death and dying we're confronting in this book.

First let's consider recent findings on health care
quality among minorities. There have been a number
of studies about whether a patient's race matters when
seeking medical care, but a major debate was ignited
in 2002 when the Institute of Medicine (IOM) released

a report, *Unequal Treatment: Confronting Racial and Ethnic Disparities in Health Care.*

Brian Smedley, with the Health Policy Institute of the Joint Center for Political and Economic Studies in Washington, D.C., writes: "What the IOM found shocked many: An overwhelming body of evidence in the peer-reviewed literature demonstrates that many minority patients receive a lower quality of health care than whites, even when access-related factors are controlled. These disparities . . . associated with poorer health outcomes . . . are unacceptable." The IOM concluded there's strong evidence that racial bias, discrimination, and stereotyping play a role in health care disparities, but other factors including politics, regional policies, and practices illuminate how such racism in the health care system operates.

The 2005 National Healthcare Quality and Disparities Report validated the observation that white patients received better quality of care than 53 percent of Hispanic, 43 percent of African American, 38 percent of American Indian/Alaska Native, and 22 percent of Asian and Pacific Islander patients. The 2010 edition of the report showed few disparities were decreasing for these ethnic groups.

One form of racial bias in medicine occurs when individuals are treated unfairly and poorly because of their membership in a minority group. We all walk into a room with preconceived attitudes toward each other, and it's no different in the health care setting. The following example shows it doesn't take much to alienate a person when faced with subtle biases, and the outcome can be dramatic:

> An elderly African American woman accompanied by her adult son showed up for her appointment with a white doctor. The doctor came into the examination room with an air of confidence and competence but he didn't seem very warm, almost unkind, and appeared stiff and tight. The patient can tell immediately that he's not comfortable around them and doesn't relate to them. The patient, having experienced prejudice in the past, is already distrustful. Both patient and physician are resistant to each other from the onset.
>
> This triggered the patient's son to be aggressive and demanding while his mother just wanted to leave. The doctor neglected a thorough examination and prescribed a medication for the patient's cough. The patient ignored what was recommended because the whole exchange was dissatisfying and she delayed medical assistance until the next day, when she was rushed to the ER and admitted to the ICU, severely dehydrated and with pneumonia.

Language and educational level can be major barriers to care, hindering communication with providers. Providers may underestimate a patient's ability to understand and limit what they tell. I've heard people say that sure, sometimes you can bump up against a doctor or other health care professional who's prejudiced or discriminates. But it's more than a "bad apple" problem. Discriminatory treatment and provider biases permeate the entire health care system.

There's institutionalized discrimination, where the health care system is unfair and inefficient because it rations care by income. "You get better care and treatment if you have the money to pay for it and good insurance coverage" or "You're likely to get more frequent visits and more time with the doctor." Among some minorities, bias and distrust affect how they're treated and regrettably interfere with getting the best care possible. There's also internalized discrimination, when some people who are discriminated against make these discriminatory beliefs part of their self-image, accepting negative stereotypes about themselves. It's hard for us to acknowledge that these things occur.

These same problems surround death and dying. Minorities can experience discrimination at end of life, raising concerns that minority patients receive inferior dying care. Here are two examples of such racial biases that show the kind of judgments we impose on each other and ourselves. Two minority patients, attended by different doctors who are both Caucasian, are diagnosed with cancer that has spread. The first-line chemotherapy proved unsuccessful.

The first patient, Mrs. R., is Hispanic. Her doctor recommends hospice because he feels it's most appropriate for her at this time, but she and her family are unfamiliar with hospice, believing it equates to less attention and care than in the hospital. She and her family have a deep distrust of the medical system and providers, and they feel the advice to end treatment is premature and an affront. While the suggestion of hospice is the best decision for her, the family fears ceasing therapeutic care and insists life-extending interventions and treatment continue.

Another patient, Mr. P., with the same prognosis as Mrs. R., is an African American. Mr. P. has a different doctor who pushes for further life-sustaining therapy, although the family isn't quite sure what to do about having a DNR and whether to continue with life-prolonging measures. This doctor wants to continue with more aggressive care, not less, because he believes such interventions are a well-considered preference of African Americans. Hospice care is more appropriate in this case than medical treatment, but the physician bases the decision of care on a false assumption about African American patient preferences with respect to health care.

The dying care Mrs. R. and Mr. P. received is the same, but Mrs. R.'s care is driven by minority suspicions of abandonment or poorer quality of care, and Mr. P.'s by a doctor's stereotypical approach to care. These examples show how we can become victims of prejudice at end of life. Our attitudes toward each other and our policies need to change so none of us receives inadequate, inferior end-of-life care or less customized care.

Each of us wants to be treated with respect and have our dying wishes honored, whatever our race, or ethnic origin. Wishes at the end of life may be strongly influenced by cultural factors, but it can't be assumed that patients' origin or race will lead them to approach decisions about their death in a culturally specified manner.

SAME-SEX COUPLES AND DISCRIMINATION

Same-sex couples are another group facing health care biases and inequalities. It's upsetting to hear stories of unmarried same-sex couples in which a partner is excluded from decisions about a partner's care. For example, a gay man was prevented from visiting his partner of 20 years by his partner's relatives, who never approved of their relationship. Consequently the medical staff was unsympathetic and treated him like a stranger. He was prevented from being by his partner's side, even when his partner was dying and passed away.

Marriage equality alleviates many of these concerns, and recognition of same-sex marriage is changing rapidly. At this time, gay couples can marry in twelve states— Massachusetts, New York, Maine, Connecticut, Iowa, Vermont, New Hampshire, Washington, Rhode Island,

Delaware, Minnesota, and Maryland plus Washington D.C.. No matter what the law, same-sex spouses should have an advance directive appointing a proxy to avoid facing discrimination and being challenged about health care decisions.

Each of us should be approached as unique, with our own perspectives regardless of sexual orientation.

WHAT IF YOU DON'T HAVE A HEALTH CARE PROXY?

What if you didn't appoint someone as your proxy? You thought, "If I don't have an advance care plan, I can rely on family to make health care decisions for me when I can't make them myself." What can happen if you choose not to choose someone?

Many states have laws that define a "priority listing of decision makers" who can make decisions for an incapacitated patient. There's an order of surrogates who can be appointed to speak for you. In such situations, you have no say in who becomes your health care surrogate. By not picking a proxy, treatment may be delayed and family may face limitations with decision making.

The person highest in priority from the surrogate list is most often the spouse, if not legally separated from the patient, or the domestic partner, then a son or daughter eighteen or older, followed by a parent, and then adult sibling(s). But you should check what the rules are in your state. The attending physician usually selects the surrogate decision maker as specified by this priority listing process.

This process can quickly get complicated when there's more than one among equal priority surrogates. In these circumstances, state requirements for decision making vary greatly, from providing no rules to requiring consensus or majority rule if there's disagreement among them. If there's a deadlock, the primary physician could be asked to decide.

For example, a patient has two adult children, the domineering son who wants all the input and the daughter who has been caregiver and feels entitled to be in charge. They don't agree, and the physician has to make the decision. Say there are five children, and they can't agree on a spokesperson. The parent's condition can't be put on hold while they dispute who's in charge.

A family may not know what the patient would want in a given situation or disagree about the best course of action. Disagreement can easily undermine family consent when no proxy is selected. Patients risk having decisions made contrary to their wishes or by persons whom they would not choose. Moreover, family members and persons close to patients experience needless agony in being forced to make life and death decisions without the patient's clear guidance.

To avoid conflict with other family members, unmarried partners should have health care directives. In states where marriage or civil unions are possible for same-sex couples, spouses or partners have priority over other family members. Most states do not include partners in their list of potential surrogate decision makers, but a few do: Arizona, New Mexico, Delaware, and Maine. New Mexico is the only state that gives priority to a long-term partner. Sometimes unmarried partners get around state priority listing by getting classified as "close friends," but only if listed family members are unavailable.

No matter what state you live in, you can save your partner a great deal of time and trouble by planning ahead. The Patients Rights Council, an organization that addresses advance directives, patients' rights, and euthanasia, describes what can happen if you don't name someone to make your health care decisions. The Council's examples are provided below with some details added to complete their stories.

BOB. Bob is a nineteen-year-old college student (and therefore, no longer a minor) seriously injured in a sports accident. His condition is stabilized. He is expected to improve, but he's not yet able to communicate, and decisions must be made about his therapy and treatment.

Bob's parents are unable to get information from his medical records and have no authority to make decisions for him, because Bob is in a state that does not have a priority listing of decision makers.

Bob's parents are distraught. The physician realizes the treatment decisions are left up to her. She decides to sit down with Bob's parents to explain what is going on. They listen, talk quietly together, and with the doctor come up with a plan of treatment they believe is in Bob's best interest. Although they aren't totally sure it's what Bob would want, they are comfortable with the plan. This was the best possible approach given the state's rules, but it would have been less difficult for all involved if Bob had talked with his parents and appointed his mom and dad as primary and secondary proxy in the first place.

JOE AND SALLY. Joe and Sally are married with three children—fifteen-year-old Richard, eighteen-year-old Tom, and twenty-year-old Mary. Driving home from a local restaurant, Joe and Sally are hit head-on by another car. Joe is killed. Sally is in critical condition. Sally's twin sister, Sue, who is very close to Sally and with whom Sally had often discussed her wishes about health care, rushes to the hospital. She attempts to get information about Sally's condition.

She is told the law prohibits disclosing such information to her. Instead, the information can be given to Tom and Mary who, under state law, have the authority to make medical decisions for their mother. Unfortunately, Tom and Mary don't get along with each other, and the law requires agreement between them before any action can be taken. This leads to a delay in authorizing treatment that could have vastly improved Sally's ability to recover fully.

To avoid further delay, Sue asks Tom and Mary to confer with her and the physician. The physician agrees, and through an open discussion, they're able to put aside personal issues and resolve what's best for Sally, but not without emotional cost and loss of precious time.

ALEX. Alex is a fifty-seven-year-old truck driver who had a heart attack while mowing the lawn. Due to a lack of oxygen, he sustained brain damage. He hasn't named anyone to make health care decisions, but he lives in a state that gives his wife, Anna, first priority in making his decisions. Anna knows that Alex wouldn't want a ventilator but would want to be tube fed if necessary. Alex is breathing on his own and being fed by tube. His brother, Dave, objects to the tube feeding. The doctor in charge of Alex's care thinks the tube feeding should be stopped.

In the state where Alex and Anna live, the attending physician or an advanced practice nurse can select a decision maker who is ranked lower in priority if, in his or her judgment, that person is "better qualified." Because Dave agrees with him, the doctor decides Dave is better qualified than Anna to make decisions for Alex. The tube is removed and twelve days later, Alex dies of dehydration.

CODE STATUS AND SLOW CODE

You've heard the term "no code" or "code blue" referring to patients requiring resuscitation on TV shows like *House*, ER, *Scrubs*, and *Grey's Anatomy*. But what are these codes and what do they have to do with DNR? And what's the problem with code status?

Code status is about resuscitation and all the life-sustaining treatments associated with CPR. A code status is assigned to tell medical staff what you want to have done if you stop breathing or your heart stops beating. It's derived from the DNR order when you are admitted to a hospital and establishes the level of treatment you will receive in a cardiac or respiratory arrest.

The problem with code status is it has potential for misinterpretation. Code status is not included in a living will or AMD. It's not a plan for your care. It refers only to resuscitation. There are three code statuses: full code (resuscitate), no code (DNR), and partial code.

DNR or no code doesn't mean "do not treat." This is a huge misunderstanding and it's a problem. You are not saying you don't want everything that can be done if you have a DNR order in place. You may want other life-sustaining treatments, just not CPR. The only thing that a DNR order means is that if you suffer a cardiac arrest you are not to have CPR.

The misinterpretation of "do not treat" is unfortunate. Where did this idea come from? Perhaps when patients say they want resuscitation attempted, full treatment is assumed and intensive care is then required. Resuscitate = full treatment. Do not resuscitate = no treatment. This logic is wrong.

Partial code is a term many doctors are not comfortable with because it's elastic. It has the potential to cover many treatments or interventions under different circumstances. It's not a universal term. Partial code says do some things related to resuscitation, but it's not always clear what those things are. Partial code must always be followed by specific mention of those things wanted or not wanted.

There's another term you may or may not know about: *slow code*. It's an almost unspoken procedure in hospital and ICU settings in which a seriously ill patient without a DNR order suffers cardiac arrest. This code is well known to the house staff in every hospital in the country, but no laws exist that cover it.

A slow code is when, in the opinion of the treating medical staff, there's no hope of successfully resuscitating the patient, and yet without a DNR order, they are obligated to do something. So they begin the motions of resuscitation slowly and without attempting a full effort. That's a slow code. This is not an official or recognized code status. It's an attempt to be "softer" or "kinder" to the family rather than refusing outright to make any attempt at resuscitation. There are often disagreements among medical staff as to whether or not this should be done.

Slow code occurs infrequently, usually with elderly patients. Why does it happen? The reasons are multiple and include difficulty in talking about the realities of the situation between medical staff and family, failure of the physicians to convey the information in an understandable way, unrealistic expectations about the patient getting better, and misunderstanding by the family about the process of resuscitation.

The medical community has a variety of opinions about slow code. Some believe that it is unethical and takes away patient rights, possibly leading to legal consequences. Others believe the complete reverse, that it is taking a patient advocacy stance, with a focus on preventing more suffering.

Slow code points to a failure on the part of the medical staff to communicate with family and a failure on our part not to have educated ourselves and our family about our wishes for dying care. It emphasizes the need for you to have a conversation based on a sound understanding of care choices and the realities you may face at the end of life.

7

EXTERNAL PROBLEMS

External problems relate to the extreme complexity arising from medical care made ever more innovative, sophisticated, and refined. It's knowing what to expect and preparing for such things as the inpatient hospital terrain, medicalization, and the possibility of medical error. You're not able to change any one of these things, but it's important to know what they're about because they certainly can affect your end of life.

How we died a hundred years ago is very different from how we die now. Care for the dying was basic and simple because so little could be done. But these days, care mostly centers on intensive care, critical care, and life support. A patient can survive injuries and maladies once uniformly fatal because of amazing technologies that in turn have led to huge changes in the hospital setting and the practice of medicine.

Medical care in the twenty-first century has provided us great success but also great failures. We can't always know if our decisions are prolonging life or postponing dying. Perhaps in some cases modern medicine has failed those of us facing the end of our lives, but I believe we actually fail ourselves by not preparing adequately. We need to understand the market forces behind health care. We need to know about this terrain of caring, curing, and dying. We need to understand that where we die matters because the whole systemic way of handling our care is predicated on where.

THE INPATIENT HOSPITAL TERRAIN

In the modern in-hospital terrain you can expect to see many more physicians. There are not only specialists but subspecialists as medicine continues to focus on critical care. A question you'll want to ask when hospitalized and seriously ill is, "Who are all these caring strangers that surround me?"

One important result of having so many different specialized physicians around you is that no single doctor will take responsibility for facilitating end-of-life choices. They won't know you and you won't know them. Your primary care doctor may or may not have privileges at the hospital where you're admitted and if not, won't be able to treat you. As a result, there's a growing trend of hospital-based physicians called "hospitalists," who assume care of hospitalized patients in the place of a patient's primary care physician. These doctors often have a group practice and their work focuses on full-time caring for inpatients. Their role is to consult with specialists and oversee your care.

Let's consider all this from your standpoint as a patient. If the hospitalist you've become familiar with is in a group practice, he or she may not be on call in an emergency situation. In such a case, an associate you don't know will treat you instead. On average, a hospitalist sees twenty to thirty patients a day, leaving little if any time to talk to the patient about an overall care plan.

A similar set of circumstances surrounds medical specialties. Specialists can also be associated with a group practice, and a different specialist within that group may come see you. So if you are very ill in the ICU, expect to see many different doctors.

A hospital's overall plan for medical care of the dying is often either nonexistent or inadequate. Listen to these words from Dr. Sherwin Nuland, a practicing surgeon for over thirty years, author of *How We Die* and *The Art of Aging*, and teacher of bioethics, history of medicine, and medicine at Yale University: "Lest anyone be deluded into thinking our present system of in-hospital care is a well-thought-out, sequentially planned model of deliberate design let me say without any possibility of refutation that it is not." It is as if all the physicians are in the same car but everyone is a back seat driver. One expert in the field of dying said, "The sicker you get, the interaction with doctors goes down." Care is nonintegrated because specialties are narrowly defined, making a total care approach nearly impossible.

A recent movement addresses this issue of the left hand not knowing what the right hand is doing. The collaborative care approach to hospital care creates a patient-centered, team-based model such as TedaCare based in Appleton, Wisconsin, tackling quality and cost issues, involving people in their care, and most importantly redefining the patient experience. It's encouraging to hear about this.

What's also happening is dying has become a medical specialty, palliative care. The average physician doesn't have practical experience with sitting by the bedside and too often doesn't know about death and dying.

Palliative care is delivered whether the goal is to cure, prolong life, or achieve a peaceful death. Many of us these days die in a hospital. If you are admitted and suffering, ask if there is a board certified palliative doctor and ask for a palliative medicine consult. This can better assure that you are kept comfortable and that pain is kept at a minimum.

The people you and your family will see most are nurses. They are the people who will come to know you and your family on a more personal basis, and you will find that they can become your confidantes and advocates.

Of course if your primary care physician doesn't have privileges at a certain hospital, he or she is still notified of your admission as a patient as part of patients rights explicitly expressed in the standards of the Joint Commission and the Centers for Medicare and Medicaid Services. It's okay for you and your family to ask hospital physicians to call and confer with your personal doctor regarding your wishes and how they affect your care. And your doctor can also come visit you in the hospital and talk with you and your family. Consequently, be sure to check with your primary care physician, nurse practitioner, or physician assistant about how they see themselves involved before an emergency or life-threatening situation occurs requiring inpatient hospital admission.

Your health information can be shared with your primary care physician, but you or your proxy must give written permission to the health care facility and/ or specialist treating you. Your personal doctor's name can be put on the HIPAA consent form. Health information cannot be shared otherwise; HIPAA gives you the rights over your medical and health records.

All of this can give you and your family peace of mind, knowing that someone who knows you is looking out for you—someone who can guide your family to stay true to your wishes.

Sadly, there are times when medical staff and family members don't agree on a patient's treatment. This often centers on discontinuation of life support when the medical staff feels treatment is not indicated, but the family wishes it to continue. In these situations medical staff may ask a hospital ethics committee or board to advise on continuation or change in treatment. It's interesting to know that such consultative bodies were almost nonexistent before the '70s because medical and moral decisions were not as integrated as they tend to be now.

While doctors may be inclined to do everything to keep a patient alive, an ethics committee will explore what's meant by "everything," weighing possible treatments against what is appropriate and beneficial. A hospital ethics committee doesn't take action or give orders. It only recommends, and the medical staff can take the recommendation or not.

Such circumstances are difficult, but there's a silver lining. With end-of-life issues, the attending physician may feel that the committee's recommendation in a sense gives "permission" to let go of his patient and stop specific medical treatment. Likewise, when the physician shares the recommendation with a family and takes action based on the recommendation, the family is helped in the process of letting go of their loved one.

Gwen's request to stop treatment is an example of this silver lining.

My sister Gwen was only fifty-four when she was diagnosed with chronic end-stage heart failure. She was not a candidate for a heart transplant and wanted to live longer. She decided to receive a left ventricular assist device, an LVAD, in 2010. Open-heart surgery is required to implant this device, which is attached to the left ventricle and the aorta. Apparently, a small pump is placed in a person's abdominal cavity and this is connected to an external battery-controlled system.

Over the next two years she suffered frequent and disabling complications. She had innumerable mini-strokes and serious infections. In 2012 she was readmitted to the hospital with yet another infection. She also could no longer walk because a hematoma or blood clot was causing nerve compression in her left leg.

Gwen asked that her device be turned off but Dr. W. wouldn't do it. He feared that this would be perceived as physician-assisted suicide. Dr. W. didn't want any part of that label.

Luckily, a hospital social worker suggested we get in touch with a Dr. M., who worked closely with the ethics committee, for a consultation. Dr. M. ascertained that Gwen knew she had heart failure and that was why the LVAD was there to keep her alive. Gwen understood that turning off the device would result in her death. Gwen talked with Dr. M. at length and told him that what was important to her was to live independently and to be able to walk. These things were no longer possible. The doctor determined "that the burdens of the device outweighed its benefits" and that Gwen was giving informed consent for the LVAD to be turned off.

This was the medical staff's way of saying she was within her rights to stop this device. My sister died soon after the machine was stopped. To me, her last breath sounded more like a sigh of relief.

If efforts to resolve differences in treatment goals fail among the physician, the bioethics committee, and the family, most hospitals have medical futility or "nonbeneficial care" policies supporting the hospital bioethics committee on decisions regarding the quality of a patient's life and the efficacy of treatment. And beginning in the 1990s, states began enacting futile-care statutes. These state laws center on a physician's determination of futility that is contrary to the request in the advance directive or the wishes of the proxy or family. Basically, futile-care statutes are designed to protect health care providers in defending their position of good medical practice when they determine further treatment would be without purpose or benefits.

In such a situation, the physician is required to inform the family that they have the option of either making arrangements for a transfer of care to a facility that will respect their wishes, or preparing for withdrawal of life support. This is very difficult for the medical staff and for the patient's family because in most cases, no time constraint is imposed to effect a transfer, and the statute specifies no procedural process to follow. Patient rights advocates contend that patient rights are violated because the statutes state that care is to be stopped after a certain period of time when care is deemed futile, and there's no formal process available to the family for appeal of the merits of the ethics committee's recommendation. However, the application of futile-care statutes may alleviate some of the guilt in letting a loved one die.

MEDICALIZATION AND SOCIETY

Ira Byock gives us a clear picture of just what medicalization is: "The medical profession commonly approaches dying as if it was a problematic medical event. From the first day in medical school, doctors are taught to approach patients by defining a set of medical problems to be solved. People come to doctors with problems. For each case a problem list must be developed through which both physical and psycho-social problems can be addressed."

It's through such a process that our human conditions and problems become defined and treated as medical conditions. Each of us is responsible in part for what drives this process due to our obsession with cure, an obsession that sprang from post-World War II scientific and technological victories that transformed American life. As medical care became more effective, we came to expect a medical cure time after time.

Many of us have also come to think of ourselves as part of an invincible society, imagining ourselves eternally young with the accompanying expectation of being eternally healthy. You and I carry this feeling of invincibility into the doctor's office, down hospital corridors, and to the bedside in critical care units. And as we grow old and find ourselves in poor health and then possibly hopeless health, we are still driven by new treatments and an overriding impulse to cure and be cured. So we ourselves become responsible for allowing medicalization to have a negative impact on our last days.

But there's more to medicalization than treating the symptoms but ignoring the whole person. The disease-treatment model is also about hospitalization and treating no matter what the cost or outcome. So many people end up in the hospital because it's the path of least resistance. Dr. Elliott Fisher, a researcher at the Dartmouth Institute for Health Policy, said, "The way we set up the system right now, primary care physicians don't have time to spend an hour with you, see how you respond if they wanted to adjust your medication. So the easiest thing for everybody up the stream is to admit you to the hospital. I think 30 percent of hospital stays in the United States are probably unnecessary given what our research looks like."

Despite this amazing figure of 30 percent unnecessary hospitalizations, most doctors feel that it's simply more efficient to manage patients in a hospital setting. So going to the hospital is what we're expected to do. We are to be treated aggressively as if there's no other option, and it's rarely about helping patients die. We appear to be caught in some kind of catch twenty-two. We're wrong to consider any other approach to dying (natural, hospice, holistic, or aid to dying) other than the conventional one. These approaches are to be avoided because they are seen as either inadequate or giving up, rationing care, not doing enough, or letting yourself or someone die.

Look at this situation about Joel, who pursued a number of approaches to dying care, all supported by his partner.

My partner Joel's idea about dying was that we don't die. We travel on to another life. So he had no fear of dying. It angered me because I felt that he didn't care he was leaving me.

Joel straddled both Eastern and Western medicine so he had surgery, sought out a healer, and then agreed to become part of a clinical drug trial for his brain tumor. This healer had him drinking so much carrot juice that he became an odd shade of orange. But his brain tumor kept growing.

He received hospice care during the last few months. The day before Joel died he said, "I'm not dying, you know; I'm not going to die." I heard what I wanted to hear. I believed we would work our way out of this hole!

Joel's always been a stoic, but it's physically and mentally agonizing to be apart because we've been soul mates forever. We've lived many lives before this one, and somehow every time we've been able to find each other. We will find each other again.

Clearly there are many views surrounding alternative medicine, and just as many if not more around a patient's right to seek aid in dying or taking one's own life. We're all different people, and I think the most difficult thing is honoring and respecting each other's choices about how to die. This story reflects these kinds of difficulties.

My papa had been diagnosed with early-stage Alzheimer's. One cool afternoon he decided to go for a swim at the lake. It was late April in Maine. He drowned that afternoon from hypothermia. We all thought he decided to end it before he got worse. He never did say goodbye.

It was awful. Devastating. But we had to respect the tough decision he'd made for himself.

The practice of medicine and how we died a century ago wouldn't work today. But what's happening now with dying care isn't working either. We hear clinicians, health policy researchers, and policymakers talking about the need to restructure hospital care for dying patients. But like us, they are coming up against the same barriers, ones David Weissman, an oncologist and palliativist, describes as follows: "The overreliance on technology: a 'never say die' attitude by patients, families, and physicians; and the fear of personally confronting the issues of death—these are the core social and cultural issues standing in the way of better care for the dying."

It may not be possible to change the social attitudes driving medicalized death. But each of us can insist on recognizing that "how to exit" is a deeply personal decision. It requires integrating the care possibilities and a cast of caring strangers with what you hold dear, finding that delicate balance between on the one hand, the benefits of medications and treatments, and on the other, dying your own death.

MEDICAL ERROR

Each of us trusts we're in good hands when hospitalized, but medical errors happen, and even the best doctors make mistakes. Medical error kills nearly 100,000 people a year in our country and injures many others. That means medical error is ranked in the top ten causes of death in the United States. Many of us are unaware of how pervasive this problem is and yet, there are others who believe these numbers underestimate the problem.

Medical errors are made every day in every hospital and can happen during any procedure, from any treatment, and to any patient. Most mistakes are repeated daily and are often avoidable. These relate to missing allergies and sensitivity to medications, spreading infection from staff to patient, operating on the wrong patient or wrong body part, and leaving things like instruments and sponges inside a patient during an operation. Other mistakes include masking symptoms with drugs, failing to obtain timely consultation, diagnosing and prescribing by phone, treating symptoms without looking for a cause, misjudging, misdiagnosing, performing unnecessary surgery, delaying treatment, and prescribing a drug either too little, too much, too soon, or too late.

The hope of course is that the mistake is corrected or caught before complications occur. Many errors are avoidable, and you can do something to avoid becoming a victim. Choose a health care proxy carefully, and do the same when choosing a doctor and hospital.

There are some other simple strategies you can use to help hospital staff avoid the avoidables such as making sure the staff checks your entire name and date of birth on your wristband and asking doctors and nurses if they washed their hands before touching you, even if they are wearing gloves. These small things can help avoid additional medical complications.

Let's also consider medical emergencies and the ER. To avoid delaying medical attention, call your physician to notify the ER that you're on the way. Always get to the ER as quickly as possible. If you believe it's truly a medical emergency, go by ambulance, because if a friend or family member drives you there, it's not giving a message of urgency.

MEDICAL MALPRACTICE

Not all medical errors rise to the level of malpractice. While malpractice must usually be determined through the legal system, it's generally said to occur when medical care fails to meet the standard of care in the community and causes damage.

Medical malpractice is a controversial topic across health care, government, malpractice insurance, and the legal system. We've all heard allegations of poor quality medical care or exploding litigation egged on by greedy lawyers and juries awarding eye-popping sums to undeserving plaintiffs. We've heard some doctors are actually leaving the field because they feel coerced to spend more than they can afford on insurance that may not even cover a suit, and some who remain are practicing in fear and silence.

Regardless of one's opinion on these issues, medical errors do happen and quality of care can improve. Examples of medical errors comprising malpractice include technical errors in the operating room, mistakes in diagnosis, and failure to recognize postoperative complications. These and other errors have to do with the complexities of modern medicine, which requires expertise, experience, judgment, and knowledge of anatomy and the infinite possibilities of doing harm.

It helps to appreciate how extremely difficult the job is. Today's medicine puts a great deal of energy into intensive care and artificial controls of failing bodies. On any given day almost 90,000 people are admitted to the ICU requiring critical care. Atul Gawande notes, "Intensive care succeeds only when we hold the odds of doing harm low enough for the odds of doing good to prevail. This is hard. There are dangers simply in lying unconscious in bed for a few days." Gawande is referring to conditions like muscle atrophy, bedsores, and clotting veins. To keep these dangerous problems at bay, every patient must be exercised, given blood thinners, and turned in bed frequently, in addition to keeping the patient, the lines, and the bed and room clean. "Add a ventilator, dialysis, and the care of open wounds, and the difficulties only accumulate."

There's so much more that has to be done right. The body can fail in 13,000 ways from diseases, syndromes, and types of injury, and there are different steps for each condition. To help fix what's wrong, there are 4,000 procedures and 6,000 drugs. Clearly, experience and judgment are important factors.

It's good to have an understanding of the tremendous burden that clinicians carry. But medical malpractice is a fact, and even with medical expertise, doctors are fallible. Mistakes are made, many avoidable, some careless, and others inexcusable. The best protection from being a victim of medical malpractice is to have a vigilant proxy, to recognize that hospital selection is a big item, and to exercise care in selecting your doctors.

COST OF CARE AT END OF LIFE, HEALTH INSURANCE, AND HOW WE DIE

The cost of care is an immense problem that we face at the end of life. This is a difficult area to discuss, as no one wants to feel they are not getting the care they deserve because of cost. Still, it's an area that we must be knowledgeable about when we make decisions about end-of-life-care. Electing to have extremely expensive treatments that have no chance of extending meaningful life is not something that most of us would intentionally choose, but there are factors that lead us into making costly choices that fail to result in the best care possible.

A friend said, "I plan to live forever because I can't afford to die." Another friend in her 80s shared this: "You know you've got to have a lot of money to grow old and to die right."

Yes, the cost of dying can be astronomical, even for those of us with health insurance. And yes, death is not an option—we all die even if we don't want to and can't afford it. But what are these costs and what about health insurance coverage? What's behind the costs and where do you fit into this picture?

Let's start with the overall price tag for health care and move toward the sticker price of the last days of patients' lives. An extraordinary amount of money is spent on medical care, with costs doubling over the past decade from $1.3 trillion to $2.6 trillion a year and expected to be nearly half again as much by 2020.

And these medical care expenses are highly concentrated, as a small percentage of heavy users consume a disproportionate amount of health resources. According to the Department of Health and Human Services, in 2009 only 1 percent of Americans accounted for 30 percent of health care expenditures, and 30 percent of Americans accounted for nearly 90 percent of expenditures. What's more, medical costs are rising faster than economic growth while our population is aging.

More than 80 percent of all deaths in the United States these days are among Medicare beneficiaries, and a large share of the rest are the results of accidents, homicide, or suicide in which medical costs are generally very low. In the last year of life, individuals consume more than a quarter of Medicare's expenditures, costing more than six times as much as other beneficiaries.

But what about you and me and health care coverage? For now, some of us have health insurance, some are covered by multiple polices, and some have no coverage. By 2022 there will be near-universal coverage, since the Affordable Care Act of 2010 will significantly expand options for Americans who now lack health care coverage. There are Medicare and wraparound or Medigap policies; there is Medicaid spend-down, the process of reducing an individual's assets to qualify for Medicaid; and there is long-term care insurance. And some people are dual eligible, covered under Medicare and Medicaid.

Without Medicare and private insurance, very few individuals can afford costly end-of-life treatments such as $10,000 a day in the ICU, where some patients remain for weeks or even months. It's amazing that as many as one-fifth of Americans end up dying costly deaths in these critical care units. Even with private insurance, most American families faced with a catastrophic illness cannot afford the cost of even deductibles and copays. And even those with generous insurance coverage may face extreme costs for medical equipment to manage health conditions and specialized needs.

Dr. Amy S. Kelley at Mount Sinai School of Medicine provides sobering information based on a recent study of Medicare data from 2003 to 2008: "A quarter of Medicare recipients (or about 13 million elderly) spend more than the total value of their assets on out-of-pocket health care expenses during the last five years of their lives."

Yet we can request what we want for care, no matter how sick or how imminent is death. Because of patients' rights, there are few restrictions in requesting what you want. Medicare, for instance, by law cannot reject a treatment based on cost. As Ira Byock told CBS News in 2009, "Medicare will pay $55,000 for patients with advanced breast cancer to receive the chemotherapy drug Avastin, even though it extends life only an average of a month and a half; it will pay $40,000 for a ninety-three-year-old man with terminal cancer to get a surgically implanted defibrillator if he happens to have heart problems too."

Clearly this has to do with patient rights, but equally important are consumer rights. Insurance disguises costs by making us insensitive to them, but there's much more to this than just insurance. We don't know the costs up front. The total amount of a health care decision is not disclosed. We are asked to make life and death decisions but are in the dark as to the price; we don't know the price of the care we are buying. The business of health care is about us, the patients, but we have no real cost information when making our health care choices.

It's hard to have a constructive conversation without the necessary data. Amanda Bennett, author of *The Cost of Hope*, shares what she confronted: "Figuring out how much all of this care will cost during the course of an illness is almost impossible." There's no way to assess the influence of costs because we don't know them. Bennett talks of clinging fiercely to hope. This leads doctors and patients to regard any reduction in treatment as a failure, even though the patient is eventually going to die. We may trust a physician to give the best advice and figure that the cost, for say one quality extra year of life, may be worth it.

We can empower ourselves to choose the care we want. That should include a transparency regarding the costs of dying, but it doesn't. For now, because we can't peel away the costs, we remain burdened with a propensity to do something to extend life without knowing all the facts.

Part 4
Learning from Other People's Experiences

*You matter because you are you. You matter to the last
moment of your life. We will do all we can, not only to
help you die peacefully, but also to live until you die.*
—Dame Cicely Saunders, founder
of the hospice movement

I have spent a lot of time with people in the process of dying—and for those who had happy relationships and loving friends and families, their efforts to leave them with a spiritual legacy as well as an example to treasure is a very real thing.
—David G. Smith, Richter Professor Emeritus of Political Science at Swarthmore College

Everyone has a story about someone, a loved one, who died. We all die differently, and some ways are gentler than others. They are reflections of choices made intentionally about dying, and dying that happened regardless of any choices.

Death and dying are inevitable, but the when and how are not highly predictable, and they're subject to internal and external obstacles. Often the best we can do is construct some scenarios and choose one that seems to make the best of an uncertain and often harsh reality.

Here are four such stories. Stories that show dying is about deciding how you want to live your last days, and your family allowing itself to experience these moments with you.

As you read these, ask yourself, "Who am I most like and why? What changes would I make in their approach or decisions?"

Dying is an event and a process, not just the end but also a leave-taking. Ask yourself about the kind of relationship you want to create between the final, physical event and the rest of the process, and with those close to you. Go back to the questions asked earlier about who you are and why you think and feel the way you do.

Preparing for a good death is a process of making decisions long before we die. There are many values to be preserved and perils to be avoided, but these preliminary and yes, preparatory exercises—knowing who you are, your choices, and the problems—will help you achieve your objectives of dying a good death on your own terms. I hope that in the midst of modern medicine and the inevitability of dying, maybe they can help bring peace back to the bedside.

8

·············

FOUR STORIES

JILL, THE GRASSHOPPER: FOOD AND WINE

A traveling companion who shared many New Orleans jazz fests talks about how Jill experienced every day, even the final ones.

Remember Aesop's fable, "The Ant and The Grasshopper," where the ant toiled all summer storing kernels of corn in his nest for the harsh winter ahead while the grasshopper chirped and hopped his way through the lazy days of summer? Winter came and the grasshopper suffered greatly without food. Jill was a grasshopper. Some people just cannot plan. Occasionally it seems they get away with it as she did, but it's dangerous and can go very wrong.

She was one of my best friends and a fabulous cook. She was one of those people who are at their happiest when cooking. She loved that. She could spend hours in the kitchen concocting all sorts of indescribable dishes, and most were grand. She enjoyed every delicacy that could be had and savored a fine wine.

Jill was diagnosed with inoperable cancer at sixty-nine and chose to do nothing but what she always knew how to do: enjoy the moment. She went home to die, and every day she dined in great fashion. Thankfully, her appetite was never affected until close to the end. Friends from all over brought her favorite meals served with a coveted pinot or malbec. Over these meals we sat and laughed so hard we were gasping for breath. She died two weeks later at home. Fortunately she remained mentally alert, and fortunately too she had so many friends to care for her the way she liked.

For many years, Jill had gone to the N'awlins jazz fest, eating everything from catfish po'boys to chicken cordon bleu. So we made sure that her funeral procession was reminiscent of Mardi Gras with musicians playing, "Oh When the Saints Go Marching In." A banner draped over her coffin read "Laissez les bon temps roulez" (let the good times roll). The celebration of this vibrant, incredibly charming woman continued on through the night and still does.

She was one of the lucky ones, a good life with a good ending without a lot of forethought. It's great when this happens but can be a disaster when lack of planning throws you into the "machine of health care" without your wishes being known or a proxy to ensure that your final wishes are honored.

CLAYT AND HIS FAMILY

A retired Navy Seal describes how he was there for his father those last days just the way his father wanted.

My father Clayt was an old codger. His elder sister said he was always that way since birth. He was a man of the deep woods, lived in Maine, and hunted yearly for long spells up in Canada with some Indian friends. He built his own home sixty years ago, where he raised his family and still lived.

Father had a strong opinion about everything and everybody. What he was most proud of was being a self-made man who valued being independent. He seldom went to visit a doctor and he never wanted to go to a hospital after, as he puts it, he erred on common sense and agreed to have an implantable cardioverter-defibrillator put in for abnormal heart rhythms at seventy. He hated it because it made him feel funny. He went and got the battery turned off.

He fought going inside those institution's walls to visit a friend in need and even his dying wife of fifty-five years. He was as clear as a man can be about his wishes for care at end of life—let me be at home with family. And he readily expressed this view to others, like what he said to his long-time friend Fred: "I'm eighty and Fred, you're seventy-nine. You've already had five open-heart surgeries and spent six months in rehab. Your bills are astronomical. I tell you, Fred, you aren't worth it. Fred's a good friend and a good listener. So far he hasn't gone for number six."

Father was as good as his word and he wrote an advance directive that said if he was seriously ill, he definitely didn't want to be hospitalized, and if he was dying, he didn't want anything done to prolong his life. He appointed me to be his medical proxy in case he was unable to speak for himself. He gave me a copy of the document appointing me as his proxy and a copy of his advance directive. While we never had any direct conversations after that regarding his wishes, I knew them clearly.

Just before Clayt's eighty-first birthday, he ended up admitted to the hospital one morning for dehydration and bronchitis. But then he checked himself out of the hospital at 10 p.m. and got a cab to take him home, the prescription for antibiotics left unfilled at his insistence.

Faye, one of the nurses at the hospital who was an old high school friend, alerted my sister, Olivia, and me. We tended him all night, making him drink water and keeping him steady and upright for the frequent trips to the bathroom. Two days passed and he admitted he was having pain in his abdomen. His urine output was negligible and he was retaining fluid. His feet were swollen and his cough no better. He fessed up, he was turning on the bathroom sink and running water so we couldn't hear whether he peed or not.

Olivia and I were full of questions for each other: Will he consent to any treatment? How do you honor his wishes and make sure he's without pain and suffering? How do we keep ourselves from crashing and burning in the meantime? We didn't know where this was going. How do you help someone who doesn't want to be helped?

Well, you know what we did for him? The only thing we could: we listened, like Fred listened to him. He stayed in his home to die but it wasn't easy because very quickly his pain intensified. He didn't have time to qualify for hospice care, but what were we to do about his pain now that he was home? His lungs were filling with fluid and his respiratory system was shutting down. We were fortunate he wasn't delirious or agitated.

We were also fortunate that he was an icon in this small town where he lived his whole life. Dr. N. and his staff, the nurse practitioner Bill, and R.N.s Brad, Helen, and Rachel, we knew them all. They came to his rescue and ours, visiting frequently and helping us to help him. They relieved his pain and other symptoms. Father's passing happened at home as he wished, but the pain would have been excruciating without the care given by these capable professionals.

He passed away how he wanted. I can hear his constant reminder even now, "I'm a person who likes home. It's where I feel comfortable."

MILDRED'S SPIRIT OF LIFE

This is a story about Mildred as told by her twin sister.

She was like MSG, an accent to every gathering, some drawn to her and others, repulsed. She and I had many discussions over the years about life and death. She of course wanted to live as long and strong as she possibly could. She wanted everything done to prolong the life she loved. She put this into writing in case she was in a situation where she could not direct everything as she usually did. She prepared a very simple but firm advance directive in which she made her wishes known. She did not appoint a proxy, she said, "No one can speak for me as well as I can!"

She's always been a fighter and that's a good thing, because Mildred was diagnosed with cancer three separate times. She was lucky, got excellent care, and her body responded well each time. Thirteen years after the last occurrence, at eighty-five, she was determined to live on.

She was then diagnosed with heart block that is sometime seen in the elderly as a result of heart disease, and that news sent her shopping around for a pacemaker. Doctor after doctor said no. My little pit bull of a sister found someone who said yes.

Within another year, her health was failing rapidly even with the pacemaker. Her life became a struggle and painful. But Mildred's not only eccentric, she's true grit. She seemed actually to believe, since she had plenty of money, that was the secret: that money could buy her time. And it did. It gave her another five months of reprieve.

Denying that you're dying isn't uncommon, but usually denial is only a temporary defense. During those five months she believed she'd get well. She was in and out of the hospital regularly, actually happy to go and get the attention and care. She spent her last days in intensive care.

Dying isn't easy, especially for Mildred who struggled so. Her doctor made her reasonably comfortable and she kept pretending that she wasn't going to die. I decided she wasn't hurting anyone with this belief and why take this away from her, especially since I had nothing to give in its place.

On one of her last days, she took my hand and whispered, "Thank you. Thank you so much for letting me be myself and fight death. I don't think I'll beat this one, but you never know." I smiled and nodded.

With Mildred, you never were quite sure whether it was the final death fight. While she was sleeping, I slipped out to make a call. When I returned, she was gone. I didn't really believe it until the nurse held me and assured me she'd passed away. I'm glad I was there for my sister the way she wanted.

DAVID AND HIS NATURE

One of my oldest friends told this story about her husband, his letting go, and her being there for him.

In early March 1999, David and I were sitting in the doctor's office waiting for the nurse to take us in to see the doctor. When we walked in, the doctor introduced himself and asked us to take a seat.

"Mr. Watson," he said, "you have bone cancer throughout your body. We will take care of getting hospice for you. I would say you have about six months."

Can you imagine that? But those were the words. He said all this in one breath. His words left us breathless. Our conversation the rest of the day and evening was without words.

David chose not to have hospice but to be at home with me. He told me he wanted to stay home if at all possible and die a natural death without machines and a lot of medicines. He wrote this out on a single sheet of paper and stated I was to be his proxy. Our neighbors Jim and Hilda were present and signed as witnesses. I knew what being his proxy was about, simply being in his presence. For the next year David taught me how to let God's love and joy have their way in our lives. He and I felt more present with each other than ever before. That year became the most precious in our fifty-nine years together.

David kept a small area of grass for his nature spot during the summer afternoons. Sometimes the temperatures soared into the nineties. The heat seemed to soothe David's bones. I often joined him. He taught me to watch for the breeze rather than feel the heat.

He would watch the birds and listen to their songs. He experienced the magic of the moment.

A year after the diagnosis he asked that hospice come to ease his pain. His time was close.

One morning our daughter, Mary, and I were with David. As always, his mind was clear; however, he was sleeping more and talking less, which made us wonder if he was near to making the transition. At one point he turned to us and said, "I got to get up there and bore holes through heaven's carpet so I can pull up people who want to die but whose family won't let them."

Mary sat on one side of David's bed, and I sat on the other. We held his hands and rubbed his arms. I said, "You're doing great." Mary reminded him that he was almost there and offered other encouraging phrases. I told him that the bridge we had built was finished, and he could walk over when he was ready. He smiled.

As his breathing became more difficult, Mary and I continued to rub his arms and whisper to him how well he was doing. At six-thirty he called us by name, lifted his eyes, took a soft breath and ascended. His passing was so gentle and loving it was as though he was carried away on angel wings.

He died on May 9, 2000. I never felt life go out of me. It was more like life came in.

It's now October 2012, and I continue to feel renewed as I rest in what life is teaching me. I rejoice that David was able to live as he wanted, to the end. My body grew weary sometimes during David's illness, but never my heart. Every day is a bit of a lifetime. Every day in itself is complete. Now, I reflect on my ponderings in the Presence over the past ninety-one years and can say David was true to himself in life and dying and taught me the same.

ACKNOWLEDGMENTS

Any book is the work of many hands and that's particularly true for this one. I knew really very little about dying and death other than my personal experiences with loved ones. Almost everything in the book reflects, however indirectly, the assistance of others.

I have many to thank for their generosity in time and spirit. Let me begin with my husband, Steve, for his patience. Countless times he'd sit and listen to details about my personal mission, to write about the new art of dying and to create the mobile health app, My Health Care Wishes. The app would never have become a reality without his help in its development.

Special thanks go to friends and others who confided their stories about loved ones who died and family controversies. Writing this book was made possible not simply by my own life and work experiences, but by an amazing collaboration of friends, relatives, caregivers,

cancer survivors, physicians, attorneys, hospice administrators, health policy analysts, palliativists, chaplains,
and bioethicists. I wish particularly to thank Michael
Holtz, M.D.; Gay Bulan; Roberta Wollons, Ph.D.; Dee
Leahman; David Cochran; Sarah Grant Schmidt, M.D.;
and Ray Adelman, M.D. I am grateful for all their help.

I owe so much to my editor, Alan Rinzler. With his
support, I found a way to express my authentic feelings
and show the power of the book's message in all its
intensity and originality. Alan helped me free myself
from years of writing in a technical and rigid style.

Judy Moore is the kind of person who brings people
together. I'm grateful she read through my book before
publication because her insights and recommendations
were right on the mark. And then she introduced me to
others so I could share my book and get more invaluable
feedback. Lastly, she has this uncanny ability of saying
just the right thing at the right time to spur you on.

And then there are these amazing people whom I was
privileged to have as critical readers, catching errors,
guiding me away from digressions and distractions, and
enriching this book with their observations and wisdom.
Thank you Les Morgan, Founder of Growth House;
Bruce Vladeck, a recognized expert in health care policy
and finance, Medicare, Medicaid, and long-term care
and senior advisor to the health care consulting firm
Nexera; Judy Peres, a palliative care and hospice expert
and owner of Supporting Successful Transitions; and
David Smith, Richter Professor Emeritus of Political

Science at Swarthmore College, for giving so generously of your knowledge and time.

I offer thanks to my brother, Chris Burnside, who has always stood beside me even when I am beside myself. I leaned heavily on him, counting on his every comment, especially thrilling to his compliments on words well said. Louise Wilson is the voice in my head that I listen to. Her words are instantly recognizable as truth and always affect my very being. Louise kept me going, her excitement and interest propped me up, and her insights made the book complete.

I am especially grateful for the support of Elwood Headley, M.D. He was my next-door neighbor in Boston, and we had many exchanges from one rooftop to the other. He graciously accepted the invitation to read the manuscript's first draft and quickly became my teacher and mentor. I couldn't have stumbled on a more wonderful guide and adviser. Working with this bright star of a man these five years, I wish we had met earlier in our careers. I am thankful for his attention to detail, his patience in explaining the complexities of the practice of medicine, and his gentle but honest way. Over the course of our association, he has become a dear friend.

Thanks to all who held me loosely in an open hand so I could find my voice to share what I saw and heard in the midst of the medical terrain of dying, and what I believe can help you define wishes for dying care consistent with your life and who you are.

—*Diane Burnside Murdock*

RESOURCES AND NEW MOVEMENTS FOR CONSUMER DISCUSSION ABOUT DYING AND FOR ADVANCE CARE PLANNING

Advance Care Planning Decisions
  http://www.acpdecisions.org

  Advance Care Planning Decisions is a non-profit
  foundation created by a group of clinicians
  offering a series of patient education videos to
  empower patients and families about advance
  care planning and medical care choices.

Caring Connections
    HelpLine: 800-658-8898
    Multilingual Line: 877-658-8896
    E-mail: caringinfo@nhpco.org
    http://www.caringinfo.org
    For state advance directives forms:
    http://www.caringinfo.org/stateaddownload

    Caring Connections is a program of the National
    Hospice and Palliative Care Organization
    (NHPCO). NHPCO is a national consumer and com-
    munity engagement initiative to improve care at
    the end of life, supported by a grant from the
    Robert Wood Johnson Foundation. You can down-
    load state forms from this site.

Caring Conversations Workbook
    See Center for Practical Bioethics

Center for Practical Bioethics
    Harzfeld Building
    1111 Main Street, Suite 500
    Kansas City, MO 64105-2116
    800-344-3829
    http://www.practicalbioethics.org/

    The Center for Practical Bioethics is a nonprofit
    organization helping others become better
    informed on ethical issues in healthcare, working

on aging and end-of-life issues, addressing end-
of-life care planning and advance directives, and
improving patient protection.

Compassion and Choices
    P.O. Box 101810
    Denver, CO 80250
    800-247-7421
    www.compassionandchoices.org

    Compassion and Choices helps people plan for
    and achieve a good death offering such services as
    end-of-life counseling and advance care planning.

The Consumer's Tool Kit for Health Care
Advance Planning
    The American Bar Association
    Commission on Law and Aging
    740 15th Street, NW
    Washington, DC 20005-1022
    202-662 8690
    E-mail: abaaging@abanet.org
    http://new.abanet.org/aging/

    This kit provides ten user-friendly tools including
    self-help worksheets, discussion guides, and
    resources. It helps you to create an advance care
    plan and to have a conversation.

The Conversation Project
    The Institute of Healthcare Improvement
    20 University Road, Cambridge, MA 02138
    617-301-4800
    http://theconversationproject.org/

    The Conversation Project, supported by the
    Institute for Healthcare Improvement, is
    dedicated to helping people talk about their
    wishes for end-of-life care by sharing their stories
    about dying. The starter kit is a tool for having
    conversations about dying.

Death Café
    http://www.deathcafe.com

    At Death Cafés, people gather in a relaxed setting
    to discuss death, drink tea, and eat cake. The
    objective is to increase awareness of death and to
    help people make the most of their (finite) lives.

Death over Dinner
    http://www.deathoverdinner.org

    A contemporary movement about "Let's have din-
    ner and talk about dying," encouraging people to
    "discuss the beauty, mystery, fears, hopes, and chal-
    lenges of end of life decision making" in a setting
    that's comfortable and comforting—over dinner."

Five Wishes
    Aging with Dignity
    P.O. Box 1661
    Tallahassee, FL 32302-1661
    888-5-WISHES or 888-594-7437
    http://www.agingwithdignity.org/
    http://www.agingwithdignity.org/five-wishes.php

    Five Wishes is a living will specifying five health
    care wishes you should talk about: your choice of
    proxy and your personal, emotional, medical, and
    spiritual wishes. Aging with Dignity is a national
    nonprofit organization.

Go Wish
    http://www.gowish.org/
    http://www.codaalliance.org/gowishcards.html

    The Coda Alliance, a collaboration of
    individuals and representatives in the San Jose
    Silicon Valley, California, presents the Go Wish
    card game as a way to think and talk about
    what's important to you.

The Good to Go Toolkit
    http://community.compassionandchoices.org/
    document.doc?id=425

    A guide published by Compassion and Choices.

Handbook for Mortals:
Guidance for People Facing Serious Illness
    Joanne Lynn, M.D., and Joan Harrold, M.D.
    Oxford University Press
    An online edition is available at: http://www.
    growthhouse.org/educate/flash/mortals/layouts/
    frameset1.html

    Handbook for Mortals is a comprehensive guide
    to dealing with terminal illness.

Growth House
    http://www.growthhouse.org

    Growth House, Inc. provides education about
    life-threatening illness and end-of-life-care giving
    free access to over 4,000 pages of related high-
    quality educational materials.

Hard Choices for Loving People:
CPR, Artificial Feeding, Comfort Care and the Patient
with a Life-Threatening Illness
    Harold Dunn
    A&A Publishers
    www.hardchoices.com

    Hard Choices is a booklet on end-of-life decisions.

Loving Conversations
>American Health Lawyer Association
>http://www.healthlawyers.org/hlresources/PI/
>InfoSeries/Pages/LovingConversations.aspx

>Loving Conversations is about a fictional family's
>process of decision making for a loved one who
>didn't have an advance directive.

Making Health Care Decisions for Others:
A Guide to Being a Health Care Proxy or Surrogate
>Division of Bioethics
>Department of Epidemiology and Social Medicine
>Montefiore Medical Center
>Albert Einstein College of Medicine
>http://www.montefiore.org

>This guide is a quick reference for physicians to help
>a proxy or substitute decision maker make decisions
>for others when they are unable to make their own.

Midwest Bioethics Center
>*See Center for Practical Bioethics*

National Healthcare Decisions Day—April 16
>http://www.nhdd.org/

>An initiative that encourages expressing wishes regard-
>ing healthcare and provides resources and materials.

On Our Own Terms: Moyers on Dying
Bill Moyers on Death and Dying,
September 10, 2000
http://billmoyers.com/content/a-death-of-ones-own/

In this program, Moyers unravels the complexities
underlying the many choices at the end of life.
Three patients, their families, and their doctors
discuss some of the hardest decisions.

Prepare
https://www.prepareforyourcare.org/

Prepare is a project to help you make medical
decisions for yourself and others and find the care
you want at end of life. The site's purpose is to
simplify the process of making decisions about
dying care.

Put It in Writing
American Hospital Association
http://www.aha.org/advocacy-issues/initiatives/
piiw/index.shtml

The Put It in Writing Web site is a resource
providing basic facts about advance directives and
care options. The site includes a link to state forms.

Shape Your Health Care Future with Health Care
Advance Directives
http://apps.americanbar.org/aging/

This is a document jointly published by the
American Bar Association, the American Medical
Association, and the American Association of
Retired Persons.

TED Talks on Death and Dying
http://www.ted.com/topics/death

TED is a nonprofit devoted to Ideas Worth
Spreading. It started out in 1984 as a conference
bringing people together from three worlds:
technology, entertainment, and design. Currently
there are twelve discussions on death and dying to
stimulate dialogue.

Your Life Your Choices—Planning for
Future Medical Decisions:
How to Prepare a Personalized Living Will
Robert Pearlman, et al., and the Veterans
Administration Medical Center, Seattle, Washington
http://www.lifeissues.org/

Your Life Your Choices is a workbook dealing with
end-of-life choices and planning for end-of-life care.

There are many local and national organizations that may be helpful with advance care planning, including the following:

Alzheimer's Association
http://www.alz.org

AARP Caregiving Resource Center
http://www.aarp.org/content/aarp/en/home/
relationships/caregiving.html

Caregiver Action Network
Also referred to as Family Caregiver Alliance (FCA)
and National Family Caregivers Association (NFCA)
http://www.caregiver.org

Get Palliative Care
http://www.getpalliativecare.org/

SELECTED BIBLIOGRAPHY

Albom, Mitch. *Tuesdays with Morrie: An Old Man, a Young Man, and Life's Greatest Lesson*. New York: Random House, Broadway Books, 1997.

Altman, Kenneth W., Gou-Pei Yu, and Steven D. Schaefer. "Consequence of Dysphagia in the Hospitalized Patient: Impact on Prognosis and Hospital Resources." *Archive of Otolaryngology—Head and Neck Surgery 136* (2010): 784–789.

American Medical Association. *Code of Medical Ethics of the American Medical Association: Current Opinions with Annotations, 2010–2011*. Chicago: American Medical Association, 2010.

Baker, Tom. *The Medical Malpractice Myth*. Chicago: University of Chicago Press, 2005.

Bartholomc, Claire. "Health Care Proxies for Same-Sex Couples." *14 Stories Blog*, February 10, 2010. http://www.14stories.com/_blog/ Weddings_Redefined/post/Health_Care_Proxies_for_Same-Sex_Couples/

Beck, Melinda. "Preparing for the Final Hours." Health Journal. *Wall Street Journal,* August 18, 2009.

Becker, Ernest. *The Denial of Death*. New York: The Free Press, 1978.

Bennett, Amanda. *The Cost of Hope: A Memoir*. New York: Random House, 2012.

Bennett, Amanda. "End-of-Life Warning at $618,616 Makes Me Wonder Was It Worth It." Bloomberg, March 4, 2010. http://www.bloomberg.com/apps/news?pid=newsarchive&sid=aVRFGNF6Qw_w

Berman, Amy. "Terminal Breast Cancer Leads Woman to Pick Palliative Care, Not Aggressive Therapy." Health and Science. *Washington Post,* April 30, 2012.

Bonifield, John, and Elizabeth Cohen. "10 Shocking Medical Mistakes." The Empowered Patient, CNN Health. *CNN*, June 10, 2012. http://www.cnn.com/2012/06/09/health/medical-mistakes

Brody, Jane. *Jane Brody's Guide to the Great Beyond: A Practical Primer to Help You and Your Loved Ones Prepare Medically, Legally, and Emotionally for the End of Life*. New York: Random House, 2009.

Brody, Jane E. "Mapping Your End-of-Life Choices." Personal Health. *New York Times*, June 18, 2012.

Brouhard, Rod. "Do Not Resuscitate (DNR) Orders: Getting Emergency Responders to Honor Your Wishes." First Aid. About.com, 2007. http://firstaid.about.com/od/medicallegal/qt/07_DNR_Orders.htm

Brownlee, Shannon. *Overtreated: Why Too Much Medicine Is Making Us Sicker and Poorer*. New York: Bloomsbury USA, 2008.

Burns, Jeffrey P., et al. "Do-Not-Resuscitate Orders after 25 Years." *Critical Care Medicine* 31 (2003): 1543–1550.

Byock, Ira. *The Best Care Possible: A Physician's Quest to Transform Care through the End of Life*. New York: Avery, Penguin Books, 2012.

Byock, Ira. *Dying Well: Peace and Possibilities at the End of Life*. New York: Riverhead Books, 1997.

Chan, P.S., et al. "Delayed Time to Defibrillation after In-Hospital Cardiac Arrest." *New England Journal of Medicine* 358 (2008): 9–17.

Collins, Lauren G., Susan M. Parks, and Laraine Winter. "The State of Advance Care Planning: One Decade after Support." *American Journal of Hospice and Palliative Care* 23 (2006): 378–384.

"Consumer's Tool Kit for Health Care Advance Planning." 2nd ed. Commission on Law and Aging, American Bar Association, 2005. http://www.americanbar.org/groups/law_aging/resources/consumer_s_toolkit_for_health_care_advance_planning.html

Coolen, Phyllis R. "Cultural Relevance in End-of-Life Care." *EthnoMed*, May 1, 2012. http://ethnomed.org/clinical/end-of-life/cultural-relevance-in-end-of-life-care

Court, Andy. "The Cost of Dying: End-of-Life Care." *60 Minutes.* CBS News, December 3, 2010.

DePalma, Judith A., et al. "'Slow' Code: Perspectives of a Physician and Critical Care Nurse." *Critical Care Nursing Quarterly* 22 (1999): 89–99.

DeSpelder, Lynne Ann, and Albert Lee Strickland. *The Last Dance: Encountering Death and Dying.* New York: McGraw-Hill, 1983.

Donley, Greer, and Marion Danis. "Making the Case for Talking to Patients about the Costs of End-of-Life Care." *Journal of Law, Medicine, and Ethics* 39 (2011): 183–193.

"Do Not Resuscitate—Advance Directives for EMS, Frequently Asked Questions and Answers." California Emergency Medical Services Authority, State of California, 2007. http://www.emsa.ca.gov/personnel/DNR_faq.asp

Dovidio, John F., and Susan T. Fiske. "Under the Radar: How Unexamined Biases in Decision-Making Processes in Clinical Interactions Can Contribute to Health Care Disparities." The Science of Research on Racial/Ethnic Discrimination. *American Journal of Public Health* 102 (2012): 945–952.

Emanuel, Ezekiel J. "Legal Aspects of End of Life Care." UpToDate. *Wolters Kluwer Health*, March 15, 2011. http://www.uptodate.com/contents/legal-aspects-of-end-of-life-care

"End-of-Life Choices: CPR & DNR." Family Caregiver Alliance, National Center on Caregiving, 2003. http://www.caregiver.org/caregiver/jsp/content_node.jsp?nodeid=397&expandnodeid=482

"End-of-Life Decisions: Honoring the Wishes of the Person with Alzheimer's Disease." Alzheimer's Association, 2012. http://www.alz.org/national/documents/brochure_ endoflifedecisions.pdf

"End-of-Life Uncertainty: Americans Need to Be More Assertive in Detailing the Medical Treatment They Want as They Age." Editorial. *Los Angeles Times,* November 29, 2010.

"The End-of-Life War." *Freakonomics,* July 27, 2010. http://www.freakonomics.com/2010/07/27/the-end-of-life-war/

Feldman, David B., and S. Andrew Lasher, Jr. *The End-of-Life Handbook: A Compassionate Guide to Connecting with and Caring for a Dying Loved One.* Oakland: New Harbinger Publications, 2007.

"Frank Sloan: Reforming Malpractice Liability to Improve Health Care." Investigator Awards in Health Policy Research. *Research in Profile* 28 (2010). http://www.investigatorawards.org/ downloads/research_in_profiles_iss28_apr2010.pdf

Gawande, Atul. *The Checklist Manifesto: How to Get Things Right,* New York: Henry Holt and Company, Metropolitan Books, 2009.

Gawande, Atul. "Letting Go: What Should Medicine Do When It Can't Save Your Life." *New Yorker,* August 2, 2010, 36–49.

Gawande, Atul. Interview by Terry Gross. "Make End of Life More Humane." *Fresh Air.* National Public Radio, July 29, 2010.

Gazelle, Gail. "The Slow Code—Should Anyone Rush to Its Defense?" *New England Journal of Medicine* 338 (1998): 467–469.

Gazelle, Gail. Interview by Noah Adams. "Slow Code." *All Things Considered.* National Public Radio, February 11, 1998.

"Giving Someone a Power of Attorney For Your Health Care: A Guide with An Easy-to-Use, Legal Form for All Adults." Commission on Law and Aging, American Bar Association, 2011. http://www.americanbar.org/content/dam/aba/ administrative/law_aging/2011/2011_aging_hcdec_ univhcpaform_4_2012_v2.authcheckdam.pdf

Goldman, Lee, and Dennis Arthur Ausiello. *Cecil Textbook of Medicine.* 23rd ed. Philadelphia: Saunders Elsevier, 2007.

Gordon, Geoffrey H. "Disclosing Error to a Patient, Vignette 1: Physician-to-Patient Communication." *American Medical Association Journal of Ethics, Virtual Mentor 7* (2005). http://virtualmentor.ama-assn.org/2005/08/pdf/ccas1-0508.pdf

Graham, Judith. "The High Cost of Out-of-Pocket Expenses." The New Old Age (blog). *New York Times,* September 21, 2012. http://newoldage.blogs.nytimes.com/2012/09/21/the-high-cost-of-out-of-pocket-expenses/

Grimmelmann, James. "The Slow Code." *Laboratorium,* January 6, 2008. http://laboratorium.net/archive/2008/01/06/the_slow_code

Grove, Andy. "Peeling Away Health Care's Sticker Shock." Business, Health Science, Commentary. *Wired,* October 16, 2012. http://www.wired.com/business/2012/10/mf-health-care-transparency/all/

Gupta, Sanjay. "More Treatment, More Mistakes." Opinion. *New York Times,* July 31, 2012.

Hobson, Katherine. "The Latest Site for Palliative Care: The Emergency Room." Health Blog. *Wall Street Journal,* August 5, 2010. http://blogs.wsj.com/health/2010/08/05/the-latest-site-for-palliative-care-the-emergency-room/

Hughes, Allison. "State Advance Directive Registries: A Survey and Assessment." Health Care Decision Making. *Bifocal: Bar Associations in Focus on Aging and the Law* 31 (2009): 23–50.

Institute of Medicine. National Research Council. *Unequal Treatment: Confronting Racial and Ethnic Disparities in Health Care.* Washington: National Academies Press, 2003.

"Isn't It Time We Talk? How to Plan for Your Care at the End of Life." The Carolinas Center for Hospice and End of Life Care. http://cchospice.org/Public_Awareness_Materials.aspx

Johnson, Tim, James Wang, and Jennifer Metz. "End-Of-Life Care at Home Can Improve Quality of Life for Patients and Families." *World News with Diane Sawyer.* ABC News, December 27, 2010.

Jonsen, Albert R., Mark Siegler, and William J. Winslade. *Clinical Ethics: A Practical Approach to Ethical Decisions in Clinical Medicine*. 6th ed. New York: McGraw-Hill, 2006.

Kass-Bartelmes, Barbara L., and Ronda Hughes. "Advance Care Planning, Preferences for Care at the End of Life." *Research in Action* 12 (2003). http://www.ahrq.gov/research/findings/factsheets/aging/endliferia/index.html

Kelley, Amy S., et al. "Out-of-Pocket Spending in the Last Five Years of Life." *Journal of General Internal Medicine* 28 (2012): 304–309.

Kenen, Joanne. "We Can't Save You: How to Tell Emergency Room Patients that They're Dying."

Kessler, Richard E., and Patrick Trese. *Bitter Medicine: What I've learned and Teach about Malpractice Lawsuits (and How to Avoid Them)*. Create Space Independent Publishing Platform, 2012.

Kiernan, Stephen P. *Last Rights: Rescuing the End of Life from the Medical System*. New York: St. Martin's Press, 2006.

Klein, Joe. "The Long Goodbye." *Time*, June 11, 2012.

Knaus, William, and Joanne Lynn. "Study to Understand Prognoses and Preferences for Outcomes and Risks of Treatment (SUPPORT) and Hospitalized Elderly Longitudinal Project (HELP), 1989–1997." Ann Arbor, MI: Inter-university Consortium for Political and Social Research, 2001.

Krishnamoorthy, Brintha, and Kevin O'Rourke. "Disagreement over Error Disclosure." *American Medical Association Journal of Ethics, Virtual Mentor* 6 (2004). http://virtualmentor.ama-assn.org/2004/03/ccas1-0403.html

Kristof, Nicholas. "A Possibly Fatal Mistake." Opinion. *New York Times*, October 14, 2012.

Kübler-Ross, Elisabeth. *On Death and Dying*. New York: Macmillan, 1969.

Kübler-Ross, Elisabeth. *Questions and Answers on Death and Dying: A Companion Volume to On Death and Dying*. New York: Simon and Schuster, 1974.

LaMie, Beth. "Overview of Ethical Wills." 2010. http://www.bethlamie.com/ethical-wills.html

Levinson, David. *Seasons of a Man's Life*. New York: Random House, 1978.

Lynn, Joanne, and Joan Harrold. *Handbook for Mortals: Guidance for People Facing Serious Illness*. New York: Oxford University Press, 1999.

Mahler, Jonathan. "A. Stone Freedberg: The Good Doctor." The Lives They Lived. Magazine. *New York Times*, December 27, 2009.

Marshall, Samuel, Kathleen M. McGarry, and Jonathan S. Skinner. "The Risk of Out-of-Pocket Health Care Expenditure at End of Life." National Bureau of Economic Research, Working Paper No. 16170, July 2010. http://www.nber.org/papers/w16170

Martensen, Robert. *A Life Worth Living: Reflections on Illness in a High-Tech Era*. New York: Farrar, Straus and Giroux, 2008.

Medical Examiner, Health and Medicine Explained. *Slate*, August 4, 2010. http://www.slate.com/articles/health_and_science/medical_examiner/2010/08/we_cant_save_you.html

Meier, Diane E., Stephen L. Isaacs, and Robert G. Hughes, eds. *Palliative Care: Transforming the Care of Serious Illness*. San Francisco. Jossey-Bass, 2010.

Mirarchi, Ferdinando L. *Understanding Your Living Will: What You Need to Know before a Medical Emergency*. Omaha: Addicus Books, 2006.

Moon, Marilyn, and Cristina Boccuti. *"Medicare and End-of-Life Care."* Urban Institute, September 2002.

Morgan, Ernest. *Dealing Creatively with Death: A Manual of Death Education and Simple Burial*. 14th ed. Hinesburg, Vt.: Upper Access, 2001.

Mukherjee, Siddhartha. *The Emperor of All Maladies: A Biography of Cancer*. New York: Scribner, 2010.

"Myths and Facts about Heath Care Advance Directives." Commission on Law and Aging, American Bar Association. http://www.americanbar.org/content/dam/aba/migrated/Commissions/myths_fact_hc_ad.authcheckdam.pdf

National Consensus Project for Quality Palliative Care. http://www.nationalconsensusproject.org/

National Healthcare Quality and Disparities Reports. Agency for Healthcare Research and Quality, Rockville, Md. http://www.ahrq.gov/research/findings/nhqrdr/index.html

National Quality Forum. http://www.qualityforum.org

Navasky, Miri, and Karen O'Connor. "Facing Death." *Frontline.* PBS, November 23, 2010.

Nuland, Sherwin B. *How We Die: Reflections on Life's Final Chapter.* New York: Random House, 1995.

"Overview of Comfort Care/DNR Order Verification Protocol." Massachusetts Office of Health and Human Services. Updated January 22, 2007. http://www.mass.gov/eohhs/ provider/guidclines-resources/clinical-treatment/comfort-care/public-health-oems-comfort-care-overview.html

"Patient Values Questionnaire." Vermont Ethics Network. http://www.vtethicsnetwork.org/patientvaluesquestionnaire.html

Patrick, Maggy. "Three Generations Gather for End-of-Life Conversation." *World News with Diane Sawyer.* ABC News, October 9, 2012. http://abcnews.go.com/Health/generations-gather-end-life-conversation/story?id=17435323#.UKASMeOe8zE

POLST: Physician Orders for Life-Sustaining Treatment Paradigm. http://www.polst.org/

Porter, Eduardo. "Rationing Health Care More Fairly." *New York Times,* August 22, 2012. http://www.nytimes.com/2012/08/22/ business/economy/rationing-health-care-more-fairly.html? pagewanted=all&_r=0

Puchalski, Christina M., et al. "Religion, Spirituality, and End of Life Care." UpToDate. *Wolters Kluwer Health,* June 11, 2012. http://www.uptodate.com/contents/religion-spirituality-and-end-of-life-care

Quach, Thu, et al. "Experiences and Perceptions of Medical Discrimination Among a Multiethnic Sample of Breast Cancer Patients in the Greater San Francisco Bay Area, California." *American Journal of Public Health* 102 (2012): 1027–1034.

Reinhardt, Uwe. "End-of-Life Care: Where Ethics Meet
Economics." Economix (blog). *The New York Times*, August 14,
2009. http://economix.blogs.nytimes.com/2009/08/14/end-
of-life-care-where-ethics-meet-economics/

Sapienza, Jerral. "Reflections on Death: A Guest Book/
Questionnaire." Lifelong Learning Excellence. Bardo of
Death Studies. http://www.bardo.org/reflects.html

"Shape Your Health Care Future with Health Care Advance
Directives." American Association of Retired Persons, ABA
Commission on Legal Problems of the Elderly, and American
Medical Association, 1995. http://apps.americanbar.org/
aging/publications/docs/shape_your.pdf

Shapiro, Susan P. "Advance Directives: The Elusive Goal of
Having the Last Word." *The National Academy of Elder Law
Attorneys Journal*, Fall 2012.

Shavers, Vickie L., William M.P. Klein, and Pebbles Fagan.
"Research on Race/Ethnicity and Health Care Discrimination:
Where We Are and Where We Need to Go." *American Journal
of Public Health* 102 (2012): 953–966.

Sloan, Frank A., and Lindsey M. Chepke. *Medical Malpractice.*
Cambridge: MIT Press, 2008.

Span, Paula. "Where the Oldest Die Now." The New Old Age
(blog). *New York Times*, April 18, 2012.
http://newoldage.blogs.nytimes.com/2012/04/18/where-the-
oldest-die-now/

Span, Paula. *When the Time Comes: Families with Aging Parents
Share Their Struggles and Solutions.* New York: Springboard
Press Hachette Book Group, 2009.

Spring, Janis A., Sue Belanger, and Charles Sabatino. Interview
by Diane Rehm. "Family Conversations about End-Of-Life
Care." *Diane Rehm Show*. National Public Radio, August 8,
2012. http://thedianerehmshow.org/shows/2012-08-08/family-
conversations-about-end-life-care

Terman, Stanley A. *The Best Way to Say Goodbye.* Carlsbad,
California: Life Transitions Publications, 2007.

Thomas, Lewis. *The Youngest Science: Notes of a Medicine-Watcher*. New York: Penguin Books, 1995.

Wachter, Robert M., and Lee Goldman. "The Emerging Role of 'Hospitalists' in the American Health Care System." *New England Journal of Medicine* 335 (1996): 514–517.

Webb, Marilyn. *The Good Death: The New American Search to Reshape the End of Life*. New York: Bantam, 1997.

Wiener, Lori, et al. "Allowing Adolescents and Young Adults to Plan Their End-of-Life Care." *Pediatrics* 130 (2012): 897–905.

Wolf, Nicole. "Self-Awareness Questionnaire." FlowNow. 2011. http://www.flow-now.com/self-awareness-questionnaire

Wyatt, Karen M. *What Really Matters: Seven Lessons for Living from the Stories of the Dying*. New York: SelectBooks, 2011.

INDEX

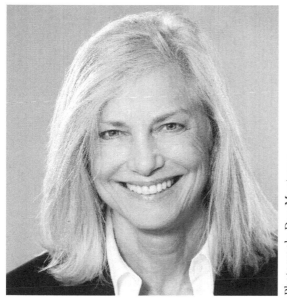

DIANE BURNSIDE MURDOCK is a writer, researcher, blogger, and mHealth app cocreator, aka Murdock Without Borders. She has worked at the Congressional Budget Office and the Prospective Payment Assessment Commission (PROPAC) and established her own consulting firm, Health Policy Research, offering services to organizations like the Institute of Medicine/National Academy of Sciences and the U.S. Government Accountability Office. She received a bachelor's degree in sociology from Tulane University and a master's degree in health services administration from the George Washington University. She lives with her family in Virginia. She is 63 years old, old to some and young to others.

MY HEALTH CARE WISHES©
APP GIVES REALITY TO
ADVANCE CARE PLANNING

A transformative iPhone and Android app
that makes your legal documents available
in a medical emergency

The My Health Care Wishes mobile health app is offered to you as a key feature of *The New Art of Dying*. This new app is a game changer designed for consumers who have had conversations about dying and are looking for a way to assure that advance care plan documents are there when most needed. The app breaks a critical barrier to anyone's dying plan by providing immediate access to PDF versions of your living will, advance medical directive, health care power of attorney or health care proxy, do-not-resuscitate order, psychiatric advance directive, and physician orders for life-sustaining treatment.

Imagine having your wishes and those belonging to your loved ones—away at college, in a retirement community or nursing home, working in a different city, or under the same roof—stored in one smartphone and a click away, just in case. Import and store them on your smartphone so they're there for medical decision making anytime, anywhere.

This app is a major improvement to anything currently available. Estimates for 2012 indicate that there are 116 million smartphone users in the United States, and 20 percent of them use health apps. Those who have smartphones can carry the wishes of those who don't, especially elderly loved ones. And it emphasizes the importance of having an advance medical directive. As a family, we can carry each other's wishes in our back pocket or in our purse 24/7, ensuring our wishes are carried out when we cannot speak for ourselves. It's about being there for each other in a way not possible before.

My Health Care Wishes is available now
at iTunes and Google play and is compatible
with iPhone, iPod touch, iPad, and Android smartphones.
You can learn more at
http://www.myhealthcarewishes.com.

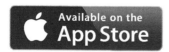
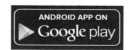

Made in the USA
San Bernardino, CA
15 February 2014

8611398R00116

SLAVE NARRATIVES

SLAVE NARRATIVES

*Narrative of the Most Remarkable Particulars in the Life
of James Albert Ukawsaw Gronniosaw*

Interesting Narrative of the Life of Olaudah Equiano

The Confessions of Nat Turner

Narrative of the Life of Frederick Douglass

Narrative of William W. Brown

Narrative of the Life and Adventures of Henry Bibb

Narrative of Sojourner Truth

Running a Thousand Miles for Freedom

Incidents in the Life of a Slave Girl

Narrative of the Life of J. D. Green

COLLEGE
EDITIONS

THE LIBRARY OF AMERICA

Distributed to the trade
in the United States by Penguin Putnam Inc.
and in Canada by Penguin Books Canada Ltd.

Library of Congress Catalog Number: 99–40360
For cataloging information, see end of Notes.
ISBN 1–931082–11–1
―――――
Originally published in hardcover by
The Library of America in 2000.

First Library of America College Edition
Spring 2002

Manufactured in the United States of America

WILLIAM L. ANDREWS
AND
HENRY LOUIS GATES JR.
SELECTED THE CONTENTS AND WROTE THE NOTES
FOR THIS VOLUME

Contents

A

NARRATIVE

OF THE

MOST REMARKABLE PARTICULARS

IN THE LIFE OF

JAMES ALBERT UKAWSAW GRONNIOSAW,

AN AFRICAN PRINCE,

As related by HIMSELF.

I will bring the Blind by a Way that they know not, I will lead them in Paths that they have not known: I will make Darkness Light before them and crooked Things straight. These Things will I do unto them and not forsake them. Isa. xlii. 16.

BATH:
Printed by W. GYE in Westgate-Street; and sold by T. MILLS, Bookseller, in King's-Mead-Square.
Price SIX-PENCE.

TO THE

RIGHT HONOURABLE

The *Countess* of HUNTINGDON;

THIS

NARRATIVE

Of my *LIFE*,

And of GOD's wonderful Dealings with me, is,

(*Through Her LADYSHIP's Permission*)

Most Humbly Dedicated,

By her LADYSHIP's

Most obliged

And obedient Servant,

JAMES ALBERT.

THE PREFACE to the READER.

THIS Account of the Life and spiritual Experience of JAMES ALBERT was taken from his own Mouth and committed to Paper by the elegant Pen of a young LADY of the Town of LEOMINSTER, for her own private Satisfaction, and without any Intention at first that it should be made public. But she has now been prevail'd on to commit it to the Press, both with a view to serve ALBERT and his distressed Family, who have the sole Profits arising from the Sale of it; and likewise as it is apprehended, this little History contains Matter well worthy the Notice and Attention of every Christian Reader.

Perhaps we have here in some Degree a Solution of that Question that has perplex'd the Minds of so many serious Persons, viz. In what Manner will God deal with those benighted Parts of the World where the Gospel of Jesus Christ hath never reach'd? Now it appears from the Experience of this remarkable Person, that God does not save without the Knowledge of the Truth; but, with Respect to those whom he hath fore-known, though born under every outward Disadvantage, and in Regions of the grossest Darkness and Ignorance, he most amazingly acts upon and influences their Minds, and in the Course of wisely and most wonderfully appointed Providences, he brings them to the Means of spiritual Information, gradually opens to their View the Light of his Truth, and gives them full Possession and Enjoyment of the inestimable Blessings of his Gospel. Who can doubt but that the Suggestion so forcibly press'd upon the Mind of ALBERT (when a Boy) that there was a Being superior to the Sun, Moon, and Stars (the Objects of African Idolatry) came from the Father of Lights, and was, with Respect to him, the First-Fruit of the Display of Gospel-Glory? His long and perilous Journey to the Coast of Guinea, where he was sold for a Slave, and so brought into a Christian Land; shall we consider this as the alone Effect of a curious and inquisitive Disposition? Shall we in accounting for it refer to nothing higher than mere Chance and accidental Circumstances? Whatever Infidels and Deists may think; I trust the Christian Reader will

3

easily discern an All-wise and Omnipotent Appointment and Direction in these Movements. He belong'd to the Redeemer of lost Sinners; he was the Purchase of his Cross; and therefore the Lord undertook to bring him by a Way that he knew not, out of Darkness into his marvellous Light, that he might lead him to a saving Heart-Acquaintance and Union with the triune God in Christ reconciling the World unto himself; and not imputing their Trespasses. As his Call was very extraordinary, so there are certain Particulars exceedingly remarkable in his Experience. God has put singular Honour upon him in the Exercise of his Faith and Patience, which in the most distressing and pitiable Trials and Calamities have been found to the Praise and Glory of God. How deeply must it affect a tender Heart, not only to be reduc'd to the last Extremity himself, but to have his Wife and Children perishing for Want before his Eyes! Yet his Faith did not fail him; he put his Trust in the Lord, and he was delivered. And at this Instant, though born in an exalted Station of Life, and now under the Pressure of various afflicting Providences, I am persuaded (for I know the Man) he would rather embrace the Dung-hill, having Christ in his Heart, than give up his spiritual Possessions and Enjoyment, to fill the Throne of Princes. It perhaps may not be amiss to observe that JAMES ALBERT left his native Country, (as near as I can guess from certain Circumstances) when he was about 15 Years old. He now appears to be turn'd of Sixty; has a good natural Understanding; is well acquainted with the Scriptures, and the Things of God, has an amiable and tender Disposition, and his Character can be well attested not only at Kidderminster, the Place of his Residence but likewise by many creditable Persons in London and other Places. Reader, recommending this Narrative to your perusal, and him who is the Subject of it to your charitable Regard,

I am your faithful and obedient Servant,

For Christ's Sake,

W. SHIRLEY.

AN

ACCOUNT

OF

JAMES ALBERT, &c.

I WAS BORN in the city BOURNOU; my mother was the eldest daughter of the reigning King there, of which BOURNOU is the chief city. I was the youngest of six children, and particularly loved by my mother, and my grand-father almost doated on me.

I had, from my infancy, a curious turn of mind; was more grave and reserved in my disposition than either of my brothers and sisters. I often teazed them with questions they could not answer: for which reason they disliked me, as they supposed that I was either foolish, or insane. 'Twas certain that I was, at times, very unhappy in myself: it being strongly impressed on my mind that there was some GREAT MAN of power which resided above the sun, moon and stars, the objects of our worship. My dear indulgent mother would bear more with me than any of my friends beside.—I often raised my hand to heaven, and asked her who lived there? was much dissatisfied when she told me the sun, moon and stars, being persuaded, in my own mind, that there must be some SUPERIOR POWER.—I was frequently lost in wonder at the works of the Creation: was afraid and uneasy and restless, but could not tell for what. I wanted to be informed of things that no person could tell me; and was always dissatisfied.— These wonderful impressions begun in my childhood, and followed me continually 'till I left my parents, which affords me matter of admiration and thankfulness.

To this moment I grew more and more uneasy every day, in so much that one saturday, (which is the day on which we keep our sabbath) I laboured under anxieties and fears that cannot be expressed; and, what is more extraordinary, I could not give a reason for it.—I rose, as our custom is, about three

o'clock, (as we are oblig'd to be at our place of worship an hour before the sun rise) we say nothing in our worship, but continue on our knees with our hands held up, observing a strict silence 'till the sun is at a certain height, which I suppose to be about 10 or 11 o'clock in England: when, at a certain sign made by the priest, we get up (our duty being over) and disperse to our different houses.—Our place of meeting is under a large palm tree; we divide ourselves into many congregations; as it is impossible for the same tree to cover the inhabitants of the whole City, though they are extremely large, high and majestic; the beauty and usefulness of them are not to be described; they supply the inhabitants of the country with meat, drink and clothes;* the body of the palm tree is very large; at a certain season of the year they tap it, and bring vessels to receive the wine, of which they draw great quantities, the quality of which is very delicious: the leaves of this tree are of a silky nature; they are large and soft; when they are dried and pulled to pieces it has much the same appearance as the English flax, and the inhabitants of BOURNOU manufacture it for cloathing &c. This tree likewise produces a plant or substance which has the appearance of a cabbage, and very like it, in taste almost the same: it grows between the branches. Also the palm tree produces a nut, something like a cocoa, which contains a kernel, in which is a large quantity of milk, very pleasant to the taste: the shell is of a hard substance, and of a very beautiful appearance, and serves for basons, bowls, &c.

I hope this digression will be forgiven.—I was going to observe that after the duty of our Sabbath was over (on the day in which I was more distressed and afflicted than ever) we were all on our way home as usual, when a remarkable black cloud arose and covered the sun; then followed very heavy rain and thunder more dreadful than ever I had heard: the heav'ns roared, and the earth trembled at it: I was highly affected and cast down; in so much that I wept sadly, and could not follow my relations and friends home.—I was obliged to

---

*It is a generally received opinion, in *England,* that the natives of *Africa* go entirely unclothed; but this supposition is very unjust: they have a kind of dress so as to appear decent, though it is very slight and thin.

stop and felt as if my legs were tied, they seemed to shake under me: so I stood still, being in great fear of the MAN of POWER that I was persuaded in myself, lived above. One of my young companions (who entertained a particular friendship for me and I for him) came back to see for me: he asked me why I stood still in such very hard rain? I only said to him that my legs were weak, and I could not come faster: he was much affected to see me cry, and took me by the hand, and said he would lead me home, which he did. My mother was greatly alarmed at my tarrying out in such terrible weather; she asked me many questions, such as what I did so for, and if I was well? My dear mother says I, pray tell me who is the great MAN of POWER that makes the thunder? She said, there was no power but the sun, moon and stars; that they made all our country.—I then enquired how all our people came? She answered me, from one another; and so carried me to many generations back.—Then says I, who made the *First Man*? and who made the first Cow, and the first Lyon, and where does the fly come from, as no one can make him? My mother seemed in great trouble; she was apprehensive that my senses were impaired, or that I was foolish. My father came in, and seeing her in grief asked the cause, but when she related our conversation to him, he was exceedingly angry with me, and told me he would punish me severely if ever I was so troublesome again; so that I resolved never to say any thing more to him. But I grew very unhappy in myself; my relations and acquaintance endeavoured by all the means they could think on, to divert me, by taking me to ride upon goats, (which is much the custom of our country) and to shoot with a bow and arrow; but I experienced no satisfaction at all in any of these things; nor could I be easy by any means whatever: my parents were very unhappy to see me so dejected and melancholy.

About this time there came a merchant from the *Gold Coast* (the third city in GUINEA) he traded with the inhabitants of our country in ivory &c. he took great notice of my unhappy situation, and enquired into the cause; he expressed vast concern for me, and said, if my parents would part with me for a little while, and let him take me home with him, it would be of more service to me than any thing they could do for me.—He told me that if I would go with him I should see houses with wings to them walk upon the water, and should also see the white folks; and that he had many sons of my age, which should be my companions; and he added to all this that he would bring me safe back again soon.—I was highly pleased with the account of this strange place, and was very desirous of going.—I seemed sensible of a secret impulse upon my mind which I could not resist that seemed to tell me I must go. When my dear mother saw that I was willing to leave them, she spoke to my father and grandfather and the rest of my relations, who all agreed that I should accompany the merchant to the Gold Coast. I was the more willing as my brothers and sisters despised me, and looked on me with contempt on the account of my unhappy disposition; and even my servants slighted me, and disregarded all I said to them. I had one sister who was always exceeding fond of me, and I loved her entirely; her name was LOGWY, she was quite white, and fair, with fine light hair though my father and mother were black.—I was truly concerned to leave my beloved sister, and she cry'd most sadly to part with me, wringing her hands, and discovered every sign of grief that can be imagined. Indeed if I could have known when I left my friends and country that I should never return to them again my misery on that occasion would have been inexpressible. All my relations were sorry to part with me; my dear mother came with me upon a camel more than three hundred miles, the first of our journey lay chiefly through woods: at night we secured ourselves from the wild beasts by making fires all around us; we and our camels kept within the circle, or we must have been torn to pieces by the Lyons, and other wild creatures, that roared terribly as soon as night came on, and continued to do so 'till morning.—There can be little said in favour of the country through which we passed; only a valley of marble that we came through which is unspeakably beautiful.—On each side of this valley are exceedingly high and almost inaccessible mountains—Some of these pieces of marble are of prodigious length and breadth but of different sizes and colour, and shaped in a variety of forms, in a wonderful manner.—It is most of it veined with gold mixed with striking and beautiful colours; so that when the sun darts upon it, it is as pleasing a sight as can be imagined.—The merchant that brought me from BOURNOU, was in partnership with another gentleman who accompanied us; he was very unwilling that he should take me from home, as, he said, he foresaw many difficulties that would attend my going with them.—He endeavoured to prevail on the merchant to throw me into a very deep pit that was in the valley, but he refused to listen to him, and said, he was resolved to take care of me: but the other was greatly dissatisfied; and when we came to a river, which we were obliged to pass through, he purpos'd throwing me in and drowning me; but the Merchant would not consent to it, so that I was preserv'd.

We travel'd 'till about four o'clock every day, and then began to make preparations for night, by cutting down large quantities of wood, to make fires to preserve us from the wild beasts.—I had a very unhappy and discontented journey, being in continual fear that the people I was with would murder me. I often reflected with extreme regret on the kind friends I had left, and the idea of my dear mother frequently drew tears from my eyes.—I cannot recollect how long we were in going from BOURNOU to the GOLD COAST; but as there is no shipping nearer to BOURNOU than that City, it was tedious in travelling so far by land, being upwards of a thousand miles.—I was heartily rejoic'd when we arriv'd at the end of our journey: I now vainly imagin'd that all my troubles and inquietudes would terminate here; but could I have looked into futurity, I should have perceiv'd that I had much more to suffer than I had before experienc'd, and that they had as yet but barely commenc'd.

I was now more than a thousand miles from home, without a friend or any means to procure one. Soon after I came to the merchant's house I heard the drums beat remarkably loud, and the trumpets blow—the persons accustom'd to this employ, are oblig'd to go upon a very high structure appointed for that purpose, that the sound might be heard at a great distance: They are higher than the steeples are in England. I was mightily pleas'd with sounds so entirely new to me, and was very inquisitive to know the cause of this re-

joicing, and ask'd many questions concerning it: I was answer'd that it was meant as a compliment to me, because I
was Grandson to the King of BOURNOU.

This account gave me a secret pleasure; but I was not suffer'd long to enjoy this satisfaction, for in the evening of the
same day, two of the merchant's sons (boys about my own
age) came running to me, and told me, that the next day I
was to die, for the King intended to behead me.—I reply'd
that I was sure it could not be true, for that I came there to
play with them, and to see houses walk upon the water with
wings to them, and the white folks; but I was soon inform'd
that their King imagined that I was sent by my father as a spy,
and would make such discoveries at my return home that
would enable them to make war with the greater advantage to
ourselves; and for these reasons he had resolved I should
never return to my native country.—When I heard this I suffered misery that cannot be described.—I wished a thousand
times that I had never left my friends and country.—But still
the ALMIGHTY was pleased to work miracles for me.

The morning I was to die, I was washed and all my gold
ornaments made bright and shining, and then carried to
the palace, where the King was to behead me himself (as is
the custom of the place).—He was seated upon a throne at
the top of an exceeding large yard, or court, which you
must go through to enter the palace, it is as wide and
spacious as a large field in England.—I had a lane of life-
guards to go through.—I guessed it to be about three hundred paces.

I was conducted by my friend, the merchant, about half
way up; then he durst proceed no further: I went up to the
KING alone—I went with an undaunted courage, and it
pleased GOD to melt the heart of the King, who sat with his
scymitar in his hand ready to behead me; yet, being himself so
affected, he dropped it out of his hand, and took me upon his
knee and wept over me. I put my right hand round his neck,
and prest him to my heart.—He sat me down and blest me;
and added that he would not kill me, and that I should not
go home, but be sold for a slave, so then I was conducted
back again to the merchant's house.

The next day he took me on board a French brig; but the

Captain did not chuse to buy me: he said I was too small; so the merchant took me home with him again.

The partner, whom I have spoken of as my enemy, was very angry to see me return, and again purposed putting an end to my life; for he represented to the other, that I should bring them into troubles and difficulties, and that I was so little that no person would buy me.

The merchant's resolution began to waver, and I was indeed afraid that I should be put to death: but however he said he would try me once more.

A few days after a Dutch ship came into the harbour, and they carried me on board, in hopes that the Captain would purchase me.—As they went, I heard them agree, that, if they could not sell me *then*, they would throw me overboard.—I was in extreme agonies when I heard this; and as soon as ever I saw the Dutch Captain, I ran to him, and put my arms round him, and said, "father, save me." (for I knew that if he did not buy me, I should be treated very ill, or, possibly, murdered) And though he did not understand my language, yet it pleased the ALMIGHTY to influence him in my behalf, and he bought me *for two yards of check*, which is of more value *there*, than in England.

When I left my dear mother I had a large quantity of gold about me, as is the custom of our country, it was made into rings, and they were linked into one another, and formed into a kind of chain, and so put round my neck, and arms and legs, and a large piece hanging at one ear almost in the shape of a pear. I found all this troublesome, and was glad when my new Master took it from me—I was now washed, and clothed in the Dutch or English manner.—My master grew very fond of me, and I loved him exceedingly. I watched every look, was always ready when he wanted me, and endeavoured to convince him, by every action, that my only pleasure was to serve him well.—I have since thought that he must have been a serious man. His actions corresponded very well with such a character.—He used to read prayers in public to the ship's crew every Sabbath day; and when first I saw him read, I was never so surprised in my whole life as when I saw the book talk to my master; for I thought it did, as I observed him to look upon it, and move his lips.—I wished it would do so to me.—As soon as my master had done reading I follow'd him to the place where he put the book, being mightily delighted with it, and when nobody saw me, I open'd it and put my ear down close upon it, in great hope that it wou'd say something to me; but was very sorry and greatly disappointed when I found it would not speak, this thought immediately presented itself to me, that every body and every thing despis'd me because I was black.

I was exceedingly sea-sick at first; but when I became more accustom'd to the sea, it wore off.—My master's ship was bound for Barbadoes. When we came there, he thought fit to speak of me to several gentlemen of his acquaintance, and one of them exprest a particular desire to see me.—He had a great mind to buy me; but the Captain could not immediately be prevail'd on to part with me; but however, as the gentleman seem'd very solicitous, he at length let me go, and I was sold for fifty dollars (*four and sixpenny-pieces in English*). My new master's name was Vanhorn, a young Gentleman; his home was in New-England in the City of New-York; to which place he took me with him. He dress'd me in his livery, and was very good to me. My chief business was to wait at table, and tea, and clean knives, and I had a very easy place; but the servants us'd to curse and swear surprizingly; which I learnt faster than any thing, 'twas almost the first English I could speak. If any of them affronted me, I was sure to call upon God to damn them immediately; but I was broke of it all at once, occasioned by the correction of an old black servant that liv'd in the family—One day I had just clean'd the knives for dinner, when one of the maids took one to cut bread and butter with; I was very angry with her, and called upon God to damn her; when this old black man told me I must not say so. I ask'd him why? He replied there was a wicked man call'd the Devil, that liv'd in hell, and would take all that said these words, and put them in the fire and burn them.—This terrified me greatly, and I was entirely broke of swearing.— Soon after this, as I was placing the china for tea, my mistress came into the room just as the maid had been cleaning it; the girl had unfortunately sprinkled the wainscot with the mop; at which my mistress was angry; the girl very foolishly answer'd her again, which made her worse, and she call'd upon God to

damn her.—I was vastly concern'd to hear this, as she was a
fine young lady, and very good to me, insomuch that I could
not help speaking to her, "Madam, says I, you must not say
so," Why, says she? Because there is a black man call'd the
Devil that lives in hell, and he will put you in the fire and
burn you, and I shall be very sorry for that. Who told you this
replied my lady? Old Ned, says I. Very well was all her answer;
but she told my master of it, and he order'd that old Ned
should be tyed up and whipp'd, and was never suffer'd to
come into the kitchen with the rest of the servants afterwards.—My mistress was not angry with me, but rather diverted with my simplicity and, by way of talk, She repeated
what I had said, to many of her acquaintance that visited her;
among the rest, Mr. Freelandhouse, a very gracious, good
Minister, heard it, and he took a great deal of notice of me,
and desired my master to part with me to him. He would not
hear of it at first, but, being greatly persuaded, he let me go,
and Mr. Freelandhouse gave £50. for me.—He took me
home with him, and made me kneel down, and put my two
hands together, and pray'd for me, and every night and
morning he did the same.—I could not make out what it was
for, nor the meaning of it, nor what they spoke to when they
talk'd—I thought it comical, but I lik'd it very well.—After I
had been a little while with my new master I grew more familiar, and ask'd him the meaning of prayer: (I could hardly
speak english to be understood) he took great pains with me,
and made me understand that he pray'd to God, who liv'd in
Heaven; that He was my Father and BEST Friend.—I told him
that this must be a mistake; that *my* father liv'd at BOURNOU,
and I wanted very much to see him, and likewise my dear
mother, and sister, and I wish'd he would be so good as to
send me home to them; and I added, all I could think of to
induce him to convey me back. I appeared in great trouble,
and my good master was so much affected that the tears ran
down his face. He told me that God was a GREAT and GOOD
SPIRIT, that He created all the world, and every person and
thing in it, in Ethiopia, Africa, and America, and every where.
I was delighted when I heard this: There, says I, I always
thought so when I liv'd at home! Now if I had wings like an
Eagle I would fly to tell my dear mother that God is greater

than the sun, moon, and stars; and that they were made by Him.

I was exceedingly pleas'd with this information of my master's, because it corresponded so well with my own opinion; I thought now if I could but get home, I should be wiser than all my country-folks, my grandfather, or father, or mother, or any of them—But though I was somewhat enlighten'd by this information of my master's, yet, I had no other knowledge of God but that He was a GOOD SPIRIT, and created every body, and every thing—I never was sensible in myself, nor had any one ever told me, that He would punish the wicked, and love the just. I was only glad that I had been told there was a God because I had always thought so.

My dear kind master grew very fond of me, as was his Lady; she put me to School, but I was uneasy at that, and did not like to go; but my master and mistress requested me to learn in the gentlest terms, and persuaded me to attend my school without any anger at all; that, at last, I came to like it better, and learnt to read pretty well. My schoolmaster was a good man, his name was Vanosdore, and very indulgent to me.—I was in this state when, one sunday, I heard my master preach from these words out of the Revelations, chap. i. v. 7. *"Behold, He cometh in the clouds and every eye shall see him and they that pierc'd Him."* These words affected me excessively; I was in great agonies because I thought my master directed them to me only; and, I fancied, that he observ'd me with unusual earnestness—I was farther confirm'd in this belief as I look'd round the church, and could see no one person beside myself in such grief and distress as I was; I began to think that my master hated me, and was very desirous to go home, to my own country; for I thought that if God did come (as he said) He would be sure to be most angry with *me*, as I did not know what He was, nor had ever heard of him before.

I went home in great trouble, but said nothing to any body.—I was somewhat afraid of my master; I thought he disliked me.—The next text I heard him preach from was, Heb. xii. 14. *"follow peace with all men, and holiness, without which no man shall see the LORD."* he preached the law so severely, that it made me tremble.—he said, that GOD would judge the whole world; ETHIOPIA, ASIA, and AFRICA, and every where.—I was now excessively perplexed, and undetermined what to do; as I had now reason to believe my situation would be equally bad to go, as to stay.—I kept these thoughts to myself, and said nothing to any person whatever.

I should have complained to my good mistress of this great trouble of mind, but she had been a little strange to me for several days before this happened, occasioned by a story told of me by one of the maids. The servants were all jealous, and envied me the regard, and favour shewn me by my master and mistress; and the Devil being always ready, and diligent in wickedness, had influenced this girl, to make a lye on me.— This happened about hay-harvest, and one day when I was unloading the waggon to put the hay into the barn, she watched an opportunity, in my absence, to take the fork out of the stick, and hide it: when I came again to my work, and could not find it, I was a good deal vexed, but I concluded it was dropt somewhere among the hay; so I went and bought another with my own money: when the girl saw that I had another, she was so malicious that she told my mistress I was very unfaithful, and not the person she took me for; and that she knew, I had, without my master's permission, order'd many things in his name, that he must pay for; and as a proof of my carelessness produc'd the fork she had taken out of the stick, and said, she had found it out of doors—My Lady, not knowing the truth of these things, was a little shy to me, till she mention'd it, and then I soon cleared myself, and convinc'd her that these accusations were false.

I continued in a most unhappy state for many days. My good mistress insisted on knowing what was the matter. When I made known my situation she gave me John Bunyan on the holy war, to read; I found his experience similar to my own, which gave me reason to suppose he must be a bad man; as I was convinc'd of my own corrupt nature, and the misery of my own heart: and as he acknowledg'd that he was likewise in the same condition, I experienc'd no relief at all in reading his work, but rather the reverse.—I took the book to my lady, and inform'd her I did not like it at all, it was concerning a wicked man as bad as myself; and I did not chuse to read it, and I desir'd her to give me another, wrote by a better man that was holy and without sin.—She assur'd me that

John Bunyan was a good man, but she could not convince me; I thought him to be too much like myself to be upright, as his experience seem'd to answer with my own.

I am very sensible that nothing but the great power and unspeakable mercies of the Lord could relieve my soul from the heavy burden it laboured under at that time.—A few days after my master gave me Baxter's *Call to the unconverted*. This was no relief to me neither; on the contrary it occasioned as much distress in me as the other had before done, *as it* invited all to come to *Christ* and I found myself so wicked and miserable that I could not come—This consideration threw me into agonies that cannot be described; insomuch that I even attempted to put an end to my life—I took one of the large case-knives, and went into the stable with an intent to destroy myself; and as I endeavoured with all my strength to force the knife into my side, it bent double. I was instantly struck with horror at the thought of my own rashness, and my conscience told me that had I succeeded in this attempt I should probably have gone to hell.

I could find no relief, nor the least shadow of comfort; the extreme distress of my mind so affected my health that I continued very ill for three Days, and Nights; and would admit of no means to be taken for my recovery, though my lady was very kind, and sent many things to me; but I rejected every means of relief and wished to die—I would not go into my own bed, but lay in the stable upon straw—I felt all the horrors of a troubled conscience, so hard to be born, and saw all the vengeance of God ready to overtake me—I was sensible that there was no way for me to be saved unless I came to *Christ*, and I could not come to Him: I thought that it was impossible He should receive such a sinner as me.

The last night that I continued in this place, in the midst of my distress these words were brought home upon my mind, *"Behold the Lamb of God."* I was something comforted at this, and began to grow easier and wished for day that I might find these words in my bible—I rose very early the following morning, and went to my school-master, Mr. Vanosdore, and communicated the situation of my mind to him; he was greatly rejoiced to find me enquiring the way to Zion, and blessed the Lord who had worked so wonderfully for me a poor heathen.—I was more familiar with this good gentleman than with my master, or any other person; and found myself more at liberty to talk to him: he encouraged me greatly, and prayed with me frequently, and I was always benefited by his discourse.

About a quarter of a mile from my Master's house stood a large remarkably fine Oak-tree, in the midst of a wood; I often used to be employed there in cutting down trees, (a work I was very fond of) I seldom failed going to this place every day; sometimes twice a day if I could be spared. It was the highest pleasure I ever experienced to set under this Oak; for there I used to pour out all my complaints to the LORD: and when I had any particular grievance I used to go there, and talk to the tree, and tell my sorrows, as if it had been to a friend.

Here I often lamented my own wicked heart, and undone state; and found more comfort and consolation than I ever was sensible of before.—Whenever I was treated with ridicule or contempt, I used to come here and find peace. I now began to relish the book my Master gave me, Baxter's *Call to the unconverted*, and took great delight in it. I was always glad to be employ'd in cutting wood, 'twas a great part of my business, and I follow'd it with delight, as I was then quite alone and my heart lifted up to GOD, and I was enabled to pray continually; and blessed for ever be his Holy Name, he faithfully answer'd my prayers. I can never be thankful enough to Almighty GOD for the many comfortable opportunities I experienced there.

It is possible the circumstance I am going to relate will not gain credit with many; but this I know, that the joy and comfort it conveyed to me, cannot be expressed and only conceived by those who have experienced the like.

I was one day in a most delightful frame of mind; my heart so overflowed with love and gratitude to the Author of all my comforts.—I was so drawn out of myself, and so fill'd and awed by the Presence of God that I saw (or thought I saw) light inexpressible dart down from heaven upon me, and shone around me for the space of a minute.—I continued on my knees, and joy unspeakable took possession of my soul.— The peace and serenity which filled my mind after this was wonderful, and cannot be told.—I would not have changed situations, or been any one but myself for the whole world. I blest God for my poverty, that I had no worldly riches or grandeur to draw my heart from Him. I wish'd at that time, if it had been possible for me, to have continued on that spot for ever. I felt an unwillingness in myself to have any thing more to do with the world, or to mix with society again. I seemed to possess a full assurance that my sins were forgiven me. I went home all my way rejoicing, and this text of scripture came full upon my mind. *"And I will make an everlasting covenant with them, that I will not turn away from them, to do them good; but I will put my fear in their hearts that they shall not depart from me."* The first opportunity that presented itself, I went to my old school-master, and made known to him the happy state of my soul who joined with me in praise to God for his mercy to me the vilest of sinners.—I was now perfectly easy, and had hardly a wish to make beyond what I possess'd, when my temporal comforts were all blasted by the death of my dear and worthy Master Mr. Freelandhouse, who was taken from this world rather suddenly: he had but a short illness, and died of a fever. I held his hand in mine when he departed; he told me he had given me my freedom. I was at liberty to go where I would.—He added that he had always pray'd for me and hop'd I should be kept unto the end. My master left me by his will ten pounds, and my freedom.

I found that if he had lived 'twas his intention to take me with him to Holland, as he had often mention'd me to some friends of his there that were desirous to see me; but I chose to continue with my Mistress who was as good to me as if she had been my mother.

The loss of Mr. Freelandhouse distress'd me greatly, but I was render'd still more unhappy by the clouded and perplex'd situation of my mind; the great enemy of my soul being ready to torment me, would present my own misery to me in such striking light, and distress me with doubts, fears, and such a deep sense of my own unworthiness, that after all the comfort and encouragement I had received, I was often tempted to believe I should be a Cast-away at last.—The more I saw of the Beauty and Glory of God, the more I was humbled under a sense of my own vileness. I often repair'd to my old place of prayer; I seldom came away without consolation. One day this Scripture was wonderfully apply'd to my mind, *"And ye are compleat in Him which is the Head of all principalities and power."*—The Lord was pleas'd to comfort me by the application of many gracious promises at times when I was ready to sink under my troubles. *"Wherefore He is able also to save them to the uttermost that come unto God by Him seeing He ever liveth to make intercession for them.* Hebrews x. ver. 14. *For by one offering He hath perfected for ever them that are sanctified."*

My kind, indulgent Mistress liv'd but two years after my Master. Her death was a great affliction to me. She left five sons, all gracious young men, and Ministers of the Gospel.— I continued with them all, one after another, till they died; they liv'd but four years after their parents. When it pleased God to take them to Himself, I was left quite destitute, without a friend in the world. But I who had so often experienced the Goodness of GOD, trusted in Him to do what He pleased with me.—In this helpless condition I went in the wood to prayer as usual; and tho' the snow was a considerable height, I was not sensible of cold, or any other inconveniency.—At times indeed when I saw the world frowning round me, I was tempted to think that the LORD had forsaken me. I found great relief from the contemplation of these words in Isaiah xlix. v. 16. *"Behold I have graven thee on the palms of my hands; thy walls are continually before me."* And very many comfortable promises were sweetly applied to me. The lxxxix. Psalm and 34th verse, *"My covenant will I not break nor alter the thing that is gone out of my lips."* Hebrews, chap. xvi. v. 17, 18. Phillipians, chap. i. v. 6; and several more.

As I had now lost all my dear and valued friends every place in the world was alike to me. I had for a great while entertain'd a desire to come to ENGLAND.—I imagined that all the Inhabitants of this Island were *Holy*; because all those that had visited my Master from thence were good, (Mr. Whitefield was his particular friend) and the authors of the books that had been given me were all English. But above all places in the world I wish'd to see Kidderminster, for I could not but think that on the spot where Mr. Baxter had liv'd, and preach'd, the people must be all *Righteous*.

The situation of my affairs requir'd that I should tarry a little longer in NEW-YORK, as I was something in debt, and was embarrass'd how to pay it.—About this time a young Gentleman that was a particular acquaintance of one of my young Master's, pretended to be a friend to me, and promis'd to pay my debts, which was three pounds; and he assur'd me he would never expect the money again.—But, in less than a month, he came and demanded it; and when I assur'd him I had nothing to pay, he threatened to sell me.—Though I knew he had no right to do that, yet as I had no friend in the world to go to, it alarm'd me greatly.—At length he purpos'd my going a Privateering, that I might by these means, be enabled to pay him, to which I agreed.—Our Captain's name was ——— ——— I went in Character of Cook to him.—Near St. Domingo we came up to five French ships, Merchant-men.— We had a very smart engagement that continued from eight in the morning till three in the afternoon; when victory declar'd on our side.—Soon after this we were met by three English ships which join'd us, and that encourag'd us to attack a fleet of 36 Ships.—We boarded the three first and then follow'd the others; and had the same success with twelve; but the rest escap'd us.—There was a great deal of blood shed, and I was near death several times, but the LORD preserv'd me.

I met with many enemies, and much persecution, among the sailors; one of them was particularly unkind to me, and studied ways to vex and teaze me.—I can't help mentioning one circumstance that hurt me more than all the rest, which was, that he snatched a book out of my hand that I was very fond of, and used frequently to amuse myself with, and threw it into the sea.—But what is remarkable he was the first that was killed in our engagement.—I don't pretend to say that this happen'd because he was not my friend: but I thought 'twas a very awful Providence to see how the enemies of the LORD are cut off.

Our Captain was a cruel hard-hearted man. I was excessively sorry for the prisoners we took in general; but the pitiable case of one young Gentleman grieved me to the heart.—He appear'd very amiable; was strikingly handsome. Our Captain took four thousand pounds from him; but that did not satisfy him, as he imagin'd he was possess'd of more, and had somewhere conceal'd it, so that the Captain threatened him with death, at which he appear'd in the deepest distress, and took the buckles out of his shoes, and untied his hair, which was very fine, and long; and in which several very valuable rings were fasten'd. He came into the Cabbin to me, and in the most obliging terms imaginable ask'd for something to eat and drink; which when I gave him, he was so thankful and pretty in his manner that my heart bled for him; and I heartily wish'd that I could have spoken in any language in which the ship's crew would not have understood me; that I might have let him know his danger; for I heard the Captain say he was resolv'd upon his death; and he put his barbarous design into execution, for he took him on shore with one of the sailors, and there they shot him.

This circumstance affected me exceedingly, I could not put him out of my mind a long while.—When we return'd to NEW-YORK the Captain divided the prize-money among us, that we had taken. When I was call'd upon to receive my part, I waited upon Mr. ——, (the Gentleman that paid my debt and was the occasion of my going abroad) to know if he chose to go with me to receive my money or if I should bring him what I owed.—He chose to go with me; and when the Captain laid my money on the table ('twas an hundred and thirty-five pounds) I desir'd Mr. —— to take what I was indebted to him; and he swept it all into his handkerchief, and would never be prevail'd on to give a farthing of money, nor any thing at all beside.—And he likewise secur'd a hogshead of sugar which was my due from the same ship. The Captain was very angry with him for this piece of cruelty to me, as was every other person that heard it.—But I have reason to believe (as he was one of the Principal Merchants in the city) that he transacted business for him and on that account did not chuse to quarrel with him.

At this time a very worthy Gentleman, a Wine Merchant, his name Dunscum, took me under his protection, and would have recovered my money for me if I had chose it; but I told him to let it alone; that I wou'd rather be quiet.—I believed that it would not prosper with him, and so it happen'd, for by a series of losses and misfortunes he became poor, and was soon after drowned, as he was on a party of pleasure.—The vessel was driven out to sea, and struck against a rock by which means every soul perished.

I was very much distress'd when I heard it, and felt greatly for his family who were reduc'd to very low circumstances.— I never knew how to set a proper value on money. If I had but a little meat and drink to supply the present necessaries of life, I never wish'd for more; and when I had any I always gave it if ever I saw an object in distress. If it was not for my dear Wife and Children I should pay as little regard to money now as I did at that time.—I continu'd some time with Mr. Dunscum as his servant; he was very kind to me.—But I had a vast inclination to visit ENGLAND, and wish'd continually that it would please Providence to make a clear way for me to see this Island. I entertain'd a notion that if I could get to ENGLAND I should never more experience either cruelty or ingratitude, so that I was very desirous to get among Christians. I knew Mr. Whitefield very well.—I had heard him preach often at NEW-YORK. In this disposition I listed in the twenty-eighth Regiment of Foot, who were design'd for Martinico in the late war.—We went in Admiral Pocock's fleet from New-York to Barbadoes; from thence to Martinico.—When that was taken we proceeded to the Havannah, and took that place likewise.—There I got discharged.

I was then worth about thirty pounds, but I never regarded money in the least, nor would I tarry to receive my prize-money least I should lose my chance of going to England.— I went with the Spanish prisoners to Spain; and came to Old-England with the English prisoners.—I cannot describe my joy when we were within sight of Portsmouth. But I was astonished when we landed to hear the inhabitants of that place curse and swear, and otherwise profane. I expected to find nothing but goodness, gentleness and meekness in this Christian Land, I then suffer'd great perplexities of mind.

I enquir'd if any serious Christian people resided there, the woman I made this enquiry of, answer'd me in the affirmative; and added that she was one of them.—I was heartily glad to hear her say so. I thought I could give her my whole heart: she kept a Public-House. I deposited with her all the money that I had not an immediate occasion for; as I thought it would be safer with her.—It was 25 guineas but 6 of them I desired her to lay out to the best advantage, to buy me some shirts, hat and some other necessaries. I made her a present of a very handsome large looking glass that I brought with me from Martinico, in order to recompence her for the trouble I had given her. I must do this woman the justice to acknowledge that she did lay out some little for my use, but the 19 guineas and part of the 6, with my watch, she would not return, but denied that I ever gave it her.

I soon perceived that I was got among bad people, who defrauded me of my money and watch; and that all my promis'd happiness was blasted, I had no friend but GOD and I pray'd to Him earnestly. I could scarcely believe it possible that the place where so many eminent Christians had lived and preached could abound with so much wickedness and deceit. I thought it worse than *Sodom* (considering the great advantages they have) I cryed like a child and that almost continually: at length GOD heard my prayers and rais'd me a friend indeed.

This publican had a brother who lived on Portsmouth-common, his wife was a very serious good woman.—When she heard of the treatment I had met with, she came and enquired into my real situation and was greatly troubled at the ill usage I had received, and took me home to her own house.—I began now to rejoice, and my prayer was turned into praise. She made use of all the arguments in her power to prevail on her who had wronged me, to return my watch and money, but it was to no purpose, as she had given me no receipt and I had nothing to show for it, I could not demand it.—My good friend was excessively angry with her and obliged her to give me back four guineas, which she said she gave me out of charity: Though in fact it was my own, and much more. She would have employed some rougher means to oblige her to give up my money, but I would not suffer her, let it go says I "My GOD is in heaven." Still I did not mind my loss in the least; all that grieved me was, that I had been disappointed in finding some Christian friends, with whom I hoped to enjoy a little sweet and comfortable society.

I thought the best method that I could take now, was to go to London, and find out Mr. Whitefield, who was the only living soul I knew in England, and get him to direct me to some way or other to procure a living without being troublesome to any Person.—I took leave of my christian friend at Portsmouth, and went in the stage to London.—A creditable tradesman in the City, who went up with me in the stage, offer'd to show me the way to Mr. Whitefield's Tabernacle. Knowing that I was a perfect stranger, I thought it very kind, and accepted his offer; but he obliged me to give him half-a-crown for going with me, and likewise insisted on my giving him five shillings more for conducting me to Dr. Gifford's Meeting.

I began now to entertain a very different idea of the inhabitants of England than what I had figur'd to myself before I came amongst them.—Mr. Whitefield receiv'd me very friendly, was heartily glad to see me, and directed me to a proper place to board and lodge in Petticoat-Lane, till he could think of some way to settle me in, and paid for my lodging, and all my expences. The morning after I came to my new lodging, as I was at breakfast with the gentlewoman of the house, I heard the noise of some looms over our heads: I enquir'd what it was; she told me a person was weaving silk.—I express'd a great desire to see it, and ask'd if I might: She told me she would go up with me; she was sure I should be very welcome. She was as good as her word, and as soon as we enter'd the room, the person that was weaving look'd about, and smiled upon us, and I loved her from that moment.—She ask'd me many questions, and I in turn talk'd a great deal to her. I found she was a member of Mr. Allen's Meeting, and I begun to entertain a good opinion of her, though I was almost afraid to indulge this inclination, least she should prove like all the rest I had met with at Portsmouth, &c. and which had almost given me a dislike to all white women.—But after a short acquaintance I had the happiness to find she was very different, and quite sincere, and I was not without hope that she entertain'd some esteem for me. We often went together to hear Dr. Gifford, and as I had always a propensity to relieve every object in distress as far as I was able, I used to give to all that complain'd to me; sometimes half a guinea at a time, as I did not understand the real value of it.—This gracious, good woman took great pains to correct and advise me in that and many other respects.

After I had been in London about six weeks I was recommended to the notice of some of my late Master Mr. Freelandhouse's acquaintance, who had heard him speak frequently of me. I was much persuaded by them to go to Holland.— My Master lived there before he bought me, and used to speak of me so respectfully among his friends there, that it raised in them a curiosity to see me; particularly the Gentlemen engaged in the Ministry, who expressed a desire to hear my experience and examine me. I found that it was my good old Master's design that I should have gone if he had lived; for which reason I resolved upon going to Holland, and informed my dear friend Mr. Whitefield of my intention; he was much averse to my going at first, but after I gave him my reasons appeared very well satisfied. I likewise informed my Betty (the good woman that I have mentioned above) of my determination to go to Holland and I told her that I believed she was to be my Wife: that if it was the LORD's Will I desired it, but not else.—She made me very little answer, but has since told me, she did not think it at that time.

I embarked at Tower-wharf at four o'clock in the morning, and arriv'd at Amsterdam the next day by three o'clock in the afternoon. I had several letters of recommendation to my old master's friends, who receiv'd me very graciously. Indeed, one of the chief Ministers was particularly good to me; he kept me at his house a long while, and took great pleasure in asking questions, which I answer'd with delight, being always ready to say, *"Come unto me all ye that fear GOD, and I will tell what he hath done for my Soul."* I cannot but admire the footsteps of Providence; astonish'd that I should be so wonderfully preserved! Though the Grandson of a King, I have wanted bread, and should have been glad of the hardest crust I ever saw. I who, at home, was surrounded and guarded by slaves, so that no indifferent person might approach me, and clothed with gold, have been inhumanly threatened with death; and frequently wanted clothing to defend me from the inclemency of the weather; yet I never murmured, nor was I discontented.—I am willing, and even desirous to be counted as nothing, a stranger in the world, and a pilgrim here; for *"I know that my* REDEEMER *liveth,"* and I'm thankful for every trial and trouble that I've met with, as I am not without hope that they have been all sanctified to me.

The Calvinist Ministers desired to hear my Experience from myself, which proposal I was very well pleased with: So I stood before 38 Ministers every Thursday for seven weeks together, and they were all very well satisfied, and persuaded I was what I pretended to be.—They wrote down my experience as I spoke it; and the LORD ALMIGHTY was with me at that time in a remarkable manner, and gave me words and enabled me to answer them; so great was his mercy to take me in hand a poor blind heathen.

At this time a very rich Merchant at AMSTERDAM offered to take me into his family in the capacity of his Butler, and I very willingly accepted it.—He was a gracious worthy Gentleman and very good to me.—He treated me more like a friend than a servant.—I tarried there a twelvemonth but was not thoroughly contented, I wanted to see my wife; (that is now) and for that reason I wished to return to ENGLAND, I wrote to her once in my absence, but she did not answer my letter; and I must acknowledge if she had, it would have given me a less opinion of her.—My Master and Mistress persuaded me much not to leave them and likewise their two Sons who entertained a good opinion of me; and if I had found my Betty married on my arrival in ENGLAND, I should have returned to them again immediately.

My Lady purposed my marrying her maid; she was an agreeable young woman, had saved a good deal of money, but I could not fancy her, though she was willing to accept of me, but I told her my inclinations were engaged in ENGLAND, and I could think of no other Person.—On my return home, I found my Betty disengaged.—She had refused several offers in my absence, and told her sister that, she thought, if ever she married I was to be her husband.

Soon after I came home, I waited on Doctor Gifford who took me into his family and was exceedingly good to me. The character of this pious worthy Gentleman is well known; my praise can be of no use or signification at all.—I hope I shall ever gratefully remember the many favours I have received from him.—Soon after I came to Doctor Gifford I expressed a desire to be admitted into their Church, and set down with them; they told me I must first be baptized; so I gave in my experience before the Church, with which they were very well satisfied, and I was baptized by Doctor Gifford with some others. I then made known my intentions of being married; but I found there were many objections against it because the person I had fixed on was poor. She was a widow, her husband had left her in debt, and with a child, so that they persuaded me against it out of real regard to me.—But I had promised and was resolved to have her; as I knew her to be a gracious woman, her poverty was no objection to me, as they had nothing else to say against her. When my friends found that they could not alter my opinion respecting her, they wrote to Mr. Allen, the Minister she attended, to persuade her to leave me; but he replied that he would not interfere at all, that we might do as we would. I was resolved that all my wife's little debt should be paid before we were married; so that I sold almost every thing I had and with all the money I could raise cleared all that she owed, and I never did any thing with a better will in all my Life, because I firmly believed that we should be very happy together, and so it prov'd, for she was given me from the LORD. And I have found her a blessed partner, and we have never repented, tho' we have gone through many great troubles and difficulties.

My wife got a very good living by weaving, and could do extremely well; but just at that time there was great disturbance among the weavers; so that I was afraid to let my wife work, least they should insist on my joining the rioters which I could not think of, and, possibly, if I had refused to do so they would have knock'd me on the head.—So that by these means my wife could get no employ, neither had I work enough to maintain my family. We had not yet been married a year before all these misfortunes overtook us.

Just at this time a gentleman, that seemed much concerned for us, advised me to go into *Essex* with him and promised to get me employed.—I accepted his kind proposal, and he spoke to a friend of his, a Quaker, a gentleman of large fortune, who resided a little way out of the town of *Colchester*; his name was *Handbarar*; he ordered his steward to set me to work.

There were several employed in the same way with myself. I was very thankful and contented though my wages were but small.—I was allowed but eight pence a day, and found myself; but after I had been in this situation for a fortnight, my Master, being told that a Black was at work for him, had an inclination to see me. He was pleased to talk to me for some time, and at last enquired what wages I had; when I told him he declared, it was too little, and immediately ordered his Steward to let me have eighteen pence a day, which he constantly gave me after; and I then did extremely well.

I did not bring my wife with me: I came first alone and it was my design, if things answered according to our wishes, to send for her—I was now thinking to desire her to come to me when I receiv'd a letter to inform me she was just brought to bed and in want of many necessaries.—This news was a great trial to me and a fresh affliction: but my GOD, *faithful and abundant in mercy*, forsook me not in this trouble.—As I could not read *English*, I was obliged to apply to some one to read the letter I received, relative to my wife. I was directed by the good Providence of GOD to a worthy young gentleman, a Quaker, and friend of my Master.—I desired he would take the trouble to read my letter for me, which he readily comply'd with and was greatly moved and affected at the contents; insomuch that he said he would undertake to make a gathering for me, which he did and was the first to contribute to it himself. The money was sent that evening to LONDON by a person who happen'd to be going there: nor was this All the goodness that I experienced from these kind friends, for, as soon as my wife came about and was fit to travel, they sent for her to me, and were at the whole expence of her coming; so evidently has the love and mercy of GOD appeared through every trouble that ever I experienced. We went on very comfortably all the summer.—We lived in a little cottage near Mr. *Handbarrar's* House; but when the winter came on I was discharged, as he had no further occasion for me. And now the prospect began to darken upon us again. We thought it most adviseable to move our habitation a little nearer to the Town, as the house we lived in was very cold, and wet, and ready to tumble down.

The boundless goodness of GOD to me has been so very great, that with the most humble gratitude I desire to prostrate myself before Him; for I have been wonderfully supported in every affliction. My GOD never left me. I perceived light *still* through the thickest darkness.

My dear wife and I were now both unemployed, we could get nothing to do. The winter prov'd remarkably severe, and we were reduc'd to the greatest distress imaginable.—I was always very shy of asking for any thing; I could never beg; neither did I chuse to make known our wants to any person, for fear of offending as we were entire strangers; but our last bit of bread was gone, and I was obliged to think of something to do for our support.—I did not mind for myself at all; but to see my dear wife and children in want pierc'd me to the heart.—I now blam'd myself for bringing her from London, as doubtless had we continued there we might have found friends to keep us from starving. The snow was at this season remarkably deep; so that we could see no prospect of being relieved. In this melancholy situation, not knowing what step to pursue, I resolved to make my case known to a Gentleman's Gardiner that lived near us, and entreat him to employ me: but when I came to him, my courage failed me, and I was ashamed to make known our real situation.—I endeavoured all I could to prevail on him to set me to work, but to no purpose: he assur'd me it was not in his power: but just as I was about to leave him, he asked me if I would accept of some Carrots? I took them with great thankfulness and carried them home: he gave me four, they were very large and fine.—We had nothing to make fire with, so consequently could not boil them: But was glad to have them to eat *raw*. Our youngest child was quite an infant; so that my wife was obliged to chew it, and fed her in that manner for several days.—We allowed ourselves but one every day, least they should not last 'till we could get some other supply. I was unwilling to eat at all myself; nor would I take any the last day that we continued in this situation, as I could not bear the thought that my dear wife and children would be in want of every means of support. We lived in this manner, 'till our carrots were all gone: then my Wife began to lament because of our poor babies: but I comforted her all I could; still hoping, and believing that *my* GOD would not let us die: but that it would please Him to relieve us, which *He* did by almost a Miracle.

We went to bed, as usual, before it was quite dark, (as we had neither fire nor candle) but had not been there long before some person knocked at the door & enquir'd if *James Albert* lived there? I answer'd in the affirmative, and rose immediately; as soon as I open'd the door I found it was the servant of an eminent Attorney who resided at *Colchester.*—He ask'd me how it was with me? if I was not almost starv'd? I burst out a crying, and told him I was indeed. He said his master suppos'd so, and that he wanted to speak with me, and I must return with him. This Gentleman's name was *Danniel*, he was a sincere, good christian. He used to stand and talk with me frequently when I work'd in the road for Mr. *Handbarrar*, and would have employed me himself, if I had wanted work.—When I came to his house he told me that he had thought a good deal about me of late, and was apprehensive that I must be in want, and could not be satisfied till he sent to enquire after me. I made known my distress to him, at which he was greatly affected; and generously gave me a guinea; and promis'd to be kind to me in future. I could not help exclaiming. *O the boundless mercies of my God!* I pray'd unto Him, and He has heard me; I trusted in Him and He has preserv'd me: where shall I begin to praise Him, or how shall I love Him enough?

I went immediately and bought some bread and cheese and coal and carried it home. My dear wife was rejoiced to see me return with something to eat. She instantly got up and dressed our Babies, while I made a fire, and the first Nobility in the land never made a more comfortable meal.—We did not forget to thank the LORD for all his goodness to us.— Soon after this, as the spring came on, Mr. Peter *Daniel* employed me in helping to pull down a house, and rebuilding it. I had then very good work, and full employ: he sent for my wife, and children to *Colchester*, and provided us a house where we lived very comfortably.—I hope I shall always gratefully acknowledge his kindness to myself and family. I worked at this house for more than a year, till it was finished; and after that I was employed by several successively, and was never so happy as when I had something to do; but perceiving the winter coming on, and work rather slack, I was apprehensive that we should again be in want or become troublesome to our friends.

I had at this time an offer made me of going to *Norwich* and having constant employ.—My wife seemed pleased with this proposal, as she supposed she might get work there in the weaving-manufactory, being the business she was brought up to, and more likely to succeed there than any other place; and we thought as we had an opportunity of moving to a Town where we could both be employ'd it was most adviseable to do so; and that probably we might settle there for our lives.— When this step was resolv'd on, I went first alone to see how it would answer; which I very much repented after, for it was not in my power immediately to send my wife any supply, as I fell into the hands of a Master that was neither kind nor considerate; and she was reduced to great distress, so that she was oblig'd to sell the few goods that we had, and when I sent for her was under the disagreeable necessity of parting with our bed.

When she came to *Norwich* I hired a room ready furnished.—I experienced a great deal of difference in the carriage of my Master from what I had been accustomed to from some of my other Masters. He was very irregular in his payments to me.—My wife hired a loom and wove all the leisure time she had and we began to do very well, till we were overtaken by fresh misfortunes. Our three poor children fell ill of the small pox; this was a great trial to us; but still I was persuaded in myself we should not be forsaken.—And I did all in my power to keep my dear partner's spirits from sinking. Her whole attention now was taken up with the children as she could mind nothing else, and all I could get was but little to support a family in such a situation, beside paying for the hire of our room, which I was obliged to omit doing for several weeks: but the woman to whom we were indebted would not excuse us, tho' I promised she should have the very first money we could get after my children came about, but she would not be satisfied and had the cruelty to threaten us that if we did not pay her immediately she would turn us all into the street.

The apprehension of this plunged me in the deepest distress, considering the situation of my poor babies: if they had been in health I should have been less sensible of this misfortune. But My GOD, *still faithful to his promise*, raised me a friend. Mr. Henry Gurdney, a Quaker, a gracious gentleman heard of our distress, he sent a servant of his own to the woman we hired the room of, paid our rent, and bought all the goods with my wife's loom and gave it us all.

Some other gentlemen, hearing of his design, were pleased to assist him in these generous acts, for which we never can be thankful enough; after this my children soon came about; we began to do pretty well again; my dear wife work'd hard and constant when she could get work, but it was upon a disagreeable footing as her employ was so uncertain, sometimes she could get nothing to do and at other times when the weavers of *Norwich* had orders from LONDON they were so excessively hurried, that the people they employ'd were often oblig'd to work on the *Sabbath-day*; but this my wife would never do, and it was matter of uneasiness to us that we could not get our living in a regular manner, though we were both diligent, industrious, and willing to work. I was far from being happy in my Master, he did not use me well. I could scarcely ever get my money from him; but I continued patient 'till it pleased GOD to alter my situation.

My worthy friend Mr. Gurdney advised me to follow the employ of chopping chaff, and bought me an instrument for that purpose. There were but few people in the town that made this their business beside myself; so that I did very well indeed and we became easy and happy.—But we did not continue long in this comfortable state: Many of the inferior people were envious and ill-natur'd and set up the same employ and work'd under price on purpose to get my business from me, and they succeeded so well that I could hardly get any thing to do, and became again unfortunate: Nor did this misfortune come alone, for just at this time we lost one of our little girls who died of a fever; this circumstance occasion'd us new troubles, for the Baptist Minister refused to bury her because we were not their members. The Parson of the parish denied us because she had never been baptized. I applied to the Quakers, but met with no success; this was one of the greatest trials I ever met with, as we did not know what to do with our poor baby.—At length I resolv'd to dig a grave in the garden behind the house, and bury her there; when the Parson of the parish sent for me to tell me he would bury the child, but did not chuse to read the burial service over her. I told him I did not mind whether he would or not, as the child could not hear it.

We met with a great deal of ill treatment after this, and found it very difficult to live.—We could scarcely get work to do, and were obliged to pawn our cloaths. We were ready to sink under our troubles.—When I purposed to my wife to go to *Kidderminster* and try if we could do there. I had always an inclination for that place, and now more than ever as I had heard *Mr. Fawcet* mentioned in the most respectful manner, as a pious worthy Gentleman; and I had seen his name in a favourite book of mine, Baxter's *Saints everlasting rest*; and as the Manufactory of *Kidderminster* seemed to promise my wife some employment, she readily came into my way of thinking.

I left her once more, and set out for *Kidderminster*, in order to judge if the situation would suit us.—As soon as I came there I waited immediately on *Mr. Fawcet*, who was pleased to receive me very kindly and recommended me to *Mr. Watson* who employed me in twisting silk and worsted together. I continued here about a fortnight, and when I thought it would answer our expectation, I returned to *Norwich* to fetch my wife; she was then near her time, and too much indisposed. So we were obliged to tarry until she was brought to bed, and as soon as she could conveniently travel we came to *Kidderminster*, but we brought nothing with us as we were obliged to sell all we had to pay our debts and the expences of my wife's illness, *&c.*

Such is our situation at present.—My wife, by hard labor at the loom, does every thing that can be expected from her towards the maintenance of our family; and GOD is pleased to incline the hearts of his People at times to yield us their charitable assistance; being myself through age and infirmity able to contribute but little to their support. As Pilgrims, and very poor Pilgrims, we are travelling through many difficulties towards our HEAVENLY HOME, and waiting patiently for his gracious call, when the LORD shall deliver us out of the evils of this present world and bring us to the EVERLASTING GLORIES of the world to come.—To HIM be PRAISE for EVER and EVER, AMEN.

FINIS.

THE
INTERESTING NARRATIVE

OF

THE LIFE

OF

OLAUDAH EQUIANO,

OR

GUSTAVUS VASSA,

THE AFRICAN.

WRITTEN BY HIMSELF.

*Behold, God is my salvation; I will trust and not be
afraid, for the Lord Jehovah is my strength and my
song; he also is become my salvation.
And in that shall ye say, Praise the Lord, call upon his
name, declare his doings among the people.* Isaiah xii.
2, 4.

LONDON:

Printed for and sold by the AUTHOR, No. 10, Union-Street,
Middlesex Hospital

Sold also by Mr. Johnson, St. Paul's Church-Yard; Mr. Murray, Fleet-Street;
Messrs. Robson and Clark, Bond-Street; Mr. Davis, opposite Gray's Inn,
Holborn; Messrs. Shepperson and Reynolds, and Mr. Jackson, Oxford-
Street; Mr. Lackington, Chiswell-Street; Mr. Mathews, Strand; Mr. Murray,
Prince's-Street, Soho; Mess. Taylor and Co. South Arch, Royal Exchange;
Mr. Button, Newington-Causeway; Mr. Parsons, Paternoster-Row; and may
be had of all the Booksellers in Town and Country.

[Entered at Stationer's Hall.]

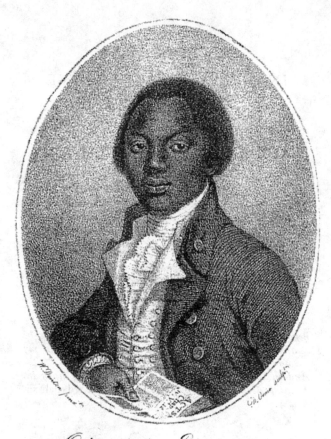

Olaudah Equiano

or

GUSTAVUS VASSA,

the African

To the Lords Spiritual and Temporal, and the Commons of the Parliament of Great Britain.

My Lords and Gentlemen,

Permit me, with the greatest deference and respect, to lay at your feet the following genuine Narrative; the chief design of which is to excite in your august assemblies a sense of compassion for the miseries which the Slave-Trade has entailed on my unfortunate countrymen. By the horrors of that trade was I first torn away from all the tender connexions that were naturally dear to my heart; but these, through the mysterious ways of Providence, I ought to regard as infinitely more than compensated by the introduction I have thence obtained to the knowledge of the Christian religion, and of a nation which, by its liberal sentiments, its humanity, the glorious freedom of its government, and its proficiency in arts and sciences, has exalted the dignity of human nature.

I am sensible I ought to entreat your pardon for addressing to you a work so wholly devoid of literary merit; but, as the production of an unlettered African, who is actuated by the hope of becoming an instrument towards the relief of his suffering countrymen, I trust that *such a man*, pleading in *such a cause*, will be acquitted of boldness and presumption.

May the God of heaven inspire your hearts with peculiar benevolence on that important day when the question of Abolition is to be discussed, when thousands, in consequence of your Determination, are to look for Happiness or Misery!

I am,

My Lords and Gentlemen,

Your most obedient,

And devoted humble Servant,

Olaudah Equiano,

or

Gustavus Vassa.

Union-Street, Mary-le-bone,
    March 24, 1789.

His Royal Highness the Prince of Wales.
His Royal Highness the Duke of York.

A

The Right Hon. the Earl of Ailesbury
Admiral Affleck
Mr. William Abington, 2 copies
Mr. John Abraham
James Adair, Esq.
Reverend Mr. Aldridge
Mr. John Almon
Mrs. Arnot
Mr. Joseph Armitage
Mr. Joseph Ashpinshaw
Mr. Samuel Atkins
Mr. John Atwood
Mr. Thomas Atwood
Mr. Ashwell
J. C. Ashworth, Esq.

B

His Grace the Duke of Bedford
Her Grace the Duchess of Buccleugh
The Right Rev. the Lord Bishop of Bangor
The Right Hon. Lord Belgrave
The Rev. Doctor Baker
Mrs. Baker
Matthew Baillie, M. D.
Mrs. Baillie
Miss Baillie
Miss J. Baillie
David Barclay, Esq.
Mr. Robert Barrett
Mr. William Barrett
Mr. John Barnes
Mr. John Basnett
Mr. Bateman
Mrs. Baynes, 2 copies
Mr. Thomas Bellamy
Mr. J. Benjafield
Mr. William Bennett
Mr. Bensley
Mr. Samuel Benson
Mrs. Benton
Reverend Mr. Bentley

Mr. Thomas Bently
Sir John Berney, Bart.
Alexander Blair, Esq.
James Bocock, Esq.
Mrs. Bond
Miss Bond
Mrs. Borckhardt
Mrs. E. Bouverie
—— Brand, Esq.
Mr. Martin Brander
F. J. Brown, Esq. M. P. 2 copies
W. Buttall, Esq.
Mr. Buxton
Mr. R. L. B.
Mr. Thomas Burton, 6 copies
Mr. W. Button

      C

The Right Hon. Lord Cathcart
The Right Hon. H. S. Conway
Lady Almiria Carpenter
James Carr, Esq.
Charles Carter, Esq.
Mr. James Chalmers
Captain John Clarkson, of the Royal Navy
The Rev. Mr. Thomas Clarkson, 2 copies
Mr. R. Clay
Mr. William Clout
Mr. George Club
Mr. John Cobb
Miss Calwell
Mr. Thomas Cooper
Richard Cosway, Esq.
Mr. James Coxe
Mr. J. C.
Mr. Croucher
Mr. Cruickshanks
Ottobah Cugoano, or John Stewart

      D

The Right Hon. the Earl of Dartmouth
The Right Hon. the Earl of Derby
Sir William Dolben, Bart.
The Reverend C. E. De Coetlogon
John Delamain, Esq.
Mrs. Delamain
Mr. Davis
Mr. William Denton
Mr. T. Dickie
Mr. William Dickson

Mr. Charles Dilly, 2 copies
Andrew Drummond, Esq.
Mr. George Durant
E
The Right Hon. the Earl of Essex
The Right Hon. the Countess of Essex
Sir Gilbert Elliot, Bart. 2 copies
Lady Ann Erskine
G. Noel Edwards, Esq. M. P. 2 copies
Mr. Durs Egg
Mr. Ebenezer Evans
The Reverend Mr. John Eyre
Mr. William Eyre
F
Mr. George Fallowdown
Mr. John Fell
F. W. Foster, Esq.
The Reverend Mr. Foster
Mr. J. Frith
W. Fuller, Esq.
G
The Right Hon. the Earl of Gainsborough
The Right Hon. the Earl of Grosvenor
The Right Hon. Viscount Gallway
The Right Hon. Viscountess Gallway
—— Gardner, Esq.
Mrs. Garrick
Mr. John Gates
Mr. Samuel Gear
Sir Philip Gibbes, Bart 6 copies
Miss Gibbes
Mr. Edward Gilbert
Mr. Jonathan Gillett
W. P. Gilliess, Esq.
Mrs. Gordon
Mr. Grange
Mr. William Grant
Mr. John Grant
Mr. R. Greening
S. Griffiths
John Grove, Esq.
Mrs. Guerin
Reverend Mr. Gwinep
H
The Right Hon. the Earl of Hopetoun
The Right Hon. Lord Hawke
Right Hon. Dowager Countess of Huntingdon
Thomas Hall, Esq.

Mr. Haley
Hugh Josiah Hansard, Esq.
Mr. Moses Hart
Mrs. Hawkins
Mr. Haysom
Mr. Hearne
Mr. William Hepburn
Mr. J. Hibbert
Mr. Jacob Higman
Sir Richard Hill, Bart.
Reverend Rowland Hill
Miss Hill
Captain John Hills, Royal Navy
Edmund Hill, Esq.
The Reverend Mr. Edward Hoare
William Hodges, Esq.
Reverend Mr. John Holmes, 3 copies
Mr. Martin Hopkins
Mr. Thomas Howell
Mr. R. Huntley
Mr. J. Hunt
Mr. Philip Hurlock, jun.
Mr. Hutson

J

Mr. T. W. J. Esq.
Mr. James Jackson
Mr. John Jackson
Reverend Mr. James
Mrs. Anne Jennings
Mr. Johnson
Mrs. Johnson
Mr. William Jones
Thomas Irving, Esq. 2 copies
Mr. William Justins

K

The Right Hon. Lord Kinnaird
William Kendall, Esq.
Mr. William Ketland
Mr. Edward King
Mr. Thomas Kingston
Reverend Dr. Kippis
Mr. William Kitchener
Mr. John Knight

L

The Right Reverend the Lord Bishop of London
Mr. John Laisne
Mr. Lackington, 6 copies

Mr. John Lamb
Bennet Langton, Esq.
Mr. S. Lee
Mr. Walter Lewis
Mr. J. Lewis
Mr. J. Lindsey
Mr. T. Litchfield
Edward Loveden Loveden, Esq. M. P.
Charles Lloyd, Esq.
Mr. William Lloyd
Mr. J. B. Lucas
Mr. James Luken
Henry Lyte, Esq.
Mrs. Lyon

M

His Grace the Duke of Marlborough
His Grace the Duke of Montague
The Right Hon. Lord Mulgrave
Sir Herbert Mackworth, Bart.
Sir Charles Middleton, Bart.
Lady Middleton
Mr. Thomas Macklane
Mr. George Markett
James Martin, Esq. M. P.
Master Martin, Hayes-Grove, Kent
Mr. William Massey
Mr. Joseph Massingham
John McIntosh, Esq.
Paul Le Mesurier, Esq. M. P.
Mr. James Mewburn
Mr. N. Middleton,
T. Mitchell, Esq.
Mrs. Montague, 2 copies
Miss Hannah More
Mr. George Morrison
Thomas Morris, Esq.
Miss Morris
Morris Morgann, Esq.

N

His Grace the Duke of Northumberland
Captain Nurse

O

Edward Ogle, Esq.
James Ogle, Esq.
Robert Oliver, Esq.

P

Mr. D. Parker,
Mr. W. Parker,
Mr. Richard Packer, jun.
Mr. Parsons, 6 copies
Mr. James Pearse
Mr. J. Pearson
J. Penn, Esq.
George Peters, Esq.
Mr. W. Phillips,
J. Philips, Esq.
Mrs. Pickard
Mr. Charles Pilgrim
The Hon. George Pitt, M. P.
Mr. Thomas Pooley
Patrick Power, Esq.
Mr. Michael Power
Joseph Pratt, Esq.

Q

Robert Quarme, Esq.

R

The Right Hon. Lord Rawdon
The Right Hon. Lord Rivers, 2 copies
Lieutenant General Rainsford
Reverend James Ramsay, 3 copies
Mr. S. Remnant, jun.
Mr. William Richards, 2 copies
Mr. J. C. Robarts
Mr. James Roberts
Dr. Robinson
Mr. Robinson
Mr. C. Robinson
George Rose, Esq. M. P.
Mr. W. Ross
Mr. William Rouse
Mr. Walter Row

S

His Grace the Duke of St. Albans
Her Grace the Duchess of St. Albans
The Right Reverend the Lord Bishop of St. David's
The Right Hon. Earl Stanhope, 3 copies
The Right Hon. the Earl of Scarbrough
William, the Son of Ignatius Sancho
Mrs. Mary Ann Sandiford
Mr. William Sawyer
Mr. Thomas Seddon
W. Seward, Esq.
Reverend Mr. Thomas Scott

Granville Sharp, Esq. 2 copies
Captain Sidney Smith, of the Royal Navy
Colonel Simcoe
Mr. John Simco
General Smith
John Smith, Esq.
Mr. George Smith
Mr. William Smith
Reverend Mr. Southgate
Mr. William Starkey
Thomas Steel, Esq. M. P.
Mr. Staples Steare
Mr. Joseph Stewardson
Mr. Henry Stone, jun. 2 copies
John Symmons, Esq.

T

Henry Thornton, Esq. M. P.
Mr. Alexander Thomson, M. D.
Reverend John Till
Mr. Samuel Townly
Mr. Daniel Trinder
Reverend Mr. C. La Trobe
Clement Tudway, Esq.
Mrs. Twisden

U

Mr. M. Underwood

V

Mr. John Vaughan
Mrs. Vendt

W

The Right Hon. Earl of Warnick
The Right Reverend the Lord Bishop of Worcester
The Hon. William Windham, Esq. M. P.
Mr. C. B. Wadstrom
Mr. George Walne
Reverend Mr. Ward
Mr. S. Warren
Mr. J. Waugh
Josiah Wedgwood, Esq.
Reverend Mr. John Wesley
Mr. J. Wheble
Samuel Whitbread, Esq. M. P.
Reverend Thomas Wigzell
Mr. W. Wilson
Reverend Mr. Wills
Mr. Thomas Wimsett
Mr. William Winchester
John Wollaston, Esq.

Mr. Charles Wood
Mr. Joseph Woods
Mr. John Wood
J. Wright, Esq.
           Y
Mr. Thomas Young
Mr. Samuel Yockney

CONTENTS

THE LIFE, &c.

CHAPTER I.

The author's account of his country, and their manners and customs—Administration of justice—Embrenche—Marriage ceremony, and public entertainments—Mode of living—Dress—Manufactures Buildings—Commerce—Agriculture—War and religion—Superstition of the natives—Funeral ceremonies of the priests or magicians—Curious mode of discovering poison—Some hints concerning the origin of the author's countrymen, with the opinions of different writers on that subject.

I BELIEVE it is difficult for those who publish their own memoirs to escape the imputation of vanity; nor is this the only disadvantage under which they labour: it is also their misfortune, that what is uncommon is rarely, if ever, believed, and what is obvious we are apt to turn from with disgust, and to charge the writer with impertinence. People generally think those memoirs only worthy to be read or remembered which abound in great or striking events, those, in short, which in a high degree excite either admiration or pity: all others they consign to contempt and oblivion. It is therefore, I confess, not a little hazardous in a private and obscure individual, and a stranger too, thus to solicit the indulgent attention of the public; especially when I own I offer here the history of neither a saint, a hero, nor a tyrant. I believe there are few events in my life, which have not happened to many: it is true the incidents of it are numerous; and, did I consider myself an European, I might say my sufferings were great: but when I compare my lot with that of most of my countrymen, I regard myself as a *particular favourite of Heaven*, and acknowledge the mercies of Providence in every occurrence of my life. If then the following narrative does not appear sufficiently interesting to engage general attention, let my motive be some excuse for its publication. I am not so foolishly vain as to expect from it either immortality or literary reputation. If it affords any satisfaction to my numerous friends, at whose request it has been written, or in the smallest degree promotes the interests of humanity, the ends for which it was undertaken will be fully attained, and every wish of my heart gratified. Let it therefore be remembered, that, in wishing to avoid censure, I do not aspire to praise.

That part of Africa, known by the name of Guinea, to which the trade for slaves is carried on, extends along the coast above 3400 miles, from the Senegal to Angola, and includes a variety of kingdoms. Of these the most considerable is the kingdom of Benen, both as to extent and wealth, the richness and cultivation of the soil, the power of its king, and the number and warlike disposition of the inhabitants. It is situated nearly under the line, and extends along the coast about 170 miles, but runs back into the interior part of Africa to a distance hitherto I believe unexplored by any traveller; and seems only terminated at length by the empire of Abyssinia, near 1500 miles from its beginning. This kingdom is divided into many provinces or districts: in one of the most remote and fertile of which, called Eboe, I was born, in the year 1745, in a charming fruitful vale, named Essaka. The distance of this province from the capital of Benin and the sea coast must be very considerable; for I had never heard of white men or Europeans, nor of the sea: and our subjection to the king of Benin was little more than nominal; for every transaction of the government, as far as my slender observation extended, was conducted by the chiefs or elders of the place. The manners and government of a people who have little commerce with other countries are generally very simple; and the history of what passes in one family or village may serve as a specimen of a nation. My father was one of those elders or chiefs I have spoken of, and was styled Embrenche; a term, as I remember, importing the highest distinction, and signifying in our language a *mark* of grandeur. This mark is conferred on the person entitled to it, by cutting the skin across at the top of the forehead, and drawing it down to the eye-brows; and while it is in this situation applying a warm hand, and rubbing it until it shrinks up into a thick *weal* across the lower part of the forehead. Most of the judges and senators were thus marked; my father had long born it: I had seen it conferred on one of my brothers, and I was also *destined* to receive it by my parents. Those Embrence, or chief men, decided disputes and punished crimes; for which purpose they always assembled together. The proceedings were generally short; and in most cases the law of retaliation prevailed. I remember a man was brought before my father, and the other judges, for kidnapping a boy; and, although he was the son of a chief or senator, he was condemned to make recompense by a man or woman slave. Adultery, however, was sometimes punished with slavery or death; a punishment which I believe is inflicted on it throughout most of the nations of Africa*: so sacred among them is the honour of the marriage bed, and so jealous are they of the fidelity of their wives. Of this I recollect an instance:—a woman was convicted before the judges of adultery, and delivered over, as the custom was, to her husband to be punished. Accordingly he determined to put her to death: but it being found, just before her execution, that she had an infant at her breast; and no woman being prevailed on to perform the part of a nurse, she was spared on account of the child. The men, however, do not preserve the same constancy to their wives, which they expect from them; for they indulge in a plurality, though seldom in more than two. Their mode of marriage is thus:— both parties are usually betrothed when young by their parents, (though I have known the males to betroth themselves). On this occasion a feast is prepared, and the bride and bridegroom stand up in the midst of all their friends, who are assembled for the purpose, while he declares she is thenceforth to be looked upon as his wife, and that no other person is to pay any addresses to her. This is also immediately proclaimed in the vicinity, on which the bride retires from the assembly. Some time after she is brought home to her husband, and then another feast is made, to which the relations of both parties are invited: her parents then deliver her to the bridegroom, accompanied with a number of blessings, and at the same time they tie round her waist a cotton string of the thickness of a goose-quill, which none but married women are permitted to wear: she is now considered as completely his

*See Benezet's "Account of Guinea" throughout.

wife; and at this time the dowry is given to the new married pair, which generally consists of portions of land, slaves, and cattle, household goods, and implements of husbandry. These are offered by the friends of both parties; besides which the parents of the bridegroom present gifts to those of the bride, whose property she is looked upon before marriage; but after it she is esteemed the sole property of her husband. The ceremony being now ended the festival begins, which is celebrated with bonefires, and loud acclamations of joy, accompanied with music and dancing.

We are almost a nation of dancers, musicians, and poets. Thus every great event, such as a triumphant return from battle, or other cause of public rejoicing is celebrated in public dances, which are accompanied with songs and music suited to the occasion. The assembly is separated into four divisions, which dance either apart or in succession, and each with a character peculiar to itself. The first division contains the married men, who in their dances frequently exhibit feats of arms, and the representation of a battle. To these succeed the married women, who dance in the second division. The young men occupy the third; and the maidens the fourth. Each represents some interesting scene of real life, such as a great achievement, domestic employment, a pathetic story, or some rural sport; and as the subject is generally founded on some recent event, it is therefore ever new. This gives our dances a spirit and variety which I have scarcely seen elsewhere*. We have many musical instruments, particularly drums of different kinds, a piece of music which resembles a guitar, and another much like a stickado. These last are chiefly used by betrothed virgins, who play on them on all grand festivals.

As our manners are simple, our luxuries are few. The dress of both sexes is nearly the same. It generally consists of a long piece of callico, or muslin, wrapped loosely round the body, somewhat in the form of a highland plaid. This is usually dyed blue, which is our favourite colour. It is extracted from a berry, and is brighter and richer than any I have seen in Eu-

---

*When I was in Smyrna I have frequently seen the Greeks dance after this manner.

rope. Besides this, our women of distinction wear golden ornaments; which they dispose with some profusion on their arms and legs. When our women are not employed with the men in tillage, their usual occupation is spinning and weaving cotton, which they afterwards dye, and make it into garments. They also manufacture earthen vessels, of which we have many kinds. Among the rest tobacco pipes, made after the same fashion, and used in the same manner, as those in Turkey*.

Our manner of living is entirely plain; for as yet the natives are unacquainted with those refinements in cookery which debauch the taste: bullocks, goats, and poultry, supply the greatest part of their food. These constitute likewise the principal wealth of the country, and the chief articles of its commerce. The flesh is usually stewed in a pan; to make it savoury we sometimes use also pepper, and other spices, and we have salt made of wood ashes. Our vegetables are mostly plantains, eadas, yams, beans, and Indian corn. The head of the family usually eats alone; his wives and slaves have also their separate tables. Before we taste food we always wash our hands: indeed our cleanliness on all occasions is extreme; but on this it is an indispensable ceremony. After washing, libation is made, by pouring out a small portion of the food, in a certain place, for the spirits of departed relations, which the natives suppose to preside over their conduct, and guard them from evil. They are totally unacquainted with strong or spirituous liquours; and their principal beverage is palm wine. This is gotten from a tree of that name by tapping it at the top, and fastening a large gourd to it; and sometimes one tree will yield three or four gallons in a night. When just drawn it is of a most delicious sweetness; but in a few days it acquires a tartish and more spirituous flavour: though I never saw any one intoxicated by it. The same tree also produces nuts and oil. Our principal luxury is in perfumes; one sort of these is an odoriferous wood of delicious fragrance: the other a kind of earth;

---

*The bowl is earthen, curiously figured, to which a long reed is fixed as a tube. This tube is sometimes so long as to be born by one, and frequently out of grandeur by two boys.

a small portion of which thrown into the fire diffuses a most powerful odour*. We beat this wood into powder, and mix it with palm oil; with which both men and women perfume themselves.

In our buildings we study convenience rather than ornament. Each master of a family has a large square piece of ground, surrounded with a moat or fence, or enclosed with a wall made of red earth tempered; which, when dry, is as hard as brick. Within this are his houses to accommodate his family and slaves; which, if numerous, frequently present the appearance of a village. In the middle stands the principal building, appropriated to the sole use of the master, and consisting of two apartments; in one of which he sits in the day with his family, the other is left apart for the reception of his friends. He has besides these a distinct apartment in which he sleeps, together with his male children. On each side are the apartments of his wives, who have also their separate day and night houses. The habitations of the slaves and their families are distributed throughout the rest of the enclosure. These houses never exceed one story in height: they are always built of wood, or stakes driven into the ground, crossed with wattles, and neatly plastered within, and without. The roof is thatched with reeds. Our day-houses are left open at the sides; but those in which we sleep are always covered, and plastered in the inside, with a composition mixed with cowdung, to keep off the different insects, which annoy us during the night. The walls and floors also of these are generally covered with mats. Our beds consist of a platform, raised three or four feet from the ground, on which are laid skins, and different parts of a spungy tree called plaintain. Our covering is calico or muslin, the same as our dress. The usual seats are a few logs of wood; but we have benches, which are generally perfumed, to accommodate strangers: these compose the greater part of our household furniture. Houses so constructed and furnished require but little skill to erect them. Every man is a sufficient architect for the purpose. The whole

---

*When I was in Smyrna I saw the same kind of earth, and brought some of it with me to England; it resembles musk in strength, but is more delicious in scent, and is not unlike the smell of a rose.

neighbourhood afford their unanimous assistance in building them and in return receive, and expect no other recompense than a feast.

As we live in a country where nature is prodigal of her favours, our wants are few and easily supplied; of course we have few manufactures. They consist for the most part of calicoes, earthern ware, ornaments, and instruments of war and husbandry. But these make no part of our commerce, the principal articles of which, as I have observed, are provisions. In such a state money is of little use; however we have some small pieces of coin, if I may call them such. They are made something like an anchor; but I do not remember either their value or denomination. We have also markets, at which I have been frequently with my mother. These are sometimes visited by stout mahogany-coloured men from the south west of us: we call them Oye-Eboe, which term signifies red men living at a distance. They generally bring us fire-arms, gunpowder, hats, beads, and dried fish. The last we esteemed a great rarity, as our waters were only brooks and springs. These articles they barter with us for odoriferous woods and earth, and our salt of wood ashes. They always carry slaves through our land; but the strictest account is exacted of their manner of procuring them before they are suffered to pass. Sometimes indeed we sold slaves to them, but they were only prisoners of war, or such among us as had been convicted of kidnapping, or adultery, and some other crimes, which we esteemed heinous. This practice of kidnapping induces me to think, that, notwithstanding all our strictness, their principal business among us was to trepan our people. I remember too they carried great sacks along with them, which not long after I had an opportunity of fatally seeing applied to that infamous purpose.

Our land is uncommonly rich and fruitful, and produces all kinds of vegetables in great abundance. We have plenty of Indian corn, and vast quantities of cotton and tobacco. Our pine apples grow without culture; they are about the size of the largest sugar-loaf, and finely flavoured. We have also spices of different kinds, particularly pepper; and a variety of delicious fruits which I have never seen in Europe; together with gums of various kinds, and honey in abundance. All our industry is exerted to improve those blessings of nature.

Agriculture is our chief employment; and every one, even the children and women, are engaged in it. Thus we are all habituated to labour from our earliest years. Every one contributes something to the common stock; and as we are unacquainted with idleness, we have no beggars. The benefits of such a mode of living are obvious. The West India planters prefer the slaves of Benin or Eboe to those of any other part of Guinea, for their hardiness, intelligence, integrity, and zeal. Those benefits are felt by us in the general healthiness of the people, and in their vigour and activity; I might have added too in their comeliness. Deformity is indeed unknown amongst us, I mean that of shape. Numbers of the natives of Eboe now in London might be brought in support of this assertion: for, in regard to complexion, ideas of beauty are wholly relative. I remember while in Africa to have seen three negro children, who were tawny, and another quite white, who were universally regarded by myself, and the natives in general, as far as related to their complexions, as deformed. Our women too were in my eyes at least uncommonly graceful, alert, and modest to a degree of bashfulness; nor do I remember to have ever heard of an instance of incontinence amongst them before marriage. They are also remarkably cheerful. Indeed cheerfulness and affability are two of the leading characteristics of our nation.

Our tillage is exercised in a large plain or common, some hours walk from our dwellings, and all the neighbours resort thither in a body. They use no beasts of husbandry; and their only instruments are hoes, axes, shovels, and beaks, or pointed iron to dig with. Sometimes we are visited by locusts, which come in large clouds, so as to darken the air, and destroy our harvest. This however happens rarely, but when it does, a famine is produced by it. I remember an instance or two wherein this happened. This common is often the theatre of war; and therefore when our people go out to till their land, they not only go in a body, but generally take their arms with them for fear of a surprise; and when they apprehend an invasion they guard the avenues to their dwellings, by driving sticks into the ground, which are so sharp at one end as to pierce the foot, and are generally dipt in poison. From what I can recollect of these battles, they appear to have been irruptions of one little state or district on the other, to obtain prisoners or booty. Perhaps they were incited to this by those traders who brought the European goods I mentioned amongst us. Such a mode of obtaining slaves in Africa is common; and I believe more are procured this way, and by kidnapping, than any other*. When a trader wants slaves, he applies to a chief for them, and tempts him with his wares. It is not extraordinary, if on this occasion he yields to the temptation with as little firmness, and accepts the price of his fellow creatures liberty with as little reluctance as the enlightened merchant. Accordingly he falls on his neighbours, and a desperate battle ensues. If he prevails and takes prisoners, he gratifies his avarice by selling them; but, if his party be vanquished, and he falls into the hands of the enemy, he is put to death: for, as he has been known to foment their quarrels, it is thought dangerous to let him survive, and no ransom can save him, though all other prisoners may be redeemed. We have firearms, bows and arrows, broad two-edged swords and javelins: we have shields also which cover a man from head to foot. All are taught the use of these weapons; even our women are warriors, and march boldly out to fight along with the men. Our whole district is a kind of militia: on a certain signal given, such as the firing of a gun at night, they all rise in arms and rush upon their enemy. It is perhaps something remarkable, that when our people march to the field a red flag or banner is borne before them. I was once a witness to a battle in our common. We had been all at work in it one day as usual, when our people were suddenly attacked. I climbed a tree at some distance, from which I beheld the fight. There were many women as well as men on both sides; among others my mother was there, and armed with a broad sword. After fighting for a considerable time with great fury, and after many had been killed our people obtained the victory, and took their enemy's Chief prisoner. He was carried off in great triumph, and, though he offered a large ransom for his life, he was put to death. A virgin of note among our enemies had been slain in the battle, and her arm was exposed in our market-place, where our trophies were always exhibited. The

*See Benezet's Account of Africa throughout.

spoils were divided according to the merit of the warriors. Those prisoners which were not sold or redeemed we kept as slaves: but how different was their condition from that of the slaves in the West Indies! With us they do no more work than other members of the community, even their masters; their food, clothing and lodging were nearly the same as theirs, (except that they were not permitted to eat with those who were free-born); and there was scarce any other difference between them, than a superior degree of importance which the head of a family possesses in our state, and that authority which, as such, he exercises over every part of his household. Some of these slaves have even slaves under them as their own property, and for their own use.

As to religion, the natives believe that there is one Creator of all things, and that he lives in the sun, and is girted round with a belt that he may never eat or drink; but, according to some, he smokes a pipe, which is our own favourite luxury. They believe he governs events, especially our deaths or captivity; but, as for the doctrine of eternity, I do not remember to have ever heard of it: some however believe in the transmigration of souls in a certain degree. Those spirits, which are not transmigrated, such as our dear friends or relations, they believe always attend them, and guard them from the bad spirits or their foes. For this reason they always before eating, as I have observed, put some small portion of the meat, and pour some of their drink, on the ground for them; and they often make oblations of the blood of beasts or fowls at their graves. I was very fond of my mother, and almost constantly with her. When she went to make these oblations at her mother's tomb, which was a kind of small solitary thatched house, I sometimes attended her. There she made her libations, and spent most of the night in cries and lamentations. I have been often extremely terrified on these occasions. The loneliness of the place, the darkness of the night, and the ceremony of libation, naturally awful and gloomy, were heightened by my mother's lamentations; and these, concuring with the cries of doleful birds, by which these places were frequented, gave an inexpressible terror to the scene.

We compute the year from the day on which the sun crosses the line, and on its setting that evening there is a general shout throughout the land; at least I can speak from my own knowledge throughout our vicinity. The people at the same time make a great noise with rattles, not unlike the basket rattles used by children here, though much larger, and hold up their hands to heaven for a blessing. It is then the greatest offerings are made; and those children whom our wise men foretel will be fortunate are then presented to different people. I remember many used to come to see me, and I was carried about to others for that purpose. They have many offerings, particularly at full moons; generally two at harvest before the fruits are taken out of the ground: and when any young animals are killed, sometimes they offer up part of them as a sacrifice. These offerings, when made by one of the heads of a family, serve for the whole. I remember we often had them at my father's and my uncle's, and their families have been present. Some of our offerings are eaten with bitter herbs. We had a saying among us to any one of a cross temper, 'That if they were to be eaten, they should be eaten with bitter herbs.'

We practised circumcision like the Jews, and made offerings and feasts on that occasion in the same manner as they did. Like them also, our children were named from some event, some circumstance, or fancied foreboding at the time of their birth. I was named *Olaudah*, which, in our language, signifies vicissitude or fortune also, one favoured, and having a loud voice and well spoken. I remember we never polluted the name of the object of our adoration; on the contrary, it was always mentioned with the greatest reverence; and we were totally unacquainted with swearing, and all those terms of abuse and reproach which find their way so readily and copiously into the languages of more civilized people. The only expressions of that kind I remember were 'May you rot, or may you swell, or may a beast take you.'

I have before remarked that the natives of this part of Africa are extremely cleanly. This necessary habit of decency was with us a part of religion, and therefore we had many purifications and washings; indeed almost as many, and used on the same occasions, if my recollection does not fail me, as the Jews. Those that touched the dead at any time were obliged to wash and purify themselves before they could enter a dwelling-house. Every woman too, at certain times, was forbidden to come into a dwelling-house, or touch any person, or any thing we ate. I was so fond of my mother I could not keep from her, or avoid touching her at some of those periods, in consequence of which I was obliged to be kept out with her, in a little house made for that purpose, till offering was made, and then we were purified.

Though we had no places of public worship, we had priests and magicians, or wise men. I do not remember whether they had different offices, or whether they were united in the same persons, but they were held in great reverence by the people. They calculated our time, and foretold events, as their name imported, for we called them Ah-affoe-way-cah, which signifies calculators or yearly men, our year being called Ah-affoe. They wore their beards, and when they died they were succeeded by their sons. Most of their implements and things of value were interred along with them. Pipes and tobacco were also put into the grave with the corpse, which was always perfumed and ornamented, and animals were offered in sacrifice to them. None accompanied their funerals but those of the same profession or tribe. These buried them after sunset, and always returned from the grave by a different way from that which they went.

These magicians were also our doctors or physicians. They practised bleeding by cupping; and were very successful in healing wounds and expelling poisons. They had likewise some extraordinary method of discovering jealousy, theft, and poisoning; the success of which no doubt they derived from their unbounded influence over the credulity and superstition of the people. I do not remember what those methods were, except that as to poisoning: I recollect an instance or two, which I hope it will not be deemed impertinent here to insert, as it may serve as a kind of specimen of the rest, and is still used by the negroes in the West Indies. A virgin had been poisoned, but it was not known by whom: the doctors ordered the corpse to be taken up by some persons, and carried to the grave. As soon as the bearers had raised it on their shoulders, they seemed seized with some * sudden impulse, and ran to and fro unable to stop themselves. At last, after having passed through a number of thorns and prickly bushes unhurt, the corpse fell from them close to a house, and defaced it in the fall; and, the owner being taken up, he immediately confessed the poisoning†.

The natives are extremely cautious about poison. When they buy any eatable the seller kisses it all round before the buyer, to shew him it is not poisoned; and the same is done when any meat or drink is presented, particularly to a stranger. We have serpents of different kinds, some of which are esteemed ominous when they appear in our houses, and these we never molest. I remember two of those ominous snakes, each of which was as thick as the calf of a man's leg, and in colour resembling a dolphin in the water, crept at different times into my mother's night-house, where I always lay with her, and coiled themselves into folds, and each time they crowed like a cock. I was desired by some of our wise men to touch these, that I might be interested in the good omens, which I did, for they were quite harmless, and would tamely suffer themselves to be handled; and then they were put into a large open earthen pan, and set on one side of the highway. Some of our snakes, however, were poisonous: one of them crossed the road one day when I was standing on it, and passed between my feet without offering to touch me, to the great surprise of many who saw it; and these incidents were

*See also Leut. Matthew's Voyage, p. 123.

†An instance of this kind happened at Montserrat in the West Indies in the year 1763. I then belonged to the Charming Sally, Capt. Doran.—The chief mate, Mr. Mansfield, and some of the crew being one day on shore, were present at the burying of a poisoned negro girl. Though they had often heard of the circumstance of the running in such cases, and had even seen it, they imagined it to be a trick of the corpse-bearers. The mate therefore desired two of the sailors to take up the coffin, and carry it to the grave. The sailors, who were all of the same opinion, readily obeyed; but they had scarcely raised it to their shoulders, before they began to run furiously about, quite unable to direct themselves, till, at last, without intention, they came to the hut of him who had poisoned the girl. The coffin then immediately fell from their shoulders against the hut, and damaged part of the wall. The owner of the hut was taken into custody on this, and confessed the poisoning.—I give this story as it was related by the mate and crew on their return to the ship. The credit which is due to it I leave with the reader.

accounted by the wise men, and therefore by my mother and the rest of the people, as remarkable omens in my favour.

Such is the imperfect sketch my memory has furnished me with of the manners and customs of a people among whom I first drew my breath. And here I cannot forbear suggesting what has long struck me very forcibly, namely, the strong analogy which even by this sketch, imperfect as it is, appears to prevail in the manners and customs of my countrymen and those of the Jews, before they reached the Land of Promise, and particularly the patriarchs while they were yet in that pastoral state which is described in Genesis—an analogy, which alone would induce me to think that the one people had sprung from the other. Indeed this is the opinion of Dr. Gill, who, in his commentary on Genesis, very ably deduces the pedigree of the Africans from Afer and Afra, the descendants of Abraham by Keturah his wife and concubine (for both these titles are applied to her). It is also conformable to the sentiments of Dr. John Clarke, formerly Dean of Sarum, in his Truth of the Christian Religion: both these authors concur in ascribing to us this original. The reasonings of these gentlemen are still further confirmed by the scripture chronology; and if any further corroboration were required, this resemblance in so many respects is a strong evidence in support of the opinion. Like the Israelites in their primitive state, our government was conducted by our chiefs or judges, our wise men and elders; and the head of a family with us enjoyed a similar authority over his household with that which is ascribed to Abraham and the other patriarchs. The law of retaliation obtained almost universally with us as with them: and even their religion appeared to have shed upon us a ray of its glory, though broken and spent in its passage, or eclipsed by the cloud with which time, tradition, and ignorance might have enveloped it; for we had our circumcision (a rule I believe peculiar to that people:) we had also our sacrifices and burnt-offerings, our washings and purifications, on the same occasions as they had.

As to the difference of colour between the Eboan Africans and the modern Jews, I shall not presume to account for it. It is a subject which has engaged the pens of men of both genius and learning, and is far above my strength. The most able and Reverend Mr. T. Clarkson, however, in his much admired Essay on the Slavery and Commerce of the Human Species, has ascertained the cause, in a manner that at once solves every objection on that account, and, on my mind at least, has produced the fullest conviction. I shall therefore refer to that performance for the theory*, contenting myself with extracting a fact as related by Dr. Mitchel†. "The Spaniards, who have inhabited America, under the torrid zone, for any time, are become as dark coloured as our native Indians of Virginia; of which *I myself have been a witness.*" There is also another instance ‡ of a Portuguese settlement at Mitomba, a river in Sierra Leona; where the inhabitants are bred from a mixture of the first Portuguese discoverers with the natives, and are now become in their complexion, and in the woolly quality of their hair, *perfect negroes*, retaining however a smattering of the Portuguese language.

These instances, and a great many more which might be adduced, while they shew how the complexions of the same persons vary in different climates, it is hoped may tend also to remove the prejudice that some conceive against the natives of Africa on account of their colour. Surely the minds of the Spaniards did not change with their complexions! Are there not causes enough to which the apparent inferiority of an African may be ascribed, without limiting the goodness of God, and supposing he forbore to stamp understanding on certainly his own image, because "carved in ebony." Might it not naturally be ascribed to their situation? When they come among Europeans, they are ignorant of their language, religion, manners, and customs. Are any pains taken to teach them these? Are they treated as men? Does not slavery itself depress the mind, and extinguish all its fire and every noble sentiment? But, above all, what advantages do not a refined people possess over those who are rude and uncultivated. Let the polished and haughty European recollect that his ancestors were once, like the Africans, uncivilized, and even barbarous. Did Nature make *them* inferior to their sons? and should *they too* have been made slaves? Every rational mind

*Page 178 to 216.
†Philos. Trans. N° 476, Sect. 4, cited by Mr. Clarkson, p. 205.
‡Same page.

answers, No. Let such reflections as these melt the pride of their superiority into sympathy for the wants and miseries of their sable brethren, and compel them to acknowledge, that understanding is not confined to feature or colour. If, when they look round the world, they feel exultation, let it be tempered with benevolence to others, and gratitude to God, "who hath made of one blood all nations of men for to dwell on all the face of the earth*; and whose wisdom is not our wisdom, neither are our ways his ways."

*Acts, c. xvii. v. 26.

CHAP. II.

The author's birth and parentage—His being kidnapped with his sister—Their separation—Surprise at meeting again—Are finally separated—Account of the different places and incidents the author met with till his arrival on the coast—The effect the sight of a slave ship had on him—He sails for the West Indies—Horrors of a slave ship—Arrives at Barbadoes, where the cargo is sold and dispersed.

I HOPE the reader will not think I have trespassed on his patience in introducing myself to him with some account of the manners and customs of my country. They had been implanted in me with great care, and made an impression on my mind, which time could not erase, and which all the adversity and variety of fortune I have since experienced served only to rivet and record; for, whether the love of one's country be real or imaginary, or a lesson of reason, or an instinct of nature, I still look back with pleasure on the first scenes of my life, though that pleasure has been for the most part mingled with sorrow.

I have already acquainted the reader with the time and place of my birth. My father, besides many slaves, had a numerous family, of which seven lived to grow up, including myself and a sister, who was the only daughter. As I was the youngest of the sons, I became, of course, the greatest favourite with my mother, and was always with her; and she used to take particular pains to form my mind. I was trained up from my earliest years in the art of war; my daily exercise was shooting and throwing javelins; and my mother adorned me with emblems, after the manner of our greatest warriors. In this way I grew up till I was turned the age of eleven, when an end was put to my happiness in the following manner:—Generally when the grown people in the neighbourhood were gone far in the fields to labour, the children assembled together in some of the neighbours' premises to play; and commonly some of us used to get up a tree to look out for any assailant, or kidnapper, that might come upon us; for they sometimes took those opportunities of our parents' absence to attack and carry off as many as they could seize. One day, as I was watching at the top of a tree in our yard, I saw one of those people come into the yard of our next neighbour but one, to kidnap, there being many stout young people in it. Immediately on this I gave the alarm of the rogue, and he was surrounded by the stoutest of them, who entangled him with cords, so that he could not escape till some of the grown people came and secured him. But alas! ere long it was my fate to be thus attacked, and to be carried off, when none of the grown people were nigh. One day, when all our people were gone out to their works as usual, and only I and my dear sister were left to mind the house, two men and a woman got over our walls, and in a moment seized us both, and, without giving us time to cry out, or make resistance, they stopped our mouths, and ran off with us into the nearest wood. Here they tied our hands, and continued to carry us as far as they could, till night came on, when we reached a small house, where the robbers halted for refreshment, and spent the night. We were then unbound, but were unable to take any food; and, being quite overpowered by fatigue and grief, our only relief was some sleep, which allayed our misfortune for a short time. The next morning we left the house, and continued travelling all the day. For a long time we had kept the woods, but at last we came into a road which I believed I knew. I had now some hopes of being delivered; for we had advanced but a little way before I discovered some people at a distance, on which I began to cry out for their assistance: but my cries had no other effect than to make them tie me faster and stop my mouth, and then they put me into a large sack. They also stopped my sister's mouth, and tied her hands; and in this manner we proceeded till we were out of the sight of these people. When we went to rest the following night they offered us some victuals; but we refused it; and the only comfort we had was in being in one another's arms all that night, and bathing each other with our tears. But alas! we were soon deprived of even the small comfort of weeping together. The next day proved a day of greater sorrow than I had yet experienced; for my sister and I were then separated, while we lay clasped in each other's arms. It was in vain that we besought them not to part us; she was torn from me, and immediately carried away, while I was left in a state of distraction not to be described. I cried and grieved continually; and for several days I did not eat any thing but what they forced into my mouth. At length, after many days travelling, during which I had often changed masters, I got into the hands of a chieftain, in a very pleasant country. This man had two wives and some children, and they all used me extremely well, and did all they could to comfort me; particularly the first wife, who was something like my mother. Although I was a great many days journey from my father's house, yet these people spoke exactly the same language with us. This first master of mine, as I may call him, was a smith, and my principal employment was working his bellows, which were the same kind as I had seen in my vicinity. They were in some respects not unlike the stoves here in gentlemen's kitchens; and were covered over with leather; and in the middle of that leather a stick was fixed, and a person stood up, and worked it, in the same manner as is done to pump water out of a cask with a hand pump. I believe it was gold he worked, for it was of a lovely bright yellow colour, and was worn by the women on their wrists and ancles. I was there I suppose about a month, and they at last used to trust me some little distance from the house. This liberty I used in embracing every opportunity to inquire the way to my own home: and I also sometimes, for the same purpose, went with the maidens, in the cool of the evenings, to bring pitchers of water from the springs for the use of the house. I had also remarked where the sun rose in the morning, and set in the evening, as I had travelled along; and I had observed that my father's house was towards the rising of the sun. I therefore determined to seize the first opportunity of making my escape, and to shape my course for that quarter; for I was quite oppressed and weighed down by grief after my mother and friends; and my love of liberty, ever great, was strengthened by the mortifying circumstance of not daring to eat with the free-born children, although I was mostly their companion. While I was projecting my escape, one day an unlucky event happened, which quite disconcerted my plan, and put an end to my hopes. I used to be sometimes employed in assisting an elderly woman slave to cook and take care of the poultry; and one morning, while I was feeding some chickens, I happened to toss a small pebble at one of them, which hit it on the middle and directly killed it. The old slave, having soon after missed the chicken, inquired after it; and on my relating the accident (for I told her the truth, because my mother would never suffer me to tell a lie) she flew into a violent passion, threatened that I should suffer for it; and, my master being out, she immediately went and told her mistress what I had done. This alarmed me very much, and I expected an instant flogging, which to me was uncommonly dreadful; for I had seldom been beaten at home. I therefore resolved to fly; and accordingly I ran into a thicket that was hard by, and hid myself in the bushes. Soon afterwards my mistress and the slave returned, and, not seeing me, they searched all the house, but not finding me, and I not making answer when they called to me, they thought I had run away, and the whole neighbourhood was raised in the pursuit of me. In that part of the country (as in ours) the houses and villages were skirted with woods, or shrubberies, and the bushes were so thick that a man could readily conceal himself in them, so as to elude the strictest search. The neighbours continued the whole day looking for me, and several times many of them came within a few yards of the place where I lay hid. I then gave myself up for lost entirely, and expected every moment, when I heard a rustling among the trees, to be found out, and punished by my master: but they never discovered me, though they were often so near that I even heard their conjectures as they were looking about for me; and I now learned from them, that any attempt to return home would be hopeless. Most of them supposed I had fled towards home; but the distance was so great, and the way so intricate, that they thought I could never reach it, and that I should be lost in the woods. When I heard this I was seized with a violent panic, and abandoned myself to despair. Night too began to approach, and aggravated all my fears. I had before entertained hopes of getting home, and I had determined when it should be dark to make the attempt; but I was now convinced it was fruitless, and I began to consider that, if possibly I could escape all other animals, I could not those of the human kind; and that, not knowing the way, I must perish in the woods. Thus was I like the hunted deer:

—"Ev'ry leaf and ev'ry whisp'ring breath
Convey'd a foe, and ev'ry foe a death."

I heard frequent rustlings among the leaves; and being pretty sure they were snakes I expected every instant to be stung by them. This increased my anguish, and the horror of my situation became now quite insupportable. I at length quitted the thicket, very faint and hungry, for I had not eaten or drank any thing all the day; and crept to my master's kitchen, from whence I set out at first, and which was an open shed, and laid myself down in the ashes with an anxious wish for death to relieve me from all my pains. I was scarcely awake in the morning when the old woman slave, who was the first up, came to light the fire, and saw me in the fire place. She was very much surprised to see me, and could scarcely believe her own eyes. She now promised to intercede for me, and went for her master, who soon after came, and, having slightly reprimanded me, ordered me to be taken care of, and not to be ill-treated.

Soon after this my master's only daughter, and child by his first wife, sickened and died, which affected him so much that for some time he was almost frantic, and really would have killed himself, had he not been watched and prevented. However, in a small time afterwards he recovered, and I was again sold. I was now carried to the left of the sun's rising, through many different countries, and a number of large woods. The people I was sold to used to carry me very often, when I was tired, either on their shoulders or on their backs. I saw many convenient well-built sheds along the roads, at proper distances, to accommodate the merchants and travellers, who lay in those buildings along with their wives, who often accompany them; and they always go well armed.

From the time I left my own nation I always found somebody that understood me till I came to the sea coast. The languages of different nations did not totally differ, nor were they so copious as those of the Europeans, particularly the English. They were therefore easily learned; and, while I was journeying thus through Africa, I acquired two or three different tongues. In this manner I had been travelling for a considerable time, when one evening, to my great surprise, whom should I see brought to the house where I was but my dear sister! As soon as she saw me she gave a loud shriek, and ran into my arms—I was quite overpowered: neither of us could speak; but, for a considerable time, clung to each other in mutual embraces, unable to do any thing but weep. Our meeting affected all who saw us; and indeed I must acknowledge, in honour of those sable destroyers of human rights, that I never met with any ill treatment, or saw any offered to their slaves, except tying them, when necessary, to keep them from running away. When these people knew we were brother and sister they indulged us together; and the man, to whom I supposed we belonged, lay with us, he in the middle, while she and I held one another by the hands across his breast all night; and thus for a while we forgot our misfortunes in the joy of being together: but even this small comfort was soon to have an end; for scarcely had the fatal morning appeared, when she was again torn from me for ever! I was now more miserable, if possible, than before. The small relief which her presence gave me from pain was gone, and the wretchedness of my situation was redoubled by my anxiety after her fate, and my apprehensions lest her sufferings should be greater than mine, when I could not be with her to alleviate them. Yes, thou dear partner of all my childish sports! thou sharer of my joys and sorrows! happy should I have ever esteemed myself to encounter every misery for you, and to procure your freedom by the sacrifice of my own. Though you were early forced from my arms, your image has been always rivetted in my heart, from which neither *time nor fortune* have been able to remove it; so that, while the thoughts of your sufferings have damped my prosperity, they have mingled with adversity and increased its bitterness. To that Heaven which protects the weak from the strong, I commit the care of your innocence and virtues, if they have not already received their full reward, and if your youth and delicacy have not long since fallen victims to the violence of the African trader, the pestilential stench of a Guinea ship, the seasoning in the European colonies, or the lash and lust of a brutal and unrelenting overseer.

I did not long remain after my sister. I was again sold, and carried through a number of places, till, after travelling a considerable time, I came to a town called Tinmah, in the most beautiful country I have yet seen in Africa. It was extremely rich, and there were many rivulets which flowed through it, and supplied a large pond in the centre of the town, where the people washed. Here I first saw and tasted cocoa-nuts, which I thought superior to any nuts I had ever tasted before; and the trees, which were loaded, were also interspersed amongst the houses, which had commodious shades adjoining, and were in the same manner as ours, the insides being neatly plastered and whitewashed. Here I also saw and tasted for the first time sugar-cane. Their money consisted of little white shells, the size of the finger nail. I was sold here for one hundred and seventy-two of them by a merchant who lived and brought me there. I had been about two or three days at his house, when a wealthy widow, a neighbour of his, came there one evening, and brought with her an only son, a young gentleman about my own age and size. Here they saw me; and, having taken a fancy to me, I was bought of the merchant, and went home with them. Her house and premises were situated close to one of those rivulets I have mentioned, and were the finest I ever saw in Africa: they were very extensive, and she had a number of slaves to attend her. The next day I was washed and perfumed, and when meal-time came I was led into the presence of my mistress, and ate and drank before her with her son. This filled me with astonishment; and I could scarce help expressing my surprise that the young gentleman should suffer me, who was bound, to eat with him who was free; and not only so, but that he would not at any time either eat or drink till I had taken first, because I was the eldest, which was agreeable to our custom. Indeed every thing here, and all their treatment of me, made me forget that I was a slave. The language of these people resembled ours so nearly, that we understood each other perfectly. They had also the very same customs as we. There were likewise slaves daily to attend us, while my young master and I with other boys sported with our darts and bows and arrows, as I had been used to do at home. In this resemblance to my former happy state I passed about two months; and I now began to think I was to be adopted into the family, and was beginning to be reconciled to my situation, and to forget by degrees my misfortunes, when all at once the delusion vanished; for, without the least previous knowledge, one morning early, while my dear master and companion was still asleep, I was wakened out of my reverie to fresh sorrow, and hurried away even amongst the uncircumcised.

Thus, at the very moment I dreamed of the greatest happiness, I found myself most miserable; and it seemed as if fortune wished to give me this taste of joy, only to render the reverse more poignant. The change I now experienced was as painful as it was sudden and unexpected. It was a change indeed from a state of bliss to a scene which is inexpressible by me, as it discovered to me an element I had never before beheld, and till then had no idea of, and wherein such instances of hardship and cruelty continually occurred as I can never reflect on but with horror.

All the nations and people I had hitherto passed through resembled our own in their manners, customs, and language: but I came at length to a country, the inhabitants of which differed from us in all those particulars. I was very much struck with this difference, especially when I came among a people who did not circumcise, and ate without washing their hands. They cooked also in iron pots, and had European cutlasses and cross bows, which were unknown to us, and fought with their fists amongst themselves. Their women were not so modest as ours, for they ate, and drank, and slept, with their men. But, above all, I was amazed to see no sacrifices or offerings among them. In some of those places the people ornamented themselves with scars, and likewise filed their teeth very sharp. They wanted sometimes to ornament me in the same manner, but I would not suffer them; hoping that I might some time be among a people who did not thus disfigure themselves, as I thought they did. At last I came to the banks of a large river, which was covered with canoes, in which the people appeared to live with their household utensils and provisions of all kinds. I was beyond measure astonished at this, as I had never before seen any water larger than a pond or a rivulet: and my surprise was mingled with no small fear when I was put into one of these canoes, and we began to paddle and move along the river. We continued going on thus till night; and when we came to land, and made fires on the banks, each family by themselves, some dragged their canoes on shore, others stayed and cooked in theirs, and laid in them all night. Those on the land had mats, of which they made tents, some in the shape of little houses: in these we slept; and after the morning meal we embarked again and proceeded as before. I was often very much astonished to see some of the women, as well as the men, jump into the water, dive to the bottom, come up again, and swim about. Thus I continued to travel, sometimes by land, sometimes by water, through different countries and various nations, till, at the end of six or seven months after I had been kidnapped, I arrived at the sea coast. It would be tedious and uninteresting to relate all the incidents which befell me during this journey, and which I have not yet forgotten; of the various hands I passed through, and the manners and customs of all the different people among whom I lived: I shall therefore only observe, that in all the places where I was the soil was exceedingly rich; the pomkins, eadas, plantains, yams, &c. &c. were in great abundance, and of incredible size. There were also vast quantities of different gums, though not used for any purpose; and every where a great deal of tobacco. The cotton even grew quite wild; and there was plenty of red wood. I saw no mechanics whatever in all the way, except such as I have mentioned. The chief employment in all these countries was agriculture, and both the males and females, as with us, were brought up to it, and trained in the arts of war.

The first object which saluted my eyes when I arrived on the coast was the sea, and a slave ship, which was then riding at anchor, and waiting for its cargo. These filled me with astonishment, which was soon converted into terror when I was carried on board. I was immediately handled and tossed up to see if I were sound by some of the crew; and I was now persuaded that I had gotten into a world of bad spirits, and that they were going to kill me. Their complexions too differing so much from ours, their long hair, and the language they spoke, (which was very different from any I had ever heard) united to confirm me in this belief. Indeed such were the horrors of my views and fears at the moment, that, if ten thousand worlds had been my own, I would have freely parted with them all to have exchanged my condition with that of the meanest slave in my own country. When I looked round the ship too and saw a large furnace or copper boiling, and a multitude of black people of every description chained together, every one of their countenances expressing dejection and sorrow, I no longer doubted of my fate; and, quite overpowered with horror and anguish, I fell motionless on the deck and fainted. When I recovered a little I found some black people about me, who I believed were some of those who brought me on board, and had been receiving their pay; they talked to me in order to cheer me, but all in vain. I asked them if we were not to be eaten by those white men with horrible looks, red faces, and loose hair. They told me I was not; and one of the crew brought me a small portion of spirituous liquor in a wine glass; but, being afraid of him, I would not take it out of his hand. One of the blacks therefore took it from him and gave it to me, and I took a little down my palate, which, instead of reviving me, as they thought it would, threw me into the greatest consternation at the strange feeling it produced, having never tasted any such liquor before. Soon after this the blacks who brought me on board went off, and left me abandoned to despair. I now saw myself deprived of all chance of returning to my native country, or even the least glimpse of hope of gaining the shore, which I now considered as friendly; and I even wished for my former slavery in preference to my present situation, which was filled with horrors of every kind, still heightened by my ignorance of what I was to undergo. I was not long suffered to indulge my grief; I was soon put down under the decks, and there I received such a salutation in my nostrils as I had never experienced in my life: so that, with the loathsomeness of the stench, and crying together, I became so sick and low that I was not able to eat, nor had I the least desire to taste any thing. I now wished for the last friend, death, to relieve me; but soon, to my grief, two of the white men offered me eatables; and, on my refusing to eat, one of them held me fast by the hands, and laid me across I think the windlass, and tied my feet, while the other flogged me severely. I had never experienced any thing of this kind before; and although, not being used to the water, I naturally feared that element the first time I saw it, yet nevertheless, could I have got over the nettings, I would have jumped over the side, but I could not; and, besides, the crew used to watch us very closely who were not chained down to the decks, lest we should leap into the water: and I have seen some of these poor African prisoners most severely cut for attempting to do so, and hourly whipped for not eating. This indeed was often the case with myself. In a little time after, amongst the poor chained men, I found some of my own nation, which in a small degree gave ease to my mind. I inquired of these what was to be done with us; they gave me to understand we were to be carried to these white people's country to work for them. I then was a little revived, and thought, if it were no worse than working, my situation was not so desperate: but still I feared I should be put to death, the white people looked and acted, as I thought, in so savage a manner; for I had never seen among any people such instances of brutal cruelty; and this not only shewn towards us blacks, but also to some of the whites themselves. One white man in particular I saw, when we were permitted to be on deck, flogged so unmercifully with a large rope near the foremast, that he died in consequence of it; and they tossed him over the side as they would have done a brute. This made me fear these people the more; and I expected nothing less than to be treated in the same manner. I could not help expressing my fears and apprehensions to some of my countrymen: I asked them if these people had no country, but lived in this hollow place (the ship): they told me they did not, but came from a distant one. 'Then,' said I, 'how comes it in all our country we never heard of them?' They told me because they lived so very far off. I then asked where were their women? had they any like themselves? I was told they had: 'and why,' said I, 'do we not see them?' they answered, because they were left behind. I asked how the vessel could go? they told me they could not tell; but that there were cloths put upon the masts by the help of the ropes I saw, and then the vessel went on; and the white men had some spell or magic they put in the water when they liked in order to stop the vessel. I was exceedingly amazed at this account, and really thought they were spirits. I therefore wished much to be from amongst them, for I expected they would sacrifice me: but my wishes were vain; for we were so quartered that it was impossible for any of us to make our escape. While we stayed on the coast I was mostly on deck; and one day, to my great astonishment, I saw one of these vessels coming in with the sails up. As soon as the whites saw it, they gave a great shout, at which we were amazed; and the more so as the vessel appeared larger by approaching nearer. At last she came to an anchor in my sight, and when the anchor was let go I and my countrymen who saw it were lost in astonishment to observe the vessel stop; and were not convinced it was done by magic. Soon after this the other ship got her boats out, and they came on board of us, and the people of both ships seemed very glad to see each other. Several of the strangers also shook hands with us black people, and made motions with their hands, signifying I suppose we were to go to their country; but we did not understand them. At last, when the ship we were in had got in all her cargo, they made ready with many fearful noises, and we were all put under deck, so that we could not see how they managed the vessel. But this disappointment was the least of my sorrow. The stench of the hold while we were on the coast was so intolerably loathsome, that it was dangerous to remain there for any time, and some of us had been permitted to stay on the deck for the fresh air; but now that the whole ship's cargo were confined together, it became absolutely pestilential. The closeness of the place, and the heat of the climate, added to the number in the ship, which was so crowded that each had scarcely room to turn himself, almost suffocated us. This produced copious perspirations, so that the air soon became unfit for respiration, from a variety of loathsome smells, and brought on a sickness among the slaves, of which many died, thus falling victims to the improvident avarice, as I may call it, of their purchasers. This wretched situation was again aggravated by the galling of the chains, now become insupportable; and the filth of the necessary tubs, into which the children often fell, and were almost suffocated. The shrieks of the women, and the groans of the dying, rendered the whole a scene of horror almost inconceivable. Happily perhaps for myself I was soon reduced so low here that it was thought necessary to keep me almost always on deck; and from my extreme youth I was not put in fetters. In this situation I expected every hour to share the fate of my companions, some of whom were almost daily brought upon deck at the point of death, which I began to hope would soon put an end to my miseries. Often did I think many of the inhabitants of the deep much more happy than myself. I envied them the freedom they enjoyed, and as often wished I could change my condition for theirs. Every circumstance I met with served only to render my state more painful, and heighten my apprehensions, and my opinion of the cruelty of the whites. One day they had taken a number of fishes; and when they had killed and satisfied themselves with as many as they thought fit, to our astonishment who were on the deck, rather than give any of them to us to eat as we expected, they tossed the remaining fish into the sea again, although we begged and prayed for some as well as we could, but in vain; and some of my countrymen, being pressed by hunger, took an opportunity, when they thought no one saw them, of trying to get a little privately; but they were discovered, and the attempt procured them some very severe floggings. One day, when we had a smooth sea and moderate wind, two of my wearied countrymen who were chained together (I was near them at the time), preferring death to such a life of misery, somehow made through the nettings and jumped into the sea: immediately another quite dejected fellow, who, on account of his illness, was suffered to be out of irons, also followed their example; and I believe many more would very soon have done the same if they had not been prevented by the ship's crew, who were instantly alarmed. Those of us that were the most active were in a moment put down under the deck, and there was such a noise and confusion amongst the people of the ship as I never heard before, to stop her, and get the boat out to go after the slaves. However two of the wretches were drowned, but they got the other, and afterwards flogged him unmercifully for thus attempting to prefer death to slavery. In this manner we continued to undergo more hardships than I can now relate, hardships which are inseparable from this accursed trade. Many a time we were near suffocation from the want of fresh air, which we were often without for whole days together. This, and the stench of the necessary tubs, carried off many. During our passage I first saw flying fishes, which surprised me very much: they used frequently to fly across the ship, and many of them fell on the deck. I also now first saw the use of the quadrant; I had often with astonishment seen the mariners make observations with it, and I could not think what it meant. They at last took notice of my surprise; and one of them, willing to increase it, as well as to gratify my curiosity, made me one day look through it. The clouds appeared to me to be land, which disappeared as they passed along. This heightened my wonder; and I was now more persuaded than ever that I was in another world, and that every thing about me was magic. At last we came in sight of the island of Barbadoes, at which the whites on board gave a great shout, and made many signs of joy to us. We did not know what to think of this; but as the vessel drew nearer we plainly saw the harbour, and other ships of different kinds and sizes; and we soon anchored amongst them off Bridge Town. Many merchants and planters now came on board, though it was in the evening. They put us in separate parcels, and examined us attentively. They also made us jump, and pointed to the land, signifying we were to go there. We thought by this we should be eaten by these ugly men, as they appeared to us; and, when soon after we were all put down under the deck again, there was much dread and trembling among us, and nothing but bitter cries to be heard all the night from these apprehensions, insomuch that at last the white people got some old slaves from the land to pacify us. They told us we were not to be eaten, but to work, and were soon to go on land, where we should see many of our country people. This report eased us much; and sure enough, soon after we were landed, there came to us Africans of all languages. We were conducted immediately to the merchant's yard, where we were all pent up together like so many sheep in a fold, without regard to sex or age. As every object was new to me every thing I saw filled me with surprise. What struck me first was that the houses were built with stories, and in every other respect different from those in Africa: but I was still more astonished on seeing people on horseback. I did not know what this could mean; and indeed I thought these people were full of nothing but magical arts. While I was in this astonishment one of my fellow prisoners spoke to a countryman of his about the horses, who said they were the same kind they had in their country. I understood them, though they were from a distant part of Africa, and I thought it odd I had not seen any horses there; but afterwards, when I came to converse with different Africans, I found they had many horses amongst them, and much larger than those I then saw. We were not many days in the merchant's custody before we were sold after their usual manner, which is this:—On a signal given, (as the beat of a drum) the buyers rush at once into the yard where the slaves are confined, and make choice of that parcel they like best. The noise and clamour with which this is attended, and the eagerness visible in the countenances of the buyers, serve not a little to increase the apprehensions of the terrified Africans, who may well be supposed to consider them as the ministers of that destruction to which they think themselves devoted. In this manner, without scruple, are relations and friends separated, most of them never to see each other again. I remember in the vessel in which I was brought over, in the men's apartment, there were several brothers, who, in the sale, were sold in different lots; and it was very moving on this occasion to see and hear their cries at parting. O, ye nominal Christians! might not an African ask you, learned you this from your God, who says unto you, Do unto all men as you would men should do unto you? Is it not enough that we are torn from our country and friends to toil for your luxury and lust of gain? Must every tender feeling be likewise sacrificed to your avarice? Are the dearest friends and relations, now rendered more dear by their separation from their kindred, still to be parted from each other, and thus prevented from cheering the gloom of slavery with the small comfort of being together and mingling their sufferings and sorrows? Why are parents to lose their children, brothers their sisters, or husbands their wives? Surely this is a new refinement in cruelty, which, while it has no advantage to atone for it, thus aggravates distress, and adds fresh horrors even to the wretchedness of slavery.

CHAP. III.

*The author is carried to Virginia—His distress—Surprise at see-
ing a picture and a watch—Is bought by Captain Pascal,
and sets out for England—His terror during the voyage—Arrives in England—His wonder at a fall of snow—Is sent to
Guernsey, and in some time goes on board a ship of war with
his master—Some account of the expedition against Louis-
bourg under the command of Admiral Boscawen, in 1758.*

I NOW totally lost the small remains of comfort I had enjoyed
in conversing with my countrymen; the women too, who
used to wash and take care of me, were all gone different
ways, and I never saw one of them afterwards.

I stayed in this island for a few days; I believe it could not
be above a fortnight; when I and some few more slaves, that
were not saleable amongst the rest, from very much fretting,
were shipped off in a sloop for North America. On the passage we were better treated than when we were coming
from Africa, and we had plenty of rice and fat pork. We were
landed up a river a good way from the sea, about Virginia
county, where we saw few or none of our native Africans, and
not one soul who could talk to me. I was a few weeks weed-
ing grass, and gathering stones in a plantation; and at last all
my companions were distributed different ways, and only myself was left. I was now exceedingly miserable, and thought
myself worse off than any of the rest of my companions; for
they could talk to each other, but I had no person to speak to
that I could understand. In this state I was constantly griev-
ing and pining, and wishing for death rather than any thing
else. While I was in this plantation the gentleman, to whom I
suppose the estate belonged, being unwell, I was one day sent
for to his dwelling house to fan him; when I came into the
room where he was I was very much affrighted at some things
I saw, and the more so as I had seen a black woman slave as I
came through the house, who was cooking the dinner, and
the poor creature was cruelly loaded with various kinds of
iron machines; she had one particularly on her head, which
locked her mouth so fast that she could scarcely speak; and

could not eat nor drink. I was much astonished and shocked at this contrivance, which I afterwards learned was called the iron muzzle. Soon after I had a fan put into my hand, to fan the gentleman while he slept; and so I did indeed with great fear. While he was fast asleep I indulged myself a great deal in looking about the room, which to me appeared very fine and curious. The first object that engaged my attention was a watch which hung on the chimney, and was going. I was quite surprised at the noise it made, and was afraid it would tell the gentleman any thing I might do amiss: and when I immediately after observed a picture hanging in the room, which appeared constantly to look at me, I was still more af- frighted, having never seen such things as these before. At one time I thought it was something relative to magic; and not seeing it move I thought it might be some way the whites had to keep their great men when they died, and offer them libation as we used to do to our friendly spirits. In this state of anxiety I remained till my master awoke, when I was dis- missed out of the room, to my no small satisfaction and relief; for I thought that these people were all made up of wonders. In this place I was called Jacob; but on board the African snow I was called Michael. I had been some time in this mis- erable, forlorn, and much dejected state, without having any one to talk to, which made my life a burden, when the kind and unknown hand of the Creator (who in very deed leads the blind in a way they know not) now began to appear, to my comfort; for one day the captain of a merchant ship, called the Industrious Bee, came on some business to my master's house. This gentleman, whose name was Michael Henry Pas- cal, was a lieutenant in the royal navy, but now commanded this trading ship, which was somewhere in the confines of the county many miles off. While he was at my master's house it happened that he saw me, and liked me so well that he made a purchase of me. I think I have often heard him say he gave thirty or forty pounds sterling for me; but I do not now re- member which. However, he meant me for a present to some of his friends in England: and I was sent accordingly from the house of my then master, one Mr. Campbell, to the place where the ship lay; I was conducted on horseback by an el- derly black man, (a mode of travelling which appeared very odd to me). When I arrived I was carried on board a fine large ship, loaded with tobacco, &c. and just ready to sail for England. I now thought my condition much mended; I had sails to lie on, and plenty of good victuals to eat; and every body on board used me very kindly, quite contrary to what I had seen of any white people before; I therefore began to think that they were not all of the same disposition. A few days after I was on board we sailed for England. I was still at a loss to conjecture my destiny. By this time, however, I could smatter a little imperfect English; and I wanted to know as well as I could where we were going. Some of the people of the ship used to tell me they were going to carry me back to my own country, and this made me very happy. I was quite rejoiced at the sound of going back; and thought if I should get home what wonders I should have to tell. But I was reserved for another fate, and was soon undeceived when we came within sight of the English coast. While I was on board this ship, my captain and master named me *Gustavus Vasa*. I at that time began to understand him a little, and refused to be called so, and told him as well as I could that I would be called Jacob; but he said I should not, and still called me Gustavus; and when I refused to answer to my new name, which at first I did, it gained me many a cuff; so at length I submitted, and was obliged to bear the present name, by which I have been known ever since. The ship had a very long passage; and on that account we had very short allowance of provisions. Towards the last we had only one pound and a half of bread per week, and about the same quantity of meat, and one quart of water a-day. We spoke with only one vessel the whole time we were at sea, and but once we caught a few fishes. In our extremities the captain and people told me in jest they would kill and eat me; but I thought them in earnest, and was depressed beyond measure, expecting every moment to be my last. While I was in this situation one evening they caught, with a good deal of trouble, a large shark, and got it on board. This gladdened my poor heart exceedingly, as I thought it would serve the people to eat instead of their eating me; but very soon, to my astonishment, they cut off a small part of the tail, and tossed the rest over the side. This renewed my consternation; and I did not know what to think of these white people, though I very much feared they would kill and eat me. There was on board the ship a young lad who had never been at sea before, about four or five years older than myself: his name was Richard Baker. He was a native of America, had received an excellent education, and was of a most amiable temper. Soon after I went on board he shewed me a great deal of partiality and attention, and in return I grew extremely fond of him. We at length became inseparable; and, for the space of two years, he was of very great use to me, and was my constant companion and instructor. Although this dear youth had many slaves of his own, yet he and I have gone through many sufferings together on shipboard; and we have many nights lain in each other's bosoms when we were in great distress. Thus such a friendship was cemented between us as we cherished till his death, which, to my very great sorrow, happened in the year 1759, when he was up the Archipelago, on board his majesty's ship the Preston: an event which I have never ceased to regret, as I lost at once a kind interpreter, an agreeable companion, and a faithful friend; who, at the age of fifteen, discovered a mind superior to prejudice; and who was not ashamed to notice, to associate with, and to be the friend and instructor of one who was ignorant, a stranger, of a different complexion, and a slave! My master had lodged in his mother's house in America: he respected him very much, and made him always eat with him in the cabin. He used often to tell him jocularly that he would kill me to eat. Sometimes he would say to me—the black people were not good to eat, and would ask me if we did not eat people in my country. I said, No: then he said he would kill Dick (as he always called him) first, and afterwards me. Though this hearing relieved my mind a little as to myself, I was alarmed for Dick and whenever he was called I used to be very much afraid he was to be killed; and I would peep and watch to see if they were going to kill him: nor was I free from this consternation till we made the land. One night we lost a man overboard; and the cries and noise were so great and confused, in stopping the ship, that I, who did not know what was the matter, began, as usual, to be very much afraid, and to think they were going to make an offering with me, and perform some magic; which

I still believed they dealt in. As the waves were very high I thought the Ruler of the seas was angry, and I expected to be offered up to appease him. This filled my mind with agony, and I could not any more that night close my eyes again to rest. However, when daylight appeared I was a little eased in my mind; but still every time I was called I used to think it was to be killed. Some time after this we saw some very large fish, which I afterwards found were called grampusses. They looked to me extremely terrible, and made their appearance just at dusk; and were so near as to blow the water on the ship's deck. I believed them to be the rulers of the sea; and, as the white people did not make any offerings at any time, I thought they were angry with them: and, at last, what confirmed my belief was, the wind just then died away, and a calm ensued, and in consequence of it the ship stopped going. I supposed that the fish had performed this, and I hid myself in the fore part of the ship, through fear of being offered up to appease them, every minute peeping and quaking: but my good friend Dick came shortly towards me, and I took an opportunity to ask him, as well as I could, what these fish were. Not being able to talk much English, I could but just make him understand my question; and not at all, when I asked him if any offerings were to be made to them: however, he told me these fish would swallow any body; which sufficiently alarmed me. Here he was called away by the captain, who was leaning over the quarter-deck railing and looking at the fish; and most of the people were busied in getting a barrel of pitch to light, for them to play with. The captain now called me to him, having learned some of my apprehensions from Dick; and having diverted himself and others for some time with my fears, which appeared ludicrous enough in my crying and trembling, he dismissed me. The barrel of pitch was now lighted and put over the side into the water: by this time it was just dark, and the fish went after it; and, to my great joy, I saw them no more.

However, all my alarms began to subside when we got sight of land; and at last the ship arrived at Falmouth, after a passage of thirteen weeks. Every heart on board seemed gladdened on our reaching the shore, and none more than mine. The captain immediately went on shore, and sent on board some fresh provisions, which we wanted very much: we made good use of them, and our famine was soon turned into feasting, almost without ending. It was about the beginning of the spring 1757 when I arrived in England, and I was near twelve years of age at that time. I was very much struck with the buildings and the pavement of the streets in Falmouth; and, indeed, any object I saw filled me with new surprise. One morning, when I got upon deck, I saw it covered all over with the snow that fell over-night: as I had never seen any thing of the kind before, I thought it was salt; so I immediately ran down to the mate and desired him, as well as I could, to come and see how somebody in the night had thrown salt all over the deck. He, knowing what it was, desired me to bring some of it down to him: accordingly I took up a handful of it, which I found very cold indeed; and when I brought it to him he desired me to taste it. I did so, and I was surprised beyond measure. I then asked him what it was; he told me it was snow: but I could not in anywise understand him. He asked me if we had no such thing in my country; and I told him, No. I then asked him the use of it, and who made it; he told me a great man in the heavens, called God: but here again I was to all intents and purposes at a loss to understand him; and the more so, when a little after I saw the air filled with it, in a heavy shower, which fell down on the same day. After this I went to church; and having never been at such a place before, I was again amazed at seeing and hearing the service. I asked all I could about it; and they gave me to understand it was worshipping God, who made us and all things. I was still at a great loss, and soon got into an endless field of inquiries, as well as I was able to speak and ask about things. However, my little friend Dick used to be my best interpreter; for I could make free with him, and he always instructed me with pleasure: and from what I could understand by him of this God, and in seeing these white people did not sell one another, as we did, I was much pleased; and in this I thought they were much happier than we Africans. I was astonished at the wisdom of the white people in all things I saw; but was amazed at their not sacrificing, or making any offerings, and eating with unwashed hands, and touching the dead. I likewise could not help remarking the particular slenderness of their women, which I did not at first like; and I thought they were not so modest and shamefaced as the African women.

I had often seen my master and Dick employed in reading; and I had a great curiosity to talk to the books, as I thought they did; and so to learn how all things had a beginning: for that purpose I have often taken up a book, and have talked to it, and then put my ears to it, when alone, in hopes it would answer me; and I have been very much concerned when I found it remained silent.

My master lodged at the house of a gentleman in Falmouth, who had a fine little daughter about six or seven years of age, and she grew prodigiously fond of me; insomuch that we used to eat together, and had servants to wait on us. I was so much caressed by this family that it often reminded me of the treatment I had received from my little noble African master. After I had been here a few days, I was sent on board of the ship; but the child cried so much after me that nothing could pacify her till I was sent for again. It is ludicrous enough, that I began to fear I should be betrothed to this young lady; and when my master asked me if I would stay there with her behind him, as he was going away with the ship, which had taken in the tobacco again, I cried immediately, and said I would not leave her. At last, by stealth, one night I was sent on board the ship again; and in a little time we sailed for Guernsey, where she was in part owned by a merchant, one Nicholas Doberry. As I was now amongst a people who had not their faces scarred, like some of the African nations where I had been, I was very glad I did not let them ornament me in that manner when I was with them. When we arrived at Guernsey, my master placed me to board and lodge with one of his mates, who had a wife and family there; and some months afterwards he went to England, and left me in care of this mate, together with my friend Dick: This mate had a little daughter, aged about five or six years, with whom I used to be much delighted. I had often observed that when her mother washed her face it looked very rosy; but when she washed mine it did not look so: I therefore tried oftentimes myself if I could not by washing make my face of the same colour as my little play-mate (Mary), but it was all in vain; and I now began to be mortified at the difference in our complexions. This woman behaved to me with great kindness and attention; and taught me every thing in the same manner as she did her own child, and indeed in every respect treated me as such. I remained here till the summer of the year 1757; when my master, being appointed first lieutenant of his majesty's ship the Roebuck, sent for Dick and me, and his old mate: on this we all left Guernsey, and set out for England in a sloop bound for London. As we were coming up towards the Nore, where the Roebuck lay, a man of war's boat came alongside to press our people; on which each man ran to hide himself. I was very much frightened at this, though I did not know what it meant, or what to think or do. However I went and hid myself also under a hencoop. Immediately afterwards the press-gang came on board with their swords drawn, and searched all about, pulled the people out by force, and put them into the boat. At last I was found out also: the man that found me held me up by the heels while they all made their sport of me, I roaring and crying out all the time most lustily: but at last the mate, who was my conductor, seeing this, came to my assistance, and did all he could to pacify me; but all to very little purpose, till I had seen the boat go off. Soon afterwards we came to the Nore, where the Roebuck lay; and, to our great joy, my master came on board to us, and brought us to the ship. When I went on board this large ship, I was amazed indeed to see the quantity of men and the guns. However my surprise began to diminish as my knowledge increased; and I ceased to feel those apprehensions and alarms which had taken such strong possession of me when I first came among the Europeans, and for some time after. I began now to pass to an opposite extreme; I was so far from being afraid of any thing new which I saw, that, after I had been some time in this ship, I even began to long for a battle. My griefs too, which in young minds are not perpetual, were now wearing away; and I soon enjoyed myself pretty well, and felt tolerably easy in my present situation. There was a number of boys on board, which still made it more agreeable; for we were always together, and a great part of our time was spent in play. I remained in this ship a considerable time, during which we made several cruises, and visited a variety of places: among others we were twice in Holland, and brought over several persons of distinction from it, whose names I do not now remember. On the passage, one day, for the diversion of those gentlemen, all the boys were called on the quarter-deck, and were paired proportionably, and then made to fight; after which the gentleman gave the combatants from five to nine shillings each. This was the first time I ever fought with a white boy; and I never knew what it was to have a bloody nose before. This made me fight most desperately; I suppose considerably more than an hour: and at last, both of us being weary, we were parted. I had a great deal of this kind of sport afterwards, in which the captain and the ship's company used very much to encourage me. Sometime afterwards the ship went to Leith in Scotland, and from thence to the Orkneys, where I was surprised in seeing scarcely any night: and from thence we sailed with a great fleet, full of soldiers, for England. All this time we had never come to an engagement, though we were frequently cruising off the coast of France: during which we chased many vessels, and took in all seventeen prizes. I had been learning many of the manœuvres of the ship during our cruise; and I was several times made to fire the guns. One evening, off Havre de Grace, just as it was growing dark, we were standing off shore, and met with a fine large French-built frigate. We got all things immediately ready for fighting; and I now expected I should be gratified in seeing an engagement, which I had so long wished for in vain. But the very moment the word of command was given to fire we heard those on board the other ship cry 'Haul down the jib;' and in that instant she hoisted English colours. There was instantly with us an amazing cry of—Avast! or stop firing; and I think one or two guns had been let off, but happily they did no mischief. We had hailed them several times; but they not hearing, we received no answer, which was the cause of our firing. The boat was then sent on board of her, and she proved to be the Ambuscade man of war, to my no small disappointment. We returned to Portsmouth, without having been in any action, just at the trial of Admiral Byng (whom I saw several times during it): and my master having left the ship, and gone to London for promotion, Dick and I were put on board the Savage sloop of war, and we went in her to assist in bringing off the St. George man of war, that had ran ashore somewhere on the coast. After staying a few weeks on board the Savage, Dick and I were sent on shore at Deal, where we remained some short time, till my master sent for us to London, the place I had long desired exceedingly to see. We therefore both with great pleasure got into a waggon, and came to London, where we were received by a Mr. Guerin, a relation of my master. This gentleman had two sisters, very amiable ladies, who took much notice and great care of me. Though I had desired so much to see London, when I arrived in it I was unfortunately unable to gratify my curiosity; for I had at this time the chilblains to such a degree that I could not stand for several months, and I was obliged to be sent to St. George's Hospital. There I grew so ill, that the doctors wanted to cut my left leg off at different times, apprehending a mortification; but I always said I would rather die than suffer it; and happily (I thank God) I recovered without the operation. After being there several weeks, and just as I had recovered, the small-pox broke out on me, so that I was again confined; and I thought myself now particularly unfortunate. However I soon recovered again; and by this time my master having been promoted to be first lieutenant of the Preston man of war of fifty guns, then new at Deptford, Dick and I were sent on board her, and soon after we went to Holland to bring over the late Duke of —— to England.—While I was in this ship an incident happened, which, though trifling, I beg leave to relate, as I could not help taking particular notice of it, and considering it then as a judgment of God. One morning a young man was looking up to the fore-top, and in a wicked tone, common on shipboard, d——d his eyes about something. Just at the moment some small particles of dirt fell into his left eye, and by the evening it was very much inflamed. The next day it grew worse; and within six or seven days he lost it. From this ship my master was appointed a lieutenant on board the Royal George. When he was going he wished me to stay on board the Preston, to learn the French horn; but the ship being ordered for Turkey I could not think of leaving my master, to whom I was very warmly attached; and I told him if he left me behind it would break my heart. This prevailed on him to take me with him; but he left Dick on board the Preston, whom I embraced at parting for the last time. The Royal George was the largest ship I had ever seen; so that when I came on board of her I was surprised at the number of people, men, women, and children, of every denomination; and the largeness of the guns, many of them also of brass, which I had never seen before. Here were also shops or stalls of every kind of goods, and people crying their different commodities about the ship as in a town. To me it appeared a little world, into which I was again cast without a friend, for I had no longer my dear companion Dick. We did not stay long here. My master was not many weeks on board before he got an appointment to be sixth lieutenant of the Namur, which was then at Spithead, fitting up for Vice-admiral Boscawen, who was going with a large fleet on an expedition against Louisburgh. The crew of the Royal George were turned over to her, and the flag of that gallant admiral was hoisted on board, the blue at the maintop-gallant mast head. There was a very great fleet of men of war of every description assembled together for this expedition, and I was in hopes soon to have an opportunity of being gratified with a sea-fight. All things being now in readiness, this mighty fleet (for there was also Admiral Cornish's fleet in company, destined for the East Indies) at last weighed anchor, and sailed. The two fleets continued in company for several days, and then parted; Admiral Cornish, in the Lenox, having first saluted our admiral in the Namur, which he returned. We then steered for America; but, by contrary winds, we were driven to Teneriffe, where I was struck with its noted peak. Its prodigious height, and its form, resembling a sugar-loaf, filled me with wonder. We remained in sight of this island some days, and then proceeded for America, which we soon made, and got into a very commodious harbour called St. George, in Halifax, where we had fish in great plenty, and all other fresh provisions. We were here joined by different men of war and transport ships with soldiers; after which, our fleet being increased to a prodigious number of ships of all kinds, we sailed for Cape Breton in Nova Scotia. We had the good and gallant General Wolfe on board our ship, whose affability made him highly esteemed and beloved by all the men. He often honoured me, as well as other boys, with marks of his notice; and saved me once a flogging for fighting with a young gentleman. We arrived at Cape Breton in the summer of 1758: and here the soldiers were to be landed, in order to make an attack upon Louisbourgh. My master had some part in superintending the landing; and here I was in a small measure gratified in seeing an encounter between our men and the enemy. The French were posted on the shore to receive us, and disputed our landing for a long time; but at last they were driven from their trenches, and a complete landing was effected. Our troops pursued them as far as the town of Louisbourgh. In this action many were killed on both sides. One thing remarkable I saw this day:—A lieutenant of the Princess Amelia, who, as well as my master, superintended the landing, was giving the word of command, and while his mouth was open a musquet ball went through it, and passed out at his cheek. I had that day in my hand the scalp of an indian king, who was killed in the engagement: the scalp had been taken off by an Highlander. I saw this king's ornaments too, which were very curious, and made of feathers.

Our land forces laid siege to the town of Louisbourgh, while the French men of war were blocked up in the harbour by the fleet, the batteries at the same time playing upon them from the land. This they did with such effect, that one day I saw some of the ships set on fire by the shells from the batteries, and I believe two or three of them were quite burnt. At another time, about fifty boats belonging to the English men of war, commanded by Captain George Balfour of the Ætna fire-ship, and another junior captain, Laforey, attacked and boarded the only two remaining French men of war in the harbour. They also set fire to a seventy-gun ship, but a sixty-four, called the Bienfaisant, they brought off. During my stay here I had often an opportunity of being near Captain Balfour, who was pleased to notice me, and liked me so much that he often asked my master to let him have me, but he would not part with me; and no consideration could have induced me to leave him. At last Louisbourgh was taken, and the English men of war came into the harbour before it, to my very great joy; for I had now more liberty of indulging myself, and I went often on shore. When the ships were in the harbour we had the most beautiful procession on the water I ever saw. All the admirals and captains of the men of war, full dressed, and in their barges, well ornamented with pendants, came alongside of the Namur. The vice-admiral then went on shore in his barge, followed by the other officers in order of seniority, to take possession, as I suppose, of the town and fort. Some time after this the French governor and his lady, and other persons of note, came on board our ship to dine. On this occasion our ships were dressed with colours of all kinds, from the topgallant-mast head to the deck; and this, with the firing of guns, formed a most grand and magnificent spectacle.

As soon as every thing here was settled Admiral Boscawen sailed with part of the fleet for England, leaving some ships behind with Rear-admirals Sir Charles Hardy and Durell. It was now winter; and one evening, during our passage home, about dusk, when we were in the channel, or near soundings, and were beginning to look for land, we descried seven sail of large men of war, which stood off shore. Several people on board of our ship said, as the two fleets were (in forty minutes from the first sight) within hail of each other, that they were English men of war; and some of our people even began to name some of the ships. By this time both fleets began to mingle, and our admiral ordered his flag to be hoisted. At that instant the other fleet, which were French, hoisted their ensigns, and gave us a broadside as they passed by. Nothing could create greater surprise and confusion among us than this: the wind was high, the sea rough, and we had our lower and middle deck guns housed in, so that not a single gun on board was ready to be fired at any of the French ships. However, the Royal William and the Somerset being our sternmost ships, became a little prepared, and each gave the French ships a broadside as they passed by. I afterwards heard this was a French squadron, commanded by Mons. Conflans; and certainly had the Frenchmen known our condition, and had a mind to fight us, they might have done us great mischief. But we were not long before we were prepared for an engagement. Immediately many things were tossed overboard; the ships were made ready for fighting as soon as possible; and about ten at night we had bent a new main sail, the old one being split. Being now in readiness for fighting, we wore ship, and stood after the French fleet, who were one or two ships in number more than we. However we gave them chase, and continued pursuing them all night; and at day-light we saw six of them, all large ships of the line, and an English East India-man, a prize they had taken. We chased them all day till between three and four o'clock in the evening, when we came up with, and passed within a musquet shot of, one seventy-four gun ship, and the Indiaman also, who now hoisted her colours, but immediately hauled them down again. On this we made a signal for the other ships to take possession of her; and, supposing the man of war would likewise strike, we cheered, but she did not; though if we had fired into her, from being so near, we must have taken her. To my utter surprise the Somerset, who was the next ship a-stern of the Namur, made way likewise; and, thinking they were sure of this French ship, they cheered in the same manner, but still continued to follow us. The French Commodore was about a gun-shot ahead of all, running from us with all speed; and about four o'clock he carried his foretopmast overboard. This caused another loud cheer with us; and a little after the top-mast came close by us; but, to our great surprise, instead of coming up with her, we found she went as fast as ever, if not faster. The sea grew now much smoother; and the wind lulling, the seventy-four gun ship we had passed came again by us in the very same direction, and so near, that we heard her people talk as she went by; yet not a shot was fired on either side; and about five or six o'clock, just as it grew dark, she joined her commodore. We chased all night; but the next day they were out of sight, so that we saw no more of them; and we only had the old Indiaman (called Carnarvon I think) for our trouble. After this we stood in for the channel, and soon made the land; and, about the close of the year 1758–9, we got safe to St. Helen's. Here the Namur ran aground; and also another large ship astern of us; but, by starting our water, and tossing many things overboard to lighten her, we got the ships off without any damage. We stayed for a short time at Spithead, and then went into Portsmouth harbour to refit; from whence the admiral went to London; and my master and I soon followed, with a press-gang, as we wanted some hands to complete our complement.

CHAP. IV.

*The author is baptized—Narrowly escapes drowning—Goes on
an expedition to the Mediterranean—Incidents he met with
there—Is witness to an engagement between some English and
French ships—A particular account of the celebrated engagement between Admiral Boscawen and Mons. Le Clue, off
Cape Logas, in August 1759—Dreadful explosion of a French
ship—The author sails for England—His master appointed to
the command of a fire-ship—Meets a negro boy, from whom he
experiences much benevolence—Prepares for an expedition
against Belle-Isle—A remarkable story of a disaster which
befel his ship—Arrives at Belle-Isle—Operations of the landing and siege—The author's danger and distress, with his
manner of extricating himself—Surrender of Belle-Isle—
Transactions afterwards on the coast of France—Remarkable
instance of kidnapping—The author returns to England—
Hears a talk of peace, and expects his freedom—His ship sails
for Deptford to be paid off, and when he arrives there he is
suddenly seized by his master and carried forcibly on board a
West India ship and sold.*

IT WAS now between two and three years since I first came to
England, a great part of which I had spent at sea; so that I became inured to that service, and began to consider myself as
happily situated; for my master treated me always extremely
well; and my attachment and gratitude to him were very
great. From the various scenes I had beheld on ship-board, I
soon grew a stranger to terror of every kind, and was, in that
respect at least, almost an Englishman. I have often reflected
with surprise that I never felt half the alarm at any of the numerous dangers I have been in, that I was filled with at the
first sight of the Europeans, and at every act of theirs, even
the most trifling, when I first came among them, and for
some time afterwards. That fear, however, which was the effect of my ignorance, wore away as I began to know them. I
could now speak English tolerably well, and I perfectly understood every thing that was said. I now not only felt myself

quite easy with these new countrymen, but relished their society and manners. I no longer looked upon them as spirits, but as men superior to us; and therefore I had the stronger desire to resemble them; to imbibe their spirit, and imitate their manners; I therefore embraced every occasion of improvement; and every new thing that I observed I treasured up in my memory. I had long wished to be able to read and write; and for this purpose I took every opportunity to gain instruction, but had made as yet very little progress. However, when I went to London with my master, I had soon an opportunity of improving myself, which I gladly embraced. Shortly after my arrival, he sent me to wait upon the Miss Guerins, who had treated me with much kindness when I was there before; and they sent me to school.

While I was attending these ladies their servants told me I could not go to Heaven unless I was baptized. This made me very uneasy; for I had now some faint idea of a future state: accordingly I communicated my anxiety to the eldest Miss Guerin, with whom I was become a favourite, and pressed her to have me baptized; when to my great joy she told me I should. She had formerly asked my master to let me be baptized, but he had refused; however she now insisted on it; and he being under some obligation to her brother complied with her request; so I was baptized in St. Margaret's church, Westminster, in February 1759, by my present name. The clergyman, at the same time, gave me a book, called a Guide to the Indians, written by the Bishop of Sodor and Man. On this occasion Miss Guerin did me the honour to stand as godmother, and afterwards gave me a treat. I used to attend these ladies about the town, in which service I was extremely happy; as I had thus many opportunities of seeing London, which I desired of all things. I was sometimes, however, with my master at his rendezvous-house, which was at the foot of Westminster-bridge. Here I used to enjoy myself in playing about the bridge stairs, and often in the watermen's wherries, with other boys. On one of these occasions there was another boy with me in a wherry, and we went out into the current of the river: while we were there two more stout boys came to us in another wherry, and, abusing us for taking the boat, desired me to get into the other wherry-boat. Accordingly I went to get out of the wherry I was in; but just as I had got one of my feet into the other boat the boys shoved it off, so that I fell into the Thames; and, not being able to swim, I should unavoidably have been drowned, but for the assistance of some watermen who providentially came to my relief.

The Namur being again got ready for sea, my master, with his gang, was ordered on board; and, to my no small grief, I was obliged to leave my school-master, whom I liked very much, and always attended while I stayed in London, to repair on board with my master. Nor did I leave my kind patronesses, the Miss Guerins, without uneasiness and regret. They often used to teach me to read, and took great pains to instruct me in the principles of religion and the knowledge of God. I therefore parted from those amiable ladies with reluctance; after receiving from them many friendly cautions how to conduct myself, and some valuable presents.

When I came to Spithead, I found we were destined for the Mediterranean, with a large fleet, which was now ready to put to sea. We only waited for the arrival of the admiral, who soon came on board; and about the beginning of the spring 1759, having weighed anchor, and got under way, sailed for the Mediterranean; and in eleven days, from the Land's End, we got to Gibraltar. While we were here I used to be often on shore, and got various fruits in great plenty, and very cheap.

I had frequently told several people, in my excursions on shore, the story of my being kidnapped with my sister, and of our being separated, as I have related before; and I had as often expressed my anxiety for her fate, and my sorrow at having never met her again. One day, when I was on shore, and mentioning these circumstances to some persons, one of them told me he knew where my sister was, and, if I would accompany him, he would bring me to her. Improbable as this story was I believed it immediately, and agreed to go with him, while my heart leaped for joy: and, indeed, he conducted me to a black young woman, who was so like my sister, that, at first sight, I really thought it was her: but I was quickly undeceived; and, on talking to her, I found her to be of another nation.

While we lay here the Preston came in from the Levant. As soon as she arrived, my master told me I should now see my old companion, Dick, who had gone in her when she sailed for Turkey. I was much rejoiced at this news, and expected every minute to embrace him; and when the captain came on board of our ship, which he did immediately after, I ran to inquire after my friend; but, with inexpressible sorrow, I learned from the boat's crew that the dear youth was dead! and that they had brought his chest, and all his other things, to my master: these he afterwards gave to me, and I regarded them as a memorial of my friend, whom I loved, and grieved for, as a brother.

While we were at Gibraltar, I saw a soldier hanging by his heels, at one of the moles*: I thought this a strange sight, as I had seen a man hanged in London by his neck. At another time I saw the master of a frigate towed to shore on a grating, by several of the men of war's boats, and discharged the fleet, which I understood was a mark of disgrace for cowardice. On board the same ship there was also a sailor hung up at the yard-arm.

After lying at Gibraltar for some time, we sailed up the Mediterranean a considerable way above the Gulf of Lyons; where we were one night overtaken with a terrible gale of wind, much greater than any I had ever yet experienced. The sea ran so high that, though all the guns were well housed, there was great reason to fear their getting loose, the ship rolled so much; and if they had it must have proved our destruction. After we had cruised here for a short time, we came to Barcelona, a Spanish sea-port, remarkable for its silk manufactures. Here the ships were all to be watered; and my master, who spoke different languages, and used often to interpret for the admiral, superintended the watering of ours. For that purpose he and the officers of the other ships, who were on the same service, had tents pitched in the bay; and the Spanish soldiers were stationed along the shore, I suppose to see that no depredations were committed by our men.

I used constantly to attend my master; and I was charmed with this place. All the time we stayed it was like a fair with the natives, who brought us fruits of all kinds, and sold them to us much cheaper than I got them in England. They used

*He had drowned himself in endeavouring to desert.

also to bring wine down to us in hog and sheep skins, which diverted me very much. The Spanish officers here treated our officers with great politeness and attention; and some of them, in particular, used to come often to my master's tent to visit him; where they would sometimes divert themselves by mounting me on the horses or mules, so that I could not fall, and setting them off at full gallop; my imperfect skill in horsemanship all the while affording them no small entertainment. After the ships were watered, we returned to our old station of cruizing off Toulon, for the purpose of intercepting a fleet of French men of war that lay there. One Sunday, in our cruise, we came off a place where there were two small French frigates lying in shore; and our admiral, thinking to take or destroy them, sent two ships in after them—the Culloden and the Conqueror. They soon came up to the Frenchmen; and I saw a smart fight here, both by sea and land: for the frigates were covered by batteries, and they played upon our ships most furiously, which they as furiously returned, and for a long time a constant firing was kept up on all sides at an amazing rate. At last one frigate sunk; but the people escaped, though not without much difficulty: and a little after some of the people left the other frigate also, which was a mere wreck. However, our ships did not venture to bring her away, they were so much annoyed from the batteries, which raked them both in going and coming: their topmasts were shot away, and they were otherwise so much shattered, that the admiral was obliged to send in many boats to tow them back to the fleet. I afterwards sailed with a man who fought in one of the French batteries during the engagement, and he told me our ships had done considerable mischief that day on shore and in the batteries.

After this we sailed for Gibraltar, and arrived there about August 1759. Here we remained with all our sails unbent, while the fleet was watering and doing other necessary things. While we were in this situation, one day the admiral, with most of the principal officers, and many people of all stations, being on shore, about seven o'clock in the evening we were alarmed by signals from the frigates stationed for that purpose; and in an instant there was a general cry that the French fleet was out, and just passing through the streights. The admiral immediately came on board with some other officers; and it is impossible to describe the noise, hurry and confusion throughout the whole fleet, in bending their sails and slipping their cables; many people and ships' boats were left on shore in the bustle. We had two captains on board of our ship who came away in the hurry and left their ships to follow. We shewed lights from the gun-whale to the main topmast-head; and all our lieutenants were employed amongst the fleet to tell the ships not to wait for their captains, but to put the sails to the yards, slip their cables and follow us; and in this confusion of making ready for fighting we set out for sea in the dark after the French fleet. Here I could have exclaimed with Ajax,

> "Oh Jove! O father! if it be thy will
> That we must perish, we thy will obey,
> But let us perish by the light of day."

They had got the start of us so far that we were not able to come up with them during the night; but at day-light we saw seven sail of the line of battle some miles ahead. We immediately chased them till about four o'clock in the evening, when our ships came up with them; and, though we were about fifteen large ships, our gallant admiral only fought them with his own division, which consisted of seven; so that we were just ship for ship. We passed by the whole of the enemy's fleet in order to come at their commander, Mons. La Clue, who was in the Ocean, an eighty-four gun ship: as we passed they all fired on us; and at one time three of them fired together, continuing to do so for some time. Notwithstanding which our admiral would not suffer a gun to be fired at any of them, to my astonishment; but made us lie on our bellies on the deck till we came quite close to the Ocean, who was ahead of them all; when we had orders to pour the whole three tiers into her at once.

The engagement now commenced with great fury on both sides: the Ocean immediately returned our fire, and we continued engaged with each other for some time; during which I was frequently stunned with the thundering of the great guns, whose dreadful contents hurried many of my companions into awful eternity. At last the French line was entirely broken, and we obtained the victory, which was immediately proclaimed with loud huzzas and acclamations. We took three prizes, La Modeste, of sixty-four guns, and Le Temeraire and Centaur, of seventy-four guns each. The rest of the French ships took to flight with all the sail they could crowd. Our ship being very much damaged, and quite disabled from pursuing the enemy, the admiral immediately quitted her, and went in the broken and only boat we had left on board the Newark, with which, and some other ships, he went after the French. The Ocean, and another large French ship, called the Redoubtable, endeavouring to escape, ran ashore at Cape Logas, on the coast of Portugal; and the French admiral and some of the crew got ashore; but we, finding it impossible to get the ships off, set fire to them both. About midnight I saw the Ocean blow up, with a most dreadful explosion. I never beheld a more awful scene. In less than a minute the midnight for a certain space seemed turned into day by the blaze, which was attended with a noise louder and more terrible than thunder, that seemed to rend every element around us.

My station during the engagement was on the middle-deck, where I was quartered with another boy, to bring powder to the aftermost gun; and here I was a witness of the dreadful fate of many of my companions, who, in the twinkling of an eye, were dashed in pieces, and launched into eternity. Happily I escaped unhurt, though the shot and splinters flew thick about me during the whole fight. Towards the latter part of it my master was wounded, and I saw him carried down to the surgeon; but though I was much alarmed for him and wished to assist him I dared not leave my post. At this station my gun-mate (a partner in bringing powder for the same gun) and I ran a very great risk for more than half an hour of blowing up the ship. For, when we had taken the cartridges out of the boxes, the bottoms of many of them proving rotten, the powder ran all about the deck, near the match tub: we scarcely had water enough at the last to throw on it. We were also, from our employment, very much exposed to the enemy's shots; for we had to go through nearly the whole length of the ship to bring the powder. I expected therefore every minute to be my last; especially when I saw our men fall so thick about me; but, wishing to guard as much against the dangers as possible, at first I thought it would be safest not to go for the powder till the Frenchmen had fired their broadside; and then, while they were charging, I could go and come with my powder: but immediately afterwards I thought this caution was fruitless; and, cheering myself with the reflection that there was a time allotted for me to die as well as to be born, I instantly cast off all fear or thought whatever of death, and went through the whole of my duty with alacrity; pleasing myself with the hope, if I survived the battle, of relating it and the dangers I had escaped to the dear Miss Guerin, and others, when I should return to London.

Our ship suffered very much in this engagement; for, besides the number of our killed and wounded, she was almost torn to pieces, and our rigging so much shattered, that our mizen-mast and main-yard, &c. hung over the side of the ship; so that we were obliged to get many carpenters, and others from some of the ships of the fleet, to assist in setting us in some tolerable order; and, notwithstanding, it took us some time before we were completely refitted; after which we left Admiral Broderick to command, and we, with the prizes, steered for England. On the passage, and as soon as my master was something recovered of his wounds, the admiral appointed him captain of the Ætna fire-ship, on which he and I left the Namur, and went on board of her at sea. I liked this little ship very much. I now became the captain's steward, in which situation I was very happy: for I was extremely well treated by all on board; and I had leisure to improve myself in reading and writing. The latter I had learned a little of before I left the Namur, as there was a school on board. When we arrived at Spithead the Ætna went into Portsmouth harbour to refit, which being done, we returned to Spithead and joined a large fleet that was thought to be intended against the Havannah; but about that time the king died: whether that prevented the expedition I know not; but it caused our ship to be stationed at Cowes, in the isle of Wight, till the beginning of the year sixty-one. Here I spent my time very pleasantly; I was much on shore all about this delightful island, and found the inhabitants very civil.

While I was here, I met with a trifling incident, which surprised me agreeably. I was one day in a field belonging to a

gentleman who had a black boy about my own size; this boy
having observed me from his master's house, was transported
at the sight of one of his own countrymen, and ran to meet
me with the utmost haste. I not knowing what he was about
turned a little out of his way at first, but to no purpose: he
soon came close to me and caught hold of me in his arms as
if I had been his brother, though we had never seen each
other before. After we had talked together for some time he
took me to his master's house, where I was treated very
kindly. This benevolent boy and I were very happy in frequently seeing each other till about the month of March 1761,
when our ship had orders to fit out again for another expedition. When we got ready, we joined a very large fleet at
Spithead, commanded by Commodore Keppel, which was
destined against Belle-Isle, and with a number of transport
ships with troops on board to make a descent on the place.
We sailed once more in quest of fame. I longed to engage in
new adventures and see fresh wonders.

I had a mind on which every thing uncommon made its full
impression, and every event which I considered as marvellous.
Every extraordinary escape, or signal deliverance, either of
myself or others, I looked upon to be effected by the interposition of Providence. We had not been above ten days at
sea before an incident of this kind happened; which, whatever
credit it may obtain from the reader, made no small impression on my mind.

We had on board a gunner, whose name was John Mondle;
a man of very indifferent morals. This man's cabin was between the decks, exactly over where I lay, abreast of the quarter-deck ladder. One night, the 20th of April, being terrified
with a dream, he awoke in so great a fright that he could not
rest in his bed any longer, nor even remain in his cabin; and
he went upon deck about four o'clock in the morning extremely agitated. He immediately told those on the deck of
the agonies of his mind, and the dream which occasioned it;
in which he said he had seen many things very awful, and had
been warned by St. Peter to repent, who told him time was
short. This he said had greatly alarmed him, and he was determined to alter his life. People generally mock the fears of
others when they are themselves in safety; and some of his

shipmates who heard him only laughed at him. However, he made a vow that he never would drink strong liquors again; and he immediately got a light, and gave away his sea-stores of liquor. After which, his agitation still continuing, he began to read the Scriptures, hoping to find some relief; and soon afterwards he laid himself down again on his bed, and endeavoured to compose himself to sleep, but to no purpose; his mind still continuing in a state of agony. By this time it was exactly half after seven in the morning: I was then under the half-deck at the great cabin door; and all at once I heard the people in the waist cry out, most fearfully—'The Lord have mercy upon us! We are all lost! The Lord have mercy upon us!' Mr. Mondle hearing the cries, immediately ran out of his cabin; and we were instantly struck by the Lynne, a forty-gun ship, Captain Clark, which nearly ran us down. This ship had just put about, and was by the wind, but had not got full headway, or we must all have perished; for the wind was brisk. However, before Mr. Mondle had got four steps from his cabin-door, she struck our ship with her cutwater right in the middle of his bed and cabin, and ran it up to the combings of the quarter-deck hatchway, and above three feet below water, and in a minute there was not a bit of wood to be seen where Mr. Mondle's cabin stood; and he was so near being killed that some of the splinters tore his face. As Mr. Mondle must inevitably have perished from this accident had he not been alarmed in the very extraordinary way I have related, I could not help regarding this as an awful interposition of Providence for his preservation. The two ships for some time swinged alongside of each other; for ours being a fireship, our grappling-irons caught the Lynne every way, and the yards and rigging went at an astonishing rate. Our ship was in such a shocking condition that we all thought she would instantly go down, and every one ran for their lives, and got as well as they could on board the Lynne; but our lieutenant being the aggressor, he never quitted the ship. However, when we found she did not sink immediately, the captain came on board again, and encouraged our people to return and try to save her. Many on this came back, but some would not venture. Some of the ships in the fleet, seeing our situation, immediately sent their boats to our assistance; but it took us the whole day to save the ship with all their help. And by using every possible means, particularly frapping her together with many hawsers, and putting a great quantity of tallow below water where she was damaged, she was kept together: but it was well we did not meet with any gales of wind, or we must have gone to pieces; for we were in such a crazy condition that we had ships to attend us till we arrived at Belle-Isle, the place of our destination; and then we had all things taken out of the ship, and she was properly repaired. This escape of Mr. Mondle, which he, as well as myself, always considered as a singular act of Providence, I believe had a great influence on his life and conduct ever afterwards.

Now that I am on this subject I beg leave to relate another instance or two which strongly raised my belief of the particular interposition of Heaven, and which might not otherwise have found a place here, from their insignificance. I belonged for a few days in the year 1758 to the Jason, of fifty-four guns, at Plymouth; and one night, when I was on board, a woman, with a child at her breast, fell from the upper-deck down into the hold, near the keel. Every one thought that the mother and child must be both dashed to pieces; but, to our great surprise, neither of them was hurt. I myself one day fell headlong from the upper-deck of the Etna down the after-hold, when the ballast was out; and all who saw me fall cried out I was killed: but I received not the least injury. And in the same ship a man fell from the mast-head on the deck without being hurt. In these, and in many more instances, I thought I could plainly trace the hand of God, without whose permission a sparrow cannot fall. I began to raise my fear from man to him alone, and to call daily on his holy name with fear and reverence: and I trust he heard my supplications, and graciously condescended to answer me according to his holy word, and to implant the seeds of piety in me, even one of the meanest of his creatures.

When we had refitted our ship, and all things were in readiness for attacking the place, the troops on board the transports were ordered to disembark; and my master, as a junior captain, had a share in the command of the landing. This was on the 8th of April. The French were drawn up on the shore, and had made every disposition to oppose the landing of our men, only a small part of them this day being able to effect it; most of them, after fighting with great bravery, were cut off; and General Crawford, with a number of others, were taken prisoners. In this day's engagement we had also our lieutenant killed.

On the 21st of April we renewed our efforts to land the men, while all the men of war were stationed along the shore to cover it, and fired at the French batteries and breastworks from early in the morning till about four o'clock in the evening, when our soldiers effected a safe landing. They immediately attacked the French; and, after a sharp encounter, forced them from the batteries. Before the enemy retreated they blew up several of them, lest they should fall into our hands. Our men now proceeded to besiege the citadel, and my master was ordered on shore to superintend the landing of all the materials necessary for carrying on the siege; in which service I mostly attended him. While I was there I went about to different parts of the island; and one day, particularly, my curiosity almost cost me my life. I wanted very much to see the mode of charging the mortars and letting off the shells, and for that purpose I went to an English battery that was but a very few yards from the walls of the citadel. There, indeed, I had an opportunity of completely gratifying myself in seeing the whole operation, and that not without running a very great risk, both from the English shells that burst while I was there, but likewise from those of the French. One of the largest of their shells bursted within nine or ten yards of me: there was a single rock close by, about the size of a butt; and I got instant shelter under it in time to avoid the fury of the shell. Where it burst the earth was torn in such a manner that two or three butts might easily have gone into the hole it made, and it threw great quantities of stones and dirt to a considerable distance. Three shot were also fired at me and another boy who was along with me, one of them in particular seemed

"Wing'd with red lightning and impetuous rage;"

for with a most dreadful sound it hissed close by me, and struck a rock at a little distance, which it shattered to pieces. When I saw what perilous circumstances I was in, I attempted to return the nearest way I could find, and thereby I got between the English and the French centinels. An English serjeant, who commanded the outposts, seeing me, and surprised how I came there, (which was by stealth along the seashore), reprimanded me very severely for it, and instantly took the centinel off his post into custody, for his negligence in suffering me to pass the lines. While I was in this situation I observed at a little distance a French horse, belonging to some islanders, which I thought I would now mount, for the greater expedition of getting off. Accordingly I took some cord which I had about me, and making a kind of bridle of it, I put it round the horse's head, and the tame beast very quietly suffered me to tie him thus and mount him. As soon as I was on the horse's back I began to kick and beat him, and try every means to make him go quick, but all to very little purpose: I could not drive him out of a slow pace. While I was creeping along, still within reach of the enemy's shot, I met with a servant well mounted on an English horse. I immediately stopped; and, crying, told him my case; and begged of him to help me, and this he effectually did; for, having a fine large whip, he began to lash my horse with it so severely, that he set off full speed with me towards the sea, while I was quite unable to hold or manage him. In this manner I went along till I came to a craggy precipice. I now could not stop my horse; and my mind was filled with apprehensions of my deplorable fate should he go down the precipice, which he appeared fully disposed to do: I therefore thought I had better throw myself off him at once, which I did immediately with a great deal of dexterity, and fortunately escaped unhurt. As soon as I found myself at liberty I made the best of my way for the ship, determined I would not be so fool-hardy again in a hurry.

We continued to besiege the citadel till June, when it surrendered. During the siege I have counted above sixty shells and carcases in the air at once. When this place was taken I went through the citadel, and in the bomb-proofs under it, which were cut in the solid rock; and I thought it a surprising place, both for strength and building: notwithstanding which our shots and shells had made amazing devastation, and ruinous heaps all around it.

After the taking of this island our ships, with some others commanded by Commodore Stanhope in the Swiftsure, went to Basse-road, where we blocked up a French fleet. Our ships were there from June till February following; and in that time I saw a great many scenes of war, and stratagems on both sides to destroy each others fleet. Sometimes we would attack the French with some ships of the line; at other times with boats; and frequently we made prizes. Once or twice the French attacked us by throwing shells with their bomb-vessels: and one day as a French vessel was throwing shells at our ships she broke from her springs, behind the isle of I de Re: the tide being complicated, she came within a gun shot of the Nassau; but the Nassau could not bring a gun to bear upon her, and thereby the Frenchman got off. We were twice attacked by their fire-floats, which they chained together, and then let them float down with the tide; but each time we sent boats with graplings, and towed them safe out of the fleet.

We had different commanders while we were at this place, Commodores Stanhope, Dennis, Lord Howe, &c. From hence, before the Spanish war began, our ship and the Wasp sloop were sent to St. Sebastian in Spain, by Commodore Stanhope; and Commodore Dennis afterwards sent our ship as a cartel to Bayonne in France*, after which † we went in February in 1762 to Belle-Isle, and there stayed till the summer, when we left it, and returned to Portsmouth.

After our ship was fitted out again for service, in September she went to Guernsey, where I was very glad to see my old

*Among others whom we brought from Bayonne, two gentlemen, who had been in the West Indies, where they sold slaves; and they confessed they had made at one time a false bill of sale, and sold two Portuguese white men among a lot of slaves.

†Some people have it, that sometimes shortly before persons die their ward has been seen; that is, some spirit exactly in their likeness, though they are themselves at other places at the same time. One day while we were at Bayonne Mr. Mondle saw one of our men, as he thought, in the gun-room; and a little after, coming on the quarter-deck, he spoke of some circumstances of this man to some of the officers. They told him that the man was then out of the ship, in one of the boats with the Lieutenant: but Mr. Mondle would not believe it, and we searched the ship, when he found the man was actually out of her; and when the boat returned some time afterwards, we found the man had been drowned at the very time Mr. Mondle thought he saw him.

hostess, who was now a widow, and my former little charming companion, her daughter. I spent some time here very happily with them, till October, when we had orders to repair to Portsmouth. We parted from each other with a great deal of affection; and I promised to return soon, and see them again, not knowing what all-powerful fate had determined for me. Our ship having arrived at Portsmouth, we went into the harbour, and remained there till the latter end of November, when we heard great talk about peace; and, to our very great joy, in the beginning of December we had orders to go up to London with our ship to be paid off. We received this news with loud huzzas, and every other demonstration of gladness; and nothing but mirth was to be seen throughout every part of the ship. I too was not without my share of the general joy on this occasion. I thought now of nothing but being freed, and working for myself, and thereby getting money to enable me to get a good education; for I always had a great desire to be able at least to read and write; and while I was on shipboard I had endeavoured to improve myself in both. While I was in the Ætna particularly, the captain's clerk taught me to write, and gave me a smattering of arithmetic as far as the rule of three. There was also one Daniel Queen, about forty years of age, a man very well educated, who messed with me on board this ship, and he likewise dressed and attended the captain. Fortunately this man soon became very much attached to me, and took very great pains to instruct me in many things. He taught me to shave and dress hair a little, and also to read in the Bible, explaining many passages to me, which I did not comprehend. I was wonderfully surprised to see the laws and rules of my country written almost exactly here; a circumstance which I believe tended to impress our manners and customs more deeply on my memory. I used to tell him of this resemblance; and many a time we have sat up the whole night together at this employment. In short, he was like a father to me; and some even used to call me after his name; they also styled me the black Christian. Indeed I almost loved him with the affection of a son. Many things I have denied myself that he might have them; and when I used to play at marbles or any other game, and won a few half-pence, or got any little money, which I sometimes did, for shaving any one, I used to buy him a little sugar or tobacco, as far as my stock of money would go. He used to say, that he and I never should part; and that when our ship was paid off, as I was as free as himself or any other man on board, he would instruct me in his business, by which I might gain a good livelihood. This gave me new life and spirits; and my heart burned within me, while I thought the time long till I obtained my freedom. For though my master had not promised it to me, yet, besides the assurances I had received that he had no right to detain me, he always treated me with the greatest kindness, and reposed in me an unbounded confidence; he even paid attention to my morals; and would never suffer me to deceive him, or tell lies, of which he used to tell me the consequences; and that if I did so God would not love me; so that, from all this tenderness, I had never once supposed, in all my dreams of freedom, that he would think of detaining me any longer than I wished.

In pursuance of our orders we sailed from Portsmouth for the Thames, and arrived at Deptford the 10th of December, where we cast anchor just as it was high water. The ship was up about half an hour, when my master ordered the barge to be manned; and all in an instant, without having before given me the least reason to suspect any thing of the matter, he forced me into the barge; saying, I was going to leave him, but he would take care I should not. I was so struck with the unexpectedness of this proceeding, that for some time I did not make a reply, only I made an offer to go for my books and chest of clothes, but he swore I should not move out of his sight; and if I did he would cut my throat, at the same time taking his hanger. I began, however, to collect myself; and, plucking up courage, I told him I was free, and he could not by law serve me so. But this only enraged him the more; and he continued to swear, and said he would soon let me know whether he would or not, and at that instant sprung himself into the barge from the ship, to the astonishment and sorrow of all on board. The tide, rather unluckily for me, had just turned downward, so that we quickly fell down the river along with it, till we came among some outward-bound West Indiamen; for he was resolved to put me on board the first vessel he could get to receive me. The boat's crew, who pulled against their will, became quite faint different times, and would have gone ashore; but he would not let them. Some of them strove then to cheer me, and told me he could not sell me, and that they would stand by me, which revived me a little; and I still entertained hopes; for as they pulled along he asked some vessels to receive me, but they could not. But, just as we had got a little below Gravesend, we came alongside of a ship which was going away the next tide for the West Indies; her name was the Charming Sally, Captain James Doran; and my master went on board and agreed with him for me; and in a little time I was sent for into the cabin. When I came there Captain Doran asked me if I knew him; I answered that I did not; 'Then,' said he 'you are now my slave.' I told him my master could not sell me to him, nor to any one else. 'Why,' said he, 'did not your master buy you?' I confessed he did. 'But I have served him,' said I, 'many years, and he has taken all my wages and prize-money, for I only got one sixpence during the war; besides this I have been baptized; and by the laws of the land no man has a right to sell me:' And I added, that I had heard a lawyer and others at different times tell my master so. They both then said that those people who told me so were not my friends; but I replied—it was very extraordinary that other people did not know the law as well as they. Upon this Captain Doran said I talked too much English; and if I did not behave myself well, and be quiet, he had a method on board to make me. I was too well convinced of his power over me to doubt what he said; and my former sufferings in the slave-ship presenting themselves to my mind, the recollection of them made me shudder. However, before I retired I told them that as I could not get any right among men here I hoped I should hereafter in Heaven; and I immediately left the cabin, filled with resentment and sorrow. The only coat I had with me my master took away with him, and said if my prize-money had been 10,000l. he had a right to it all, and would have taken it. I had about nine guineas, which, during my long sea-faring life, I had scraped together from trifling perquisites and little ventures; and I hid it that instant, lest my master should take that from me likewise, still hoping that by some means or other I should make my escape to the shore; and indeed some of my old shipmates told me not to despair, for they would get me back again; and that, as soon as they could get their pay, they would immediately come to Portsmouth to me, where this ship was going: but, alas! all my hopes were baffled, and the hour of my deliverance was yet far off. My master, having soon concluded his bargain with the captain, came out of the cabin, and he and his people got into the boat and put off; I followed them with aching eyes as long as I could, and when they were out of sight I threw myself on the deck, while my heart was ready to burst with sorrow and anguish.

CHAP. V.

The author's reflections on his situation—Is deceived by a
  promise of being delivered—His despair at sailing for the
  West Indies—Arrives at Montserrat, where he is sold to Mr.
  King—Various interesting instances of oppression, cruelty,
  and extortion, which the author saw practised upon the slaves
  in the West Indies during his captivity from the year 1763 to
  1766—Address on it to the planters.

Thus, at the moment I expected all my toils to end, was I
plunged, as I supposed, in a new slavery; in comparison of
which all my service hitherto had been 'perfect freedom;' and
whose horrors, always present to my mind, now rushed on it
with tenfold aggravation. I wept very bitterly for some time:
and began to think that I must have done something to dis-
please the Lord, that he thus punished me so severely. This
filled me with painful reflections on my past conduct; I recollected that on the morning of our arrival at Deptford I had
rashly sworn that as soon as we reached London I would
spend the day in rambling and sport. My conscience smote
me for this unguarded expression: I felt that the Lord was
able to disappoint me in all things, and immediately considered my present situation as a judgment of Heaven on account of my presumption in swearing: I therefore, with
contrition of heart, acknowledged my transgression to God,
and poured out my soul before him with unfeigned repentance, and with earnest supplications I besought him not to
abandon me in my distress, nor cast me from his mercy for
ever. In a little time my grief, spent with its own violence,
began to subside; and after the first confusion of my thoughts
was over I reflected with more calmness on my present condition: I considered that trials and disappointments are sometimes for our good, and I thought God might perhaps have
permitted this in order to teach me wisdom and resignation;
for he had hitherto shadowed me with the wings of his mercy,
and by his invisible but powerful hand brought me the way I
knew not. These reflections gave me a little comfort, and I
rose at last from the deck with dejection and sorrow in my

countenance, yet mixed with some faint hope that the *Lord would appear* for my deliverance.

Soon afterwards, as my new master was going ashore, he called me to him, and told me to behave myself well, and do the business of the ship the same as any of the rest of the boys, and that I should fare the better for it; but I made him no answer. I was then asked if I could swim, and I said, No. However I was made to go under the deck, and was well watched. The next tide the ship got under way, and soon after arrived at the Mother Bank, Portsmouth; where she waited a few days for some of the West India convoy. While I was here I tried every means I could devise amongst the people of the ship to get me a boat from the shore, as there was none suffered to come alongside of the ship; and their own, whenever it was used, was hoisted in again immediately. A sailor on board took a guinea from me on pretence of getting me a boat; and promised me, time after time, that it was hourly to come off. When he had the watch upon deck I watched also; and looked long enough, but all in vain; I could never see either the boat or my guinea again. And what I thought was still the worst of all, the fellow gave information, as I afterwards found, all the while to the mates, of my intention to go off, if I could in any way do it; but, rogue like, he never told them he had got a guinea from me to procure my escape. However, after we had sailed, and his trick was made known to the ship's crew, I had some satisfaction in seeing him detested and despised by them all for his behaviour to me. I was still in hopes that my old shipmates would not forget their promise to come for me to Portsmouth: and, indeed, at last, but not till the day before we sailed, some of them did come there, and sent me off some oranges, and other tokens of their regard. They also sent me word they would come off to me themselves the next day or the day after; and a lady also, who lived in Gosport, wrote to me that she would come and take me out of the ship at the same time. This lady had been once very intimate with my former master: I used to sell and take care of a great deal of property for her, in different ships; and in return she always shewed great friendship for me, and used to tell my master that she would take me away to live with her: but, unfortunately for me, a disagreement soon afterwards took place between them; and she was succeeded in my master's good graces by another lady, who appeared sole mistress of the Ætna, and mostly lodged on board. I was not so great a favourite with this lady as with the former; she had conceived a pique against me on some occasion when she was on board, and she did not fail to instigate my master to treat me in the manner he did*.

However, the next morning, the 30th of December, the wind being brisk and easterly, the Œolus frigate, which was to escort the convoy, made a signal for sailing. All the ships then got up their anchors; and, before any of my friends had an opportunity to come off to my relief, to my inexpressible anguish our ship had got under way. What tumultuous emotions agitated my soul when the convoy got under sail, and I a prisoner on board, now without hope! I kept my swimming eyes upon the land in a state of unutterable grief; not knowing what to do, and despairing how to help myself. While my mind was in this situation the fleet sailed on, and in one day's time I lost sight of the wished-for land. In the first expressions of my grief I reproached my fate, and wished I had never been born. I was ready to curse the tide that bore us, the gale that wafted my prison, and even the ship that conducted us; and I called on death to relieve me from the horrors I felt and dreaded, that I might be in that place

> "Where slaves are free, and men oppress no more.
> Fool that I was, inur'd so long to pain,
> To trust to hope, or dream of joy again.
>
> *   *   *   *   *   *   *   *   *   *   *   *
>
> Now dragg'd once more beyond the western main,
> To groan beneath some dastard planter's chain;
> Where my poor countrymen in bondage wait
> The long enfranchisement of ling'ring fate:
> Hard ling'ring fate! while, ere the dawn of day,

---

*Thus was I sacrificed to the envy and resentment of this woman for knowing that the lady whom she had succeeded in my master's good graces designed to take me into her service; which, had I once got on shore, she would not have been able to prevent. She felt her pride alarmed at the superiority of her rival in being attended by a black servant: it was not less to prevent this than to be revenged on me, that she caused the captain to treat me thus cruelly.

> Rous'd by the lash they go their cheerless way;
> And as their souls with shame and anguish burn,
> Salute with groans unwelcome morn's return,
> And, chiding ev'ry hour the slow-pac'd sun,
> Pursue their toils till all his race is run.
> No eye to mark their suff'rings with a tear;
> No friend to comfort, and no hope to cheer:
> Then, like the dull unpity'd brutes, repair
> To stalls as wretched, and as coarse a fare;
> Thank heaven one day of mis'ry was o'er,
> Then sink to sleep, and wish to wake no more*."

The turbulence of my emotions however naturally gave way to calmer thoughts, and I soon perceived what fate had decreed no mortal on earth could prevent. The convoy sailed on without any accident, with a pleasant gale and smooth sea, for six weeks, till February, when one morning the Œolus ran down a brig, one of the convoy, and she instantly went down and was ingulfed in the dark recesses of the ocean. The convoy was immediately thrown into great confusion till it was day-light; and the Œolus was illumined with lights to prevent any farther mischief. On the 13th of February 1763, from the mast-head, we descried our destined island Montserrat; and soon after I beheld those

> "Regions of sorrow, doleful shades, where peace
> And rest can rarely dwell. Hope never comes
> That comes to all, but torture without end
> Still urges."

At the sight of this land of bondage, a fresh horror ran through all my frame, and chilled me to the heart. My former slavery now rose in dreadful review to my mind, and displayed nothing but misery, stripes, and chains; and, in the first paroxysm of my grief, I called upon God's thunder, and his avenging

---

*"The Dying Negro," a poem originally published in 1773. Perhaps it may not be deemed impertinent here to add, that this elegant and pathetic little poem was occasioned, as appears by the advertisement prefixed to it, by the following incident. "A black, who, a few days before had ran away from his master, and got himself christened, with intent to marry a white woman his fellow-servant, being taken and sent on board a ship in the Thames, took an opportunity of shooting himself through the head."

power, to direct the stroke of death to me, rather than permit me to become a slave, and be sold from lord to lord.

In this state of my mind our ship came to an anchor, and soon after discharged her cargo. I now knew what it was to work hard; I was made to help to unload and load the ship. And, to comfort me in my distress in that time, two of the sailors robbed me of all my money, and ran away from the ship. I had been so long used to an European climate that at first I felt the scorching West India sun very painful, while the dashing surf would toss the boat and the people in it frequently above high water mark. Sometimes our limbs were broken with this, or even attended with instant death, and I was day by day mangled and torn.

About the middle of May, when the ship was got ready to sail for England, I all the time believing that Fate's blackest clouds were gathering over my head, and expecting their bursting would mix me with the dead, Captain Doran sent for me ashore one morning, and I was told by the messenger that my fate was then determined. With fluttering steps and trembling heart I came to the captain, and found with him one Mr. Robert King, a quaker, and the first merchant in the place. The captain then told me my former master had sent me there to be sold; but that he had desired him to get me the best master he could, as he told him I was a very deserving boy, which Captain Doran said he found to be true; and if he were to stay in the West Indies he would be glad to keep me himself; but he could not venture to take me to London, for he was very sure that when I came there I would leave him. I at that instant burst out a crying, and begged much of him to take me to England with him, but all to no purpose. He told me he had got me the very best master in the whole island, with whom I should be as happy as if I were in England, and for that reason he chose to let him have me, though he could sell me to his own brother-in-law for a great deal more money than what he got from this gentleman. Mr. King, my new master, then made a reply, and said the reason he had bought me was on account of my good character; and, as he had not the least doubt of my good behaviour, I should be very well off with him. He also told me he did not live in the West Indies, but at Philadelphia, where he was going soon; and, as I understood something of the rules of arithmetic, when we got there he would put me to school, and fit me for a clerk. This conversation relieved my mind a little, and I left those gentlemen considerably more at ease in myself than when I came to them; and I was very grateful to Captain Doran, and even to my old master, for the character they had given me; a character which I afterwards found of infinite service to me. I went on board again, and took leave of all my shipmates; and the next day the ship sailed. When she weighed anchor I went to the waterside and looked at her with a very wishful and aching heart, and followed her with my eyes and tears until she was totally out of sight. I was so bowed down with grief that I could not hold up my head for many months; and if my new master had not been kind to me I believe I should have died under it at last. And indeed I soon found that he fully deserved the good character which Captain Doran had given me of him; for he possessed a most amiable disposition and temper, and was very charitable and humane. If any of his slaves behaved amiss he did not beat or use them ill, but parted with them. This made them afraid of disobliging him; and as he treated his slaves better than any other man on the island, so he was better and more faithfully served by them in return. By his kind treatment I did at last endeavour to compose myself; and with fortitude, though moneyless, determined to face whatever fate had decreed for me. Mr. King soon asked me what I could do; and at the same time said he did not mean to treat me as a common slave. I told him I knew something of seamanship, and could shave and dress hair pretty well; and I could refine wines, which I had learned on shipboard, where I had often done it; and that I could write, and understood arithmetic tolerably well as far as the Rule of Three. He then asked me if I knew any thing of gauging; and, on my answering that I did not, he said one of his clerks should teach me to gauge.

Mr. King dealt in all manner of merchandize, and kept from one to six clerks. He loaded many vessels in a year; particularly to Philadelphia, where he was born, and was connected with a great mercantile house in that city. He had besides many vessels and droggers, of different sizes, which used to go about the island; and others to collect rum, sugar, and other goods. I understood pulling and managing those boats very well; and this hard work, which was the first that he set me to, in the sugar seasons used to be my constant employment. I have rowed the boat, and slaved at the oars, from one hour to sixteen in the twenty-four; during which I had fifteen pence sterling per day to live on, though sometimes only ten pence. However this was considerably more than was allowed to other slaves that used to work with me, and belonged to other gentlemen on the island: those poor souls had never more than nine pence per day, and seldom more than six pence, from their masters or owners, though they earned them three or four pisterines*: for it is a common practice in the West Indies for men to purchase slaves though they have not plantations themselves, in order to let them out to planters and merchants at so much a piece by the day, and they give what allowance they chuse out of this produce of their daily work to their slaves for subsistence; this allowance is often very scanty. My master often gave the owners of these slaves two and a half of these pieces per day, and found the poor fellows in victuals himself, because he thought their owners did not feed them well enough according to the work they did. The slaves used to like this very well; and, as they knew my master to be a man of feeling, they were always glad to work for him in preference to any other gentleman; some of whom, after they had been paid for these poor people's labours, would not give them their allowance out of it. Many times have I even seen these unfortunate wretches beaten for asking for their pay; and often severely flogged by their owners if they did not bring them their daily or weekly money exactly to the time; though the poor creatures were obliged to wait on the gentlemen they had worked for sometimes for more than half the day before they could get their pay; and this generally on Sundays, when they wanted the time for themselves. In particular, I knew a countryman of mine who once did not bring the weekly money directly that it was earned; and though he brought it the same day to his master, yet he was staked to the ground for this pretended negli-

*These pisterines are of the value of a shilling.

gence, and was just going to receive a hundred lashes, but for a gentleman who begged him off fifty. This poor man was very industrious; and, by his frugality, had saved so much money by working on shipboard, that he had got a white man to buy him a boat, unknown to his master. Some time after he had this little estate the governor wanted a boat to bring his sugar from different parts of the island; and, knowing this to be a negro-man's boat, he seized upon it for himself, and would not pay the owner a farthing. The man on this went to his master, and complained to him of this act of the governor; but the only satisfaction he received was to be damned very heartily by his master, who asked him how dared any of his negroes to have a boat. If the justly-merited ruin of the governor's fortune could be any gratification to the poor man he had thus robbed, he was not without consolation. Extortion and rapine are poor providers; and some time after this the governor died in the King's Bench in England, as I was told, in great poverty. The last war favoured this poor negro-man, and he found some means to escape from his Christian master: he came to England; where I saw him afterwards several times. Such treatment as this often drives these miserable wretches to despair, and they run away from their masters at the hazard of their lives. Many of them, in this place, unable to get their pay when they have earned it, and fearing to be flogged, as usual, if they return home without it, run away where they can for shelter, and a reward is often offered to bring them in dead or alive. My master used sometimes, in these cases, to agree with their owners, and to settle with them himself; and thereby he saved many of them a flogging.

Once, for a few days, I was let out to fit a vessel, and I had no victuals allowed me by either party; at last I told my master of this treatment, and he took me away from it. In many of the estates, on the different islands where I used to be sent for rum or sugar, they would not deliver it to me, or any other negro; he was therefore obliged to send a white man along with me to those places; and then he used to pay him from six to ten pisterines a day. From being thus employed, during the time I served Mr. King, in going about the different estates on the island, I had all the opportunity I could wish for to see the dreadful usage of the poor men; usage that reconciled me to my situation, and made me bless God for the hands into which I had fallen.

I had the good fortune to please my master in every department in which he employed me; and there was scarcely any part of his business, or household affairs, in which I was not occasionally engaged. I often supplied the place of a clerk, in receiving and delivering cargoes to the ships, in tending stores, and delivering goods: and, besides this, I used to shave and dress my master when convenient, and take care of his horse; and when it was necessary, which was very often, I worked likewise on board of different vessels of his. By these means I became very useful to my master; and saved him, as he used to acknowledge, above a hundred pounds a year. Nor did he scruple to say I was of more advantage to him than any of his clerks; though their usual wages in the West Indies are from sixty to a hundred pounds current a year.

I have sometimes heard it asserted that a negro cannot earn his master the first cost; but nothing can be further from the truth. I suppose nine tenths of the mechanics throughout the West Indies are negro slaves; and I well know the coopers among them earn two dollars a day; the carpenters the same, and oftentimes more; as also the masons, smiths, and fishermen, &c. and I have known many slaves whose masters would not take a thousand pounds current for them. But surely this assertion refutes itself; for, if it be true, why do the planters and merchants pay such a price for slaves? And, above all, why do those who make this assertion exclaim the most loudly against the abolition of the slave trade? So much are men blinded, and to such inconsistent arguments are they driven by mistaken interest! I grant, indeed, that slaves are some times, by half-feeding, half-clothing, over-working and stripes, reduced so low, that they are turned out as unfit for service, and left to perish in the woods, or expire on a dunghill.

My master was several times offered by different gentlemen one hundred guineas for me; but he always told them he would not sell me, to my great joy: and I used to double my diligence and care for fear of getting into the hands of those men who did not allow a valuable slave the common support of life. Many of them even used to find fault with my master for feeding his slaves so well as he did; although I often went hungry, and an Englishman might think my fare very indifferent; but he used to tell them he always would do it, because the slaves thereby looked better and did more work.

While I was thus employed by my master I was often a witness to cruelties of every kind, which were exercised on my unhappy fellow slaves. I used frequently to have different cargoes of new negroes in my care for sale; and it was almost a constant practice with our clerks, and other whites, to commit violent depredations on the chastity of the female slaves; and these I was, though with reluctance, obliged to submit to at all times, being unable to help them. When we have had some of these slaves on board my master's vessels to carry them to other islands, or to America, I have known our mates to commit these acts most shamefully, to the disgrace, not of Christians only, but of men. I have even known them gratify their brutal passion with females not ten years old; and these abominations some of them practised to such scandalous excess, that one of our captains discharged the mate and others on that account. And yet in Montserrat I have seen a negro man staked to the ground, and cut most shockingly, and then his ears cut off bit by bit, because he had been connected with a white woman who was a common prostitute: as if it were no crime in the whites to rob an innocent African girl of her virtue; but most heinous in a black man only to gratify a passion of nature, where the temptation was offered by one of a different colour, though the most abandoned woman of her species. Another negro man was half hanged, and then burnt, for attempting to poison a cruel overseer. Thus by repeated cruelties are the wretched first urged to despair, and then murdered, because they still retain so much of human nature about them as to wish to put an end to their misery, and retaliate on their tyrants! These overseers are indeed for the most part persons of the worst character of any denomination of men in the West Indies. Unfortunately, many humane gentlemen, by not residing on their estates, are obliged to leave the management of them in the hands of these human butchers, who cut and mangle the slaves in a shocking manner on the most trifling occasions, and altogether treat them in every respect like brutes. They pay no regard to the situation of pregnant women, nor the least attention to the lodging of the field negroes. Their huts, which ought to be well covered, and the place dry where they take their little repose, are often open sheds, built in damp places; so that, when the poor creatures return tired from the toils of the field, they contract many disorders, from being exposed to the damp air in this uncomfortable state, while they are heated, and their pores are open. This neglect certainly conspires with many others to cause a decrease in the births as well as in the lives of the grown negroes. I can quote many instances of gentlemen who reside on their estates in the West Indies, and then the scene is quite changed; the negroes are treated with lenity and proper care, by which their lives are prolonged, and their masters are profited. To the honour of humanity, I knew several gentlemen who managed their estates in this manner; and they found that benevolence was their true interest. And, among many I could mention in several of the islands, I knew one in Montserrat* whose slaves looked remarkably well, and never needed any fresh supplies of negroes; and there are many other estates, especially in Barbadoes, which, from such judicious treatment, need no fresh stock of negroes at any time. I have the honour of knowing a most worthy and humane gentleman, who is a native of Barbadoes, and has estates there†. This gentleman has written a treatise on the usage of his own slaves. He allows them two hours for refreshment at mid-day; and many other indulgencies and comforts, particularly in their lying; and, besides this, he raises more provisions on his estate than they can destroy; so that by these attentions he saves the lives of his negroes, and keeps them healthy, and as happy as the condition of slavery can admit. I myself, as shall appear in the sequel, managed an estate, where, by those attentions, the negroes were uncommonly cheerful and healthy, and did more work by half than by the common mode of treatment they usually do. For want, therefore, of such care and attention to the poor negroes, and otherwise oppressed as they are, it is no wonder that the decrease should require 20,000 new negroes annually to fill up the vacant places of the dead.

*Mr. Dubury, and many others, Montserrat.
†Sir Philip Gibbes, Baronet, Barbadoes.

Even in Barbadoes, notwithstanding those humane exceptions which I have mentioned, and others I am acquainted with, which justly make it quoted as a place where slaves meet with the best treatment, and need fewest recruits of any in the West Indies, yet this island requires 1000 negroes annually to keep up the original stock, which is only 80,000. So that the whole term of a negro's life may be said to be there but sixteen years!* And yet the climate here is in every respect the same as that from which they are taken, except in being more wholesome. Do the British colonies decrease in this manner? And yet what a prodigious difference is there between an English and West India climate?

While I was in Montserrat I knew a negro man, named Emanuel Sankey, who endeavoured to escape from his miserable bondage, by concealing himself on board of a London ship: but fate did not favour the poor oppressed man; for, being discovered when the vessel was under sail, he was delivered up again to his master. This *Christian master* immediately pinned the wretch down to the ground at each wrist and ancle, and then took some sticks of sealing wax, and lighted them, and droped it all over his back. There was another master who was noted for cruelty; and I believe he had not a slave but what had been cut, and had pieces fairly taken out of the flesh: and, after they had been punished thus, he used to make them get into a long wooden box or case he had for that purpose, in which he shut them up during pleasure. It was just about the height and breadth of a man; and the poor wretches had no room, when in the case, to move.

It was very common in several of the islands, particularly in St. Kitt's, for the slaves to be branded with the initial letters of their master's name; and a load of heavy iron hooks hung about their necks. Indeed on the most trifling occasions they were loaded with chains; and often instruments of torture were added. The iron muzzle, thumb-screws, &c. are so well known, as not to need a description, and were sometimes applied for the slightest faults. I have seen a negro beaten till some of his bones were broken, for even letting a pot boil over. Is it surprising that usage like this should drive the poor

*Benezet's Account of Guinea, p. 16.

creatures to despair, and make them seek a refuge in death from those evils which render their lives intolerable—while,

> "With shudd'ring horror pale, and eyes aghast,
> They view their lamentable lot, and find
> No rest!"

This they frequently do. A negro-man on board a vessel of my master, while I belonged to her, having been put in irons for some trifling misdemeanor, and kept in that state for some days, being weary of life, took an opportunity of jumping overboard into the sea; however, he was picked up without being drowned. Another, whose life was also a burden to him, resolved to starve himself to death, and refused to eat any victuals; this procured him a severe flogging: and he also, on the first occasion which offered, jumped overboard at Charles Town, but was saved.

Nor is there any greater regard shewn to the little property than there is to the persons and lives of the negroes. I have already related an instance or two of particular oppression out of many which I have witnessed; but the following is frequent in all the islands. The wretched field-slaves, after toiling all the day for an unfeeling owner, who gives them but little victuals, steal sometimes a few moments from rest or refreshment to gather some small portion of grass, according as their time will admit. This they commonly tie up in a parcel; (either a bit, worth six pence; or half a bit's-worth) and bring it to town, or to the market, to sell. Nothing is more common than for the white people on this occasion to take the grass from them without paying for it; and not only so, but too often also, to my knowledge, our clerks, and many others, at the same time have committed acts of violence on the poor, wretched, and helpless females; whom I have seen for hours stand crying to no purpose, and get no redress or pay of any kind. Is not this one common and crying sin enough to bring down God's judgment on the islands? He tells us the oppressor and the oppressed are both in his hands; and if these are not the poor, the broken-hearted, the blind, the captive, the bruised, which our Saviour speaks of, who are they? One of these depredators once, in St. Eustatia, came on board of our vessel, and bought some fowls and pigs of me; and a whole day after his departure with the things he returned again and wanted his money back: I refused to give it; and, not seeing my captain on board, he began the common pranks with me; and swore he would even break open my chest and take my money. I therefore expected, as my captain was absent, that he would be as good as his word: and he was just proceeding to strike me, when fortunately a British seaman on board, whose heart had not been debauched by a West India climate, interposed and prevented him. But had the cruel man struck me I certainly should have defended myself at the hazard of my life; for what is life to a man thus oppressed? He went away, however, swearing; and threatened that whenever he caught me on shore he would shoot me, and pay for me afterwards.

The small account in which the life of a negro is held in the West Indies is so universally known, that it might seem impertinent to quote the following extract, if some people had not been hardy enough of late to assert that negroes are on the same footing in that respect as Europeans. By the 329th Act, page 125, of the Assembly of Barbadoes, it is enacted 'That if any negro, or other slave, under punishment by his master, or his order, for running away, or any other crime or misdemeanor towards his said master, unfortunately shall suffer in life or member, no person whatsoever shall be liable to a fine; but if any man shall out of *wantonness, or only of bloody-mindedness, or cruel intention, wilfully kill a negro, or other slave, of his own, he shall pay into the public treasury fifteen pounds sterling.*' And it is the same in most, if not all, of the West India islands. Is not this one of the many acts of the islands which call loudly for redress? And do not the assembly which enacted it deserve the appellation of savages and brutes rather than of Christians and men? It is an act at once unmerciful, unjust, and unwise; which for cruelty would disgrace an assembly of those who are called barbarians; and for its injustice and *insanity* would shock the morality and common sense of a Samaide or a Hottentot.

Shocking as this and many more acts of the bloody West India code at first view appear, how is the iniquity of it heightened when we consider to whom it may be extended! Mr. James Tobin, a zealous labourer in the vineyard of slavery, gives an account of a French planter of his acquaintance, in the island of Martinico, who shewed him many mulattoes working in the fields like beasts of burden; and he told Mr. Tobin these were all the produce of his own loins! And I myself have known similar instances. Pray, reader, are these sons and daughters of the French planter less his children by being begotten on a black woman? And what must be the virtue of those legislators, and the feelings of those fathers, who estimate the lives of their sons, however begotten, at no more than fifteen pounds; though they should be murdered, as the act says, *out of wantonness and bloody-mindedness!* But is not the slave trade entirely a war with the heart of man? And surely that which is begun by breaking down the barriers of virtue involves in its continuance destruction to every principle, and buries all sentiments in ruin!

I have often seen slaves, particularly those who were meagre, in different islands, put into scales and weighed; and then sold from three pence to six pence or nine pence a pound. My master, however, whose humanity was shocked at this mode, used to sell such by the lump. And at or after a sale it was not uncommon to see negroes taken from their wives, wives taken from their husbands, and children from their parents, and sent off to other islands, and wherever else their merciless lords chose; and probably never more during life to see each other! Oftentimes my heart has bled at these partings; when the friends of the departed have been at the water side, and, with sighs and tears, have kept their eyes fixed on the vessel till it went out of sight.

A poor Creole negro I knew well, who, after having been often thus transported from island to island, at last resided in Montserrat. This man used to tell me many melancholy tales of himself. Generally, after he had done working for his master, he used to employ his few leisure moments to go a fishing. When he had caught any fish, his master would frequently take them from him without paying him; and at other times some other white people would serve him in the same manner. One day he said to me, very movingly, 'Sometimes when a white man take away my fish I go to my maser, and he get me my right; and when my maser by strength take away my fishes, what me must do? I can't go to any body to be righted; then' said the poor man, looking up above 'I must look up to God Mighty in the top for right.' This artless tale moved me much, and I could not help feeling the just cause Moses had in redressing his brother against the Egyptian. I exhorted the man to look up still to the God on the top, since there was no redress below. Though I little thought then that I myself should more than once experience such imposition, and read the same exhortation hereafter, in my own transactions in the islands; and that even this poor man and I should some time after suffer together in the same manner, as shall be related hereafter.

Nor was such usage as this confined to particular places or individuals; for, in all the different islands in which I have been (and I have visited no less than fifteen) the treatment of the slaves was nearly the same; so nearly indeed, that the history of an island, or even a plantation, with a few such exceptions as I have mentioned, might serve for a history of the whole. Such a tendency has the slave-trade to debauch men's minds, and harden them to every feeling of humanity! For I will not suppose that the dealers in slaves are born worse than other men—No; it is the fatality of this mistaken avarice, that it corrupts the milk of human kindness and turns it into gall. And, had the pursuits of those men been different, they might have been as generous, as tender-hearted and just, as they are unfeeling, rapacious and cruel. Surely this traffic cannot be good, which spreads like a pestilence, and taints what it touches! which violates that first natural right of mankind, equality and independency, and gives one man a dominion over his fellows which God could never intend! For it raises the owner to a state as far above man as it depresses the slave below it; and, with all the presumption of human pride, sets a distinction between them, immeasurable in extent, and endless in duration! Yet how mistaken is the avarice even of the planters? Are slaves more useful by being thus humbled to the condition of brutes, than they would be if suffered to enjoy the privileges of men? The freedom which diffuses health and prosperity throughout Britain answers you—No. When you make men slaves you deprive them of half their virtue, you set them in your own conduct an example of fraud, rapine, and cruelty, and compel them to live with you in a state of war;

and yet you complain that they are not honest or faithful! You stupify them with stripes, and think it necessary to keep them in a state of ignorance; and yet you assert that they are incapable of learning; that their minds are such a barren soil or moor, that culture would be lost on them; and that they come from a climate, where nature, though prodigal of her bounties in a degree unknown to yourselves, has left man alone scant and unfinished, and incapable of enjoying the treasures she has poured out for him!—An assertion at once impious and absurd. Why do you use those instruments of torture? Are they fit to be applied by one rational being to another? And are ye not struck with shame and mortification, to see the partakers of your nature reduced so low? But, above all, are there no dangers attending this mode of treatment? Are you not hourly in dread of an insurrection? Nor would it be surprising: for when

> "——No peace is given
>   To us enslav'd, but custody severe;
>   And stripes and arbitrary punishment
>   Inflicted—What peace can we return?
>   But to our power, hostility and hate;
>   Untam'd reluctance, and revenge, though slow,
>   Yet ever plotting how the conqueror least
>   May reap his conquest, and may least rejoice
>   In doing what we most in suffering feel."

But by changing your conduct, and treating your slaves as men, every cause of fear would be banished. They would be faithful, honest, intelligent and vigorous; and peace, prosperity, and happiness, would attend you.

CHAP. VI.

Some account of Brimstone-Hill in Montserrat—Favourable change in the author's situation—He commences merchant with three pence—His various success in dealing in the different islands, and America, and the impositions he meets with in his transactions with Europeans—A curious imposition on human nature—Danger of the surfs in the West Indies—Remarkable instance of kidnapping a free mulatto —The author is nearly murdered by Doctor Perkins in Savannah.

In the preceding chapter I have set before the reader a few of those many instances of oppression, extortion, and cruelty, which I have been a witness to in the West Indies: but, were I to enumerate them all, the catalogue would be tedious and disgusting. The punishments of the slaves on every trifling occasion are so frequent, and so well known, together with the different instruments with which they are tortured, that it cannot any longer afford novelty to recite them; and they are too shocking to yield delight either to the writer or the reader. I shall therefore hereafter only mention such as incidentally befel myself in the course of my adventures.

In the variety of departments in which I was employed by my master, I had an opportunity of seeing many curious scenes in different islands; but, above all, I was struck with a celebrated curiosity called Brimstone-Hill, which is a high and steep mountain, some few miles from the town of Plymouth in Montserrat. I had often heard of some wonders that were to be seen on this hill, and I went once with some white and black people to visit it. When we arrived at the top, I saw under different cliffs great flakes of brimstone, occasioned by the steams of various little ponds, which were then boiling naturally in the earth. Some of these ponds were as white as milk, some quite blue, and many others of different colours. I had taken some potatoes with me, and I put them into different ponds, and in a few minutes they were well boiled. I tasted some of them, but they were very sulphurous; and the silver shoe buckles, and all the other things of that metal we had among us, were, in a little time, turned as black as lead.

Some time in the year 1763 kind Providence seemed to appear rather more favourable to me. One of my master's vessels, a Bermudas sloop, about sixty tons, was commanded by one Captain Thomas Farmer, an Englishman, a very alert and active man, who gained my master a great deal of money by his good management in carrying passengers from one island to another; but very often his sailors used to get drunk and run away from the vessel, which hindered him in his business very much. This man had taken a liking to me; and many different times begged of my master to let me go a trip with him as a sailor; but he would tell him he could not spare me, though the vessel sometimes could not go for want of hands, for sailors were generally very scarce in the island. However, at last, from necessity or force, my master was prevailed on, though very reluctantly, to let me go with this captain; but he gave great charge to him to take care that I did not run away, for if I did he would make him pay for me. This being the case, the captain had for some time a sharp eye upon me whenever the vessel anchored; and as soon as she returned I was sent for on shore again. Thus was I slaving as it were for life, sometimes at one thing, and sometimes at another; so that the captain and I were nearly the most useful men in my master's employment. I also became so useful to the captain on shipboard, that many times, when he used to ask for me to go with him, though it should be but for twenty-four hours, to some of the islands near us, my master would answer he could not spare me, at which the captain would swear, and would not go the trip; and tell my master I was better to him on board than any three white men he had; for they used to behave ill in many respects, particularly in getting drunk; and then they frequently got the boat stove, so as to hinder the vessel from coming back as soon as she might have done. This my master knew very well; and at last, by the captain's constant entreaties, after I had been several times with him, one day, to my great joy, my master told me the captain would not let him rest, and asked me whether I would go aboard as a sailor, or stay on shore and mind the stores, for he could not bear any longer to be plagued in this manner. I was very happy at this proposal, for I immediately thought I might in time stand some chance by being on board to get a little money, or possibly make my escape if I should be used ill: I also expected to get better food, and in greater abundance; for I had felt much hunger oftentimes, though my master treated his slaves, as I have observed, uncommonly well. I therefore, without hesitation, answered him, that I would go and be a sailor if he pleased. Accordingly I was ordered on board directly. Nevertheless, between the vessel and the shore, when she was in port, I had little or no rest, as my master always wished to have me along with him. Indeed he was a very pleasant gentleman, and but for my expectations on shipboard I should not have thought of leaving him. But the captain liked me also very much, and I was entirely his right-hand man. I did all I could to deserve his favour, and in return I received better treatment from him than any other I believe ever met with in the West Indies in my situation.

After I had been sailing for some time with this captain, at length I endeavoured to try my luck and commence merchant. I had but a very small capital to begin with; for one single half bit, which is equal to three pence in England, made up my whole stock. However I trusted to the Lord to be with me; and at one of our trips to St. Eustatia, a Dutch island, I bought a glass tumbler with my half bit, and when I came to Montserrat I sold it for a bit, or sixpence. Luckily we made several successive trips to St. Eustatia (which was a general mart for the West Indies, about twenty leagues from Montserrat); and in our next, finding my tumbler so profitable, with this one bit I bought two tumblers more; and when I came back I sold them for two bits, equal to a shilling sterling. When we went again I bought with these two bits four more of these glasses, which I sold for four bits on our return to Montserrat; and in our next voyage to St. Eustatia I bought two glasses with one bit, and with the other three I bought a jug of Geneva, nearly about three pints in measure. When we came to Montserrat I sold the gin for eight bits, and the tumblers for two, so that my capital now amounted in all to a dollar, well husbanded and acquired in the space of a month or six weeks, when I blessed the Lord that I was so rich. As we sailed to different islands, I laid this money out in various things occasionally, and it used to turn out to very good account, especially when we went to Guadaloupe, Grenada, and the rest of the French islands. Thus was I going all about the islands upwards of four years, and ever trading as I went, during which I experienced many instances of ill usage, and have seen many injuries done to other negroes in our dealings with Europeans: and, amidst our recreations, when we have been dancing and merry-making, they, without cause, have molested and insulted us. Indeed I was more than once obliged to look up to God on high, as I had advised the poor fisherman some time before. And I had not been long trading for myself in the manner I have related above, when I experienced the like trial in company with him as follows: This man being used to the water, was upon an emergency put on board of us by his master to work as another hand, on a voyage to Santa Cruz; and at our sailing he had brought his little all for a venture, which consisted of six bits' worth of limes and oranges in a bag; I had also my whole stock, which was about twelve bits' worth of the same kind of goods, separate in two bags; for we had heard these fruits sold well in that island. When we came there, in some little convenient time he and I went ashore with our fruits to sell them; but we had scarcely landed when we were met by two white men, who presently took our three bags from us. We could not at first guess what they meant to do; and for some time we thought they were jesting with us; but they too soon let us know otherwise, for they took our ventures immediately to a house hard by, and adjoining the fort, while we followed all the way begging of them to give us our fruits, but in vain. They not only refused to return them, but swore at us, and threatened if we did not immediately depart they would flog us well. We told them these three bags were all we were worth in the world, and that we brought them with us to sell when we came from Montserrat, and shewed them the vessel. But this was rather against us, as they now saw we were strangers as well as slaves. They still therefore swore, and desired us to be gone, and even took sticks to beat us; while we, seeing they meant what they said, went off in the greatest confusion and despair. Thus, in the very minute of gaining more by three times than I ever did by any venture in my life before, was I deprived of every farthing I was worth. An insupportable misfortune! but how to help ourselves we knew not. In our consternation we went to the commanding officer of the fort and told him how we had been served by some of his people; but we obtained not the least redress: he answered our complaints only by a volley of imprecations against us, and immediately took a horse-whip, in order to chastise us, so that we were obliged to turn out much faster than we came in. I now, in the agony of distress and indignation, wished that the ire of God in his forked lightning might transfix these cruel oppressors among the dead. Still however we persevered; went back again to the house, and begged and besought them again and again for our fruits, till at last some other people that were in the house asked if we would be contented if they kept one bag and gave us the other two. We, seeing no remedy whatever, consented to this; and they, observing one bag to have both kinds of fruit in it, which belonged to my companion, kept that; and the other two, which were mine, they gave us back. As soon as I got them, I ran as fast as I could, and got the first negro man I could to help me off; my companion, however, stayed a little longer to plead; he told them the bag they had was his, and likewise all that he was worth in the world; but this was of no avail, and he was obliged to return without it. The poor old man, wringing his hands, cried bitterly for his loss; and, indeed, he then did look up to God on high, which so moved me with pity for him, that I gave him nearly one third of my fruits. We then proceeded to the markets to sell them; and Providence was more favourable to us than we could have expected, for we sold our fruits uncommonly well; I got for mine about thirty-seven bits. Such a surprising reverse of fortune in so short a space of time seemed like a dream to me, and proved no small encouragement for me to trust the Lord in any situation. My captain afterwards frequently used to take my part, and get me my right, when I have been plundered or used ill by these tender Christian depredators; among whom I have shuddered to observe the unceasing blasphemous execrations which are wantonly thrown out by persons of all ages and conditions, not only without occasion, but even as if they were indulgences and pleasure.

At one of our trips to St. Kitt's I had eleven bits of my own; and my friendly captain lent me five bits more, with which I bought a Bible. I was very glad to get this book, which I scarcely could meet with any where. I think there was none sold in Montserrat; and, much to my grief, from being forced out of the Ætna in the manner I have related, my Bible, and the Guide to the Indians, the two books I loved above all others, were left behind.

While I was in this place, St. Kitt's, a very curious imposition on human nature took place:—A white man wanted to marry in the church a free black woman that had land and slaves in Montserrat: but the clergyman told him it was against the law of the place to marry a white and a black in the church. The man then asked to be married on the water, to which the parson consented, and the two lovers went in one boat, and the parson and clerk in another, and thus the ceremony was performed. After this the loving pair came on board our vessel, and my captain treated them extremely well, and brought them safe to Montserrat.

The reader cannot but judge of the irksomeness of this situation to a mind like mine, in being daily exposed to new hardships and impositions, after having seen many better days, and having been as it were in a state of freedom and plenty; added to which, every part of the world I had hitherto been in seemed to me a paradise in comparison of the West Indies. My mind was therefore hourly replete with inventions and thoughts of being freed, and, if possible, by honest and honourable means; for I always remembered the old adage; and I trust it has ever been my ruling principle, that honesty is the best policy; and likewise that other golden precept—to do unto all men as I would they should do unto me. However, as I was from early years a predestinarian, I thought whatever fate had determined must ever come to pass; and therefore, if ever it were my lot to be freed nothing could prevent me, although I should at present see no means or hope to obtain my freedom; on the other hand, if it were my fate not to be freed I never should be so, and all my endeavours for that purpose would be fruitless. In the midst of these thoughts I therefore looked up with prayers anxiously to God for my liberty; and at the same time I used every honest means, and endeavoured all that was possible on my part to obtain it. In process of time I became master of a few pounds, and in a fair way of making more, which my friendly captain knew very well; this occasioned him sometimes to take liberties with me: but whenever he treated me waspishly I used plainly to tell him my mind, and that I would die before I would be imposed on as other negroes were, and that to me life had lost its relish when liberty was gone. This I said although I foresaw my then well-being or future hopes of freedom (humanly speaking) depended on this man. However, as he could not bear the thoughts of my not sailing with him, he always became mild on my threats. I therefore continued with him; and, from my great attention to his orders and his business, I gained him credit, and through his kindness to me I at last procured my liberty. While I thus went on, filled with the thoughts of freedom, and resisting oppression as well as I was able, my life hung daily in suspense, particularly in the surfs I have formerly mentioned, as I could not swim. These are extremely violent throughout the West Indies, and I was ever exposed to their howling rage and devouring fury in all the islands. I have seen them strike and toss a boat right up an end, and maim several on board. Once in the Grenada islands, when I and about eight others were pulling a large boat with two puncheons of water in it, a surf struck us, and drove the boat and all in it about half a stone's throw, among some trees, and above the high water mark. We were obliged to get all the assistance we could from the nearest estate to mend the boat, and launch it into the water again. At Montserrat one night, in pressing hard to get off the shore on board, the punt was overset with us four times; the first time I was very near being drowned; however the jacket I had on kept me up above water a little space of time, while I called on a man near me who was a good swimmer, and told him I could not swim; he then made haste to me, and, just as I was sinking, he caught hold of me, and brought me to sounding, and then he went and brought the punt also. As soon as we had turned the water out of her, lest we should be used ill for being absent, we attempted again three times more, and as often the horrid surfs served us as at first; but at last, the fifth time we attempted, we gained our point, at the imminent hazard of our lives. One day also, at Old Road in Montserrat, our captain, and three men besides myself, were going in a large canoe in quest of rum and sugar, when a single surf tossed the canoe an amazing distance from the water, and some of us even a stone's throw from each other: most of us were very much bruised; so that I and many more often said, and really thought, that there was not such another place under the heavens as this. I longed therefore much to leave it, and daily wished to see my master's promise performed of going to Philadelphia. While we lay in this place a very cruel thing happened on board of our sloop which filled me with horror; though I found afterwards such practices were frequent. There was a very clever and decent free young mulatto-man who sailed a long time with us: he had a free woman for his wife, by whom he had a child; and she was then living on shore, and all very happy. Our captain and mate, and other people on board, and several elsewhere, even the natives of Bermudas, all knew this young man from a child that he was always free, and no one had ever claimed him as their property: however, as might too often overcomes right in these parts, it happened that a Bermudas captain, whose vessel lay there for a few days in the road, came on board of us, and seeing the mulatto-man, whose name was Joseph Clipson, he told him he was not free, and that he had orders from his master to bring him to Bermudas. The poor man could not believe the captain to be in earnest; but he was very soon undeceived, his men laying violent hands on him: and although he shewed a certificate of his being born free in St. Kitt's, and most people on board knew that he served his time to boatbuilding, and always passed for a free man, yet he was taken forcibly out of our vessel. He then asked to be carried ashore before the secretary or magistrates, and these infernal invaders of human rights promised him he should; but, instead of that, they carried him on board of the other vessel: and the next day, without giving the poor man any hearing on shore, or suffering him even to see his wife or child, he was carried away, and probably doomed never more in this world to see them again. Nor was this the only instance of this kind of barbarity I was a witness to. I have since often seen in Jamaica and other islands free men, whom I have known in America, thus villainously trepanned and held in bondage. I have heard of two similar practices even in Philadelphia: and were it not for the benevolence of the quakers in that city many of the sable race, who now breathe the air of liberty, would, I believe, be groaning indeed under some planter's chains. These things opened my mind to a new scene of horror to which I had been before a stranger. Hitherto I had thought only slavery dreadful; but the state of a free negro appeared to me now equally so at least, and in some respects even worse, for they live in constant alarm for their liberty; and even this is but nominal, for they are universally insulted and plundered without the possibility of redress; for such is the equity of the West Indian laws, that no free negro's evidence will be admitted in their courts of justice. In this situation is it surprising that slaves, when mildly treated, should prefer even the misery of slavery to such a mockery of freedom? I was now completely disgusted with the West Indies, and thought I never should be entirely free until I had left them.

> "With thoughts like these my anxious boding mind
> Recall'd those pleasing scenes I left behind;
> Scenes where fair Liberty in bright array
> Makes darkness bright, and e'en illumines day;
> Where nor complexion, wealth, or station, can
> Protect the wretch who makes a slave of man."

I determined to make every exertion to obtain my freedom, and to return to Old England. For this purpose I thought a knowledge of navigation might be of use to me; for, though I did not intend to run away unless I should be ill used, yet, in such a case, if I understood navigation, I might attempt my escape in our sloop, which was one of the swiftest sailing vessels in the West Indies, and I could be at no loss for hands to join me: and if I should make this attempt, I had intended to have gone for England; but this, as I said, was only to be in the event of my meeting with any ill usage. I therefore employed the mate of our vessel to teach me navigation, for which I agreed to give him twenty-four dollars, and actually paid him part of the money down; though when the captain, some time after, came to know that the mate was to have such a sum for teaching me, he rebuked him, and said it was a shame for him to take any money from me. However, my progress in this useful art was much retarded by the constancy of our work. Had I wished to run away I did not want opportunities, which frequently presented themselves; and particularly at one time, soon after this. When we were at the island of Gaurdeloupe there was a large fleet of merchantmen bound for Old France; and, seamen then being very scarce, they gave from fifteen to twenty pounds a man for the run. Our mate, and all the white sailors, left our vessel on this account, and went on board of the French ships. They would have had me also to go with them, for they regarded me; and they swore to protect me, if I would go: and, as the fleet was to sail the next day, I really believe I could have got safe to Europe at that time. However, as my master was kind, I would not attempt to leave him; and, remembering the old maxim, that 'honesty is the best policy,' I suffered them to go without me. Indeed my captain was much afraid of my leaving him and the vessel at that time, as I had so fair an opportunity: but, I thank God, this fidelity of mine turned out much to my advantage hereafter, when I did not in the least think of it; and made me so much in favour with the captain, that he used now and then to teach me some parts of navigation himself: but some of our passengers, and others, seeing this, found much fault with him for it, saying it was a very dangerous thing to let a negro know navigation; thus I was hindered again in my pursuits. About the latter end of the year 1764 my master bought a larger sloop, called the Providence, about seventy or eighty tons, of which my captain had the command. I went with him into this vessel, and we took a load of new slaves for Georgia and Charles Town. My master now left me entirely to the captain, though he still wished for me to be with him; but I, who always much wished to lose sight of the West Indies, was not a little rejoiced at the thoughts of seeing any other country. Therefore, relying on the goodness of my captain, I got ready all the little venture I could; and, when the vessel was ready, we sailed, to my great joy. When we got to our destined places, Georgia and Charles Town, I expected I should have an opportunity of selling my little property to advantage: but here, particularly in Charles Town, I met with buyers, white men, who imposed on me as in other places. Notwithstanding, I was resolved to have fortitude; thinking no lot or trial is too hard when kind Heaven is the rewarder. We soon got loaded again, and returned to Montserrat; and there, amongst the rest of the islands, I sold my goods well; and in this manner I continued trading during the year 1764; meeting with various scenes of imposition, as usual. After this, my master fitted out his vessel for Philadelphia, in the year 1765; and during the time we were loading her, and getting ready for the voyage, I worked with redoubled alacrity, from the hope of getting money enough by these voyages to buy my freedom in time, if it should please God; and also to see the town of Philadelphia, which I had heard a great deal about for some years past; besides which, I had always longed to prove my master's promise the first day I came to him. In the midst of these elevated ideas, and while I was about getting my little merchandize in readiness, one Sunday my master sent for me to his house. When I came there I found him and the captain together; and, on my going in, I was struck with astonishment at his telling me he heard that I meant to run away from him when I got to Philadelphia: 'And therefore,' said he, 'I must sell you again: you cost me a great deal of money, no less than forty pounds sterling; and it will not do to lose so much. You are a valuable fellow,' continued he; 'and I can get any day for you one hundred guineas, from many gentlemen in this island.' And then he told me of Captain Doran's brother-in-law, a severe master, who ever wanted to buy me to make me his overseer. My captain also said he could get much more than a hundred guineas for me in Carolina. This I knew to be a fact; for the gentleman that wanted to buy me came off several times on board of us, and spoke to me to live with him, and said he would use me well. When I asked what work he would put me to he said, as I was a sailor, he would make me a captain of one of his rice vessels. But I refused: and fearing, at the same time, by a sudden turn I saw in the captain's temper, he might mean to sell me, I told the gentleman I would not live with him on any condition, and that I certainly would run away with his vessel: but he said he did not fear that, as he would catch me again; and then he told me how cruelly he would serve me if I should do so. My captain, however, gave him to understand that I knew something of navigation: so he thought better of it; and, to my great joy, he went away. I now told my master I did not say I would run away in Philadelphia; neither did I mean it, as he did not use me ill, nor yet the captain: for if they did I certainly would have made some attempts before now; but as I thought that if it were God's will I ever should be freed it would be so, and, on the contrary, if it was not his will it would not happen; so I hoped, if ever I were freed, whilst I was used well, it should be by honest means; but, as I could not help myself, he must do as he pleased; I could only hope and trust to the God of Heaven; and at that instant my mind was big with inventions and full of schemes to escape. I then appealed to the captain whether he ever saw any sign of my making the least attempt to run away; and asked him if I did not always come on board according to the time for which he gave me liberty; and, more particularly, when all our men left us at Gaurdeloupe and went on board of the French fleet, and advised me to go with them, whether I might not, and that he could not have got me again. To my no small surprise, and very great joy, the captain confirmed every syllable that I had said: and even more; for he said he had tried different times to see if I would make any attempt of this kind, both at St. Eustatia and in America, and he never found that I made the smallest; but, on the contrary, I always came on board according to his orders; and he did really believe, if I ever meant to run away, that, as I could never have had a better opportunity, I would have done it the night the mate and all the people left our vessel at Gaurdeloupe. The captain then informed my master, who had been thus imposed on by our mate, though I did not know who was my enemy, the reason the mate had for imposing this lie upon him; which was, because I had acquainted the captain of the provisions the mate had given away or taken out of the vessel. This speech of the captain was like life to the dead to me, and instantly my soul glorified God; and still more so on hearing my master immediately say that I was a sensible fellow, and he never did intend to use me as a common slave; and that but for the entreaties of the captain, and his character of me, he would not have let me go from the stores about as I had done; that also, in so doing, he thought by carrying one little thing or other to different places to sell I might make money. That he also intended to encourage me in this by crediting me with half a puncheon of rum and half a hogshead of sugar at a time; so that, from being careful, I might have money enough, in some time, to purchase my freedom; and, when that was the case, I might depend upon it he would let me have it for forty pounds sterling money, which was only the same price he gave for me. This sound gladdened my poor heart beyond measure; though indeed it was no more than the very idea I had formed in my mind of my master long before, and I immediately made him this reply: 'Sir, I always had that very thought of you, indeed I had, and that made me so diligent in serving you.' He then gave me a large piece of silver coin, such as I never had seen or had before, and told me to get ready for the voyage, and he would credit me with a tierce of sugar, and another of rum; he also said that he had two amiable sisters in Philadelphia, from whom I might get some necessary things. Upon this my noble captain desired me to go aboard; and, knowing the African metal, he charged me not to say any thing of this matter to any body; and he promised that the lying mate should not go with him any more. This was a change indeed; in the same hour to feel the most exquisite pain, and in the turn of a moment the fullest joy. It caused in me such sensations as I was only able to express in my looks; my heart was so overpowered with gratitude that I could have kissed both of their feet. When I left the room I immediately went, or rather flew, to the vessel, which being loaded, my master, as good as his word, trusted me with a tierce of rum, and another of sugar, when we sailed, and arrived safe at the elegant town of Philadelphia. I soon sold my goods here pretty well; and in this charming place I found every thing plentiful and cheap.

While I was in this place a very extraordinary occurrence befell me. I had been told one evening of a *wise* woman, a Mrs. Davis, who revealed secrets, foretold events, &c. I put little faith in this story at first, as I could not conceive that any mortal could foresee the future disposals of Providence, nor did I believe in any other revelation than that of the Holy Scriptures; however, I was greatly astonished at seeing this woman in a dream that night, though a person I never before beheld in my life; this made such an impression on me, that I could not get the idea the next day out of my mind, and I then became as anxious to see her as I was before indifferent; accordingly in the evening, after we left off working, I inquired where she lived, and being directed to her, to my inexpressible surprise, beheld the very woman in the very same dress she appeared to me to wear in the vision. She immediately told me I had dreamed of her the preceding night; related to me many things that had happened with a correctness that astonished me; and finally told me I should not be long a slave: this was the more agreeable news, as I believed it the more readily from her having so faithfully related the past incidents of my life. She said I should be twice in very great danger of my life within eighteen months, which, if I escaped, I should afterwards go on well; so, giving me her blessing, we parted. After staying here some time till our vessel was loaded, and I had bought in my little traffic, we sailed from this agreeable spot for Montserrat, once more to encounter the raging surfs.

We arrived safe at Montserrat, where we discharged our cargo; and soon after that we took slaves on board for St. Eustatia, and from thence to Georgia. I had always exerted myself and did double work, in order to make our voyages as short as possible; and from thus overworking myself while we were at Georgia I caught a fever and ague. I was very ill for eleven days and near dying; eternity was now exceedingly impressed on my mind, and I feared very much that awful event. I prayed the Lord therefore to spare me; and I made a promise in my mind to God, that I would be good if ever I should recover. At length, from having an eminent doctor to attend me, I was restored again to health; and soon after we got the vessel loaded, and set off for Montserrat. During the passage, as I was perfectly restored, and had much business of the vessel to mind, all my endeavours to keep up my integrity, and perform my promise to God, began to fail; and, in spite of all I could do, as we drew nearer and nearer to the islands, my resolutions more and more declined, as if the very air of that country or climate seemed fatal to piety. When we were safe arrived at Montserrat, and I had got ashore, I forgot my former resolutions.—Alas! how prone is the heart to leave that God it wishes to love! and how strongly do the things of this world strike the senses and captivate the soul!—After our vessel was discharged, we soon got her ready, and took in, as usual, some of the poor oppressed natives of Africa, and other negroes; we then set off again for Georgia and Charlestown. We arrived at Georgia, and, having landed part of our cargo, proceeded to Charlestown with the remainder. While we were there I saw the town illuminated; the guns were fired, and bonfires and other demonstrations of joy shewn, on account of the repeal of the stamp act. Here I disposed of some goods on my own account; the white men buying them with smooth promises and fair words, giving me however but very indifferent payment. There was one gentleman particularly who bought a puncheon of rum of me, which gave me a great deal of trouble; and, although I used the interest of my friendly captain, I could not obtain any thing for it; for, being a negro man, I could not oblige him to pay me. This vexed me much, not knowing how to act; and I lost some time in seeking after this Christian; and though, when the Sabbath came (which the negroes usually make their holiday) I was much inclined to go to public worship, I was obliged to hire some black men to help to pull a boat across the water to God in quest of this gentleman. When I found him, after much entreaty, both from myself and my worthy captain, he at last paid me in dollars; some of them, however, were copper, and of consequence of no value; but he took advantage of my being a negro man, and obliged me to put up with those or none, although I objected to them. Immediately after, as I was trying to pass them in the market, amongst other white men, I was abused for offering to pass bad coin; and, though I shewed them the man I got them from, I was within one minute of being tied up and flogged without either judge or jury; however, by the help of a good pair of heels, I ran off, and so escaped the bastinadoes I should have received. I got on board as fast as I could, but still continued in fear of them until we sailed, which I thanked God we did not long after; and I have never been amongst them since.

We soon came to Georgia, where we were to complete our lading; and here worse fate than ever attended me: for one

Sunday night, as I was with some negroes in their master's yard in the town of Savannah, it happened that their master, one Doctor Perkins, who was a very severe and cruel man, came in drunk; and, not liking to see any strange negroes in his yard, he and a ruffian of a white man he had in his service beset me in an instant, and both of them struck me with the first weapons they could get hold of. I cried out as long as I could for help and mercy; but, though I gave a good account of myself, and he knew my captain, who lodged hard by him, it was to no purpose. They beat and mangled me in a shameful manner, leaving me near dead. I lost so much blood from the wounds I received, that I lay quite motionless, and was so benumbed that I could not feel any thing for many hours. Early in the morning they took me away to the jail. As I did not return to the ship all night, my captain, not knowing where I was, and being uneasy that I did not then make my appearance, he made inquiry after me; and, having found where I was, immediately came to me. As soon as the good man saw me so cut and mangled, he could not forbear weeping; he soon got me out of jail to his lodgings, and immediately sent for the best doctors in the place, who at first declared it as their opinion that I could not recover. My captain on this went to all the lawyers in the town for their advice, but they told him they could do nothing for me as I was a negro. He then went to Doctor Perkins, the hero who had vanquished me, and menaced him, swearing he would be revenged of him, and challenged him to fight.—But cowardice is ever the companion of cruelty—and the Doctor refused. However, by the skilfulness of one Doctor Brady of that place, I began at last to amend; but, although I was so sore and bad with the wounds I had all over me that I could not rest in any posture, yet I was in more pain on account of the captain's uneasiness about me than I otherwise should have been. The worthy man nursed and watched me all the hours of the night; and I was, through his attention and that of the doctor, able to get out of bed in about sixteen or eighteen days. All this time I was very much wanted on board, as I used frequently to go up and down the river for rafts, and other parts of our cargo, and stow them when the mate was sick or absent. In about four weeks I was able to go on duty;

and in a fortnight after, having got in all our lading, our vessel set sail for Montserrat; and in less than three weeks we arrived there safe towards the end of the year. This ended my adventures in 1764; for I did not leave Montserrat again till the beginning of the following year.

END OF THE FIRST VOLUME.

They ran the ship aground: and the fore part stuck fast, and remained unmoveable, but the hinder part was broken with the violence of the waves. ACTS xxvii. 41.

Howbeit, we must be cast upon a certain island;
Wherefore, sirs, be of good cheer: for I believe God, that it shall be even as it was told me. ACTS xxvii. 26, 25.

Now a thing was secretly brought to me, and mine ear received a little thereof.
In thoughts from the visions of the night, when deep sleep falleth on men. JOB iv. 12, 13.

Lo, all these *things* worketh God oftentimes with man,
To bring back his soul from the pit, to be enlightened with the light of the living. JOB xxxiii. 29, 30.

CHAP. VII.

*The author's disgust at the West Indies—Forms schemes to ob-
tain his freedom—Ludicrous disappointment he and his Captain meet with in Georgia—At last, by several successful
voyages, he acquires a sum of money sufficient to purchase it—
Applies to his master, who accepts it, and grants his manumission, to his great joy—He afterwards enters as a freeman
on board one of Mr. King's ships, and sails for Georgia—Impositions on free negroes as usual—His venture of turkies—
Sails for Montserrat, and on his passage his friend, the Captain, falls ill and dies.*

EVERY DAY now brought me nearer my freedom, and I was
impatient till we proceeded again to sea, that I might have an
opportunity of getting a sum large enough to purchase it. I
was not long ungratified; for, in the beginning of the year
1766, my master bought another sloop, named the Nancy, the
largest I had ever seen. She was partly laden, and was to proceed to Philadelphia; our Captain had his choice of three, and
I was well pleased he chose this, which was the largest; for,
from his having a large vessel, I had more room, and could
carry a larger quantity of goods with me. Accordingly, when
we had delivered our old vessel, the Prudence, and completed
the lading of the Nancy, having made near three hundred per
cent. by four barrels of pork I brought from Charlestown, I
laid in as large a cargo as I could, trusting to God's providence to prosper my undertaking. With these views I sailed
for Philadelphia. On our passage, when we drew near the
land, I was for the first time surprised at the sight of some
whales, having never seen any such large sea monsters before;
and as we sailed by the land one morning I saw a puppy whale
close by the vessel; it was about the length of a wherry boat,
and it followed us all the day till we got within the Capes. We
arrived safe and in good time at Philadelphia, and I sold my
goods there chiefly to the quakers. They always appeared to

be a very honest discreet sort of people, and never attempted to impose on me; I therefore liked them, and ever after chose to deal with them in preference to any others. One Sunday morning while I was here, as I was going to church, I chanced to pass a meeting-house. The doors being open, and the house full of people, it excited my curiosity to go in. When I entered the house, to my great surprise, I saw a very tall woman standing in the midst of them, speaking in an audible voice something which I could not understand. Having never seen anything of this kind before, I stood and stared about me for some time, wondering at this odd scene. As soon as it was over I took an opportunity to make inquiry about the place and people, when I was informed they were called Quakers. I particularly asked what that woman I saw in the midst of them had said, but none of them were pleased to satisfy me; so I quitted them, and soon after, as I was returning, I came to a church crowded with people; the church-yard was full likewise, and a number of people were even mounted on ladders, looking in at the windows. I thought this a strange sight, as I had never seen churches, either in England or the West Indies, crowded in this manner before. I therefore made bold to ask some people the meaning of all this, and they told me the Rev. Mr. George Whitfield was preaching. I had often heard of this gentleman, and had wished to see and hear him; but I had never before had an opportunity. I now therefore resolved to gratify myself with the sight, and I pressed in amidst the multitude. When I got into the church I saw this pious man exhorting the people with the greatest fervour and earnestness, and sweating as much as I ever did while in slavery on Montserrat beach. I was very much struck and impressed with this; I thought it strange I had never seen divines exert themselves in this manner before, and I was no longer at a loss to account for the thin congregations they preached to. When we had discharged our cargo here, and were loaded again, we left this fruitful land once more, and set sail for Montserrat. My traffic had hitherto succeeded so well with me, that I thought, by selling my goods when we arrived at Montserrat, I should have enough to purchase my freedom. But, as soon as our vessel arrived there, my master came on board, and gave orders for us to go to St. Eustatia, and discharge our cargo there, and from thence proceed for Georgia. I was much disappointed at this; but thinking, as usual, it was of no use to encounter with the decrees of fate, I submitted without repining, and we went to St. Eustatia. After we had discharged our cargo there we took in a live cargo, as we call a cargo of slaves. Here I sold my goods tolerably well; but, not being able to lay out all my money in this small island to as much advantage as in many other places, I laid out only part, and the remainder I brought away with me neat. We sailed from hence for Georgia, and I was glad when we got there, though I had not much reason to like the place from my last adventure in Savannah; but I longed to get back to Montserrat and procure my freedom, which I expected to be able to purchase when I returned. As soon as we arrived here I waited on my careful doctor, Mr. Brady, to whom I made the most grateful acknowledgments in my power for his former kindness and attention during my illness. While we were here an odd circumstance happened to the Captain and me, which disappointed us both a good deal. A silversmith, whom we had brought to this place some voyages before, agreed with the Captain to return with us to the West Indies, and promised at the same time to give the Captain a great deal of money, having pretended to take a liking to him, and being, as we thought, very rich. But while we stayed to load our vessel this man was taken ill in a house where he worked, and in a week's time became very bad. The worse he grew the more he used to speak of giving the Captain what he had promised him, so that he expected something considerable from the death of this man, who had no wife or child, and he attended him day and night. I used also to go with the Captain, at his own desire, to attend him; especially when we saw there was no appearance of his recovery: and, in order to recompense me for my trouble, the Captain promised me ten pounds, when he should get the man's property. I thought this would be of great service to me, although I had nearly money enough to purchase my freedom, if I should get safe this voyage to Montserrat. In this expectation I laid out above eight pounds of my money for a suit of superfine clothes to dance with at my freedom, which I hoped was then at hand. We still continued to attend this man, and were with him even on the last day he lived, till very late at night, when we went on board. After we were got to bed, about one or two o'clock in the morning, the Captain was sent for, and informed the man was dead. On this he came to my bed, and, waking me, informed me of it, and desired me to get up and procure a light, and immediately go to him. I told him I was very sleepy, and wished he would take somebody else with him; or else, as the man was dead, and could want no farther attendance, to let all things remain as they were till the next morning. 'No, no,' said he, 'we will have the money to-night, I cannot wait till to-morrow; so let us go.' Accordingly I got up and struck a light, and away we both went and saw the man as dead as we could wish. The Captain said he would give him a grand burial, in gratitude for the promised treasure; and desired that all the things belonging to the deceased might be brought forth. Among others, there was a nest of trunks of which he had kept the keys whilst the man was ill, and when they were produced we opened them with no small eagerness and expectation; and as there were a great number within one another, with much impatience we took them one out of the other. At last, when we came to the smallest, and had opened it, we saw it was full of papers, which we supposed to be notes; at the sight of which our hearts leapt for joy; and that instant the Captain, clapping his hands, cried out, 'Thank God, here it is.' But when we took up the trunk, and began to examine the supposed treasure and long-looked-for bounty, (alas! alas! how uncertain and deceitful are all human affairs!) what had we found! While we thought we were embracing a substance we grasped an empty nothing. The whole amount that was in the nest of trunks was only one dollar and a half; and all that the man possessed would not pay for his coffin. Our sudden and exquisite joy was now succeeded by a sudden and exquisite pain; and my Captain and I exhibited, for some time, most ridiculous figures—pictures of chagrin and disappointment! We went away greatly mortified, and left the deceased to do as well as he could for himself, as we had taken so good care of him when alive for nothing. We set sail once more for Montserrat, and arrived there safe; but much out of humour with our friend the silversmith. When we had unladen the vessel, and I had sold my venture, finding myself master of about forty-seven pounds, I consulted my true friend, the Captain, how I should proceed in offering my master the money for my freedom. He told me to come on a certain morning, when he and my master would be at breakfast together. Accordingly, on that morning I went, and met the Captain there, as he had appointed. When I went in I made my obeisance to my master, and with my money in my hand, and many fears in my heart, I prayed him to be as good as his offer to me, when he was pleased to promise me my freedom as soon as I could purchase it. This speech seemed to confound him; he began to recoil: and my heart that instant sunk within me. 'What,' said he, 'give you your freedom? Why, where did you get the money? Have you got forty pounds sterling?' 'Yes, sir,' I answered. 'How did you get it?' replied he. I told him, very honestly. The Captain then said he knew I got the money very honestly and with much industry, and that I was particularly careful. On which my master replied, I got money much faster than he did; and said he would not have made me the promise he did if he had thought I should have got money so soon. 'Come, come,' said my worthy Captain, clapping my master on the back, 'Come, Robert, (which was his name) I think you must let him have his freedom; you have laid your money out very well; you have received good interest for it all this time, and here is now the principal at last. I know Gustavus has earned you more than an hundred a-year, and he will still save you money, as he will not leave you:—Come, Robert, take the money.' My master then said, he would not be worse than his promise; and, taking the money, told me to go to the Secretary at the Register Office, and get my manumission drawn up. These words of my master were like a voice from heaven to me: in an instant all my trepidation was turned into unutterable bliss; and I most reverently bowed myself with gratitude, unable to express my feelings, but by the overflowing of my eyes, while my true and worthy friend, the Captain, congratulated us both with a peculiar degree of heart-felt pleasure. As soon as the first transports of my joy were over, and that I had expressed my thanks to these my worthy friends in the best manner I was able, I rose with a heart full of affection and reverence, and left the room, in order to obey my master's joyful mandate of going to the Register Office.

As I was leaving the house I called to mind the words of the Psalmist, in the 126th Psalm, and like him, 'I glorified God in my heart, in whom I trusted.' These words had been impressed on my mind from the very day I was forced from Deptford to the present hour, and I now saw them, as I thought, fulfilled and verified. My imagination was all rapture as I flew to the Register Office, and, in this respect, like the apostle Peter,* (whose deliverance from prison was so sudden and extraordinary, that he thought he was in a vision) I could scarcely believe I was awake. Heavens! who could do justice to my feelings at this moment! Not conquering heroes themselves, in the midst of a triumph—Not the tender mother who has just regained her long-lost infant, and presses it to her heart—Not the weary hungry mariner, at the sight of the desired friendly port—Not the lover, when he once more embraces his beloved mistress, after she had been ravished from his arms!—All within my breast was tumult, wildness, and delirium! My feet scarcely touched the ground, for they were winged with joy, and, like Elijah, as he rose to Heaven, they 'were with lightning sped as I went on.' Every one I met I told of my happiness, and blazed about the virtue of my amiable master and captain.

When I got to the office and acquainted the Register with my errand he congratulated me on the occasion, and told me he would draw up my manumission for half price, which was a guinea. I thanked him for his kindness; and, having received it and paid him, I hastened to my master to get him to sign it, that I might be fully released. Accordingly he signed the manumission that day, so that, before night, I who had been a slave in the morning, trembling at the will of another, was become my own master, and completely free. I thought this was the happiest day I had ever experienced; and my joy was still heightened by the blessings and prayers of the sable race, particularly the aged, to whom my heart had ever been attached with reverence.

---

*Acts, chap. xii. ver. 9.

As the form of my manumission has something peculiar in it, and expresses the absolute power and dominion one man claims over his fellow, I shall beg leave to present it before my readers at full length:

Montserrat.—To all men unto whom these presents shall come: I Robert King, of the parish of St. Anthony in the said island, merchant, send greeting: Know ye, that I the aforesaid Robert King, for and in consideration of the sum of seventy pounds current money of the said island, to me in hand paid, and to the intent that a negro man-slave, named Gustavus Vassa, shall and may become free, have manumitted, emancipated, enfranchised, and set free, and by these presents do manumit, emancipate, enfranchise, and set free, the aforesaid negro man-slave, named Gustavus Vassa, for ever, hereby giving, granting, and releasing unto him, the said Gustavus Vassa, all right, title, dominion, sovereignty, and property, which, as lord and master over the aforesaid Gustavus Vassa, I had, or now I have, or by any means whatsoever I may or can hereafter possibly have over him the aforesaid negro, for ever. In witness whereof I the abovesaid Robert King have unto these presents set my hand and seal, this tenth day of July, in the year of our Lord one thousand seven hundred and sixty-six.

ROBERT KING.

Signed, sealed, and delivered in the presence of Terrylegay, Montserrat.

Registered the within manumission at full length, this eleventh day of July, 1766, in liber D.

TERRYLEGAY, Register.

———

In short, the fair as well as black people immediately styled me by a new appellation, to me the most desirable in the world, which was Freeman, and at the dances I gave my Georgia superfine blue clothes made no indifferent appearance, as I thought. Some of the sable females, who formerly stood aloof, now began to relax and appear less coy; but my heart was still fixed on London, where I hoped to be ere long. So that my worthy captain and his owner, my late master, finding that the bent of my mind was towards London, said to me, 'We hope you won't leave us, but that you will still be with the vessels.' Here gratitude bowed me down; and none but the generous mind can judge of my feelings, struggling between inclination and duty. However, notwithstanding my wish to be in London, I obediently answered my benefactors that I would go in the vessel, and not leave them; and from that day I was entered on board as an able-bodied sailor, at thirty-six shillings per month, besides what perquisites I could make. My intention was to make a voyage or two, entirely to please these my honoured patrons; but I determined that the year following, if it pleased God, I would see Old England once more, and surprise my old master, Capt. Pascal, who was hourly in my mind; for I still loved him, notwithstanding his usage of me, and I pleased myself with thinking of what he would say when he saw what the Lord had done for me in so short a time, instead of being, as he might perhaps suppose, under the cruel yoke of some planter. With these kind of reveries I used often to entertain myself, and shorten the time till my return; and now, being as in my original free African state, I embarked on board the Nancy, after having got all things ready for our voyage. In this state of serenity we sailed for St. Eustatia; and, having smooth seas and calm weather, we soon arrived there: after taking our cargo on board, we proceeded to Savannah in Georgia, in August, 1766. While we were there, as usual, I used to go for the cargo up the rivers in boats; and on this business I have been frequently beset by alligators, which were very numerous on that coast, and I have shot many of them when they have been near getting into our boats; which we have with great difficulty sometimes prevented, and have been very much frightened at them. I have seen a young one sold in Georgia alive for six pence. During our stay at this place, one evening a slave belonging to Mr. Read, a merchant of Savannah, came near our vessel, and began to use me very ill. I entreated him, with all the patience I was master of, to desist, as I knew there was little or no law for a free negro here; but the fellow, instead of taking my advice, persevered in his insults, and even struck me. At this I lost all temper, and I fell on him and beat him soundly. The next morning his master came to our vessel as we lay alongside the wharf, and desired me to come ashore that he might have me flogged all round the town, for beating his negro slave. I told him he had insulted me, and had given the provocation, by first striking me. I had told my captain also the whole affair that morning, and wished him to have gone along with me to Mr. Read, to prevent bad consequences; but he said that it did not signify, and if Mr. Read said any thing he would make matters up, and had desired me to go to work, which I accordingly did. The Captain being on board when Mr. Read came, he told him I was a free man; and when Mr. Read applied to him to deliver me up, he said he knew nothing of the matter. I was astonished and frightened at this, and thought I had better keep where I was than go ashore and be flogged round the town, without judge or jury. I therefore refused to stir; and Mr. Read went away, swearing he would bring all the constables in the town, for he would have me out of the vessel. When he was gone, I thought his threat might prove too true to my sorrow; and I was confirmed in this belief, as well by the many instances I had seen of the treatment of free negroes, as from a fact that had happened within my own knowledge here a short time before. There was a free black man, a carpenter, that I knew, who, for asking a gentleman that he worked for for the money he had earned, was put into gaol; and afterwards this oppressed man was sent from Georgia, with false accusations, of an intention to set the gentleman's house on fire, and run away with his slaves. I was therefore much embarrassed, and very apprehensive of a flogging at least. I dreaded, of all things, the thoughts of being striped, as I never in my life had the marks of any violence of that kind. At that instant a rage seized my soul, and for a little I determined to resist the first man that should offer to lay violent hands on me, or basely use me without a trial; for I would sooner die like a free man, than suffer myself to be scourged by the hands of ruffians, and my blood drawn like a slave. The captain and others, more cautious, advised me to make haste and conceal myself; for they said Mr. Read was a very spiteful man, and he would soon come on board with constables and take me. At first I refused this counsel, being determined to stand my ground;

but at length, by the prevailing entreaties of the captain and
Mr. Dixon, with whom he lodged, I went to Mr. Dixon's
house, which was a little out of town, at a place called Yea-
ma-chra. I was but just gone when Mr. Read, with the constables, came for me, and searched the vessel; but, not finding
me there, he swore he would have me dead or alive. I was secreted about five days; however, the good character which my
captain always gave me as well as some other gentlemen who
also knew me, procured me some friends. At last some of
them told my captain that he did not use me well, in suffering me thus to be imposed upon, and said they would see me
redressed, and get me on board some other vessel. My captain, on this, immediately went to Mr. Read, and told him,
that ever since I eloped from the vessel his work had been neglected, and he could not go on with her loading, himself and
mate not being well; and, as I had managed things on board
for them, my absence must retard his voyage, and consequently hurt the owner; he therefore begged of him to forgive me, as he said he never had any complaint of me before,
for the many years that I had been with him. After repeated
entreaties, Mr. Read said I might go to hell, and that he
would not meddle with me; on which my captain came immediately to me at his lodging, and, telling me how pleasantly
matters had gone on, he desired me to go on board. Some of
my other friends then asked him if he had got the constable's
warrant from them; the captain said, No. On this I was desired by them to stay in the house; and they said they would
get me on board of some other vessel before the evening.
When the captain heard this he became almost distracted. He
went immediately for the warrant, and, after using every exertion in his power, he at last got it from my hunters; but I
had all the expenses to pay. After I had thanked all my friends
for their attention, I went on board again to my work, of
which I had always plenty. We were in haste to complete our
lading, and were to carry twenty head of cattle with us to the
West Indies, where they are a very profitable article. In order
to encourage me in working, and to make up for the time I
had lost, my captain promised me the privilege of carrying
two bullocks of my own with me; and this made me work
with redoubled ardour. As soon as I had got the vessel

loaded, in doing which I was obliged to perform the duty of
the mate as well as my own work, and that the bullocks were
near coming on board, I asked the captain leave to bring my
two, according to his promise; but, to my great surprise, he
told me there was no room for them. I then asked him to permit me to take one; but he said he could not. I was a good
deal mortified at this usage, and told him I had no notion
that he intended thus to impose on me; nor could I think well
of any man that was so much worse than his word. On this we
had some disagreement, and I gave him to understand, that I
intended to leave the vessel. At this he appeared to be very
much dejected; and our mate, who had been very sickly, and
whose duty had long devolved upon me, advised him to persuade me to stay: in consequence of which he spoke very
kindly to me, making many fair promises, telling me that, as
the mate was so sickly, he could not do without me, and that,
as the safety of the vessel and cargo depended greatly upon
me, he therefore hoped that I would not be offended at what
had passed between us, and swore he would make up all matters when we arrived in the West Indies; so I consented to
slave on as before. Soon after this, as the bullocks were coming on board, one of them ran at the captain, and butted him
so furiously in the breast, that he never recovered of the blow.
In order to make me some amends for his treatment about
the bullocks, the captain now pressed me very much to take
some turkeys, and other fowls, with me, and gave me liberty
to take as many as I could find room for; but I told him he
knew very well I had never carried any turkeys before, as I always thought they were such tender birds that they were not
fit to cross the seas. However, he continued to press me to
buy them for once; and, what was very surprising to me, the
more I was against it, the more he urged my taking them, insomuch that he ensured me from all losses that might happen
by them, and I was prevailed on to take them; but I thought
this very strange, as he had never acted so with me before.
This, and not being able to dispose of my paper-money in any
other way, induced me at length to take four dozen. The
turkeys, however, I was so dissatisfied about that I determined
to make no more voyages to this quarter, nor with this captain; and was very apprehensive that my free voyage would be

the worst I had ever made. We set sail for Montserrat. The captain and mate had been both complaining of sickness when we sailed, and as we proceeded on our voyage they grew worse. This was about November, and we had not been long at sea before we began to meet with strong northerly gales and rough seas; and in about seven or eight days all the bullocks were near being drowned, and four or five of them died. Our vessel, which had not been tight at first, was much less so now; and, though we were but nine in the whole, including five sailors and myself, yet we were obliged to attend to the pumps every half or three quarters of an hour. The captain and mate came on deck as often as they were able, which was now but seldom; for they declined so fast, that they were not well enough to make observations above four or five times the whole voyage. The whole care of the vessel rested, therefore, upon me, and I was obliged to direct her by my former experience, not being able to work a traverse. The captain was now very sorry he had not taught me navigation, and protested, if ever he should get well again, he would not fail to do so; but in about seventeen days his illness increased so much, that he was obliged to keep his bed, continuing sensible, however, till the last, constantly having the owner's interest at heart; for this just and benevolent man ever appeared much concerned about the welfare of what he was intrusted with. When this dear friend found the symptoms of death approaching, he called me by my name; and, when I came to him, he asked (with almost his last breath) if he had ever done me any harm? 'God forbid I should think so,' I replied, 'I should then be the most ungrateful of wretches to the best of benefactors.' While I was thus expressing my affection and sorrow by his bedside, he expired without saying another word; and the day following we committed his body to the deep. Every man on board loved this man, and regretted his death; but I was exceedingly affected at it, and I found that I did not know, till he was gone, the strength of my regard for him. Indeed I had every reason in the world to be attached to him; for, besides that he was in general mild, affable, generous, faithful, benevolent, and just, he was to me a friend and a father; and, had it pleased Providence that he had died but five months before, I verily believe I should not have obtained my freedom when I did; and it is not improbable that I might not have been able to get it at any rate afterwards. The captain being dead, the mate came on the deck, and made such observations as he was able, but to no purpose. In the course of a few days more, the few bullocks that remained were found dead; but the turkies I had, though on the deck, and exposed to so much wet and bad weather, did well, and I afterwards gained near three hundred per cent. on the sale of them; so that in the event it proved a happy circumstance for me that I had not bought the bullocks I intended, for they must have perished with the rest; and I could not help looking on this, otherwise trifling circumstance, as a particular providence of God, and I was thankful accordingly. The care of the vessel took up all my time, and engaged my attention entirely. As we were now out of the variable winds, I thought I should not be much puzzled to hit upon the islands. I was persuaded I steered right for Antigua, which I wished to reach, as the nearest to us; and in the course of nine or ten days we made this island, to our great joy; and the next day after we came safe to Montserrat. Many were surprised when they heard of my conducting the sloop into the port, and I now obtained a new appellation, and was called Captain. This elated me not a little, and it was quite flattering to my vanity to be thus styled by as high a title as any free man in this place possessed. When the death of the captain became known, he was much regretted by all who knew him; for he was a man universally respected. At the same time the sable captain lost no fame; for the success I had met with increased the affection of my friends in no small measure.

CHAP. VIII.

The author, to oblige Mr. King, once more embarks for Georgia in one of his vessels—A new captain is appointed—They sail, and steer a new course—Three remarkable dreams—The vessel is shipwrecked on the Bahama bank, but the crew are preserved, principally by means of the author—He sets out from the island with the captain, in a small boat, in quest of a ship—Their distress—Meet with a wrecker—Sail for Providence—Are overtaken again by a terrible storm, and are all near perishing—Arrive at New Providence—The author, after some time, sails from thence to Georgia—Meets with another storm, and is obliged to put back and refit—Arrives at Georgia—Meets new impositions—Two white men attempt to kidnap him—Officiates as a parson at a funeral ceremony—Bids adieu to Georgia, and sails for Martinico.

As I had now, by the death of my captain, lost my great benefactor and friend, I had little inducement to remain longer in the West Indies, except my gratitude to Mr. King, which I thought I had pretty well discharged in bringing back his vessel safe, and delivering his cargo to his satisfaction. I began to think of leaving this part of the world, of which I had been long tired, and returning to England, where my heart had always been; but Mr. King still pressed me very much to stay with his vessel; and he had done so much for me that I found myself unable to refuse his requests, and consented to go another voyage to Georgia, as the mate, from his ill state of health, was quite useless in the vessel. Accordingly a new captain was appointed, whose name was William Phillips, an old acquaintance of mine; and, having refitted our vessel, and taken several slaves on board, we set sail for St. Eustatia, where we stayed but a few days; and on the 30th of January 1767 we steered for Georgia. Our new captain boasted strangely of his skill in navigating and conducting a vessel; and in consequence of this he steered a new course, several points more to the westward than we ever did before; this appeared to me very extraordinary.

On the fourth of February, which was soon after we had

got into our new course, I dreamt the ship was wrecked amidst the surfs and rocks, and that I was the means of saving every one on board; and on the night following I dreamed the very same dream. These dreams however made no impression on my mind; and the next evening, it being my watch below, I was pumping the vessel a little after eight o'clock, just before I went off the deck, as is the custom; and being weary with the duty of the day, and tired at the pump, (for we made a good deal of water) I began to express my impatience, and I uttered with an oath, 'Damn the vessel's bottom out.' But my conscience instantly smote me for the expression. When I left the deck I went to bed, and had scarcely fallen asleep when I dreamed the same dream again about the ship that I had dreamt the two preceeding nights. At twelve o'clock the watch was changed; and, as I had always the charge of the captain's watch, I then went upon deck. At half after one in the morning the man at the helm saw something under the lee-beam that the sea washed against, and he immediately called to me that there was a grampus, and desired me to look at it. Accordingly I stood up and observed it for some time; but, when I saw the sea wash up against it again and again, I said it was not a fish but a rock. Being soon certain of this, I went down to the captain, and, with some confusion, told him the danger we were in, and desired him to come upon deck immediately. He said it was very well, and I went up again. As soon as I was upon deck the wind, which had been pretty high, having abated a little, the vessel began to be carried sideways towards the rock, by means of the current. Still the captain did not appear. I therefore went to him again, and told him the vessel was then near a large rock, and desired he would come up with speed. He said he would, and I returned to the deck. When I was upon the deck again I saw we were not above a pistol shot from the rock, and I heard the noise of the breakers all around us. I was exceedingly alarmed at this; and the captain having not yet come on the deck I lost all patience; and, growing quite enraged, I ran down to him again, and asked him why he did not come up, and what he could mean by all this? 'The breakers,' said I, 'are round us, and the vessel is almost on the rock.' With that he came on the deck with me, and we tried to put the vessel about, and get her out of the current, but all to no purpose, the wind being very small. We then called all hands up immediately; and after a little we got up one end of a cable, and fastened it to the anchor. By this time the surf was foaming round us, and made a dreadful noise on the breakers, and the very moment we let the anchor go the vessel struck against the rocks. One swell now succeeded another, as it were one wave calling on its fellow: the roaring of the billows increased, and, with one single heave of the swells, the sloop was pierced and transfixed among the rocks! In a moment a scene of horror presented itself to my mind, such as I never had conceived or experienced before. All my sins stared me in the face; and especially, I thought that God had hurled his direful vengeance on my guilty head for cursing the vessel on which my life depended. My spirits at this forsook me, and I expected every moment to go to the bottom: I determined if I should still be saved that I would never swear again. And in the midst of my distress, while the dreadful surfs were dashing with unremitting fury among the rocks, I remembered the Lord, though fearful that I was undeserving of forgiveness, and I thought that as he had often delivered he might yet deliver; and, calling to mind the many mercies he had shewn me in times past, they gave me some small hope that he might still help me. I then began to think how we might be saved; and I believe no mind was ever like mine so replete with inventions and confused with schemes, though how to escape death I knew not. The captain immediately ordered the hatches to be nailed down on the slaves in the hold, where there were above twenty, all of whom must unavoidably have perished if he had been obeyed. When he desired the man to nail down the hatches I thought that my sin was the cause of this, and that God would charge me with these people's blood. This thought rushed upon my mind that instant with such violence, that it quite overpowered me, and I fainted. I recovered just as the people were about to nail down the hatches; perceiving which, I desired them to stop. The captain then said it must be done: I asked him why? He said that every one would endeavour to get into the boat, which was but small, and thereby we should be drowned; for it would not have carried above ten at the most. I could no longer restrain my emotion, and I told him he deserved drowning for not knowing how to navigate the vessel; and I believe the people would have tossed him overboard if I had given them the least hint of it. However the hatches were not nailed down; and, as none of us could leave the vessel then on account of the darkness, and as we knew not where to go, and were convinced besides that the boat could not survive the surfs, we all said we would remain on the dry part of the vessel, and trust to God till daylight appeared, when we should know better what to do.

I then advised to get the boat prepared against morning, and some of us began to set about it; but some abandoned all care of the ship and themselves, and fell to drinking. Our boat had a piece out of her bottom near two feet long, and we had no materials to mend her; however, necessity being the mother of invention, I took some pump leather and nailed it to the broken part, and plastered it over with tallow-grease. And, thus prepared, with the utmost anxiety of mind we watched for day-light, and thought every minute an hour till it appeared. At last it saluted our longing eyes, and kind Providence accompanied its approach with what was no small comfort to us; for the dreadful swell began to subside; and the next thing that we discovered to raise our drooping spirits, was a small key or island, about five or six miles off; but a barrier soon presented itself; for there was not water enough for our boat to go over the reefs, and this threw us again into a sad consternation; but there was no alternative, we were therefore obliged to put but few in the boat at once; and, what is still worse, all of us were frequently under the necessity of getting out to drag and lift it over the reefs. This cost us much labour and fatigue; and, what was yet more distressing, we could not avoid having our legs cut and torn very much with the rocks. There were only four people that would work with me at the oars; and they consisted of three black men and a Dutch creole sailor; and, though we went with the boat five times that day, we had no others to assist us. But, had we not worked in this manner, I really believe the people could not have been saved; for not one of the white men did any thing to preserve their lives; and indeed they soon got so drunk that they were not able, but lay about the deck like swine, so that we were at last obliged to lift them into the boat and carry them on shore by force. This want of assistance made our labour intolerably severe; insomuch, that, by putting on shore so often that day, the skin was entirely stript off my hands.

However, we continued all the day to toil and strain our exertions, till we had brought all on board safe to the shore; so that out of thirty-two people we lost not one. My dream now returned upon my mind with all its force; it was fulfilled in every part; for our danger was the same I had dreamt of: and I could not help looking on myself as the principal instrument in effecting our deliverance; for, owing to some of our people getting drunk, the rest of us were obliged to double our exertions; and it was fortunate we did, for in a very little time longer the patch of leather on the boat would have been worn out, and she would have been no longer fit for service. Situated as we were, who could think that men should be so careless of the danger they were in? for, if the wind had but raised the swell as it was when the vessel struck, we must have bid a final farewell to all hopes of deliverance; and though, I warned the people who were drinking and entreated them to embrace the moment of deliverance, nevertheless they persisted, as if not possessed of the least spark of reason. I could not help thinking, that, if any of these people had been lost, God would charge me with their lives, which, perhaps, was one cause of my labouring so hard for their preservation, and indeed every one of them afterwards seemed so sensible of the service I had rendered them; and while we were on the key I was a kind of chieftain amongst them. I brought some limes, oranges, and lemons ashore; and, finding it to be a good soil where we were, I planted several of them as a token to any one that might be cast away hereafter. This key, as we afterwards found, was one of the Bahama islands, which consist of a cluster of large islands, with smaller ones or keys, as they are called, interspersed among them. It was about a mile in circumference, with a white sandy beach running in a regular order along it. On that part of it where we first attempted to land there stood some very large birds, called flamingoes: these, from the reflection of the sun, appeared to us at a little distance as large as men; and, when they walked backwards and forwards, we could not conceive what they were: our captain swore they were cannibals. This created a great panic among us; and we held a consultation how to act. The captain wanted to go to a key that was within sight, but a great way off; but I was against it, as in so doing we should not be able to save all the people; 'And therefore,' said I, 'let us go on shore here, and perhaps these cannibals may take to the water.' Accordingly we steered towards them; and when we approached them, to our very great joy and no less wonder, they walked off one after the other very deliberately; and at last they took flight and relieved us entirely from our fears. About the key there were turtles and several sorts of fish in such abundance that we caught them without bait, which was a great relief to us after the salt provisions on board. There was also a large rock on the beach, about ten feet high, which was in the form of a punch-bowl at the top; this we could not help thinking Providence had ordained to supply us with rainwater; and it was something singular that, if we did not take the water when it rained, in some little time after it would turn as salt as sea-water.

Our first care, after refreshment, was to make ourselves tents to lodge in, which we did as well as we could with some sails we had brought from the ship. We then began to think how we might get from this place, which was quite uninhabited; and we determined to repair our boat, which was very much shattered, and to put to sea in quest of a ship or some inhabited island. It took us up however eleven days before we could get the boat ready for sea in the manner we wanted it, with a sail and other necessaries. When we had got all things prepared the captain wanted me to stay on shore while he went to sea in quest of a vessel to take all the people off the key; but this I refused; and the captain and myself, with five more, set off in the boat towards New Providence. We had no more than two musket load of gun-powder with us if any thing should happen; and our stock of provisions consisted of three gallons of rum, four of water, some salt beef, some biscuit; and in this manner we proceeded to sea.

On the second day of our voyage we came to an island called Obbico, the largest of the Bahama islands. We were much in want of water; for by this time our water was expended, and we were exceedingly fatigued in pulling two days in the heat of the sun; and it being late in the evening, we hauled the boat ashore to try for water and remain during the night: when we came ashore we searched for water, but could find none. When it was dark, we made a fire around us for fear of the wild beasts, as the place was an entire thick wood, and we took it by turns to watch. In this situation we found very little rest, and waited with impatience for the morning. As soon as the light appeared we set off again with our boat, in hopes of finding assistance during the day. We were now much dejected and weakened by pulling the boat; for our sail was of no use, and we were almost famished for want of fresh water to drink. We had nothing left to eat but salt beef, and that we could not use without water. In this situation we toiled all day in sight of the island, which was very long; in the evening, seeing no relief, we made ashore again, and fastened our boat. We then went to look for fresh water, being quite faint for the want of it; and we dug and searched about for some all the remainder of the evening, but could not find one drop, so that our dejection at this period became excessive, and our terror so great, that we expected nothing but death to deliver us. We could not touch our beef, which was as salt as brine, without fresh water; and we were in the greatest terror from the apprehension of wild beasts. When unwelcome night came we acted as on the night before; and the next morning we set off again from the island in hopes of seeing some vessel. In this manner we toiled as well as we were able till four o'clock, during which we passed several keys, but could not meet with a ship; and, still famishing with thirst, went ashore on one of those keys again in hopes of finding some water. Here we found some leaves with a few drops of water in them, which we lapped with much eagerness; we then dug in several places, but without success. As we were digging holes in search of water there came forth some very thick and black stuff; but none of us could touch it, except the poor Dutch Creole, who drank above a quart of it as eagerly as if it had been wine. We tried to catch fish, but could not; and we now began to repine at our fate, and abandon ourselves to despair; when, in the midst of our murmuring, the captain all at once cried out 'A sail! a sail! a sail!' This gladdening sound was like a reptieve to a convict, and we all instantly turned to look at it; but in a little time some of us began to be afraid it was not a sail. However, at a venture, we embarked and steered after it; and, in half an hour, to our unspeakable joy, we plainly saw that it was a vessel. At this our drooping spirits revived, and we made towards her with all the speed imaginable. When we came near to her, we found she was a little sloop, about the size of a Gravesend hoy, and quite full of people; a circumstance which we could not make out the meaning of. Our captain, who was a Welchman, swore that they were pirates, and would kill us. I said, be that as it might, we must board her if we were to die for it; and, if they should not receive us kindly, we must oppose them as well as we could; for there was no alternative between their perishing and ours. This counsel was immediately taken; and I really believe that the captain, myself, and the Dutchman, would then have faced twenty men. We had two cutlasses and a musquet, that I brought in the boat; and, in this situation, we rowed alongside, and immediately boarded her. I believe there were about forty hands on board; but how great was our surprise, as soon as we got on board, to find that the major part of them were in the same predicament as ourselves!

They belonged to a whaling schooner that was wrecked two days before us about nine miles to the north of our vessel. When she was wrecked some of them had taken to their boats and had left some of their people and property on a key, in the same manner as we had done; and were going, like us, to New Providence in quest of a ship, when they met with this little sloop, called a wrecker; their employment in those seas being to look after wrecks. They were then going to take the remainder of the people belonging to the schooner; for which the wrecker was to have all things belonging to the vessel, and likewise their people's help to get what they could out of her, and were then to carry the crew to New Providence.

We told the people of the wrecker the condition of our vessel, and we made the same agreement with them as the schooner's people; and, on their complying, we begged of them to go to our key directly, because our people were in want of water. They agreed, therefore, to go along with us first; and in two days we arrived at the key, to the inexpressible joy of the people that we had left behind, as they had been reduced to great extremities for want of water in our absence. Luckily for us, the wrecker had now more people on board than she could carry or victual for any moderate length of time; they therefore hired the schooner's people to work on our wreck, and we left them our boat, and embarked for New Providence.

Nothing could have been more fortunate than our meeting with this wrecker, for New Providence was at such a distance that we never could have reached it in our boat. The island of Abbico was much longer than we expected; and it was not till after sailing for three or four days that we got safe to the farther end of it, towards New Providence. When we arrived there we watered, and got a good many lobsters and other shellfish; which proved a great relief to us, as our provisions and water were almost exhausted. We then proceeded on our voyage; but the day after we left the island, late in the evening, and whilst we were yet amongst the Bahama keys, we were overtaken by a violent gale of wind, so that we were obliged to cut away the mast. The vessel was very near foundering; for she parted from her anchors, and struck several times on the shoals. Here we expected every minute that she would have gone to pieces, and each moment to be our last; so much so that my old captain and sickly useless mate, and several others, fainted; and death stared us in the face on every side. All the swearers on board now began to call on the God of Heaven to assist them: and, sure enough, beyond our comprehension he did assist us, and in a miraculous manner delivered us! In the very height of our extremity the wind lulled for a few minutes; and, although the swell was high beyond expression, two men, who were expert swimmers, attempted to go to the buoy of the anchor, which we still saw on the water, at some distance, in a little punt that belonged to the wrecker, which was not large enough to carry more than two. She filled different times in their endeavours to get into her alongside of our vessel; and they saw nothing but death before them, as well as we; but they said they might as well die that way as any other. A coil of very small rope, with a little buoy, was put in along with them; and, at last, with great hazard, they got the punt clear from the vessel; and these two intrepid water heroes paddled away for life towards the buoy of the anchor. The eyes of us all were fixed on them all the time, expecting every minute to be their last: and the prayers of all those that remained in their senses were offered up to God, on their behalf, for a speedy deliverance; and for our own, which depended on them; and he heard and answered us! These two men at last reached the buoy; and, having fastened the punt to it, they tied one end of their rope to the small buoy that they had in the punt, and sent it adrift towards the vessel. We on board observing this threw out boat-hooks and leads fastened to lines, in order to catch the buoy: at last we caught it, and fastened a hawser to the end of the small rope; we then gave them a sign to pull, and they pulled the hawser to them, and fastened it to the buoy: which being done we hauled for our lives; and, through the mercy of God, we got again from the shoals into deep water, and the punt got safe to the vessel. It is impossible for any to conceive our heart-felt joy at this second deliverance from ruin, but those who have suffered the same hardships. Those whose strength and senses were gone came to themselves, and were now as elated as they were before depressed. Two days after this the wind ceased, and the water became smooth. The punt then went on shore, and we cut down some trees; and having found our mast and mended it we brought it on board, and fixed it up. As soon as we had done this we got up the anchor, and away we went once more for New Providence, which in three days more we reached safe, after having been above three weeks in a situation in which we did not expect to escape with life. The inhabitants here were very kind to us; and, when they learned our situation, shewed us a great deal of hospitality and friendship. Soon after this every one of my old fellow-sufferers that were free parted from us, and shaped their course where their inclination led them. One merchant, who had a large sloop, seeing our condition, and knowing we wanted to go to Georgia, told four of us that his vessel was going there; and, if we would work on board and load her, he would give us our passage free. As we could not get any wages whatever, and found it very hard to get off the place, we were obliged to consent to his proposal; and we went on board and helped to load the sloop, though we had only our victuals allowed us. When she was entirely loaded he told us she was going to Jamaica first, where we must go if we went in her. This, however, I refused; but my fellow-sufferers not having any money to help themselves with, necessity obliged them to accept of the offer, and to steer that course, though they did not like it.

We stayed in New Providence about seventeen or eighteen days; during which time I met with many friends, who gave me encouragement to stay there with them: but I declined it; though, had not my heart been fixed on England, I should have stayed, as I liked the place extremely, and there were some free black people here who were very happy, and we passed our time pleasantly together, with the melodious sound of the catguts, under the lime and lemon trees. At length Captain Phillips hired a sloop to carry him and some of the slaves that he could not sell to Georgia; and I agreed to go with him in this vessel, meaning now to take my farewell of that place. When the vessel was ready we all embarked; and I took my leave of New Providence, not without regret. We sailed about four o'clock in the morning, with a fair wind, for Georgia; and about eleven o'clock the same morning a short and sudden gale sprung up and blew away most of our sails; and, as we were still amongst the keys, in a very few minutes it dashed the sloop against the rocks. Luckily for us the water was deep; and the sea was not so angry but that, after having for some time laboured hard, and being many in number, we were saved through God's mercy; and, by using our greatest exertions, we got the vessel off. The next day we returned to Providence, where we soon got her again refitted. Some of the people swore that we had spells set upon us by somebody in Montserrat; and others that we had witches and wizzards amongst the poor helpless slaves; and that we never should arrive safe at Georgia. But these things did not deter me; I said, 'Let us again face the winds and seas, and swear not, but trust to God, and he will deliver us.' We therefore once more set sail; and, with hard labour, in seven day's time arrived safe at Georgia.

After our arrival we went up to the town of Savannah; and the same evening I went to a friend's house to lodge, whose name was Mosa, a black man. We were very happy at meeting each other; and after supper we had a light till it was between nine and ten o'clock at night. About that time the watch or patrol came by; and, discerning a light in the house, they knocked at the door: we opened it; and they came in and sat down, and drank some punch with us: they also begged some limes of me, as they understood I had some, which I readily gave them. A little after this they told me I must go to the watch-house with them: this surprised me a good deal, after our kindness to them; and I asked them, Why so? They said that all negroes who had light in their houses after nine o'clock were to be taken into custody, and either pay some dollars or be flogged. Some of those people knew that I was a free man; but, as the man of the house was not free, and had his master to protect him, they did not take the same liberty with him they did with me. I told them that I was a free man, and just arrived from Providence; that we were not making any noise, and that I was not a stranger in that place, but was very well known there: 'Besides,' said I, 'what will you do with me?'—'That you shall see,' replied they, 'but you must go to the watch-house with us.' Now whether they meant to get money from me or not I was at a loss to know; but I thought immediately of the oranges and limes at Santa Cruz: and seeing that nothing would pacify them I went with them to the watch-house, where I remained during the night. Early the the next morning these imposing ruffians flogged a negro-man and woman that they had in the watch-house, and then they told me that I must be flogged too. I asked why? and if there was no law for free men? And told them if there was I would have it put in force against them. But this only exasperated them the more; and instantly they swore they would serve me as Doctor Perkins had done; and they were going to lay violent hands on me; when one of them, more humane than the rest, said that as I was a free man they could not justify stripping me by law. I then immediately sent for Doctor Brady, who was known to be an honest and worthy man; and on his coming to my assistance they let me go.

This was not the only disagreeable incident I met with while I was in this place; for, one day, while I was a little way out of the town of Savannah, I was beset by two white men,

who meant to play their usual tricks with me in the way of
kidnapping. As soon as these men accosted me, one of them
said to the other, 'This is the very fellow we are looking for
that you lost:' and the other swore immediately that I was the
identical person. On this they made up to me, and were about
to handle me; but I told them to be still and keep off; for I
had seen those kind of tricks played upon other free blacks,
and they must not think to serve me so. At this they paused a
little, and one said to the other—it will not do; and the other
answered that I talked too good English. I replied, I believed
I did; and I had also with me a revengeful stick equal to the
occasion; and my mind was likewise good. Happily however it
was not used; and, after we had talked together a little in this
manner, the rogues left me. I stayed in Savannah some time,
anxiously trying to get to Montserrat once more to see Mr.
King, my old master, and then to take a final farewell of the
American quarter of the globe. At last I met with a sloop
called the Speedwell, Captain John Bunton, which belonged
to Grenada, and was bound to Martinico, a French island,
with a cargo of rice, and I shipped myself on board of her. Before I left Georgia a black woman, who had a child lying
dead, being very tenacious of the church burial service, and
not able to get any white person to perform it, applied to me
for that purpose. I told her I was no parson; and besides, that
the service over the dead did not affect the soul. This however did not satisfy her; she still urged me very hard: I
therefore complied with her earnest entreaties, and at last
consented to act the parson for the first time in my life. As she
was much respected, there was a great company both of white
and black people at the grave. I then accordingly assumed my
new vocation, and performed the funeral ceremony to the satisfaction of all present; after which I bade adieu to Georgia,
and sailed for Martinico.

CHAP. IX

The author arrives at Martinico—Meets with new difficulties—Gets to Montserrat, where he takes leave of his old master, and sails for England—Meets Capt. Pascal—Learns the French horn—Hires himself with Doctor Irving, where he learns to freshen sea water—Leaves the doctor, and goes a voyage to Turkey and Portugal; and afterwards goes a voyage to Grenada, and another to Jamaica—Returns to the Doctor, and they embark together on a voyage to the North Pole, with the Hon. Capt. Phipps—Some account of that voyage, and the dangers the author was in—He returns to England.

I THUS took a final leave of Georgia; for the treatment I had received in it disgusted me very much against the place; and when I left it and sailed for Martinico I determined never more to revisit it. My new captain conducted his vessel safer than my former one; and, after an agreeable voyage, we got safe to our intended port. While I was on this island I went about a good deal, and found it very pleasant: in particular I admired the town of St. Pierre, which is the principal one in the island, and built more like an European town than any I had seen in the West Indies. In general also, slaves were better treated, had more holidays, and looked better than those in the English islands. After we had done our business here, I wanted my discharge, which was necessary; for it was then the month of May, and I wished much to be at Montserrat to bid farewell to Mr. King, and all my other friends there, in time to sail for Old England in the July fleet. But, alas! I had put a great stumbling block in my own way, by which I was near losing my passage that season to England. I had lent my captain some money, which I now wanted to enable me to prosecute my intentions. This I told him; but when I applied for it, though I urged the necessity of my occasion, I met with so much shuffling from him, that I began at last to be afraid of losing my money, as I could not recover it by law: for I have already mentioned, that throughout the West Indies no black man's testimony is admitted, on any occasion, against any white person whatever, and therefore my own oath would

have been of no use. I was obliged, therefore, to remain with
him till he might be disposed to return it to me. Thus we
sailed from Martinico for the Grenades. I frequently pressing
the captain for my money to no purpose; and, to render my
condition worse, when we got there, the captain and his owners quarrelled; so that my situation became daily more irksome: for besides that we on board had little or no victuals
allowed us, and I could not get my money nor wages, I could
then have gotten my passage free to Montserrat had I been
able to accept it. The worst of all was, that it was growing late
in July, and the ships in the islands must sail by the 26th of
that month. At last, however, with a great many entreaties, I
got my money from the captain, and took the first vessel I
could meet with for St. Eustatia. From thence I went in another to Basseterre in St. Kitts, where I arrived on the 19th of
July. On the 22d, having met with a vessel bound to Montserrat, I wanted to go in her; but the captain and others would
not take me on board until I should advertise myself, and give
notice of my going off the island. I told them of my haste to
be in Montserrat, and that the time then would not admit of
advertising, it being late in the evening, and the captain about
to sail; but he insisted it was necessary, and otherwise he said
he would not take me. This reduced me to great perplexity;
for if I should be compelled to submit to this degrading necessity, which every black freeman is under, of advertising
himself like a slave, when he leaves an island, and which I
thought a gross imposition upon any freeman, I feared I
should miss that opportunity of going to Montserrat, and
then I could not get to England that year. The vessel was just
going off, and no time could be lost; I immediately therefore
set about, with a heavy heart, to try who I could get to befriend me in complying with the demands of the captain.
Luckily I found, in a few minutes, some gentlemen of
Montserrat whom I knew; and, having told them my situation, I requested their friendly assistance in helping me off the
island. Some of them, on this, went with me to the captain,
and satisfied him of my freedom; and, to my very great joy, he
desired me to go on board. We then set sail, and the next day,
the 23d, I arrived at the wished-for place, after an absence of
six months, in which I had more than once experienced the

delivering hand of Providence, when all human means of escaping destruction seemed hopeless. I saw my friends with a gladness of heart which was increased by my absence and the dangers I had escaped, and I was received with great friendship by them all, but particularly by Mr. King, to whom I related the fate of his sloop, the Nancy, and the causes of her being wrecked. I now learned with extreme sorrow, that his house was washed away during my absence, by the bursting of a pond at the top of a mountain that was opposite the town of Plymouth. It swept great part of the town away, and Mr. King lost a great deal of property from the inundation, and nearly his life. When I told him I intended to go to London that season, and that I had come to visit him before my departure, the good man expressed a great deal of affection for me, and sorrow that I should leave him, and warmly advised me to stay there; insisting, as I was much respected by all the gentlemen in the place, that I might do very well, and in a short time have land and slaves of my own. I thanked him for this instance of his friendship; but, as I wished very much to be in London, I declined remaining any longer there, and begged he would excuse me. I then requested he would be kind enough to give me a certificate of my behaviour while in his service, which he very readily complied with, and gave me the following:

Montserrat, January 26, 1767.

'The bearer hereof, Gustavus Vassa, was my slave for upwards of three years, during which he has always behaved himself well, and discharged his duty with honesty and assiduity.

'ROBERT KING.

'To all whom this may concern.'

Having obtained this, I parted from my kind master, after many sincere professions of gratitude and regard, and prepared for my departure for London. I immediately agreed to go with one Capt. John Hamer, for seven guineas, the passage to London, on board a ship called the Andromache; and on the 24th and 25th I had free dances, as they are called, with some of my countrymen, previous to my setting off; after which I took leave of all my friends, and on the 26th I embarked for London, exceedingly glad to see myself once more on board of a ship; and still more so, in steering the course I had long wished for. With a light heart I bade Montserrat farewell, and never had my feet on it since; and with it I bade adieu to the sound of the cruel whip, and all other dreadful instruments of torture; adieu to the offensive sight of the violated chastity of the sable females, which has too often accosted my eyes; adieu to oppressions (although to me less severe than most of my countrymen); and adieu to the angry howling, dashing surfs. I wished for a grateful and thankful heart to praise the Lord God on high for all his mercies!

We had a most prosperous voyage, and, at the end of seven weeks, arrived at Cherry-Garden stairs. Thus were my longing eyes once more gratified with a sight of London, after having been absent from it above four years. I immediately received my wages, and I never had earned seven guineas so quick in my life before; I had thirty-seven guineas in all, when I got cleared of the ship. I now entered upon a scene, quite new to me, but full of hope. In this situation my first thoughts were to look out for some of my former friends, and amongst the first of those were the Miss Guerins. As soon, therefore, as I had regaled myself I went in quest of those kind ladies, whom I was very impatient to see; and with some difficulty and perseverance, I found them at May's-hill, Greenwich. They were most agreeably surprised to see me, and I quite overjoyed at meeting with them. I told them my history, at which they expressed great wonder, and freely acknowledged it did their cousin, Capt. Pascal, no honour. He then visited there frequently; and I met him four or five days after in Greenwich park. When he saw me he appeared a good deal surprised, and asked me how I came back? I answered, 'In a ship.' To which he replied dryly, 'I suppose you did not walk back to London on the water.' As I saw, by his manner, that he did not seem to be sorry for his behaviour to me, and that I had not much reason to expect any favour from him, I told him that he had used me very ill, after I had been such a faithful servant to him for so many years; on which, without saying any more, he turned about and went away. A few days after this I met Capt. Pascal at Miss Guerin's house, and asked him for my prize-money. He said there was none due to me; for, if my prize money had been 10,000l. he had a right to it all. I told him I was informed otherwise; on which he bade me defiance; and, in a bantering tone, desired me to commence a lawsuit against him for it: 'There are lawyers enough,' said he, 'that will take the cause in hand, and you had better try it.' I told him then that I would try it, which enraged him very much; however, out of regard to the ladies, I remained still, and never made any farther demand of my right. Some time afterwards these friendly ladies asked me what I meant to do with myself, and how they could assist me. I thanked them, and said, if they pleased, I would be their servant; but if not, as I had thirty-seven guineas, which would support me for some time, I would be much obliged to them to recommend me to some person who would teach me a business whereby I might earn my living. They answered me very politely, that they were sorry it did not suit them to take me as their servant, and asked me what business I should like to learn? I said, hair-dressing. They then promised to assist me in this; and soon after they recommended me to a gentleman whom I had known before, one Capt. O'Hara, who treated me with much kindness, and procured me a master, a hair-dresser, in Coventry-court, Haymarket, with whom he placed me. I was with this man from September till the February following. In that time we had a neighbour in the same court who taught the French horn. He used to blow it so well that I was charmed with it, and agreed with him to teach me to blow it. Accordingly he took me in hand, and began to instruct me, and I soon learned all the three parts. I took great delight in blowing on this instrument, the evenings being long; and besides that I was fond of it, I did not like to be idle, and it filled up my vacant hours innocently. At this time also I agreed with the Rev. Mr. Gregory, who lived in the same court, where he kept an academy and an evening-school, to improve me in arithmetic. This he did as far as barter and alligation; so that all the time I was there I was entirely employed. In February 1768 I hired myself to Dr. Charles Irving, in Pall-mall, so celebrated for his successful experiments in making sea water fresh; and here I had plenty of hair-dressing to improve my hand. This gentleman was an excellent master; he was ex-

ceedingly kind and good tempered; and allowed me in the
evenings to attend my schools, which I esteemed a great
blessing; therefore I thanked God and him for it, and used all
my diligence to improve the opportunity. This diligence and
attention recommended me to the notice and care of my
three preceptors, who on their parts bestowed a great deal of
pains in my instruction, and besides were all very kind to me.
My wages, however, which were by two thirds less than I ever
had in my life (for I had only 12l. per annum) I soon found
would not be sufficient to defray this extraordinary expense of
masters, and my own necessary expenses; my old thirty-seven
guineas had by this time worn all away to one. I thought it
best, therefore, to try the sea again in quest of more money,
as I had been bred to it, and had hitherto found the profession of it successful. I had also a very great desire to see
Turkey, and I now determined to gratify it. Accordingly, in
the month of May, 1768, I told the doctor my wish to go to
sea again, to which he made no opposition; and we parted on
friendly terms. The same day I went into the city in quest of
a master. I was extremely fortunate in my inquiry; for I soon
heard of a gentleman who had a ship going to Italy and
Turkey, and he wanted a man who could dress hair well. I was
overjoyed at this, and went immediately on board of his ship,
as I had been directed, which I found to be fitted up with
great taste, and I already foreboded no small pleasure in sailing in her. Not finding the gentleman on board, I was directed to his lodgings, where I met with him the next day,
and gave him a specimen of my dressing. He liked it so well
that he hired me immediately, so that I was perfectly happy;
for the ship, master, and voyage, were entirely to my mind.
The ship was called the Delawar, and my master's name was
John Jolly, a neat smart good humoured man, just such an
one as I wished to serve. We sailed from England in July following, and our voyage was extremely pleasant. We went to
Villa Franca, Nice, and Leghorn; and in all these places I was
charmed with the richness and beauty of the countries, and
struck with the elegant buildings with which they abound. We
had always in them plenty of extraordinary good wines and
rich fruits, which I was very fond of; and I had frequent occasions of gratifying both my taste and curiosity; for my cap-

tain always lodged on shore in those places, which afforded me opportunities to see the country around. I also learned navigation of the mate, which I was very fond of. When we left Italy we had delightful sailing among the Archipelago islands, and from thence to Smyrna in Turkey. This is a very ancient city; the houses are built of stone, and most of them have graves adjoining to them; so that they sometimes present the appearance of church-yards. Provisions are very plentiful in this city, and good wine less than a penny a pint. The grapes, pomegranates, and many other fruits, were also the richest and largest I ever tasted. The natives are well looking and strong made, and treated me always with great civility. In general I believe they are fond of black people; and several of them gave me pressing invitations to stay amongst them, although they keep the franks, or Christians, separate, and do not suffer them to dwell immediately amongst them. I was astonished in not seeing women in any of their shops, and very rarely any in the streets; and whenever I did they were covered with a veil from head to foot, so that I could not see their faces, except when any of them out of curiosity uncovered them to look at me, which they sometimes did. I was surprised to see how the Greeks are, in some measure, kept under by the Turks, as the negroes are in the West Indies by the white people. The less refined Greeks, as I have already hinted, dance here in the same manner as we do in my nation. On the whole, during our stay here, which was about five months, I liked the place and the Turks extremely well. I could not help observing one very remarkable circumstance there: the tails of the sheep are flat, and so very large, that I have known the tail even of a lamb to weigh from eleven to thirteen pounds. The fat of them is very white and rich, and is excellent in puddings, for which it is much used. Our ship being at length richly loaded with silk, and other articles, we sailed for England.

In May 1769, soon after our return from Turkey, our ship made a delightful voyage to Oporto in Portugal, where we arrived at the time of the carnival. On our arrival, there were sent on board to us thirty-six articles to observe, with very heavy penalties if we should break any of them; and none of us even dared to go on board any other vessel or on shore till the Inquisition had sent on board and searched for every thing illegal, especially bibles. Such as were produced, and certain other things, were sent on shore till the ships were going away; and any person in whose custody a bible was found concealed was to be imprisoned and flogged, and sent into slavery for ten years. I saw here many very magnificent sights, particularly the garden of Eden, where many of the clergy and laity went in procession in their several orders with the host, and sung Te Deum. I had a great curiosity to go into some of their churches, but could not gain admittance without using the necessary sprinkling of holy water at my entrance. From curiosity, and a wish to be holy, I therefore complied with this ceremony, but its virtues were lost on me, for I found myself nothing the better for it. This place abounds with plenty of all kinds of provisions. The town is well built and pretty, and commands a fine prospect. Our ship having taken in a load of wine, and other commodities, we sailed for London, and arrived in July following. Our next voyage was to the Mediterranean. The ship was again got ready, and we sailed in September for Genoa. This is one of the finest cities I ever saw; some of the edifices were of beautiful marble, and made a most noble appearance; and many had very curious fountains before them. The churches were rich and magnificent, and curiously adorned both in the inside and out. But all this grandeur was in my eyes disgraced by the galley slaves, whose condition both there and in other parts of Italy is truly piteous and wretched. After we had stayed there some weeks, during which we bought many different things which we wanted, and got them very cheap, we sailed to Naples, a charming city, and remarkably clean. The bay is the most beautiful I ever saw; the moles for shipping are excellent. I thought it extraordinary to see grand operas acted here on Sunday nights, and even attended by their majesties. I too, like these great ones, went to those sights, and vainly served God in the day while I thus served mammon effectually at night. While we remained here there happened an eruption of mount Vesuvius, of which I had a perfect view. It was extremely awful; and we were so near that the ashes from it used to be thick on our deck. After we had transacted our business at Naples we sailed with a fair wind once more for

Smyrna, where we arrived in December. A seraskier or officer took a liking to me here, and wanted me to stay, and offered me two wives; however I refused the temptation. The merchants here travel in caravans or large companies. I have seen many caravans from India, with some hundreds of camels, laden with different goods. The people of these caravans are quite brown. Among other articles, they brought with them a great quantity of locusts, which are a kind of pulse, sweet and pleasant to the palate, and in shape resembling French beans, but longer. Each kind of goods is sold in a street by itself, and I always found the Turks very honest in their dealings. They let no Christians into their mosques or churches, for which I was very sorry; as I was always fond of going to see the different modes of worship of the people wherever I went. The plague broke out while we were in Smyrna, and we stopped taking goods into the ship till it was over. She was then richly laden, and we sailed in about March 1770 for England. One day in our passage we met with an accident which was near burning the ship. A black cook, in melting some fat, overset the pan into the fire under the deck, which immediately began to blaze, and the flame went up very high under the foretop. With the fright the poor cook became almost white, and altogether speechless. Happily however we got the fire out without doing much mischief. After various delays in this passage, which was tedious, we arrived in Standgate creek in July; and, at the latter end of the year, some new event occurred, so that my noble captain, the ship, and I all separated.

In April 1771 I shipped myself as a steward with Capt. Wm. Robertson of the ship Grenada Planter, once more to try my fortune in the West Indies; and we sailed from London for Madeira, Barbadoes, and the Grenades. When we were at this last place, having some goods to sell, I met once more with my former kind of West India customers. A white man, an islander, bought some goods of me to the amount of some pounds, and made me many fair promises as usual, but without any intention of paying me. He had likewise bought goods from some more of our people, whom he intended to serve in the same manner; but he still amused us with promises. However, when our ship was loaded, and near sailing, this honest buyer discovered no intention or sign of paying for any thing he had bought of us; but on the contrary, when I asked him for my money he threatened me and another black man he had bought goods of, so that we found we were like to get more blows than payment. On this we went to complain to one Mr. M'Intosh, a justice of the peace; we told his worship of the man's villainous tricks, and begged that he would be kind enough to see us redressed: but being negroes, although free, we could not get any remedy; and our ship being then just upon the point of sailing, we knew not how to help ourselves, though we thought it hard to lose our property in this manner. Luckily for us however, this man was also indebted to three white sailors, who could not get a farthing from him; they therefore readily joined us, and we all went together in search of him. When we found where he was, I took him out of a house and threatened him with vengeance; on which, finding he was likely to be handled roughly, the rogue offered each of us some small allowance, but nothing near our demands. This exasperated us much more; and some were for cutting his ears off; but he begged hard for mercy, which was at last granted him, after we had entirely stripped him. We then let him go, for which he thanked us, glad to get off so easily, and ran into the bushes, after having wished us a good voyage. We then repaired on board, and shortly after set sail for England. I cannot help remarking here a very narrow escape we had from being blown up, owing to a piece of negligence of mine. Just as our ship was under sail, I went down into the cabin to do some business, and had a lighted candle in my hand, which, in my hurry, without thinking, I held in a barrel of gunpowder. It remained in the powder until it was near catching fire, when fortunately I observed it and snatched it out in time, and providentially no harm happened; but I was so overcome with terror that I immediately fainted at this deliverance.

In twenty-eight days time we arrived in England, and I got clear of this ship. But, being still of a roving disposition, and desirous of seeing as many different parts of the world as I could, I shipped myself soon after, in the same year, as steward on board of a fine large ship, called the Jamaica, Captain David Watt; and we sailed from England in December 1771 for Nevis and Jamaica. I found Jamaica to be a very fine large

island, well peopled, and the most considerable of the West
India islands. There was a vast number of negroes here,
whom I found as usual exceedingly imposed upon by the
white people, and the slaves punished as in the other islands.
There are negroes whose business it is to flog slaves; they go
about to different people for employment, and the usual pay
is from one to four bits. I saw many cruel punishments inflicted on the slaves in the short time I stayed here. In particular I was present when a poor fellow was tied up and kept
hanging by the wrists at some distance from the ground, and
then some half hundred weights were fixed to his ancles, in
which posture he was flogged most unmercifully. There were
also, as I heard, two different masters noted for cruelty on the
island, who had staked up two negroes naked, and in two
hours the vermin stung them to death. I heard a gentleman I
well knew tell my captain that he passed sentence on a negro
man to be burnt alive for attempting to poison an overseer. I
pass over numerous other instances, in order to relieve the
reader by a milder scene of roguery. Before I had been long
on the island, one Mr. Smith at Port Morant bought goods of
me to the amount of twenty-five pounds sterling; but when I
demanded payment from him, he was going each time to beat
me, and threatened that he would put me in goal. One time
he would say I was going to set his house on fire, at another
he would swear I was going to run away with his slaves. I was
astonished at this usage from a person who was in the situation of a gentleman, but I had no alternative; I was therefore
obliged to submit. When I came to Kingston, I was surprised
to see the number of Africans who were assembled together
on Sundays; particularly at a large commodious place, called
Spring Path. Here each different nation of Africa meet and
dance after the manner of their own country. They still retain
most of their native customs: they bury their dead, and put
victuals, pipes and tobacco, and other things, in the grave
with the corps, in the same manner as in Africa. Our ship having got her loading we sailed for London, where we arrived in
the August following. On my return to London, I waited on
my old and good master, Dr. Irving, who made me an offer
of his service again. Being now tired of the sea I gladly accepted it. I was very happy in living with this gentleman once

more; during which time we were daily employed in reducing old Neptune's dominions by purifying the briny element and making it fresh. Thus I went on till May 1773, when I was roused by the sound of fame, to seek new adventures, and to find, towards the north pole, what our Creator never intended we should, a passage to India. An expedition was now fitting out to explore a north-east passage, conducted by the Honourable John Constantine Phipps, since Lord Mulgrave, in his Majesty's sloop of war the Race Horse. My master being anxious for the reputation of this adventure, we therefore prepared every thing for our voyage, and I attended him on board the Race Horse, the 24th day of May 1773. We proceeded to Sheerness, where we were joined by his Majesty's sloop the Carcass, commanded by Captain Lutwidge. On the 4th of June we sailed towards our destined place, the pole; and on the 15th of the same month we were off Shetland. On this day I had a great and unexpected deliverance from an accident which was near blowing up the ship and destroying the crew, which made me ever after during the voyage uncommonly cautious. The ship was so filled that there was very little room on board for any one, which placed me in a very aukward situation. I had resolved to keep a journal of this singular and interesting voyage; and I had no other place for this purpose but a little cabin, or the doctor's store-room, where I slept. This little place was stuffed with all manner of combustibles, particularly with tow and aquafortis, and many other dangerous things. Unfortunately it happened in the evening as I was writing my journal, that I had occasion to take the candle out of the lanthorn, and a spark having touched a single thread of the tow, all the rest caught the flame, and immediately the whole was in a blaze. I saw nothing but present death before me, and expected to be the first to perish in the flames. In a moment the alarm was spread, and many people who were near ran to assist in putting out the fire. All this time I was in the very midst of the flames; my shirt, and the handkerchief on my neck, were burnt, and I was almost smothered with the smoke. However, through God's mercy, as I was nearly giving up all hopes, some people brought blankets and mattresses and threw them on the flames, by which means in a short time the fire was put out. I was severely reprimanded and menaced by such of the officers who knew it, and strictly charged never more to go there with a light: and, indeed, even my own fears made me give heed to this command for a little time; but at last, not being able to write my journal in any other part of the ship, I was tempted again to venture by stealth with a light in the same cabin, though not without considerable fear and dread on my mind. On the 20th of June we began to use Dr. Irving's apparatus for making salt water fresh; I used to attend the distillery: I frequently purified from twenty-six to forty gallons a day. The water thus distilled was perfectly pure, well tasted, and free from salt; and was used on various occasions on board the ship. On the 28th of June, being in lat. 78, we made Greenland, where I was surprised to see the sun did not set. The weather now became extremely cold; and as we sailed between north and east, which was our course, we saw many very high and curious mountains of ice; and also a great number of very large whales, which used to come close to our ship, and blow the water up to a very great height in the air. One morning we had vast quantities of sea-horses about the ship, which neighed exactly like any other horses. We fired some harpoon guns amongst them, in order to take some, but we could not get any. The 30th, the captain of a Greenland ship came on board, and told us of three ships that were lost in the ice; however we still held on our course till July the 11th, when we were stopt by one compact impenetrable body of ice. We ran along it from east to west above ten degrees; and on the 27th we got as far north as 80, 37; and in 19 or 20 degrees east longitude from London. On the 29th and 30th of July we saw one continued plain of smooth unbroken ice, bounded only by the horizon; and we fastened to a piece of ice that was eight yards eleven inches thick. We had generally sunshine, and constant daylight; which gave cheerfulness and novelty to the whole of this striking, grand, and uncommon scene; and, to heighten it still more, the reflection of the sun from the ice gave the clouds a most beautiful appearance. We killed many different animals at this time, and among the rest nine bears. Though they had nothing in their paunches but water yet they were all very fat. We used to decoy them to the ship sometimes by burning feathers or skins. I thought them coarse eating, but some of the ship's company relished them very much. Some of our people once, in the boat, fired at and wounded a sea-horse, which dived immediately; and, in a little time after, brought up with it a number of others. They all joined in an attack upon the boat, and were with difficulty prevented from staving or oversetting her; but a boat from the Carcass having come to assist ours, and joined it, they dispersed, after having wrested an oar from one of the men. One of the ship's boats had before been attacked in the same manner, but happily no harm was done. Though we wounded several of these animals we never got but one. We remained hereabouts until the 1st of August; when the two ships got completely fastened in the ice, occasioned by the loose ice that set in from the sea. This made our situation very dreadful and alarming; so that on the 7th day we were in very great apprehension of having the ships squeezed to pieces. The officers now held a council to know what was best for us to do in order to save our lives; and it was determined that we should endeavour to escape by dragging our boats along the ice towards the sea; which, however, was farther off than any of us thought. This determination filled us with extreme dejection, and confounded us with despair; for we had very little prospect of escaping with life. However, we sawed some of the ice about the ships to keep it from hurting them; and thus kept them in a kind of pond. We then began to drag the boats as well as we could towards the sea; but, after two or three days labour, we made very little progress; so that some of our hearts totally failed us, and I really began to give up myself for lost, when I saw our surrounding calamities. While we were at this hard labour I once fell into a pond we had made amongst some loose ice, and was very near being drowned; but providentially some people were near who gave me immediate assistance, and thereby I escaped drowning. Our deplorable condition, which kept up the constant apprehension of our perishing in the ice, brought me gradually to think of eternity in such a manner as I never had done before. I had the fears of death hourly upon me, and shuddered at the thoughts of meeting the grim king of terrors in the *natural* state I then was in, and was exceedingly doubtful of a happy eternity if I should die in it. I had no hopes of my life being prolonged for any time; for we saw that our existence could not be long on the ice after leaving the ships, which were now out of sight, and some miles from the boats. Our appearance now became truly lamentable; pale dejection seized every countenance; many, who had been before blasphemers, in this our distress began to call on the good God of heaven for his help; and in the time of our utter need he heard us, and against hope or human probability delivered us! It was the eleventh day of the ships being thus fastened, and the fourth of our drawing the boats in this manner, that the wind changed to the E. N. E. The weather immediately became mild, and the ice broke towards the sea, which was to the S. W. of us. Many of us on this got on board again, and with all our might we hove the ships into every open water we could find, and made all the sail on them in our power; and now, having a prospect of success, we made signals for the boats and the remainder of the people. This seemed to us like a reprieve from death; and happy was the man who could first get on board of any ship, or the first boat he could meet. We then proceeded in this manner till we got into the open water again, which we accomplished in about thirty hours, to our infinite joy and gladness of heart. As soon as we were out of danger we came to anchor and refitted; and on the 19th of August we sailed from this uninhabited extremity of the world, where the inhospitable climate affords neither food nor shelter, and not a tree or shrub of any kind grows amongst its barren rocks; but all is one desolate and expanded waste of ice, which even the constant beams of the sun for six months in the year cannot penetrate or dissolve. The sun now being on the decline the days shortened as we sailed to the southward; and, on the 28th, in latitude 73, it was dark by ten o'clock at night. September the 10th, in latitude 58–59, we met a very severe gale of wind and high seas, and shipped a great deal of water in the space of ten hours. This made us work exceedingly hard at all our pumps a whole day; and one sea, which struck the ship with more force than any thing I ever met with of the kind before, laid her under water for some time, so that we thought she would have gone down. Two boats were washed from the booms, and the long-boat from the chucks: all other moveable things on the deck were also washed away, among which were many curious things of different kinds which we had brought from Greenland; and we were obliged, in order to lighten the ship, to toss some of our guns overboard. We saw a ship, at the same time, in very great distress, and her masts were gone; but we were unable to assist her. We now lost sight of the Carcass till the 26th, when we saw land about Orfordness, off which place she joined us. From thence we sailed for London, and on the 30th came up to Deptford. And thus ended our Arctic voyage, to the no small joy of all on board, after having been absent four months; in which time, at the imminent hazard of our lives, we explored nearly as far towards the Pole as 81 degrees north, and 20 degrees east longitude; being much farther, by all accounts, than any navigator had ever ventured before; in which we fully proved the impracticability of finding a passage that way to India.

CHAP. X.

The author leaves Doctor Irving and engages on board a Turkey ship—Account of a black man's being kidnapped on board and sent to the West Indies, and the author's fruitless endeavours to procure his freedom—Some account of the manner of the author's conversion to the faith of Jesus Christ.

OUR voyage to the North Pole being ended, I returned to London with Doctor Irving, with whom I continued for some time, during which I began seriously to reflect on the dangers I had escaped, particularly those of my last voyage, which made a lasting impression on my mind, and, by the grace of God, proved afterwards a mercy to me; it caused me to reflect deeply on my eternal state, and to seek the Lord with full purpose of heart ere it was too late. I rejoiced greatly; and heartily thanked the Lord for directing me to London, where I was determined to work out my own salvation, and in so doing procure a title to heaven, being the result of a mind blended by ignorance and sin.

In process of time I left my master, Doctor Irving, the purifier of waters, and lodged in Coventry-court, Haymarket, where I was continually oppressed and much concerned about the salvation of my soul, and was determined (in my own strength) to be a first-rate Christian. I used every means for this purpose; and, not being able to find any person amongst my acquaintance that agreed with me in point of religion, or, in scripture language, 'that would shew me any good;' I was much dejected, and knew not where to seek relief; however, I first frequented the neighbouring churches, St. James's, and others, two or three times a day, for many weeks: still I came away dissatisfied; something was wanting that I could not obtain, and I really found more heartfelt relief in reading my bible at home than in attending the church; and, being resolved to be saved, I pursued other methods still. First I went among the quakers, where the word of God was neither read or preached, so that I remained as much in the dark as ever. I then searched into the Roman catholic principles, but was not in the least satisfied. At length I had recourse to the Jews, which availed me nothing, for the fear of eternity daily harassed my mind, and I knew not where to seek shelter from the wrath to come. However this was my conclusion, at all events, to read the four evangelists, and whatever sect or party I found adhering thereto such I would join. Thus I went on heavily without any guide to direct me the way that leadeth to eternal life. I asked different people questions about the manner of going to heaven, and was told different ways. Here I was much staggered, and could not find any at that time more righteous than myself, or indeed so much inclined to devotion. I thought we should not all be saved (this is agreeable to the holy scriptures), nor would all be damned. I found none among the circle of my acquaintance that kept wholly the ten commandments. So righteous was I in my own eyes, that I was convinced I excelled many of them in that point, by keeping eight out of ten; and finding those who in general termed themselves Christians not so honest or so good in their morals as the Turks, I really thought the Turks were in a safer way of salvation than my neighbours: so that between hopes and fears I went on, and the chief comforts I enjoyed were in the musical French horn, which I then practised, and also dressing of hair. Such was my situation some months, experiencing the dishonesty of many people here. I determined at last to set out for Turkey, and there to end my days. It was now early in the spring 1774. I sought for a master, and found a captain John Hughes, commander of a ship called Anglicania, fitting out in the river Thames, and bound to Smyrna in Turkey. I shipped myself with him as a steward; at the same time I recommended to him a very clever black man, John Annis, as a cook. This man was on board the ship near two months doing his duty: he had formerly lived many years with Mr. William Kirkpatrick, a gentleman of the island of St. Kitts, from whom he parted by consent, though he afterwards tried many schemes to inveigle the poor man. He had applied to many captains who traded to St. Kitts to trepan him; and when all their attempts and schemes of kidnapping proved abortive, Mr. Kirkpatrick came to our ship at Union Stairs on Easter Monday, April the fourth, with two wherry boats and six men, having learned that the man was on board; and tied, and forcibly took him away from the ship, in the presence of the crew and the chief mate, who had detained him after he had notice to come away. I believe that this was a combined piece of business: but, at any rate, it certainly reflected great disgrace on the mate and captain also, who, although they had desired the oppressed man to stay on board, yet he did not in the least assist to recover him, or pay me a farthing of his wages, which was about five pounds. I proved the only friend he had, who attempted to regain him his liberty if possible, having known the want of liberty myself. I sent as soon as I could to Gravesend, and got knowledge of the ship in which he was; but unluckily she had sailed the first tide after he was put on board. My intention was then immediately to apprehend Mr. Kirkpatrick, who was about setting off for Scotland; and, having obtained a *habeas corpus* for him, and got a tipstaff to go with me to St. Paul's church-yard, where he lived, he, suspecting something of this kind, set a watch to look out. My being known to them occasioned me to use the following deception: I whitened my face, that they might not know me, and this had its desired effect. He did not go out of his house that night, and next morning I contrived a well plotted stratagem notwithstanding he had a gentleman in his house to personate him. My direction to the tipstaff, who got admittance into the house, was to conduct him to a judge, according to the writ. When he came there, his plea was, that he had not the body in custody, on which he was admitted to bail. I proceeded immediately to that philanthropist, Granville Sharp, Esq. who received me with the utmost kindness, and gave me every instruction that was needful on the occasion. I left him in full hope that I should gain the unhappy man his liberty, with the warmest sense of gratitude towards Mr. Sharp for his kindness; but, alas! my attorney proved unfaithful; he took my money, lost me many months employ, and did not do the least good in the cause: and when the poor man arrived at St. Kitts, he was, according to custom, staked to the ground with four pins through a cord, two on his wrists, and two on his ancles, was cut and flogged most unmercifully, and afterwards loaded cruelly with irons about his neck. I had two very moving letters from him, while he was in this situation; and also was told of it by some very respectable families now in London, who saw him in St. Kitts, in the same state in which he remained till kind death released him out of the hands of his tyrants. During this disagreeable business I was under strong convictions of sin, and thought that my state was worse than any man's; my mind was unaccountably disturbed; I often wished for death, though at the same time convinced I was altogether unprepared for that awful summons. Suffering much by villains in the late cause, and being much concerned about the state of my soul, these things (but particularly the latter) brought me very low; so that I became a burden to myself, and viewed all things around me as emptiness and vanity, which could give no satisfaction to a troubled conscience. I was again determined to go to Turkey, and resolved, at that time, never more to return to England. I engaged as steward on board a Turkeyman (the Wester Hall, Capt. Linna); but was prevented by means of my late captain, Mr. Hughes, and others. All this appeared to be against me, and the only comfort I then experienced was, in reading the holy scriptures, where I saw that 'there is no new thing under the sun,' Eccles. i. 9; and what was appointed for me I must submit to. Thus I continued to travel in much heaviness, and frequently murmured against the Almighty, particularly in his providential dealings; and, awful to think! I began to blaspheme, and wished often to be any thing but a human being. In these severe conflicts the Lord answered me by awful 'visions of the night, when deep sleep falleth upon men, in slumberings upon the bed,' Job xxxiii. 15. He was pleased, in much mercy, to give me to see, and in some measure to understand, the great and awful scene of the judgment-day, that 'no unclean person, no unholy thing, can enter into the kingdom of God,' Eph. v. 5. I would then, if it had been possible, have changed my nature with the meanest worm on the earth; and was ready to say to the mountains and rocks 'fall on me,' Rev. vi. 16; but all in vain. I then requested the divine Creator that he would grant me a small space of time to repent of my follies and vile iniquities, which I felt were grievous. The Lord, in his manifold mercies, was pleased to grant my request, and being yet in a state of time, the sense of God's mercies was so great on my mind when I awoke, that my strength entirely failed me for many minutes, and I was exceedingly weak. This was the first spiritual mercy I ever was sensible of, and being on praying ground, as soon as I recovered a little strength, and got out of bed and dressed myself, I invoked Heaven from my inmost soul, and fervently begged that God would never again permit me to blaspheme his most holy name. The Lord, who is long-suffering, and full of compassion to such poor rebels as we are, condescended to hear and answer. I felt that I was altogether unholy, and saw clearly what a bad use I had made of the faculties I was endowed with; they were given me to glorify God with; I thought, therefore, I had better want them here, and enter into life eternal, than abuse them and be cast into hell fire. I prayed to be directed, if there were any holier than those with whom I was acquainted, that the Lord would point them out to me. I appealed to the Searcher of hearts, whether I did not wish to love him more, and serve him better. Notwithstanding all this, the reader may easily discern, if he is a believer, that I was still in nature's darkness. At length I hated the house in which I lodged, because God's most holy name was blasphemed in it; then I saw the word of God verified, viz. 'Before they call, I will answer; and while they are yet speaking, I will hear.'

I had a great desire to read the bible the whole day at home; but not having a convenient place for retirement, I left the house in the day, rather than stay amongst the wicked ones; and that day as I was walking, it pleased God to direct me to a house where there was an old sea-faring man, who experienced much of the love of God shed abroad in his heart. He began to discourse with me; and, as I desired to love the Lord, his conversation rejoiced me greatly; and indeed I had never heard before the love of Christ to believers set forth in such a manner, and in so clear a point of view. Here I had more questions to put to the man than his time would permit him to answer; and in that memorable hour there came in a dissenting minister; he joined our discourse, and asked me some few questions; among others, where I heard the gospel preached. I knew not what he meant by hearing the gospel; I told him I had read the gospel: and he asked where I went to church, or whether I went at all or not. To which I replied, 'I attended St. James's, St. Martin's, and

St. Ann's, Soho;'—'So,' said he, 'you are a churchman.' I answered, I was. He then invited me to a love-feast at his chapel
that evening. I accepted the offer, and thanked him; and soon
after he went away, I had some further discourse with the old
Christian, added to some profitable reading, which made me
exceedingly happy. When I left him he reminded me of coming to the feast; I assured him I would be there. Thus we
parted, and I weighed over the heavenly conversation that
had passed between these two men, which cheered my then
heavy and drooping spirit more than any thing I had met with
for many months. However, I thought the time long in going
to my supposed banquet. I also wished much for the company
of these friendly men; their company pleased me much; and I
thought the gentlemen very kind, in asking me, a stranger, to
a feast; but how singular did it appear to me, to have it in a
chapel! When the wished-for hour came I went, and happily
the old man was there, who kindly seated me, as he belonged
to the place. I was much astonished to see the place filled with
people, and no signs of eating and drinking. There were many
ministers in the company. At last they began by giving out
hymns, and between the singing the minister engaged in
prayer; in short, I knew not what to make of this sight, having never seen any thing of the kind in my life before now.
Some of the guests began to speak their experience, agreeable
to what I read in the Scriptures; much was said by every
speaker of the providence of God, and his unspeakable mercies, to each of them. This I knew in a great measure, and
could most heartily join them. But when they spoke of a future state, they seemed to be altogether certain of their calling and election of God; and that no one could ever separate
them from the love of Christ, or pluck them out of his hands.
This filled me with utter consternation, intermingled with admiration. I was so amazed as not to know what to think of
the company; my heart was attracted and my affections were
enlarged. I wished to be as happy as them, and was persuaded
in my mind that they were different from the world 'that lieth
in wickedness,' 1 John v. 19. Their language and singing, &c.
did well harmonize; I was entirely overcome, and wished to
live and die thus. Lastly, some persons in the place produced
some neat baskets full of buns, which they distributed about;

and each person communicated with his neighbour, and sipped water out of different mugs, which they handed about to all who were present. This kind of Christian fellowship I had never seen, nor ever thought of seeing on earth; it fully reminded me of what I had read in the holy scriptures, of the primitive Christians, who loved each other and broke bread. In partaking of it, even from house to house, this entertainment (which lasted about four hours) ended in singing and prayer. It was the first soul feast I ever was present at. This last twenty-four hours produced me things, spiritual and temporal, sleeping and waking, judgment and mercy, that I could not but admire the goodness of God, in directing the blind, blasphemous sinner in the path that he knew not of, even among the just; and instead of judgment he has shewed mercy, and will hear and answer the prayers and supplications of every returning prodigal:

> O! to grace how great a debtor
> Daily I'm constrain'd to be!

After this I was resolved to win Heaven if possible; and if I perished I thought it should be at the feet of Jesus, in praying to him for salvation. After having been an eye-witness to some of the happiness which attended those who feared God, I knew not how, with any propriety, to return to my lodgings, where the name of God was continually profaned, at which I felt the greatest horror. I paused in my mind for some time, not knowing what to do; whether to hire a bed elsewhere, or go home again. At last, fearing an evil report might arise, I went home, with a farewell to card-playing and vain jesting, &c. I saw that time was very short, eternity long, and very near, and I viewed those persons alone blessed who were found ready at midnight call, or when the Judge of all, both quick and dead, cometh.

The next day I took courage, and went to Holborn, to see my new and worthy acquaintance, the old man, Mr. C——; he, with his wife, a gracious woman, were at work at silk weaving; they seemed mutually happy, and both quite glad to see me, and I more so to see them. I sat down, and we conversed much about soul matters, &c. Their discourse was amazingly delightful, edifying, and pleasant. I knew not at last how to leave this agreeable pair, till time summoned me away. As I was going they lent me a little book, entitled "The Conversion of an Indian." It was in questions and answers. The poor man came over the sea to London, to inquire after the Christian's God, who, (through rich mercy) he found, and had not his journey in vain. The above book was of great use to me, and at that time was a means of strengthening my faith; however, in parting, they both invited me to call on them when I pleased. This delighted me, and I took care to make all the improvement from it I could; and so far I thanked God for such company and desires. I prayed that the many evils I felt within might be done away, and that I might be weaned from my former carnal acquaintances. This was quickly heard and answered, and I was soon connected with those whom the scripture calls the excellent of the earth. I heard the gospel preached, and the thoughts of my heart and actions were laid open by the preachers, and the way of salvation by Christ alone was evidently set forth. Thus I went on happily for near two months; and I once heard, during this period, a reverend gentleman speak of a man who had departed this life in full assurance of his going to glory. I was much astonished at the assertion; and did very deliberately inquire how he could get at this knowledge. I was answered fully, agreeable to what I read in the oracles of truth; and was told also, that if I did not experience the new birth, and the pardon of my sins, through the blood of Christ, before I died, I could not enter the kingdom of heaven. I knew not what to think of this report, as I thought I kept eight commandments out of ten; then my worthy interpreter told me I did not do it, nor could I; and he added, that no man ever did or could keep the commandments, without offending in one point. I thought this sounded very strange, and puzzled me much for many weeks; for I thought it a hard saying. I then asked my friend, Mr. L——d, who was a clerk in a chapel, why the commandments of God were given, if we could not be saved by them? To which he replied, 'The law is a schoolmaster to bring us to Christ,' who alone could and did keep the commandments, and fulfilled all their requirements for his elect people, even those to whom he had given a living faith, and the sins of those chosen vessels *were already* atoned for and forgiven them whilst living; and if I did not experience the same before my exit, the Lord would say at that great day to me 'Go ye cursed,' &c. &c. for God would appear faithful in his judgments to the wicked, as he would be faithful in shewing mercy to those who were ordained to it before the world was; therefore Christ Jesus seemed to be all in all to that man's soul. I was much wounded at this discourse, and brought into such a dilemma as I never expected. I asked him, if *he* was to die that moment, whether he was sure to enter the kingdom of God? and added, 'Do you *know* that your sins are forgiven you?' He answered in the affirmative. Then confusion, anger, and discontent seized me, and I staggered much at this sort of doctrine; it brought me to a stand, not knowing which to believe, whether salvation by works or by faith only in Christ. I requested him to tell me how I might know when my sins were forgiven me. He assured me he could not, and that none but God alone could do this. I told him it was very mysterious; but he said it was really matter of fact, and quoted many portions of scripture immediately to the point, to which I could make no reply. He then desired me to pray to God to shew me these things. I answered, that I prayed to God every day He said, 'I perceive you are a churchman.' I answered I was. He then entreated me to beg of God to shew me what I was, and the true state of my soul. I thought the prayer very short and odd; so we parted for that time. I weighed all these things well over, and could not help thinking how it was possible for a man to know that his sins were forgiven him in this life. I wished that God would reveal this self same thing unto me. In a short time after this I went to Westminster chapel; the Rev. Mr. P—— preached, from Lam. iii. 39. It was a wonderful sermon; he clearly shewed that a living man had no cause to complain for the punishment of his sins; he evidently justified the Lord in all his dealings with the sons of men; he also shewed the justice of God in the eternal punishment of the wicked and impenitent. The discourse seemed to me like a two-edged sword cutting all ways; it afforded me much joy, intermingled with many fears, about my soul; and when it was ended, he gave it out that he intended, the ensuing week, to examine all those who meant to attend the Lord's table. Now

I thought much of my good works, and at the same time was doubtful of my being a proper object to receive the sacrament; I was full of meditation till the day of examining. However, I went to the chapel, and, though much distressed, I addressed the reverend gentleman, thinking, if I was not right, he would endeavour to convince me of it. When I conversed with him, the first thing he asked me was, what I knew of Christ? I told him I believed in him, and had been baptized in his name. 'Then,' said he, 'when were you brought to the knowledge of God? and how were you convinced of sin?' I knew not what he meant by these questions; I told him I kept eight commandments out of ten; but that I sometimes swore on board ship, and sometimes when on shore, and broke the sabbath. He then asked me if I could read? I answered, 'Yes.'—'Then,' said he, 'do you not read in the bible, he that offends in one point is guilty of all?' I said, 'Yes.' Then he assured me, that one sin unatoned for was as sufficient to damn a soul as one leak was to sink a ship. Here I was struck with awe; for the minister exhorted me much, and reminded me of the shortness of time, and the length of eternity, and that no unregenerate soul, or any thing unclean, could enter the kingdom of Heaven. He did not admit me as a communicant; but recommended me to read the scriptures, and hear the word preached, not to neglect fervent prayer to God, who has promised to hear the supplications of those who seek him in godly sincerity; so I took my leave of him, with many thanks, and resolved to follow his advice, so far as the Lord would condescend to enable me. During this time I was out of employ, nor was I likely to get a situation suitable for me, which obliged me to go once more to sea. I engaged as steward of a ship called the Hope, Capt. Richard Strange, bound from London to Cadiz in Spain. In a short time after I was on board I heard the name of God much blasphemed, and I feared greatly, lest I should catch the horrible infection. I thought if I sinned again, after having life and death set evidently before me, I should certainly go to hell. My mind was uncommonly chagrined, and I murmured much at God's providential dealings with me, and was discontented with the commandments, that I could not be saved by what I had done; I hated all things, and wished I had never been born;

confusion seized me, and I wished to be annihilated. One day I was standing on the very edge of the stern of the ship, thinking to drown myself; but this scripture was instantly impressed on my mind—'that no murderer hath eternal life abiding in him,' 1 John iii. 15. Then I paused, and thought myself the unhappiest man living. Again I was convinced that the Lord was better to me than I deserved, and I was better off in the world than many. After this I began to fear death; I fretted, mourned, and prayed, till I became a burden to others, but more so to myself. At length I concluded to beg my bread on shore rather than go again to sea amongst a people who feared not God, and I entreated the captain three different times to discharge me; he would not, but each time gave me greater and greater encouragement to continue with him, and all on board shewed me very great civility: notwithstanding all this I was unwilling to embark again. At last some of my religious friends advised me, by saying it was my lawful calling, consequently it was my duty to obey, and that God was not confined to place, &c. &c. particularly Mr. G. S. the governor of Tothil-fields Bridewell, who pitied my case, and read the eleventh chapter of the Hebrews to me, with exhortations. He prayed for me, and I believed that he prevailed on my behalf, as my burden was then greatly removed, and I found a heartfelt resignation to the will of God. The good man gave me a pocket Bible and Allen's Alarm to the unconverted. We parted, and the next day I went on board again. We sailed for Spain, and I found favour with the captain. It was the fourth of the month of September when we sailed from London; we had a delightful voyage to Cadiz, where we arrived the twenty-third of the same month. The place is strong, commands a fine prospect, and is very rich. The Spanish galloons frequent that port, and some arrived whilst we were there. I had many opportunities of reading the scriptures. I wrestled hard with God in fervent prayer, who had declared in his word that he would hear the groanings and deep sighs of the poor in spirit. I found this verified to my utter astonishment and comfort in the following manner:

On the morning of the 6th of October, (I pray you to attend) or all that day, I thought that I should either see or hear something supernatural. I had a secret impulse on my mind of something that was to take place, which drove me continually for that time to a throne of grace. It pleased God to enable me to wrestle with him, as Jacob did: I prayed that if sudden death were to happen, and I perished, it might be at Christ's feet.

In the evening of the same day, as I was reading and meditating on the fourth chapter of the Acts, twelfth verse, under the solemn apprehensions of eternity, and reflecting on my past actions, I began to think I had lived a moral life, and that I had a proper ground to believe I had an interest in the divine favour; but still meditating on the subject, not knowing whether salvation was to be had partly for our own good deeds, or solely as the sovereign gift of God; in this deep consternation the Lord was pleased to break in upon my soul with his bright beams of heavenly light; and in an instant as it were, removing the veil, and letting light into a dark place, I saw clearly with the eye of faith the crucified Saviour bleeding on the cross on mount Calvary: the scriptures became an unsealed book, I saw myself a condemned criminal under the law, which came with its full force to my conscience, and when 'the commandment came sin revived, and I died,' I saw the Lord Jesus Christ in his humiliation, loaded and bearing my reproach, sin, and shame. I then clearly perceived that by the deeds of the law no flesh living could be justified. I was then convinced that by the first Adam sin came, and by the second Adam (the Lord Jesus Christ) all that are saved must be made alive. It was given me at that time to know what it was to be born again, John iii. 5. I saw the eighth chapter to the Romans, and the doctrines of God's decrees, verified agreeable to his eternal, everlasting, and unchangeable purposes. The word of God was sweet to my taste, yea sweeter than honey and the honeycomb. Christ was revealed to my soul as the chiefest among ten thousand. These heavenly moments were really as life to the dead, and what John calls an earnest of the Spirit*. This was indeed unspeakable, and I firmly believe undeniable by many. Now every leading providential circumstance that happened to me, from the day I was taken from my parents to that hour, was then in my view, as

*John xvi. 13, 14. &c.

if it had but just then occurred. I was sensible of the invisible hand of God, which guided and protected me when in truth I knew it not: still the Lord pursued me although I slighted and disregarded it; this mercy melted me down. When I considered my poor wretched state I wept, seeing what a great debtor I was to sovereign free grace. Now the Ethiopian was willing to be saved by Jesus Christ, the sinner's only surety, and also to rely on none other person or thing for salvation. Self was obnoxious, and good works he had none, for it is God that worketh in us both to will and to do. The amazing things of that hour can never be told—it was joy in the Holy Ghost! I felt an astonishing change; the burden of sin, the gaping jaws of hell, and the fears of death, that weighed me down before, now lost their horror; indeed I thought death would now be the best earthly friend I ever had. Such were my grief and joy as I believe are seldom experienced. I was bathed in tears, and said, What am I that God should thus look on me the vilest of sinners? I felt a deep concern for my mother and friends, which occasioned me to pray with fresh ardour; and, in the abyss of thought, I viewed the unconverted people of the world in a very awful state, being without God and without hope.

It pleased God to pour out on me the Spirit of prayer and the grace of supplication, so that in loud acclamations I was enabled to praise and glorify his most holy name. When I got out of the cabin, and told some of the people what the Lord had done for me, alas, who could understand me or believe my report!—None but to whom the arm of the Lord was revealed. I became a barbarian to them in talking of the love of Christ: his name was to me as ointment poured forth; indeed it was sweet to my soul, but to them a rock of offence. I thought my case singular, and every hour a day until I came to London, for I much longed to be with some to whom I could tell of the wonders of God's love towards me, and join in prayer to him whom my soul loved and thirsted after. I had uncommon commotions within, such as few can tell aught about. Now the bible was my only companion and comfort; I prized it much, with many thanks to God that I could read it for myself, and was not left to be tossed about or led by man's devices and notions. The worth of a soul cannot be told.—

May the Lord give the reader an understanding in this. Whenever I looked in the bible I saw things new, and many texts were immediately applied to me with great comfort, for I knew that to me was the word of salvation sent. Sure I was that the Spirit which indited the word opened my heart to receive the truth of it as it is in Jesus—that the same Spirit enabled me to act faith upon the promises that were so precious to me, and enabled me to believe to the salvation of my soul. By free grace I was persuaded that I had a part in the first resurrection, and was 'enlightened with the light of the living,' Job xxxiii. 30. I wished for a man of God with whom I might converse: my soul was like the chariots of Aminidab, Canticles vi. 12. These, among others, were the precious promises that were so powerfully applied to me: 'All things whatsoever ye shall ask in prayer, believing, ye shall receive,' Mat. xxi. 22. 'Peace I leave with you, my peace I give unto you,' John xiv. 27. I saw the blessed Redeemer to be the fountain of life, and the well of salvation. I experienced him all in all; he had brought me by a way that I knew not, and he had made crooked paths straight. Then in his name I set up my Ebenezer, saying, Hitherto he hath helped me: and could say to the sinners about me, Behold what a Saviour I have! Thus I was, by the teaching of that all-glorious Deity, the great One in Three, and Three in One, confirmed in the truths of the bible, those oracles of everlasting truth, on which every soul living must stand or fall eternally, agreeable to Acts iv. 12. 'Neither is there salvation in any other, for there is none other name under heaven given among men whereby we must be saved, but only Christ Jesus.' May God give the reader a right understanding in these facts! To him that believeth all things are possible, but to them that are unbelieving nothing is pure, Titus i. 15. During this period we remained at Cadiz until our ship got laden. We sailed about the fourth of November; and, having a good passage, we arrived in London the month following, to my comfort, with heartfelt gratitude to God for his rich and unspeakable mercies. On my return I had but one text which puzzled me, or that the devil endeavoured to buffet me with, viz. Rom. xi. 6. and, as I had heard of the Reverend Mr. Romaine, and his great knowledge in the scriptures, I wished much to hear him preach. One day I went to Blackfriars church, and, to my great satisfaction and surprise, he preached from that very text. He very clearly shewed the difference between human works and free election, which is according to God's sovereign will and pleasure. These glad tidings set me entirely at liberty, and I went out of the church rejoicing, seeing my spots were those of God's children. I went to Westminster Chapel, and saw some of my old friends, who were glad when they perceived the wonderful change that the Lord had wrought in me, particularly Mr. G— S—, my worthy acquaintance, who was a man of a choice spirit, and had great zeal for the Lord's service. I enjoyed his correspondence till he died in the year 1784. I was again examined at that same chapel, and was received into church fellowship amongst them: I rejoiced in spirit, making melody in my heart to the God of all my mercies. Now my whole wish was to be dissolved, and to be with Christ—but, alas! I must wait mine appointed time.

MISCELLANEOUS VERSES,
OR.
Reflections on the State of my mind during my first Convictions; of the Necessity of believing the Truth, and experiencing the inestimable Benefits of Christianity.

Well may I say my life has been
One scene of sorrow and of pain;
From early days I griefs have known,
And as I grew my griefs have grown:

Dangers were always in my path;
And fear of wrath, and sometimes death;
While pale dejection in me reign'd
I often wept, by grief constrain'd.

When taken from my native land,
By an unjust and cruel band,
How did uncommon dread prevail!
My sighs no more I could conceal.

'To ease my mind I often strove,
And tried my trouble to remove:
I sung, and utter'd sighs between—
Assay'd to stifle guilt with sin.

'But O! not all that I could do
Would stop the current of my woe;
Conviction still my vileness shew'd;
How great my guilt—how lost from God!

'Prevented, that I could not die,
Nor might to one kind refuge fly;
An orphan state I had to mourn,—
Forsook by all, and left forlorn.'

Those who beheld my downcast mien
Could not guess at my woes unseen:
They by appearance could not know
The troubles that I waded through.

'Lust, anger, blasphemy, and pride,
With legions of such ills beside,
Troubled my thoughts,' while doubts and fears
Clouded and darken'd most my years.

'Sighs now no more would be confin'd—
They breath'd the trouble of my mind:
I wish'd for death, but check'd the word,
And often pray'd unto the Lord.'

Unhappy, more than some on earth,
I thought the place that gave me birth—
Strange thoughts oppress'd—while I replied
"Why not in Ethiopia died?"

And why thus spared, nigh to hell?—
God only knew—I could not tell!
'A tott'ring fence, a bowing wall
thought myself ere since the fall.'

'Oft times I mused, nigh despair,
While birds melodious fill'd the air:
Thrice happy songsters, ever free,
How bless'd were they compar'd to me!'

Thus all things added to my pain,
While grief compell'd me to complain;
When sable clouds began to rise
My mind grew darker than the skies.

The English nation call'd to leave,
How did my breast with sorrows heave!
I long'd for rest—cried "Help me, Lord!
Some mitigation, Lord, afford!"

Yet on, dejected, still I went—
Heart-throbbing woes within were pent;
Nor land, nor sea, could comfort give,
Nothing my anxious mind relieve.

Weary with travail, yet unknown
To all but God and self alone,
Numerous months for peace I strove,
And numerous foes I had to prove.

Inur'd to dangers, griefs, and woes,
Train'd up 'midst perils, deaths, and foes,
I said "Must it thus ever be?—
No quiet is permitted me."

Hard hap, and more than heavy lot!
I pray'd to God "Forget me not—
What thou ordain'st willing I'll bear;
But O! deliver from despair!"

Strivings and wrestlings seem'd in vain;
Nothing I did could ease my pain:
Then gave I up my works and will,
Confess'd and own'd my doom was hell!

Like some poor pris'ner at the bar,
Conscious of guilt, of sin and fear,
Arraign'd, and self-condemned, I stood—
'Lost in the world, and in my blood!'

Yet here, 'midst blackest clouds confin'd,
A beam from Christ, the day-star, shin'd;
Surely, thought I, if Jesus please,
He can at once sign my release.

I, ignorant of his righteousness,
Set up my labours in its place;
'Forgot for why his blood was shed,
And pray'd and fasted in its stead.'

He dy'd for sinners—I am one!
Might not his blood for me atone?
Tho' I am nothing else but sin,
Yet surely he can make me clean!

Thus light came in, and I believ'd;
Myself forgot, and help receiv'd!
My Saviour then I know I found,
For, eas'd from guilt, no more I groan'd.

O, happy hour, in which I ceas'd
To mourn, for then I found a rest!
My soul and Christ were now as one—
Thy light, O Jesus, in me shone!

Bless'd be thy name, for now I know
I and my works can nothing do;
"The Lord alone can ransom man—
For this the spotless Lamb was slain!"

When sacrifices, works, and pray'r,
Prov'd vain, and ineffectual were,
"Lo, then I come!" the Saviour cry'd,
And, bleeding, bow'd his head and dy'd!

He dy'd for all who ever saw
No help in them, nor by the law:—
I this have seen; and gladly own
"Salvation is by Christ alone*!"

*Acts iv. 12.

CHAP. XI.

*The author embarks on board a ship bound for Cadiz—Is near
being shipwrecked—Goes to Malaga—Remarkable fine cathe-
dral there—The author disputes with a popish priest—Picking
up eleven miserable men at sea in returning to England—
Engages again with Doctor Irving to accompany him to Jamaica and the Mosquito Shore—Meets with an Indian prince
on board—The author attempts to instruct him in the truths
of the Gospel—Frustrated by the bad example of some in the
ship—They arrive on the Mosquito Shore with some slaves they
purchased at Jamaica, and begin to cultivate a plantation—
Some account of the manners and customs of the Mosquito Indians—Successful device of the author's to quell a riot among
them—Curious entertainment given by them to Doctor
Irving and the author, who leaves the shore and goes for
Jamaica—Is barbarously treated by a man with whom he engaged for his passage—Escapes and goes to the Mosquito admiral, who treats him kindly—He gets another vessel and goes
on board—Instances of bad treatment—Meets Doctor Irving—Gets to Jamaica—Is cheated by his captain—Leaves the
Doctor and goes for England.*

WHEN our ship was got ready for sea again, I was entreated
by the captain to go in her once more; but, as I felt myself
now as happy as I could wish to be in this life, I for some time
refused; however, the advice of my friends at last prevailed;
and, in full resignation to the will of God, I again embarked
for Cadiz in March 1775. We had a very good passage, without any material accident, until we arrived off the Bay of
Cadiz; when one Sunday, just as we were going into the harbour, the ship struck against a rock and knocked off a gar-
board plank, which is the next to the keel. In an instant all
hands were in the greatest confusion, and began with loud
cries to call on God to have mercy on them. Although I could
not swim, and saw no way of escaping death, I felt no dread
in my then situation, having no desire to live. I even rejoiced
in spirit, thinking this death would be sudden glory. But the
fulness of time was not yet come. The people near to me were

much astonished in seeing me thus calm and resigned; but I told them of the peace of God, which through sovereign grace I enjoyed, and these words were that instant in my mind:

"Christ is my pilot wise, my compass is his word;
My soul each storm defies, while I have such a Lord.
I trust his faithfulness and power,
To save me in the trying hour.
Though rocks and quicksands deep through all my
passage lie,
Yet Christ shall safely keep and guide me with his eye.
How can I sink with such a prop,
That bears the world and all things up?"

At this time there were many large Spanish flukers or passage-vessels full of people crossing the channel; who seeing our condition, a number of them came alongside of us. As many hands as could be employed began to work; some at our three pumps, and the rest unloading the ship as fast as possible. There being only a single rock called the Porpus on which we struck, we soon got off it, and providentially it was then high water, we therefore run the ship ashore at the nearest place to keep her from sinking. After many tides, with a great deal of care and industry, we got her repaired again. When we had dispatched our business at Cadiz, we went to Gibraltar, and from thence to Malaga, a very pleasant and rich city, where there is one of the finest cathedrals I had ever seen. It had been above fifty years in building, as I heard, though it was not then quite finished; great part of the inside, however, was completed and highly decorated with the richest marble columns and many superb paintings; it was lighted occasionally by an amazing number of wax tapers of different sizes, some of which were as thick as a man's thigh; these, however, were only used on some of their grand festivals.

I was very much shocked at the custom of bull-baiting, and other diversions which prevailed here on Sunday evenings, to the great scandal of Christianity and morals. I used to express my abhorrence of it to a priest whom I met with. I had frequent contests about religion with the reverend father, in which he took great pains to make a proselyte of me to his church; and I no less to convert him to mine. On these occasions I used to produce my Bible, and shew him in what points his church erred. He then said he had been in England, and that every person there read the Bible, which was very wrong; but I answered him that Christ desired us to search the Scriptures. In his zeal for my conversion, he solicited me to go to one of the universities in Spain, and declared that I should have my education free; and told me, if I got myself made a priest, I might in time become even pope; and that Pope Benedict was a black man. As I was ever desirous of learning, I paused for some time upon this temptation; and thought by being crafty I might catch some with guile; but I began to think that it would be only hypocrisy in me to embrace his offer, as I could not in conscience conform to the opinions of his church. I was therefore enabled to regard the word of God, which says, 'Come out from amongst them,' and refused Father Vincent's offer. So we parted without conviction on either side.

Having taken at this place some fine wines, fruits, and money, we proceeded to Cadiz, where we took about two tons more of money, &c. and then sailed for England in the month of June. When we were about the north latitude 42, we had contrary wind for several days, and the ship did not make in that time above six or seven miles straight course. This made the captain exceeding fretful and peevish: and I was very sorry to hear God's most holy name often blasphemed by him. One day, as he was in that impious mood, a young gentleman on board, who was a passenger, reproached him, and said he acted wrong; for we ought to be thankful to God for all things, as we were not in want of any thing on board; and though the wind was contrary for us, yet it was fair for some others, who, perhaps, stood in more need of it than we. I immediately seconded this young gentleman with some boldness, and said we had not the least cause to murmur, for that the Lord was better to us than we deserved, and that he had done all things well. I expected that the captain would be very angry with me for speaking, but he replied not a word. However, before that time on the following day, being the 21st of June, much to our great joy and astonishment, we saw the providential hand of our benign Creator, whose ways with his blind creatures are past finding out. The preceding night I dreamed that I saw a boat immediately off the starboard main shrouds; and exactly at half past one o'clock, the following day at noon, while I was below, just as we had dined in the cabin, the man at the helm cried out, A boat! which brought my dream that instant into my mind. I was the first man that jumped on the deck; and, looking from the shrouds onward, according to my dream, I descried a little boat at some distance; but, as the waves were high, it was as much as we could do sometimes to discern her; we however stopped the ship's way, and the boat, which was extremely small, came alongside with eleven miserable men, whom we took on board immediately. To all human appearance, these people must have perished in the course of one hour or less, the boat being small, it barely contained them. When we took them up they were half drowned, and had no victuals, compass, water, or any other necessary whatsoever, and had only one bit of an oar to steer with, and that right before the wind; so that they were obliged to trust entirely to the mercy of the waves. As soon as we got them all on board, they bowed themselves on their knees, and, with hands and voices lifted up to heaven, thanked God for their deliverance; and I trust that my prayers were not wanting amongst them at the same time. This mercy of the Lord quite melted me, and I recollected his words, which I saw thus verified in the 107th Psalm 'O give thanks unto the Lord, for he is good, for his mercy endureth for ever. Hungry and thirsty, their souls fainted in them. They cried unto Lord in their trouble, and he delivered them out of their distresses. And he led them forth by the right way, that they might go to a city of habitation. O that men would praise the Lord for his goodness and for his wonderful works to the children of men! For he satisfieth the longing soul, and filleth the hungry soul with goodness.

'Such as sit in darkness and in the shadow of death:

'Then they cried unto the Lord in their trouble, and he saved them out of their distresses. They that go down to the sea in ships; that do business in great waters: these see the works of the Lord, and his wonders in the deep. Whoso is wise and will observe these things, even they shall understand the loving kindness of the Lord.'

The poor distressed captain said, 'that the Lord is good; for, seeing that I am not fit to die, he therefore gave me a space of time to repent.' I was very glad to hear this expression, and took an opportunity when convenient of talking to him on the providence of God. They told us they were Portuguese, and were in a brig loaded with corn, which shifted that morning at five o'clock, owing to which the vessel sunk that instant with two of the crew; and how these eleven got into the boat (which was lashed to the deck) not one of them could tell. We provided them with every necessary, and brought them all safe to London: and I hope the Lord gave them repentance unto life eternal.

I was happy once more amongst my friends and brethren, till November, when my old friend, the celebrated Doctor Irving, bought a remarkable fine sloop, about 150 tons. He had a mind for a new adventure in cultivating a plantation at Jamaica and the Musquito Shore; asked me to go with him, and said that he would trust me with his estate in preference to any one. By the advice, therefore, of my friends, I accepted of the offer, knowing that the harvest was fully ripe in those parts, and hoped to be the instrument, under God, of bringing some poor sinner to my well beloved master, Jesus Christ. Before I embarked, I found with the Doctor four Musquito Indians, who were chiefs in their own country, and were brought here by some English traders for some selfish ends. One of them was the Musquito king's son; a youth of about eighteen years of age; and whilst he was here he was baptized by the name of George. They were going back at the government's expense, after having been in England about twelve months, during which they learned to speak pretty good English. When I came to talk to them about eight days before we sailed, I was very much mortified in finding that they had not frequented any churches since they were here, to be baptized, nor was any attention paid to their morals. I was very sorry for this mock Christianity, and had just an opportunity to take some of them once to church before we sailed. We embarked in the month of November 1775, on board of the sloop Morning Star, Captain David Miller, and sailed for Jamaica. In our passage, I took all the pains that I could to instruct the Indian prince in the doctrines of Christianity, of which he was entirely ignorant; and, to my great joy, he was quite attentive, and received with gladness the truths that the Lord enabled me to set forth to him. I taught him in the compass of eleven days all the letters, and he could put even two or three of them together and spell them. I had Fox's Martyrology with cuts, and he used to be very fond of looking into it, and would ask many questions about the papal cruelties he saw depicted there, which I explained to him. I made such progress with this youth, especially in religion, that when I used to go to bed at different hours of the night, if he was in his bed, he would get up on purpose to go to prayer with me, without any other clothes than his shirt; and before he would eat any of his meals amongst the gentlemen in the cabin, he would first come to me to pray, as he called it. I was well pleased at this, and took great delight in him, and used much supplication to God for his conversion. I was in full hope of seeing daily every appearance of that change which I could wish; not knowing the devices of satan, who had many of his emissaries to sow his tares as fast as I sowed the good seed, and pull down as fast as I built up. Thus we went on nearly four fifths of our passage, when satan at last got the upper hand. Some of his messengers, seeing this poor heathen much advanced in piety, began to ask him whether I had converted him to Christianity, laughed, and made their jest at him, for which I rebuked them as much as I could; but this treatment caused the prince to halt between two opinions. Some of the true sons of Belial, who did not believe that there was any hereafter, told him never to fear the devil, for there was none existing; and if ever he came to the prince, they desired he might be sent to them. Thus they teazed the poor innocent youth, so that he would not learn his book any more! He would not drink nor carouse with these ungodly actors, nor would he be with me, even at prayers. This grieved me very much. I endeavoured to persuade him as well as I could, but he would not come; and entreated him very much to tell me his reasons for acting thus. At last he asked me, 'How comes it that all the white men on board who can read and write, and observe the sun, and know all things, yet swear, lie, and get drunk, only excepting yourself?' I answered him, the reason was, that they did not fear God; and that if any one of them died so they could not go to, or be happy with God. He replied, that if these persons went to hell he would go to hell too. I was sorry to hear this; and, as he sometimes had the tooth-ach, and also some other persons in the ship at the same time, I asked him if their toothach made his easy: he said, No. Then I told him if he and these people went to hell together, their pains would not make his any lighter. This answer had great weight with him: it depressed his spirits much; and he became ever after, during the passage, fond of being alone. When we were in the latitude of Martinico, and near making the land, one morning we had a brisk gale of wind, and, carrying too much sail, the main-mast went over the side. Many people were then all about the deck, and the yards, masts, and rigging, came tumbling all about us, yet there was not one of us in the least hurt, although some were within a hair's breadth of being killed: and, particularly, I saw two men then, by the providential hand of God, most miraculously preserved from being smashed to pieces. On the fifth of January we made Antigua and Montserrat, and ran along the rest of the islands: and on the fourteenth we arrived at Jamaica. One Sunday while we were there I took the Musquito Prince George to church, where he saw the sacrament administered. When we came out we saw all kinds of people, almost from the church door for the space of half a mile down to the waterside, buying and selling all kinds of commodities: and these acts afforded me great matter of exhortation to this youth, who was much astonished. Our vessel being ready to sail for the Musquito shore, I went with the Doctor on board a Guinea-man, to purchase some slaves to carry with us, and cultivate a plantation; and I chose them all my own countrymen. On the twelfth of February we sailed from Jamaica, and on the eighteenth arrived at the Musquito shore, at a place called Dupeupy. All our Indian guests now, after I had admonished them and a few cases of liquor given them by the Doctor, took an affectionate leave of us, and went ashore, where they were met by the Musquito king, and we never saw one of them afterwards. We then sailed to the southward of the shore, to a place called Cape Gracias a Dios, where there was a large lagoon or lake, which received the emptying of two or three very fine large rivers, and abounded much in fish and land tortoise. Some of the native Indians came on board of us here; and we used them well, and told them we were come to dwell amongst them, which they seemed pleased at. So the Doctor and I, with some others, went with them ashore; and they took us to different places to view the land, in order to choose a place to make a plantation of. We fixed on a spot near a river's bank, in a rich soil; and, having got our necessaries out of the sloop, we began to clear away the woods, and plant different kinds of vegetables, which had a quick growth. While we were employed in this manner, our vessel went northward to Black River to trade. While she was there, a Spanish guarda costa met with and took her. This proved very hurtful, and a great embarrassment to us. However, we went on with the culture of the land. We used to make fires every night all around us, to keep off wild beasts, which, as soon as it was dark, set up a most hideous roaring. Our habitation being far up in the woods, we frequently saw different kinds of animals; but none of them ever hurt us, except poisonous snakes, the bite of which the Doctor used to cure by giving to the patient, as soon as possible, about half a tumbler of strong rum, with a good deal of Cayenne pepper in it. In this manner he cured two natives and one of his own slaves. The Indians were exceedingly fond of the Doctor, and they had good reason for it; for I believe they never had such an useful man amongst them. They came from all quarters to our dwelling; and some *woolwow*, or flat-headed Indians, who lived fifty or sixty miles above our river, and this side of the South Sea, brought us a good deal of silver in exchange for our goods. The principal articles we could get from our neighbouring Indians, were turtle oil, and shells, little silk grass, and some provisions; but they would not work at any thing for us, except fishing; and a few times they assisted to cut some trees down, in order to build us houses; which they did exactly like the Africans, by the joint labour of men, women, and children. I do not recollect any of them to have had more than two wives. These always accompanied their husbands when they came to our dwelling; and then they generally carried whatever they brought to us, and always squatted down behind their husbands. Whenever we gave them any thing to eat, the men and their wives ate it separate.

I never saw the least sign of incontinence amongst them. The women are ornamented with beads, and fond of painting themselves; the men also paint, even to excess, both their faces and shirts: their favourite colour is red. The women generally cultivate the ground, and the men are all fishermen and canoe makers. Upon the whole, I never met any nation that were so simple in their manners as these people, or had so little ornament in their houses. Neither had they, as I ever could learn, one word expressive of an oath. The worst word I ever heard amongst them when they were quarreling, was one that they had got from the English, which was, 'you rascal.' I never saw any mode of worship among them; but in this they were not worse than their European brethren or neighbours: for I am sorry to say that there was not one white person in our dwelling, nor any where else that I saw in different places I was at on the shore, that was better or more pious than those unenlightened Indians; but they either worked or slept on Sundays: and, to my sorrow, working was too much Sunday's employment with ourselves; so much so, that in some length of time we really did not know one day from another. This mode of living laid the foundation of my decamping at last. The natives are well made and warlike; and they particu larly boast of having never been conquered by the Spaniards. They are great drinkers of strong liquors when they can get them. We used to distil rum from pine apples, which were very plentiful here; and then we could not get them away from our place. Yet they seemed to be singular, in point of honesty, above any other nation I was ever amongst. The country being hot, we lived under an open shed, where we had all kinds of goods, without a door or a lock to any one article; yet we slept in safety, and never lost any thing, or were disturbed. This surprised us a good deal; and the Doctor, myself, and others, used to say, if we were to lie in that manner in Europe we should have our throats cut the first night. The Indian governor goes once in a certain time all about the province or district, and has a number of men with him as attendants and assistants. He settles all the differences among the people, like the judge here, and is treated with very great respect. He took care to give us timely notice before he came to our habitation, by sending his stick as a token, for rum, sugar, and gunpowder, which we did not refuse sending; and at the same time we made the utmost preparation to receive his honour and his train. When he came with his tribe, and all our neighbouring chieftains, we expected to find him a grave reverend judge, solid and sagacious; but instead of that, before he and his gang came in sight, we heard them very clamorous; and they even had plundered some of our good neighbouring Indians, having intoxicated themselves with our liquor. When they arrived we did not know what to make of our new guests, and would gladly have dispensed with the honour of their company. However, having no alternative, we feasted them plentifully all the day till the evening; when the governor, getting quite drunk, grew very unruly, and struck one of our most friendly chiefs, who was our nearest neighbour, and also took his gold-laced hat from him. At this a great commotion taken place; and the Doctor interfered to make peace, as we could all understand one another, but to no purpose; and at last they became so outrageous that the Doctor, fearing he might get into trouble, left the house, and made the best of his way to the nearest wood, leaving me to do as well as I could among them. I was so enraged with the Governor, that I could have wished to have seen him tied fast to a tree and flogged for his behaviour; but I had not people enough to cope with his party. I therefore thought of a stratagem to appease the riot. Recollecting a passage I had read in the life of Columbus, when he was amongst the Indians in Mexico or Peru, where, on some occasion, he frightened them, by telling them of certain events in the heavens, I had recourse to the same expedient; and it succeeded beyond my most sanguine expectations. When I had formed my determination, I went in the midst of them; and, taking hold of the Governor, I pointed up to the heavens. I menaced him and the rest: I told them God lived there, and that he was angry with them, and they must not quarrel so; that they were all brothers, and if they did not leave off, and go away quietly, I would take the book (pointing to the Bible), read, and *tell* God to make them dead. This was something like magic. The clamour immediately ceased, and I gave them some rum and a few other things; after which they went away peaceably; and the Governor afterwards gave our neighbour, who was called Captain Plasmyah, his hat again. When the Doctor returned, he was exceedingly glad at my success in thus getting rid of our troublesome guests. The Musquito people within our vicinity, out of respect to the Doctor, myself and his people, made entertainments of the grand kind, called in their tongue *tourrie* or *dryckbot*. The English of this expression is, a feast of drinking about, of which it seems a corruption of language. The drink consisted of pine apples roasted, and casades chewed or beaten in mortars; which, after lying some time, ferments, and becomes so strong as to intoxicate, when drank in any quantity. We had timely notice given to us of the entertainment. A white family, within five miles of us, told us how the drink was made, and I and two others went before the time to the village, where the mirth was appointed to be held; and there we saw the whole art of making the drink, and also the kind of animals that were to be eaten there. I cannot say the sight of either the drink or the meat were enticing to me. They had some thousands of pine apples roasting, which they squeezed, dirt and all, into a canoe they had there for the purpose. The casade drink was in beef barrels and other vessels, and looked exactly like hog-wash. Men, women, and children, were thus employed in roasting the pine apples, and squeezing them with their hands. For food they had many land torpins or tortoises, some dried turtle, and three large alligators alive, and tied fast to the trees. I asked the people what they were going to do with these alligators; and I was told they were to be eaten. I was much surprised at this, and went home, not a little disgusted at the preparations. When the day of the feast was come, we took some rum with us, and went to the appointed place, where we found a great assemblage of these people, who received us very kindly. The mirth had begun before we came; and they were dancing with music: and the musical instruments were nearly the same as those of any other sable people; but, as I thought, much less melodious than any other nation I ever knew. They had many curious gestures in dancing, and a variety of motions and postures of their bodies, which to me were in no wise attracting. The males danced by themselves,

and the females also by themselves, as with us. The Doctor
shewed his people the example, by immediately joining the
women's party, though not by their choice. On perceiving
the women disgusted, he joined the males. At night there
were great illuminations, by setting fire to many pine trees,
while the dryckbot went round merrily by calabashes or
gourds: but the liquor might more justly be called eating than
drinking. One Owden, the oldest father in the vicinity, was
dressed in a strange and terrifying form. Around his body
were skins adorned with different kinds of feathers, and he
had on his head a very large and high head-piece, in the form
of a grenadier's cap, with prickles like a porcupine; and he
made a certain noise which resembled the cry of an alligator.
Our people skipped amongst them out of complaisance,
though some could not drink of their tourrie; but our rum
met with customers enough, and was soon gone. The alligators were killed and some of them roasted. Their manner of
roasting is by digging a hole in the earth, and filling it with
wood, which they burn to coal, and then they lay sticks
across, on which they set the meat. I had a raw piece of the
alligator in my hand: it was very rich: I thought it looked like
fresh salmon, and it had a most fragrant smell, but I could
not eat any of it. This merry-making at last ended without
the least discord in any person in the company, although it
was made up of different nations and complexions. The rainy
season came on here about the latter end of May, which continued till August very heavily; so that the rivers were overflowed, and our provisions then in the ground were washed
away. I thought this was in some measure a judgment upon
us for working on Sundays, and it hurt my mind very much.
I often wished to leave this place and sail for Europe; for our
mode of procedure and living in this heathenish form was
very irksome to me. The word of God saith, 'What does it
avail a man if he gain the whole world, and lose his own
soul?' This was much and heavily impressed on my mind;
and, though I did not know how to speak to the Doctor for
my discharge, it was disagreeable for me to stay any longer.
But about the middle of June I took courage enough to ask
him for it. He was very unwilling at first to grant my request;
but I gave him so many reasons for it, that at last he con-

sented to my going, and gave me the following certificate of my behaviour:

> 'The bearer, Gustavus Vassa, has served me several years with strict honesty, sobriety, and fidelity. I can, therefore, with justice recommend him for these qualifications; and indeed in every respect I consider him as an excellent servant. I do hereby certify that he always behaved well, and that he is perfectly trust-worthy.
>
> 'CHARLES IRVING.'
>
> *Musquito Shore, June 15, 1776.*

Though I was much attached to the doctor, I was happy when he consented. I got every thing ready for my departure, and hired some Indians, with a large canoe, to carry me off. All my poor countrymen, the slaves, when they heard of my leaving them, were very sorry, as I had always treated them with care and affection, and did every thing I could to comfort the poor creatures, and render their condition easy. Having taken leave of my old friends and companions, on the 18th of June, accompanied by the doctor, I left that spot of the world, and went southward above twenty miles along the river. There I found a sloop, the captain of which told me he was going to Jamaica. Having agreed for my passage with him and one of the owners, who was also on board, named Hughes, the doctor and I parted, not without shedding tears on both sides. The vessel then sailed along the river till night, when she stopped in a lagoon within the same river. During the night a schooner belonging to the same owners came in, and, as she was in want of hands, Hughes, the owner of the sloop, asked me to go in the schooner as a sailor, and said he would give me wages. I thanked him; but I said I wanted to go to Jamaica. He then immediately changed his tone, and swore, and abused me very much, and asked how I came to be freed. I told him, and said that I came into that vicinity with Dr. Irving, whom he had seen that day. This account was of no use; he still swore exceedingly at me, and cursed the master for a fool that sold me my freedom, and the doctor for another in letting me go from him. Then he desired me to go in the schooner, or else I should not go out of the sloop as a freeman. I said this was very hard, and begged to be put on shore again; but he swore that I should not. I said I had been twice amongst the Turks, yet had never seen any such usage with them, and much less could I have expected any thing of this kind amongst Christians. This incensed him exceedingly; and, with a volley of oaths and imprecations, he replied, 'Christians! Damn you, you are one of St. Paul's men; but by G——, except you have St. Paul's or St. Peter's faith, and walk upon the water to the shore, you shall not go out of the vessel;' which I now found was going amongst the Spaniards towards Carthagena, where he swore he would sell me. I simply asked him what right he had to sell me? but, without another word, he made some of his people tie ropes round each of my ancles, and also to each wrist, and another rope round my body, and hoisted me up without letting my feet touch or rest upon any thing. Thus I hung, without any crime committed, and without judge or jury; merely because I was a free man, and could not by the law get any redress from a white person in those parts of the world. I was in great pain from my situation, and cried and begged very hard for some mercy; but all in vain. My tyrant, in a great rage, brought a musquet out of the cabin, and loaded it before me and the crew, and swore that he would shoot me if I cried any more. I had now no alternative; I therefore remained silent, seeing not one white man on board who said a word on my behalf. I hung in that manner from between ten and eleven o'clock at night till about one in the morning; when, finding my cruel abuser fast asleep, I begged some of his slaves to slack the rope that was round my body, that my feet might rest on something. This they did at the risk of being cruelly used by their master, who beat some of them severely at first for not tying me when he commanded them. Whilst I remained in this condition, till between five and six o'clock next morning, I trust I prayed to God to forgive this blasphemer, who cared not what he did, but when he got up out of his sleep in the morning was of the very same temper and disposition as when he left me at night. When they got up the anchor, and the vessel was getting under way, I once more cried and begged to be released; and now, being fortunately in the way of their hoisting the sails, they released me. When I was let down, I spoke to one Mr.

Cox, a carpenter, whom I knew on board, on the impropriety of this conduct. He also knew the doctor, and the good opinion he ever had of me. This man then went to the captain, and told him not to carry me away in that manner; that I was the doctor's steward, who regarded me very highly, and would resent this usage when he should come to know it. On which he desired a young man to put me ashore in a small canoe I brought with me. This sound gladdened my heart, and I got hastily into the canoe and set off, whilst my tyrant was down in the cabin; but he soon spied me out, when I was not above thirty or forty yards from the vessel, and, running upon the deck with a loaded musket in his hand, he presented it at me, and swore heavily and dreadfully, that he would shoot me that instant, if I did not come back on board. As I knew the wretch would have done as he said, without hesitation, I put back to the vessel again; but, as the good Lord would have it, just as I was alongside he was abusing the captain for letting me go from the vessel; which the captain returned, and both of them soon got into a very great heat. The young man that was with me now got out of the canoe; the vessel was sailing on fast with a smooth sea: and I then thought it was neck or nothing, so at that instant I set off again, for my life, in the canoe, towards the shore; and fortunately the confusion was so great amongst them on board, that I got out of the reach of the musquet shot unnoticed, while the vessel sailed on with a fair wind a different way; so that they could not overtake me without tacking: but even before that could be done I should have been on shore, which I soon reached, with many thanks to God for this unexpected deliverance. I then went and told the other owner, who lived near that shore (with whom I had agreed for my passage) of the usage I had met with. He was very much astonished, and appeared very sorry for it. After treating me with kindness, he gave me some refreshment, and three heads of roasted Indian corn, for a voyage of about eighteen miles south, to look for another vessel. He then directed me to an Indian chief of a district, who was also the Musquito admiral, and had once been at our dwelling; after which I set off with the canoe across a large lagoon alone (for I could not get any one to assist me), though I was much jaded, and had pains in my bowels, by means of the rope I had hung by the night before. I was therefore at different times unable to manage the canoe, for the paddling was very laborious. However, a little before dark I got to my destined place, where some of the Indians knew me, and received me kindly. I asked for the admiral; and they conducted me to his dwelling. He was glad to see me, and refreshed me with such things as the place afforded; and I had a hammock to sleep in. They acted towards me more like Christians than those whites I was amongst the last night, though they had been baptized. I told the admiral I wanted to go to the next port to get a vessel to carry me to Jamaica; and requested him to send the canoe back which I then had, for which I was to pay him. He agreed with me, and sent five able Indians with a large canoe to carry my things to my intended place, about fifty miles; and we set off the next morning. When we got out of the lagoon and went along shore, the sea was so high that the canoe was oftentimes very near being filled with water. We were obliged to go ashore and drag across different necks of land; we were also two nights in the swamps, which swarmed with musquito flies, and they proved troublesome to us. This tiresome journey of land and water ended, however, on the third day, to my great joy; and I got on board of a sloop commanded by one Captain Jenning. She was then partly loaded, and he told me he was expecting daily to sail for Jamaica; and having agreed with me to work my passage, I went to work accordingly. I was not many days on board before we sailed; but to my sorrow and disappointment, though used to such tricks, we went to the southward along the Musquito shore, instead of steering for Jamaica. I was compelled to assist in cutting a great deal of mahogany wood on the shore as we coasted along it, and load the vessel with it, before she sailed. This fretted me much; but, as I did not know how to help myself among these deceivers, I thought patience was the only remedy I had left, and even that was forced. There was much hard work and little victuals on board, except by good luck we happened to catch turtles. On this coast there was also a particular kind of fish called manatee, which is most excellent eating, and the flesh is more like beef than fish; the scales are as large as a shilling, and the skin thicker than I ever saw that of any other fish. Within the brackish waters along shore there were likewise vast numbers of alligators, which made the fish scarce. I was on board this sloop sixteen days, during which, in our coasting, we came to another place, where there was a smaller sloop called the Indian Queen, commanded by one John Baker. He also was an Englishman, and had been a long time along the shore trading for turtle shells and silver, and had got a good quantity of each on board. He wanted some hands very much; and, understanding I was a free man, and wanted to go to Jamaica, he told me if he could get one or two, that he would sail immediately for that island: he also pretended to me some marks of attention and respect, and promised to give me forty-five shillings sterling a month if I would go with him. I thought this much better than cutting wood for nothing. I therefore told the other captain that I wanted to go to Jamaica in the other vessel; but he would not listen to me: and, seeing me resolved to go in a day or two, he got the vessel to sail, intending to carry me away against my will. This treatment mortified me extremely. I immediately, according to an agreement I had made with the captain of the Indian Queen, called for her boat, which was lying near us, and it came alongside; and, by the means of a north-pole shipmate which I met with in the sloop I was in, I got my things into the boat, and went on board of the Indian Queen, July the 10th. A few days after I was there, we got all things ready and sailed: but again, to my great mortification, this vessel still went to the south, nearly as far as Carthagena, trading along the coast, instead of going to Jamaica, as the captain had promised me: and, what was worst of all, he was a very cruel and bloody-minded man, and was a horrid blasphemer. Among others he had a white pilot, one Stoker, whom he beat often as severely as he did some negroes he had on board. One night in particular, after he had beaten this man most cruelly, he put him into the boat, and made two negroes row him to a desolate key, or small island; and he loaded two pistols, and swore bitterly that he would shoot the negroes if they brought Stoker on board again. There was not the least doubt but that he would do as he said, and the two poor fellows were obliged to obey the cruel mandate; but, when the captain was asleep, the two negroes took a blanket and carried it to the unfortunate Stoker, which I believe was the means of saving his life from the annoyance of insects. A great deal of entreaty was used with the captain the next day, before he would consent to let Stoker come on board; and when the poor man was brought on board he was very ill, from his situation during the night, and he remained so till he was drowned a little time after. As we sailed southward we came to many uninhabited islands, which were overgrown with fine large cocoa nuts. As I was very much in want of provisions, I brought a boat load of them on board, which lasted me and others for several weeks, and afforded us many a delicious repast in our scarcity. One day, before this, I could not help observing the providential hand of God, that ever supplies all our wants, though in the ways and manner we know not. I had been a whole day without food, and made signals for boats to come off, but in vain. I therefore earnestly prayed to God for relief in my need; and at the close of the evening I went off the deck. Just as I laid down I heard a noise on the deck; and, not knowing what it meant, I went directly on the the deck again, when what should I see but a fine large fish about seven or eight pounds, which had jumped aboard! I took it, and admired, with thanks, the good hand of God; and, what I considered as not less extraordinary, the captain, who was very avaricious, did not attempt to take it from me, there being only him and I on board; for the rest were all gone ashore trading. Sometimes the people did not come off for some days: this used to fret the captain, and then he would vent his fury on me by beating me, or making me feel in other cruel ways. One day especially, in his wild, wicked, and mad career, after striking me several times with different things, and once across my mouth, even with a red burning stick out of the fire, he got a barrel of gunpowder on the deck, and swore that he would blow up the vessel. I was then at my wit's end, and earnestly prayed to God to direct me. The head was out of the barrel; and the captain took a lighted stick out of the fire to blow himself and me up, because there was a vessel then in sight coming in, which he supposed was a Spaniard, and he was afraid of falling into their hands. Seeing this I got an axe, unnoticed by him, and placed myself between him and the powder, having resolved in myself as soon as he attempted to put the fire in the barrel to chop him down that instant. I was more than an hour in this situation; during which he struck me often, still keeping the fire in his hand for this wicked purpose. I really should have thought myself justifiable in any other part of the world if I had killed him, and prayed to God, who gave me a mind which rested solely on himself. I prayed for resignation, that his will might be done; and the following two portions of his holy word, which occurred to my mind, buoyed up my hope, and kept me from taking the life of this wicked man. 'He hath determined the times before appointed, and set bounds to our habitations,' Acts xvii. 26. And, 'Who is there amongst you that feareth the Lord, that obeyeth the voice of his servant, that walketh in darkness and hath no light? let him trust in the name of the Lord, and stay upon his God,' Isaiah l. 10. And thus by the grace of God I was enabled to do. I found him a present help in the time of need, and the captain's fury began to subside as the night approached: but I found,

"That he who cannot stem his anger's tide
Doth a wild horse without a bridle ride."

The next morning we discovered that the vessel which had caused such a fury in the captain was an English sloop. They soon came to an anchor where we were, and, to my no small surprise, I learned that Doctor Irving was on board of her on his way from the Musquito shore to Jamaica. I was for going immediately to see this old master and friend, but the captain would not suffer me to leave the vessel. I then informed the doctor, by letter, how I was treated, and begged that he would take me out of the sloop: but he informed me that it was not in his power, as he was a passenger himself; but he sent me some rum and sugar for my own use. I now learned that after I had left the estate which I managed for this gentleman on the Musquito shore, during which the slaves were well fed and comfortable, a white overseer had supplied my place: this man, through inhumanity and ill-judged avarice, beat and cut the poor slaves most unmercifully; and the consequence was, that every one got into a large Puriogua canoe, and endeavoured to escape; but not knowing where to go, or how to manage the canoe, they were all drowned; in consequence of which the doctor's plantation was left uncultivated, and he was now returning to Jamaica to purchase more slaves and stock it again. On the 14th of October the Indian Queen arrived at Kingston in Jamaica. When we were unloaded I demanded my wages, which amounted to eight pounds and five shillings sterling; but Captain Baker refused to give me one farthing, although it was the hardest-earned money I ever worked for in my life. I found out Doctor Irving upon this, and acquainted him of the captain's knavery. He did all he could to help me to get my money; and we went to every magistrate in Kingston (and there were nine), but they all refused to do any thing for me, and said my oath could not be admitted against a white man. Nor was this all; for Baker threatened that he would beat me severely if he could catch me for attempting to demand my money; and this he would have done, but that I got, by means of Dr. Irving, under the protection of Captain Douglas of the Squirrel man of war. I thought this exceedingly hard usage; though indeed I found it to be too much the practice there to pay free men for their labour in this manner. One day I went with a free negroe taylor, named Joe Diamond, to one Mr. Cochran, who was indebted to him some trifling sum; and the man, not being able to get his money, began to murmur. The other immediately took a horse-whip to pay him with it; but, by the help of a good pair of heels, the taylor got off. Such oppressions as these made me seek for a vessel to get off the island as fast as I could; and by the mercy of God I found a ship in November bound for England, when I embarked with a convoy, after having taken a last farewell of Doctor Irving. When I left Jamaica he was employed in refining sugars; and some months after my arrival in England I learned, with much sorrow, that this my amiable friend was dead, owing to his having eaten some poisoned fish. We had many very heavy gales of wind in our passage; in the course of which no material incident occurred, except that an American privateer, falling in with the fleet, was captured and set fire to by his Majesty's ship the Squirrel. On January the seventh, 1777, we arrived at Plymouth. I was happy once more to tread upon English ground; and, after passing some little time at Plymouth and Exeter among some pious friends, whom I was happy to see, I went to London with a heart replete with thanks to God for all past mercies.

CHAP. XII.

Different transactions of the author's life till the present time—His application to the late Bishop of London to be appointed a missionary to Africa—Some account of his share in the conduct of the late expedition to Sierra Leona—Petition to the Queen—Conclusion.

SUCH were the various scenes which I was a witness to, and the fortune I experienced until the year 1777. Since that period my life has been more uniform, and the incidents of it fewer, than in any other equal number of years preceding; I therefore hasten to the conclusion of a narrative, which I fear the reader may think already sufficiently tedious.

I had suffered so many impositions in my commercial transactions in different parts of the world, that I became heartily disgusted with the seafaring life, and I was determined not to return to it, at least for some time. I therefore once more engaged in service shortly after my return, and continued for the most part in this situation until 1784.

Soon after my arrival in London, I saw a remarkable circumstance relative to African complexion, which I thought so extraordinary, that I beg leave just to mention it: A white negro woman, that I had formerly seen in London and other parts, had married a white man, by whom she had three boys, and they were every one mulattoes, and yet they had fine light hair. In 1779 I served Governor Macnamara, who had been a considerable time on the coast of Africa. In the time of my service, I used to ask frequently other servants to join me in family prayers; but this only excited their mockery. However, the Governor, understanding that I was of a religious turn, wished to know of what religion I was; I told him I was a protestant of the church of England, agreeable to the thirty-nine articles of that church, and that whomsoever I found to preach according to that doctrine, those I would hear. A few days after this, we had some more discourse on the same subject: the Governor spoke to me on it again, and said that he would, if I chose, as he thought I might be of service in converting my countrymen to the Gospel faith, get me sent out as a missionary to Africa. I at first refused going, and told him how I had been served on a like occasion by some white people the last voyage I went to Jamaica, when I attempted (if it were the will of God) to be the means of converting the Indian prince; and I said I supposed they would serve me worse than Alexander the coppersmith did St. Paul, if I should attempt to go amongst them in Africa. He told me not to fear, for he would apply to the Bishop of London to get me ordained. On these terms I consented to the Governor's proposal to go to Africa, in hope of doing good if possible amongst my countrymen; so, in order to have me sent out properly, we immediately wrote the following letters to the late Bishop of London:

To the Right Reverend Father in God,
    ROBERT, Lord Bishop of London:
        The MEMORIAL of GUSTAVUS VASSA
SHEWETH,
        THAT your memorialist is a native of Africa, and has a knowledge of the manners and customs of the inhabitants of that country.

That your memorialist has resided in different parts of Europe for twenty-two years last past, and embraced the Christian faith in the year 1759.

That your memorialist is desirous of returning to Africa as a missionary, if encouraged by your Lordship, in hopes of being able to prevail upon his countrymen to become Christians; and your memorialist is the more induced to undertake the same, from the success that has attended the like undertakings when encouraged by the Portuguese through their different settlements on the coast of Africa, and also by the Dutch: both governments encouraging the blacks, who, by their education are qualified to undertake the same, and are found more proper than European clergymen, unacquainted with the language and customs of the country.

Your memorialist's only motive for soliciting the office of a missionary is, that he may be a means, under God, of reforming his countrymen and persuading them to embrace the

Christian religion. Therefore your memorialist humbly prays your Lordship's encouragement and support in the undertaking.

GUSTAVUS VASSA.

At Mr. Guthrie's, taylor,
  No. 17, Hedge-lane.

MY LORD,

I HAVE resided near seven years on the coast of Africa, for most part of the time as commanding officer. From the knowledge I have of the country and it's inhabitants, I am inclined to think that the within plan will be attended with great success, if countenanced by your Lordship. I beg leave further to represent to your Lordship, that the like attempts, when encouraged by other governments, have met with uncommon success; and at this very time I know a very respectable character a black priest at Cape Coast Castle. I know the within named Gustavus Vassa, and believe him a moral good man.

I have the honour to be,
My Lord,
Your Lordship's
Humble and obedient servant,
MATT. MACNAMARA.

Grove, 11th March 1779.

This letter was also accompanied by the following from Doctor Wallace, who had resided in Africa for many years, and whose sentiments on the subject of an African mission were the same with Governor Macnamara's.

March 13, 1779.

MY LORD,

I have resided near five years on Senegambia on the coast of Africa, and have had the honour of filling very considerable employments in that province. I do approve of the within plan, and think the undertaking very laudable and proper, and that it deserves your Lordship's protection and encouragement, in which case it must be attended with the intended success.

I am,
My Lord,
Your Lordship's
Humble and obedient servant,
THOMAS WALLACE.

With these letters, I waited on the Bishop by the Governor's desire, and presented them to his Lordship. He received me with much condescension and politeness; but, from some certain scruples of delicacy, declined to ordain me.

My sole motive for thus dwelling on this transaction, or inserting these papers, is the opinion which gentlemen of sense and education, who are acquainted with Africa, entertain of the probability of converting the inhabitants of it to the faith of Jesus Christ, if the attempt were countenanced by the legislature.

Shortly after this I left the Governor, and served a nobleman in the Devonshire militia, with whom I was encamped at Coxheath for some time; but the operations there were too minute and uninteresting to make a detail of.

In the year 1783 I visited eight counties in Wales, from motives of curiosity. While I was in that part of the country I was led to go down into a coal-pit in Shropshire, but my curiosity nearly cost me my life; for while I was in the pit the coals fell in, and buried one poor man, who was not far from me: upon this I got out as fast as I could, thinking the surface of the earth the safest part of it.

In the spring 1784 I thought of visiting old ocean again. In consequence of this I embarked as steward on board a fine new ship called the London, commanded by Martin Hopkin, and sailed for New-York. I admired this city very much; it is large and well-built, and abounds with provisions of all kinds. While we lay here a circumstance happened which I thought extremely singular:—One day a malefactor was to be executed on a gallows; but with a condition that if any woman, having nothing on but her shift, married the man under the gallows, his life was to be saved. This extraordinary privilege was claimed; a woman presented herself; and the marriage cere-

mony was performed. Our ship having got laden we returned
to London in January 1785. When she was ready again for another voyage, the captain being an agreeable man, I sailed
with him from hence in the spring, March 1785, for Philadelphia. On the fifth of April we took our departure from the
Land's-end, with a pleasant gale; and about nine o'clock that
night the moon shone bright, and the sea was smooth, while
our ship was going free by the wind, at the rate of about four
or five miles an hour. At this time another ship was going
nearly as fast as we on the opposite point, meeting us right in
the teeth, yet none on board observed either ship until we
struck each other forcibly head and head, to the astonishment
and consternation of both crews. She did us much damage,
but I believe we did her more; for when we passed by each
other, which we did very quickly, they called to us to bring to,
and hoist out our boat, but we had enough to do to mind
ourselves; and in about eight minutes we saw no more of her.
We refitted as well as we could the next day, and proceeded
on our voyage, and in May arrived at Philadelphia. I was very
glad to see this favourite old town once more; and my pleasure was much increased in seeing the worthy quakers freeing
and easing the burthens of many of my oppressed African
brethren. It rejoiced my heart when one of these friendly people took me to see a free-school they had erected for every
denomination of black people, whose minds are cultivated
here and forwarded to virtue; and thus they are made useful
members of the community. Does not the success of this
practice say loudly to the planters in the language of scripture—"Go ye and do likewise?"

In October 1785 I was accompanied by some of the
Africans, and presented this address of thanks to the gentlemen called Friends or Quakers, in Gracechurch-Court Lombard-Street:

GENTLEMEN,
            By reading your book, entitled a Caution to Great
Britain and her Colonies, concerning the Calamitous State of
the enslaved Negroes: We the poor, oppressed, needy, and
much-degraded negroes, desire to approach you with this address of thanks, with our inmost love and warmest acknowl-

edgment; and with the deepest sense of your benevolence, unwearied labour, and kind interposition, towards breaking the yoke of slavery, and to administer a little comfort and ease to thousands and tens of thousands of very grievously afflicted, and too heavy burthened negroes.

Gentlemen, could you, by perseverance, at last be enabled, under God, to lighten in any degree the heavy burthen of the afflicted, no doubt it would, in some measure, be the possible means, under God, of saving the souls of many of the oppressors; and, if so, sure we are that the God, whose eyes are ever upon all his creatures, and always rewards every true act of virtue, and regards the prayers of the oppressed, will give to you and yours those blessings which it is not in our power to express or conceive, but which we, as a part of those captived, oppressed, and afflicted people, most earnestly wish and pray for.

These gentlemen received us very kindly, with a promise to exert themselves on behalf of the oppressed Africans, and we parted.

While in town I chanced once to be invited to a quaker's wedding. The simple and yet expressive mode used at their solemnizations is worthy of note. The following is the true form of it:

After the company have met they have seasonable exhortations by several of the members; the bride and bridegroom stand up, and, taking each other by the hand in a solemn manner, the man audily declares to this purpose:

"Friends, in the fear of the Lord, and in the presence of this assembly, whom I desire to be my witnesses, I take this my friend, M. N. to be my wife; promising, through divine assistance, to be unto her a loving and faithful husband till death separate us:" and the woman makes the like declaration. Then the two first sign their names to the record, and as many more witnesses as have a mind. I had the honour to subscribe mine to a register in Gracechurch-Court, Lombard-Street.

We returned to London in August; and our ship not going immediately to sea, I shipped as a steward in an American ship called the Harmony, Captain John Willet, and left London in March 1786, bound to Philadelphia. Eleven days after sailing we carried our foremast away. We had a nine weeks passage, which caused our trip not to succeed well, the market for our goods proving bad; and, to make it worse, my commander began to play me the like tricks as others too often practise on free negroes in the West Indies. But I thank God I found many friends here, who in some measure prevented him. On my return to London in August I was very agreeably surprised to find that the benevolence of government had adopted the plan of some philanthropic individuals to send the Africans from hence to their native quarter; and that some vessels were then engaged to carry them to Sierra Leone; an act which redounded to the honour of all concerned in its promotion, and filled me with prayers and much rejoicing. There was then in the city a select committee of gentlemen for the black poor, to some of whom I had the honour of being known; and, as soon as they heard of my arrival they sent for me to the committee. When I came there they informed me of the intention of government; and as they seemed to think me qualified to superintend part of the undertaking, they asked me to go with the black poor to Africa. I pointed out to them many objections to my going; and particularly I expressed some difficulties on the account of the slave dealers, as I would certainly oppose their traffic in the human species by every means in my power. However these objections were over-ruled by the gentlemen of the committee, who prevailed on me to go, and recommended me to the honourable Commissioners of his Majesty's Navy as a proper person to act as commissary for government in the intended expedition; and they accordingly appointed me in November 1786 to that office, and gave me sufficient power to act for the government in the capacity of commissary, having received my warrant and the following order.

By the principal Officers and Commissioners of
his Majesty's Navy.

WHEREAS you were directed, by our warrant of the 4th of last month, to receive into your charge from Mr. Irving the surplus provisions remaining of what was provided for the voyage, as well as the provisions for the support of the black poor, after the landing at Sierra Leone, with the cloathing, tools, and all other articles provided at government's expense; and as the provisions were laid in at the rate of two months for the voyage, and for four months after the landing, but the number embarked being so much less than was expected, whereby there may be a considerable surplus of provisions, cloathing, &c. These are, in addition to former orders, to direct and require you to appropriate or dispose of such surplus to the best advantage you can for the benefit of government, keeping and rendering to us a faithful account of what you do herein. And for your guidance in preventing any white persons going, who are not intended to have the indulgences of being carried thither, we send you herewith a list of those recommended by the Committee for the black poor as proper persons to be permitted to embark, and acquaint you that you are not to suffer any others to go who do not produce a certificate from the committee for the black poor, of their having their permission for it. For which this shall be your warrant. Dated at the Navy Office, January 16, 1787.

J. HINSLOW,
GEO. MARSH,
W. PALMER.

To Mr. Gustavus Vassa,
    Commissary of Provisions and
    Stores for the Black Poor
    going to Sierra Leone.

I proceeded immediately to the execution of my duty on board the vessels destined for the voyage, where I continued till the March following.

During my continuance in the employment of government, I was struck with the flagrant abuses committed by the agent, and endeavoured to remedy them, but without effect. One instance, among many which I could produce, may serve as a specimen. Government had ordered to be provided all necessaries (slops, as they are called, included) for 750 persons; however, not being able to muster more than 426, I was ordered to send the superfluous slops, &c. to the king's stores at Portsmouth; but, when I demanded them for that purpose from the agent, it appeared they had never been bought, though paid for by government. But that was not all, government were not the only objects of peculation; these poor people suffered infinitely more; their accommodations were most wretched; many of them wanted beds, and many more cloathing and other necessaries. For the truth of this, and much more, I do not seek credit from my own assertion. I appeal to the testimony of Capt. Thompson, of the Nautilus, who convoyed us, to whom I applied in February 1787 for a remedy, when I had remonstrated to the agent in vain, and even brought him to be a witness of the injustice and oppression I complained of. I appeal also to a letter written by these wretched people, so early as the beginning of the preceding January, and published in the Morning Herald of the 4th of that month, signed by twenty of their chiefs.

I could not silently suffer government to be thus cheated, and my countrymen plundered and oppressed, and even left destitute of the necessaries for almost their existence. I therefore informed the Commissioners of the Navy of the agent's proceeding; but my dismission was soon after procured, by means of a gentleman in the city, whom the agent, conscious of his peculation, had deceived by letter, and whom, moreover, empowered the same agent to receive on board, at the government expense, a number of persons as passengers, contrary to the orders I received. By this I suffered a considerable loss in my property: however, the commissioners were satisfied with my conduct, and wrote to Capt. Thompson, expressing their approbation of it.

Thus provided, they proceeded on their voyage; and at last, worn out by treatment, perhaps not the most mild, and wasted by sickness, brought on by want of medicine, cloaths, bedding, &c. they reached Sierra Leone just at the commencement of the rains. At that season of the year it is impossible to cultivate the lands; their provisions therefore were exhausted before they could derive any benefit from agriculture; and it is not surprising that many, especially the lascars, whose constitutions are very tender, and who had been cooped up in ships from October to June, and accommodated in the manner I have mentioned, should be so wasted by their confinement as not long to survive it.

Thus ended my part of the long-talked-of expedition to Sierra Leone; an expedition which, however unfortunate in the event, was humane and politic in its design, nor was its failure owing to government: every thing was done on their part; but there was evidently sufficient mismanagement attending the conduct and execution of it to defeat its success.

I should not have been so ample in my account of this transaction, had not the share I bore in it been made the subject of partial animadversion, and even my dismission from my employment thought worthy of being made by some a matter of public triumph*. The motives which might influence any person to descend to a petty contest with an obscure African, and to seek gratification by his depression, perhaps it is not proper here to inquire into or relate, even if its detection were necessary to my vindication; but I thank Heaven it is not. I wish to stand by my own integrity, and not to shelter myself under the impropriety of another; and I trust the behaviour of the Commissioners of the Navy to me entitle me to make this assertion; for after I had been dismissed, March 24, I drew up a memorial thus:

To the Right Honourable the Lords Commissioners of his Majesty's Treasury:
The Memorial and Petition of GUSTAVUS VASSA *a black Man, late Commissary to the black Poor going to* AFRICA.
HUMBLY SHEWETH,

THAT your Lordships' memorialist was, by the Honourable the Commissioners of his Majesty's Navy, on the 4th of December last, appointed to the above employment by warrant from that board;

That he accordingly proceeded to the execution of his duty on board of the Vernon, being one of the ships appointed to proceed to Africa with the above poor;

That your memorialist, to his great grief and astonishment, received a letter of dismission from the Honourable Commissioners of the Navy, by your Lordships' orders;

That, conscious of having acted with the most perfect fidelity and the greatest assiduity in discharging the trust reposed in him, he is altogether at a loss to conceive the reasons

---

*See the Public Advertiser, July 14, 1787.

of your Lordships' having altered the favourable opinion you were pleased to conceive of him, sensible that your Lordships would not proceed to so severe a measure without some apparent good cause; he therefore has every reason to believe that his conduct has been grossly misrepresented to your Lordships; and he is the more confirmed in his opinion, because, by opposing measures of others concerned in the same expedition, which tended to defeat your Lordships' humane intentions, and to put the government to a very considerable additional expense, he created a number of enemies, whose misrepresentations, he has too much reason to believe, laid the foundation of his dismission. Unsupported by friends, and unaided by the advantages of a liberal education, he can only hope for redress from the justice of his cause, in addition to the mortification of having been removed from his employment, and the advantage which he reasonably might have expected to have derived therefrom. He has had the misfortune to have sunk a considerable part of his little property in fitting himself out, and in other expenses arising out of his situation, an account of which he here annexes. Your memorialist will not trouble your Lordships with a vindication of any part of his conduct, because he knows not of what crimes he is accused; he, however, earnestly entreats that you will be pleased to direct an inquiry into his behaviour during the time he acted in the public service; and, if it be found that his dismission arose from false representations, he is confident that in your Lordships' justice he shall find redress.

Your petitioner therefore humbly prays that your Lordships will take his case into consideration, and that you will be pleased to order payment of the above referred-to account, amounting to 32l. 4s. and also the wages intended, which is most humbly submitted.

London, May 12, 1787.

The above petition was delivered into the hands of their Lordships, who were kind enough, in the space of some few months afterwards, without hearing, to order me 50l. sterling —that is, 18l. wages for the time (upwards of four months) I acted a faithful part in their service. Certainly the sum is more than a free negro would have had in the western colonies!!!

March the 21st, 1788, I had the honour of presenting the Queen with a petition on behalf of my African brethren, which was received most graciously by her Majesty*:

To the QUEEN's *most Excellent Majesty.*

MADAM,

YOUR Majesty's well known benevolence and humanity emboldens me to approach your royal presence, trusting that the obscurity of my situation will not prevent your Majesty from attending to the sufferings for which I plead.

Yet I do not solicit your royal pity for my own distress; my sufferings, although numerous, are in a measure forgotten. I supplicate your Majesty's compassion for millions of my African countrymen, who groan under the lash of tyranny in the West Indies.

The oppression and cruelty exercised to the unhappy negroes there, have at length reached the British legislature, and they are now deliberating on its redress; even several persons of property in slaves in the West Indies, have petitioned parliament against its continuance, sensible that it is as impolitic as it is unjust—and what is inhuman must ever be unwise.

Your Majesty's reign has been hitherto distinguished by private acts of benevolence and bounty; surely the more extended the misery is, the greater claim it has to your Majesty's compassion, and the greater must be your Majesty's pleasure in administering to its relief.

I presume, therefore, gracious Queen, to implore your interposition with your royal consort, in favour of the wretched Africans; that, by your Majesty's benevolent influence, a period may now be put to their misery; and that they may be raised from the condition of brutes, to which they are at present degraded, to the rights and situation of freemen, and admitted to partake of the blessings of your Majesty's happy government; so shall your Majesty enjoy the heart-felt plea-

---

*At the request of some of my most particular friends, I take the liberty of inserting it here.

sure of procuring happiness to millions, and be rewarded in the grateful prayers of themselves, and of their posterity.

And may the all-bountiful Creator shower on your Majesty, and the Royal Family, every blessing that this world can afford, and every fulness of joy which divine revelation has promised us in the next.

I am your Majesty's most dutiful and devoted servant to command,

GUSTAVUS VASSA,
The Oppressed Ethiopean.
No. 53, Baldwin's Gardens.

The negro consolidated act, made by the assembly of Jamaica last year, and the new act of amendment now in agitation there, contain a proof of the existence of those charges that have been made against the planters relative to the treatment of their slaves.

I hope to have the satisfaction of seeing the renovation of liberty and justice resting on the British government, to vindicate the honour of our common nature. These are concerns which do not perhaps belong to any particular office: but, to speak more seriously to every man of sentiment, actions like these are the just and sure foundation of future fame; a reversion, though remote, is coveted by some noble minds as a substantial good. It is upon these grounds that I hope and expect the attention of gentlemen in power. These are designs consonant to the elevation of their rank, and the dignity of their stations: they are ends suitable to the nature of a free and generous government; and, connected with views of empire and dominion, suited to the benevolence and solid merit of the legislature. It is a pursuit of substantial greatness.— May the time come—at least the speculation to me is pleasing—when the sable people shall gratefully commemorate the auspicious æra of extensive freedom. Then shall those persons* particularly be named with praise and honour, who generously proposed and stood forth in the cause of humanity,

*Grenville Sharp, Esq; the Reverend Thomas Clarkson; the Reverend James Ramsay; our approved friends, men of virtue, are an honour to their country, ornamental to human nature, happy in themselves, and benefactors to mankind!

liberty, and good policy; and brought to the ear of the legislature designs worthy of royal patronage and adoption. May
Heaven make the British senators the dispersers of light, liberty, and science, to the uttermost parts of the earth: then will
be glory to God on the highest, on earth peace, and good-
will to men:—Glory, honour, peace, &c. to every soul of man
that worketh good, to the Britons first, (because to them the
Gospel is preached) and also to the nations. 'Those that honour their Maker have mercy on the poor.' 'It is righteousness
exalteth a nation; but sin is a reproach to any people; destruction shall be to the workers of iniquity, and the wicked
shall fall by their own wickedness.' May the blessings of the
Lord be upon the heads of all those who commiserated the
cases of the oppressed negroes, and the fear of God prolong
their days; and may their expectations be filled with gladness!
'The liberal devise liberal things, and by liberal things shall
stand,' Isaiah xxxii. 8. They can say with pious Job, 'Did not
I weep for him that was in trouble? was not my soul grieved
for the poor?' Job xxx. 25.

As the inhuman traffic of slavery is to be taken into the
consideration of the British legislature, I doubt not, if a system of commerce was established in Africa, the demand for
manufactures would most rapidly augment, as the native inhabitants will insensibly adopt the British fashions, manners,
customs, &c. In proportion to the civilization, so will be the
consumption of British manufactures.

The wear and tear of a continent, nearly twice as large as
Europe, and rich in vegetable and mineral productions, is
much easier conceived than calculated.

A case in point.—It cost the Aborigines of Britain little or
nothing in clothing, &c. The difference between their fore-
fathers and the present generation, in point of consumption,
is literally infinite. The supposition is most obvious. It will be
equally immense in Africa—The same cause, viz. civilization,
will ever have the same effect.

It is trading upon safe grounds. A commercial intercourse
with Africa opens an inexhaustible source of wealth to the
manufacturing interests of Great Britain, and to all which the
slave trade is an objection.

If I am not misinformed, the manufacturing interest is

equal, if not superior, to the landed interest, as to the value, for reasons which will soon appear. The abolition of slavery, so diabolical, will give a most rapid extension of manufactures, which is totally and diametrically opposite to what some interested people assert.

The manufacturers of this country must and will, in the nature and reason of things, have a full and constant employ by supplying the African markets.

Population, the bowels and surface of Africa, abound in valuable and useful returns; the hidden treasures of centuries will be brought to light and into circulation. Industry, enterprize, and mining, will have their full scope, proportionably as they civilize. In a word, it lays open an endless field of commerce to the British manufactures and merchant adventurer. The manufacturing interest and the general interests are synonymous. The abolition of slavery would be in reality an universal good.

Tortures, murder, and every other imaginable barbarity and iniquity, are practised upon the poor slaves with impunity. I hope the slave trade will be abolished. I pray it may be an event at hand. The great body of manufacturers, uniting in the cause, will considerably facilitate and expedite it; and, as I have already stated, it is most substantially their interest and advantage, and as such the nation's at large, (except those persons concerned in the manufacturing neck-yokes, collars, chains, hand-cuffs, leg-bolts, drags, thumb-screws, iron muzzles, and coffins; cats, scourges, and other instruments of torture used in the slave trade). In a short time one sentiment alone will prevail, from motives of interest as well as justice and humanity. Europe contains one hundred and twenty millions of inhabitants. Query—How many millions doth Africa contain? Supposing the Africans, collectively and individually, to expend 5l. a head in raiment and furniture yearly when civilized, &c. an immensity beyond the reach of imagination!

This I conceive to be a theory founded upon facts, and therefore an infallible one. If the blacks were permitted to remain in their own country, they would double themselves every fifteen years. In proportion to such increase will be the demand for manufactures. Cotton and indigo grow spontaneously in most parts of Africa; a consideration this of no small consequence to the manufacturing towns of Great Britain. It opens a most immense, glorious, and happy prospect—the clothing, &c. of a continent ten thousand miles in circumference, and immensely rich in productions of every denomination in return for manufactures.

I have only therefore to request the reader's indulgence and conclude. I am far from the vanity of thinking there is any merit in this narrative: I hope censure will be suspended, when it is considered that it was written by one who was as unwilling as unable to adorn the plainness of truth by the colouring of imagination. My life and fortune have been extremely chequered, and my adventures various. Even those I have related are considerably abridged. If any incident in this little work should appear uninteresting and trifling to most readers, I can only say, as my excuse for mentioning it, that almost every event of my life made an impression on my mind and influenced my conduct. I early accustomed myself to look for the hand of God in the minutest occurrence, and to learn from it a lesson of morality and religion; and in this light every circumstance I have related was to me of importance. After all, what makes any event important, unless by its observation we become better and wiser, and learn 'to do justly, to love mercy, and to walk humbly before God?' To those who are possessed of this spirit, there is scarcely any book or incident so trifling that does not afford some profit, while to others the experience of ages seems of no use; and even to pour out to them the treasures of wisdom is throwing the jewels of instruction away.

THE END.

THE

CONFESSIONS

OF

NAT TURNER,

THE LEADER OF THE LATE

INSURRECTIONS IN SOUTHAMPTON, VA.

As fully and voluntarily made to

THOMAS R. GRAY,

In the prison where he was confined, and acknowledged by
him to be such when read before the Court of Southampton; with the certificate, under seal of
the Court convened at Jerusalem,
Nov. 5, 1831, for his trial.

ALSO, AN AUTHENTIC

ACCOUNT OF THE WHOLE INSURRECTION,

WITH LISTS OF THE WHITES WHO WERE MURDERED,

AND OF THE NEGROES BROUGHT BEFORE THE COURT OF SOUTHAMPTON, AND THERE SENTENCED, &c.

Baltimore:
PUBLISHED BY THOMAS R. GRAY.
Lucas & Deaver, print.
1831.

DISTRICT OF COLUMBIA, TO WIT:

Be it remembered, That on this tenth day of November, Anno Domini, eighteen hundred and thirty-one, Thomas R. Gray of the said District, deposited in this office the title of a book, which is in the words as following:

"The Confessions of Nat Turner, the leader of the late insurrection in Southampton, Virginia, as fully and voluntarily made to Thomas R. Gray, in the prison where he was confined, and acknowledged by him to be such when read before the Court of Southampton; with the certificate, under seal, of the Court convened at Jerusalem, November 5, 1831, for his trial. Also, an authentic account of the whole insurrection, with lists of the whites who were murdered, and of the negroes brought before the Court of Southampton, and there sentenced, &c." the right whereof he claims as proprietor, in conformity with an Act of Congress, entitled "An act to amend the several acts respecting Copy Rights."

EDMUND J. LEE, Clerk of the District.

(Seal.)

In testimony that the above is a true copy, from the record of the District Court for the District of Columbia, I, Edmund I. Lee, the Clerk thereof, have hereunto set my hand and affixed the seal of my office, this 10th day of November, 1831.

EDMUND J. LEE, C. D. C.

TO THE PUBLIC.

THE late insurrection in Southampton has greatly excited the public mind, and led to a thousand idle, exaggerated and mischievous reports. It is the first instance in our history of an open rebellion of the slaves, and attended with such atrocious circumstances of cruelty and destruction, as could not fail to leave a deep impression, not only upon the minds of the community where this fearful tragedy was wrought, but throughout every portion of our country, in which this population is to be found. Public curiosity has been on the stretch to understand the origin and progress of this dreadful conspiracy, and the motives which influences its diabolical actors. The insurgent slaves had all been destroyed, or apprehended, tried and executed, (with the exception of the leader,) without revealing any thing at all satisfactory, as to the motives which governed them, or the means by which they expected to accomplish their object. Every thing connected with this sad affair was wrapt in mystery, until Nat Turner, the leader of this ferocious band, whose name has resounded throughout our widely extended empire, was captured. This "great Bandit" was taken by a single individual, in a cave near the residence of his late owner, on Sunday, the thirtieth of October, without attempting to make the slightest resistance, and on the following day safely lodged in the jail of the County. His captor was Benjamin Phipps, armed with a shot gun well charged. Nat's only weapon was a small light sword which he immediately surrendered, and begged that his life might be spared. Since his confinement, by permission of the Jailor, I have had ready access to him, and finding that he was willing to make a full and free confession of the origin, progress and consummation of the insurrectory movements of the slaves of which he was the contriver and head; I determined for the gratification of public curiosity to commit his statements to writing, and publish them, with little or no variation, from his own words. That this is a faithful record of his confessions, the annexed certificate of the County Court of Southampton, will attest. They certainly bear one stamp of truth and sincerity. He makes no attempt (as all the other insurgents who were examined did,) to exculpate himself, but frankly acknowledges his full participation in all the guilt of the transaction. He was not only the contriver of the conspiracy, but gave the first blow towards its execution.

It will thus appear, that whilst every thing upon the surface of society wore a calm and peaceful aspect; whilst not one note of preparation was heard to warn the devoted inhabitants of woe and death, a gloomy fanatic was revolving in the recesses of his own dark, bewildered, and overwrought mind, schemes of indiscriminate massacre to the whites. Schemes too fearfully executed as far as his fiendish band proceeded in their desolating march. No cry for mercy penetrated their flinty bosoms. No acts of remembered kindness made the least impression upon these remorseless murderers. Men, women and children, from hoary age to helpless infancy were involved in the same cruel fate. Never did a band of savages do their work of death more unsparingly. Apprehension for their own personal safety seems to have been the only principle of restraint in the whole course of their bloody proceedings. And it is not the least remarkable feature in this horrid transaction, that a band actuated by such hellish purposes, should have resisted so feebly, when met by the whites in arms. Desperation alone, one would think, might have led to greater efforts. More than twenty of them attacked Dr. Blunt's house on Tuesday morning, a little before day-break, defended by two men and three boys. They fled precipitately at the first fire; and their future plans of mischief, were entirely disconcerted and broken up. Escaping thence, each individual sought his own safety either in concealment, or by returning home, with the hope that his participation might escape detection, and all were shot down in the course of a few days, or captured and brought to trial and punishment. Nat has survived all his followers, and the gallows will speedily close his career. His own account of the conspiracy is submitted to the public, without comment. It reads an awful, and it is hoped, a useful lesson, as to the operations of a mind like his, endeavoring to grapple with things beyond its reach. How it first became bewildered and confounded, and finally corrupted and led to the conception and perpetration of the most atrocious and heart-rending deeds. It is calculated also to demonstrate the policy of our laws in restraint of this class of our population, and to induce all those entrusted with their execution, as well as our citizens generally, to see that they are strictly and rigidly enforced. Each particular community should look to its own safety, whilst the general guardians of the laws, keep a watchful eye over all. If Nat's statements can be relied on, the insurrection in this county was entirely local, and his designs confided but to a few, and these in his immediate vicinity. It was not instigated by motives of revenge or sudden anger, but the results of long deliberation, and a settled purpose of mind. The offspring of gloomy fanaticism, acting upon materials but too well prepared for such impressions. It will be long remembered in the annals of our country, and many a mother as she presses her infant darling to her bosom, will shudder at the recollection of Nat Turner, and his band of ferocious miscreants.

Believing the following narrative, by removing doubts and conjectures from the public mind which otherwise must have remained, would give general satisfaction, it is respectfully submitted to the public by their ob't serv't,

T. R. GRAY.

Jerusalem, Southampton, Va. Nov. 5, 1831.

We the undersigned, members of the Court convened at Jerusalem, on Saturday, the 5th day of Nov. 1831, for the trial of Nat, *alias* Nat Turner, a negro slave, late the property of Putnam Moore, deceased, do hereby certify, that the confessions of Nat, to Thomas R. Gray, was read to him in our presence, and that Nat acknowledged the same to be full, free, and voluntary; and that furthermore, when called upon by the presiding Magistrate of the Court, to state if he had any thing to say, why sentence of death should not be passed upon him, replied he had nothing further than he had communicated to Mr. Gray. Given under our hands and seals at Jerusalem, this 5th day of November, 1831.

JEREMIAH COBB,	[*Seal.*]
THOMAS PRETLOW,	[*Seal.*]
JAMES W. PARKER,	[*Seal.*]
CARR BOWERS,	[*Seal.*]
SAMUEL B. HINES,	[*Seal.*]
ORRIS A. BROWNE,	[*Seal.*]

State of Virginia, Southampton County, to wit:

I, James Rochelle, Clerk of the County Court of Southampton in the State of Virginia, do hereby certify, that Jeremiah Cobb, Thomas Pretlow, James W. Parker, Carr Bowers, Samuel B. Hines, and Orris A. Browne, esqr's are acting Justices of the Peace, in and for the County aforesaid, and were members of the Court which convened at Jerusalem, on Saturday the 5th day of November, 1831, for the trial of Nat *alias* Nat Turner, a negro slave, late the property of Putnam Moore, deceased, who was tried and convicted, as an insurgent in the late insurrection in the county of Southampton aforesaid, and that full faith and credit are due, and ought to be given to their acts as Justices of the peace aforesaid.

In testimony whereof, I have hereunto set my hand and caused the seal of the Court
[Seal.]   aforesaid, to be affixed this 5th day of
November, 1831.
JAMES ROCHELLE, C. S. C. C.

CONFESSION.

AGREEABLE to his own appointment, on the evening he was committed to prison, with permission of the jailer, I visited NAT on Tuesday the 1st November, when, without being questioned at all, he commenced his narrative in the following words:—

SIR,—You have asked me to give a history of the motives which induced me to undertake the late insurrection, as you call it—To do so I must go back to the days of my infancy, and even before I was born. I was thirty-one years of age the 2d of October last, and born the property of Benj. Turner, of this county. In my childhood a circumstance occurred which made an indelible impression on my mind, and laid the ground work of that enthusiasm, which has terminated so fatally to many, both white and black, and for which I am about to atone at the gallows. It is here necessary to relate this circumstance—trifling as it may seem, it was the commencement of that belief which has grown with time, and even now, sir, in this dungeon, helpless and forsaken as I am, I cannot divest myself of. Being at play with other children, when three or four years old, I was telling them something, which my mother overhearing, said it had happened before I was born—I stuck to my story, however, and related somethings which went, in her opinion, to confirm it—others being called on were greatly astonished, knowing that these things had happened, and caused them to say in my hearing, I surely would be a prophet, as the Lord had shewn me things that had happened before my birth. And my father and mother strengthened me in this my first impression, saying in my presence, I was intended for some great purpose, which they had always thought from certain marks on my head and breast—[a parcel of excrescences which I believe are not at all uncommon, particularly among negroes, as I have seen several with the same. In this case he has either cut them off or they have nearly disappeared]—My grand mother, who was very religious, and to whom I was much attached—my master, who belonged to the church, and other religious persons who visited the house, and whom I often saw at prayers, noticing the singularity of my manners, I suppose, and my uncommon intelligence for a child, remarked I had too much sense to be raised, and if I was, I would never be of any service to any one as a slave—To a mind like mine, restless, inquisitive and observant of every thing that was passing, it is easy to suppose that religion was the subject to which it would be directed, and although this subject principally occupied my thoughts—there was nothing that I saw or heard of to which my attention was not directed—The manner in which I learned to read and write, not only had great influence on my own mind, as I acquired it with the most perfect ease, so much so, that I have no recollection whatever of learning the alphabet—but to the astonishment of the family, one day, when a book was shewn me to keep me from crying, I began spelling the names of different objects—this was a source of wonder to all in the neighborhood, particularly the blacks—and this learning was constantly improved at all opportunities—when I got large enough to go to work, while employed, I was reflecting on many things that would present themselves to my imagination, and whenever an opportunity occurred of looking at a book, when the school children were getting their lessons, I would find many things that the fertility of my own imagination had depicted to me before; all my time, not devoted to my master's service, was spent either in prayer, or in making experiments in casting different things in moulds made of earth, in attempting to make paper, gunpowder, and many other experiments, that although I could not perfect, yet convinced me of its practicability if I had the means.* I was not addicted to stealing in my youth, nor have ever been—Yet such was the confidence of the negroes in the neighborhood, even at this early period of my life, in my superior judgment, that they would often carry me with them when they were going on any roguery, to plan for them. Growing up among them, with this confidence in my superior judgment, and when this, in their opinions, was perfected by

*When questioned as to the manner of manufacturing those different articles, he was found well informed on the subject.

Divine inspiration, from the circumstances already alluded to in my infancy, and which belief was ever afterwards zealously inculcated by the austerity of my life and manners, which became the subject of remark by white and black.—Having soon discovered to be great, I must appear so, and therefore studiously avoided mixing in society, and wrapped myself in mystery, devoting my time to fasting and prayer—By this time, having arrived to man's estate, and hearing the scriptures commented on at meetings, I was struck with that particular passage which says: "Seek ye the kingdom of Heaven and all things shall be added unto you." I reflected much on this passage, and prayed daily for light on this subject—As I was praying one day at my plough, the spirit spoke to me, saying, "Seek ye the kingdom of Heaven and all things shall be added unto you." *Question*—what do you mean by the Spirit. *Ans.* The Spirit that spoke to the prophets in former days—and I was greatly astonished, and for two years prayed continually, whenever my duty would permit—and then again I had the same revelation, which fully confirmed me in the impression that I was ordained for some great purpose in the hands of the Almighty. Several years rolled round, in which many events occurred to strengthen me in this my belief. At this time I reverted in my mind to the remarks made of me in my childhood, and the things that had been shewn me—and as it had been said of me in my childhood by those by whom I had been taught to pray, both white and black, and in whom I had the greatest confidence, that I had too much sense to be raised, and if I was, I would never be of any use to any one as a slave. Now finding I had arrived to man's estate, and was a slave, and these revelations being made known to me, I began to direct my attention to this great object, to fulfil the purpose for which, by this time, I felt assured I was intended. Knowing the influence I had obtained over the minds of my fellow servants, (not by the means of conjuring and such like tricks—for to them I always spoke of such things with contempt) but by the communion of the Spirit whose revelations I often communicated to them, and they believed and said my wisdom came from God. I now began to prepare them for my purpose, by telling them something was about to happen that would terminate in fulfilling the great promise that had been made to me—About this time I was placed under an overseer, from whom I ran away—and after remaining in the woods thirty days, I returned, to the astonishment of the negroes on the plantation, who thought I had made my escape to some other part of the country, as my father had done before. But the reason of my return was, that the Spirit appeared to me and said I had my wishes directed to the things of this world, and not to the kingdom of Heaven, and that I should return to the service of my earthly master—"For he who knoweth his Master's will, and doeth it not, shall be beaten with many stripes, and thus have I chastened you." And the negroes found fault, and murmured against me, saying that if they had my sense they would not serve any master in the world. And about this time I had a vision—and I saw white spirits and black spirits engaged in battle, and the sun was darkened—the thunder rolled in the Heavens, and blood flowed in streams—and I heard a voice saying, "Such is your luck, such you are called to see, and let it come rough or smooth, you must surely bare it." I now withdrew myself as much as my situation would permit, from the intercourse of my fellow servants, for the avowed purpose of serving the Spirit more fully—and it appeared to me, and reminded me of the things it had already shown me, and that it would then reveal to me the knowledge of the elements, the revolution of the planets, the operation of tides, and changes of the seasons. After this revelation in the year 1825, and the knowledge of the elements being made known to me, I sought more than ever to obtain true holiness before the great day of judgment should appear, and then I began to receive the true knowledge of faith. And from the first steps of righteousness until the last, was I made perfect; and the Holy Ghost was with me, and said, "Behold me as I stand in the Heavens"—and I looked and saw the forms of men in different attitudes—and there were lights in the sky to which the children of darkness gave other names than what they really were—for they were the lights of the Saviour's hands, stretched forth from east to west, even as they were extended on the cross on Calvary for the redemption of sinners. And I wondered greatly at these miracles, and prayed to be informed of a certainty of the meaning thereof— and shortly afterwards, while laboring in the field, I discovered drops of blood on the corn as though it were dew from heaven—and I communicated it to many, both white and black, in the neighborhood—and I then found on the leaves in the woods hieroglyphic characters, and numbers, with the forms of men in different attitudes, portrayed in blood, and representing the figures I had seen before in the heavens. And now the Holy Ghost had revealed itself to me, and made plain the miracles it had shown me—For as the blood of Christ had been shed on this earth, and had ascended to heaven for the salvation of sinners, and was now returning to earth again in the form of dew—and as the leaves on the trees bore the impression of the figures I had seen in the heavens, it was plain to me that the Saviour was about to lay down the yoke he had borne for the sins of men, and the great day of judgment was at hand. About this time I told these things to a white man, (Etheldred T. Brantley) on whom it had a wonderful effect—and he ceased from his wickedness, and was attacked immediately with a cutaneous eruption, and blood ozed from the pores of his skin, and after praying and fasting nine days, he was healed, and the Spirit appeared to me again, and said, as the Saviour had been baptised so should we be also—and when the white people would not let us be baptised by the church, we went down into the water together, in the sight of many who reviled us, and were baptised by the Spirit—After this I rejoiced greatly, and gave thanks to God. And on the 12th of May, 1828, I heard a loud noise in the heavens, and the Spirit instantly appeared to me and said the Serpent was loosened, and Christ had laid down the yoke he had borne for the sins of men, and that I should take it on and fight against the Serpent, for the time was fast approaching when the first should be last and the last should be first. *Ques.* Do you not find yourself mistaken now? *Ans.* Was not Christ crucified. And by signs in the heavens that it would make known to me when I should commence the great work—and until the first sign appeared, I should conceal it from the knowledge of men—And on the appearance of the sign, (the eclipse of the sun last February) I should arise and prepare myself, and slay my enemies with their own weapons. And immediately on the sign appearing in the heavens, the seal was removed from my lips, and I communicated the great work laid out for me to do, to four in whom I had the greatest confidence, (Henry, Hark, Nelson, and Sam)—It was intended by us to have begun the work of death on the 4th July last—Many were the plans formed and rejected by us, and it affected my mind to such a degree, that I fell sick, and the time passed without our coming to any determination how to commence—Still forming new schemes and rejecting them, when the sign appeared again, which determined me not to wait longer.

Since the commencement of 1830, I had been living with Mr. Joseph Travis, who was to me a kind master, and placed the greatest confidence in me; in fact, I had no cause to complain of his treatment to me. On Saturday evening, the 20th of August, it was agreed between Henry, Hark and myself, to prepare a dinner the next day for the men we expected, and then to concert a plan, as we had not yet determined on any. Hark, on the following morning, brought a pig, and Henry brandy, and being joined by Sam, Nelson, Will and Jack, they prepared in the woods a dinner, where, about three o'clock, I joined them.

Q. Why were you so backward in joining them.

A. The same reason that had caused me not to mix with them for years before.

I saluted them on coming up, and asked Will how came he there, he answered, his life was worth no more than others, and his liberty as dear to him. I asked him if he thought to obtain it? He said he would, or loose his life. This was enough to put him in full confidence. Jack, I knew, was only a tool in the hands of Hark, it was quickly agreed we should commence at home (Mr. J. Travis') on that night, and until we had armed and equipped ourselves, and gathered sufficient force, neither age nor sex was to be spared, (which was invariably adhered to.) We remained at the feast, until about two hours in the night, when we went to the house and found Austin; they all went to the cider press and drank, except myself. On returning to the house, Hark went to the door with an axe, for the purpose of breaking it open, as we knew we were strong enough to murder the family, if they were awaked by the noise; but reflecting that it might create an alarm in the neighborhood, we determined to enter the house secretly, and murder them whilst sleeping. Hark got a ladder and set it against the chimney, on which I ascended, and hoisting a window, entered and came down stairs, unbarred the door, and removed the guns from their places. It was then observed that I must spill the first blood. On which, armed with a hatchet, and accompanied by Will, I entered my master's chamber, it being dark, I could not give a death blow, the hatchet glanced from his head, he sprang from the bed and called his wife, it was his last word, Will laid him dead, with a blow of his axe, and Mrs. Travis shared the same fate, as she lay in bed. The murder of this family, five in number, was the work of a moment, not one of them awoke; there was a little infant sleeping in a cradle, that was forgotten, until we had left the house and gone some distance, when Henry and Will returned and killed it; we got here, four guns that would shoot, and several old muskets, with a pound or two of powder. We remained some time at the barn, where we paraded; I formed them in a line as soldiers, and after carrying them through all the manœuvres I was master of, marched them off to Mr. Salathul Francis', about six hundred yards distant. Sam and Will went to the door and knocked. Mr. Francis asked who was there, Sam replied it was him, and he had a letter for him, on which he got up and came to the door; they immediately seized him, and dragging him out a little from the door, he was dispatched by repeated blows on the head; there was no other white person in the family. We started from there for Mrs. Reese's, maintaining the most perfect silence on our march, where finding the door unlocked, we entered, and murdered Mrs. Reese in her bed, while sleeping; her son awoke, but it was only to sleep the sleep of death, he had only time to say who is that, and he was no more. From Mrs. Reese's we went to Mrs. Turner's, a mile distant, which we reached about sunrise, on Monday morning. Henry, Austin, and Sam, went to the still, where, finding Mr. Peebles, Austin shot him, and the rest of us went to the house; as we approached, the family discovered us, and shut the door. Vain hope! Will, with one stroke of his axe, opened it, and we entered and found Mrs. Turner and Mrs. Newsome in the middle of a room, almost frightened to death. Will immediately killed Mrs. Turner, with one blow of his axe. I took Mrs. Newsome by the hand, and with the sword I had when I was apprehended, I struck her several blows over the head, but not being able to kill her, as the sword was dull. Will turning around and discovering it, despatched her also. A general destruction of property and search for money and ammunition, always succeeded the murders. By this time my company amounted to fifteen, and nine men mounted, who started for Mrs. Whitehead's, (the other six were to go through a by way to Mr. Bryant's, and rejoin us at Mrs. Whitehead's,) as we approached the house we discovered Mr. Richard Whitehead standing in the cotton patch, near the lane fence; we called him over into the lane, and Will, the executioner, was near at hand, with his fatal axe, to send him to an untimely grave. As we pushed on to the house, I discovered some one run round the garden, and thinking it was some of the white family, I pursued them, but finding it was a servant girl belonging to the house, I returned to commence the work of death, but they whom I left, had not been idle; all the family were already murdered, but Mrs. Whitehead and her daughter Margaret. As I came round to the door I saw Will pulling Mrs. Whitehead out of the house, and at the step he nearly severed her head from her body, with his broad axe. Miss Margaret, when I discovered her, had concealed herself in the corner, formed by the projection of the cellar cap from the house; on my approach she fled, but was soon overtaken, and after repeated blows with a sword, I killed her by a blow on the head, with a fence rail. By this time, the six who had gone by Mr. Bryant's, rejoined us, and informed me they had done the work of death assigned them. We again divided, part going to Mr. Richard Porter's, and from thence to Nathaniel Francis', the others to Mr. Howell Harris', and Mr. T. Doyles. On my reaching Mr. Porter's, he had escaped with his family. I understood there, that the alarm had already spread, and I immediately returned to bring up those sent to Mr. Doyles, and Mr. Howell Harris'; the party I left going on to Mr. Francis', having told them I would join them in that neighborhood. I met these sent to Mr. Doyles' and Mr. Harris' returning, having met Mr. Doyle on the road and killed him; and learning from some who joined them, that Mr. Harris was from home, I immediately pursued the course taken by the party gone on before; but knowing they would complete the work of death and pillage, at Mr. Francis' before I could get there, I went to Mr. Peter Edwards', expecting to find them there, but they had been here also. I then went to Mr. John T. Barrow's, they had been here and murdered him. I pursued on their track to Capt. Newit Harris', where I found the greater part mounted, and ready to start; the men now amounting to about forty, shouted and hurraed as I rode up, some were in the yard, loading their guns, others drinking. They said Captain Harris and his family had escaped, the property in the house they destroyed, robbing him of money and other valuables. I ordered them to mount and march instantly, this was about nine or ten o'clock, Monday morning. I proceeded to Mr. Levi Waller's, two or three miles distant. I took my station in the rear, and as it 'twas my object to carry terror and devastation wherever we went, I placed fifteen or twenty of the best armed and most to be relied on, in front, who generally approached the houses as fast as their horses could run; this was for two purposes, to prevent their escape and strike terror to the inhabitants—on this account I never got to the houses, after leaving Mrs. Whitehead's, until the murders were committed, except in one case. I sometimes got in sight in time to see the work of death completed, viewed the mangled bodies as they lay, in silent satisfaction, and immediately started in quest of other victims Having murdered Mrs. Waller and ten children, we started for Mr. William Williams'—having killed him and two little boys that were there; while engaged in this, Mrs. Williams fled and got some distance from the house, but she was pursued, overtaken, and compelled to get up behind one of the company, who brought her back, and after showing her the mangled body of her lifeless husband, she was told to get down and lay by his side, where she was shot dead. I then started for Mr. Jacob Williams, where the family were murdered—Here we found a young man named Drury, who had come on business with Mr. Williams—he was pursued, overtaken and shot. Mrs. Vaughan was the next place we visited— and after murdering the family here, I determined on starting for Jerusalem—Our number amounted now to fifty or sixty, all mounted and armed with guns, axes, swords and clubs— On reaching Mr. James W. Parkers' gate, immediately on the road leading to Jerusalem, and about three miles distant, it was proposed to me to call there, but I objected, as I knew he was gone to Jerusalem, and my object was to reach there as soon as possible; but some of the men having relations at Mr. Parker's it was agreed that they might call and get his people. I remained at the gate on the road, with seven or eight; the others going across the field to the house, about half a mile off. After waiting some time for them, I became impatient, and started to the house for them, and on our return we were met by a party of white men, who had pursued our blood-stained track, and who had fired on those at the gate, and dispersed them, which I new nothing of, not having been at that time rejoined by any of them—Immediately on discovering the whites, I ordered my men to halt and form, as they appeared to be alarmed—The white men, eighteen in number, approached us in about one hundred yards, when one of them fired, (this was against the positive orders of Captain Alexander P. Peete, who commanded, and who had directed the men to reserve their fire until within thirty paces) And I discovered about half of them retreating, I then ordered my men to fire and rush on them; the few remaining stood their ground until we approached within fifty yards, when they fired and retreated. We pursued and overtook some of them who we thought we left dead; (they were not killed) after pursuing them about two hundred yards, and rising a little hill, I discovered they were met by another party, and had haulted, and were re-loading their guns, (this was a small party from Jerusalem who knew the negroes were in the field, and had just tied their horses to await their return to the road, knowing that Mr. Parker and family were in Jerusalem, but knew nothing of the party that had gone in with Captain Peete; on hearing the firing they immediately rushed to the spot and arrived just in time to arrest the progress of these barbarous villians, and save the lives of their friends and fellow citizens.) Thinking that those who retreated first, and the party who fired on us at fifty or sixty yards distant, had all only fallen back to meet others with amunition. As I saw them re-loading their guns, and more coming up than I saw at first, and several of my bravest men being wounded, the others became panick struck and squandered over the field; the white men pursued and fired on us several times. Hark had his horse shot under him, and I caught another for him as it was running by me; five or six of my men were wounded, but none left on the field; finding myself defeated here I instantly determined to go through a private way, and cross the Nottoway river at the Cypress Bridge, three miles below Jerusalem, and attack that place in the rear, as I expected they would look for me on the other road, and I had a great desire to get there to procure arms and amunition. After going a short distance in this private way, accompanied by about twenty men, I overtook two or three who told me the others were dispersed in every direction. After trying in vain to collect a sufficient force to proceed to Jerusalem, I determined to return, as I was sure they would make back to their old neighborhood, where they would rejoin me, make new recruits, and come down again. On my way back, I called at Mrs. Thomas's, Mrs. Spencer's, and several other places, the white families having fled, we found no more victims to gratify our thirst for blood, we stopped at Majr. Ridley's quarter for the night, and being joined by four of his men, with the recruits made since my defeat, we mustered now about forty strong. After placing out sentinels, I laid down to sleep, but was quickly roused by a great racket; starting up, I found some mounted, and others in great confusion; one of the sentinels having given the alarm that we were about to be attacked, I ordered some to ride round and reconnoitre, and on their return the others being more alarmed, not knowing who they were, fled in different ways, so that I was reduced to about twenty again; with this I determined to attempt to recruit, and proceed on to rally in the neighborhood, I had left. Dr. Blunt's was the nearest house, which we reached just before day; on riding up the yard, Hark fired a gun. We expected Dr. Blunt and his family were at Maj. Ridley's, as I knew there was a company of men there; the gun was fired to ascertain if any of the family were at home; we were immediately fired upon and retreated, leaving several of my men. I do not know what became of them, as I never saw them afterwards. Pursuing our course back and coming in sight of Captain Harris', where we had been the day before, we discovered a party of white men at the house, on which all deserted me but two,

(Jacob and Nat,) we concealed ourselves in the woods until
near night, when I sent them in search of Henry, Sam, Nelson, and Hark, and directed them to rally all they could, at
the place we had had our dinner the Sunday before, where
they would find me, and I accordingly returned there as soon
as it was dark and remained until Wednesday evening, when
discovering white men riding around the place as though they
were looking for some one, and none of my men joining me,
I concluded Jacob and Nat had been taken, and compelled to
betray me. On this I gave up all hope for the present; and on
Thursday night after having supplied myself with provisions
from Mr. Travis's, I scratched a hole under a pile of fence rails
in a field, where I concealed myself for six weeks, never leaving my hiding place but for a few minutes in the dead of night
to get water which was very near; thinking by this time I
could venture out, I began to go about in the night and eaves
drop the houses in the neighborhood; pursuing this course
for about a fortnight and gathering little or no intelligence,
afraid of speaking to any human being, and returning every
morning to my cave before the dawn of day. I know not how
long I might have led this life, if accident had not betrayed
me, a dog in the neighborhood passing by my hiding place
one night while I was out, was attracted by some meat I had
in my cave, and crawled in and stole it, and was coming out
just as I returned. A few nights after, two negroes having
started to go hunting with the same dog, and passed that way,
the dog came again to the place, and having just gone out to
walk about, discovered me and barked, on which thinking
myself discovered, I spoke to them to beg concealment. On
making myself known they fled from me. Knowing then they
would betray me, I immediately left my hiding place, and was
pursued almost incessantly until I was taken a fortnight afterwards by Mr. Benjamin Phipps, in a little hole I had dug out
with my sword, for the purpose of concealment, under the
top of a fallen tree. On Mr. Phipps' discovering the place of
my concealment, he cocked his gun and aimed at me. I requested him not to shoot and I would give up, upon which
he demanded my sword. I delivered it to him, and he brought
me to prison. During the time I was pursued, I had many hair
breadth escapes, which your time will not permit you to re-

late. I am here loaded with chains, and willing to suffer the fate that awaits me.

I here proceeded to make some inquiries of him, after assuring him of the certain death that awaited him, and that concealment would only bring destruction on the innocent as well as guilty, of his own color, if he knew of any extensive or concerted plan. His answer was, I do not. When I questioned him as to the insurrection in North Carolina happening about the same time, he denied any knowledge of it; and when I looked him in the face as though I would search his inmost thoughts, he replied, "I see sir, you doubt my word; but can you not think the same ideas, and strange appearances about this time in the heaven's might prompt others, as well as myself, to this undertaking." I now had much conversation with and asked him many questions, having forborne to do so previously, except in the cases noted in parenthesis; but during his statement, I had, unnoticed by him, taken notes as to some particular circumstances, and having the advantage of his statement before me in writing, on the evening of the third day that I had been with him, I began a cross examination, and found his statement corroborated by every circumstance coming within my own knowledge or the confessions of others whom had been either killed or executed, and whom he had not seen nor had any knowledge since 22d of August last, he expressed himself fully satisfied as to the impracticability of his attempt. It has been said he was ignorant and cowardly, and that his object was to murder and rob for the purpose of obtaining money to make his escape. It is notorious, that he was never known to have a dollar in his life; to swear an oath, or drink a drop of spirits. As to his ignorance, he certainly never had the advantages of education, but he can read and write, (it was taught him by his parents,) and for natural intelligence and quickness of apprehension, is surpassed by few men I have ever seen. As to his being a coward, his reason as given for not resisting Mr. Phipps, shews the decision of his character. When he saw Mr. Phipps present his gun, he said he knew it was impossible for him to escape as the woods were full of men; he therefore thought it was better to surrender, and trust to fortune for his escape. He is a complete fanatic, or plays his part most admirably. On other subjects he possesses an uncommon share of intelligence, with a mind capable of attaining any thing; but warped and perverted by the influence of early impressions. He is below the ordinary stature, though strong and active, having the true negro face, every feature of which is strongly marked. I shall not attempt to describe the effect of his narrative, as told and commented on by himself, in the condemned hole of the prison. The calm, deliberate composure with which he spoke of his late deeds and intentions, the expression of his fiend-like face when excited by enthusiasm, still bearing the stains of the blood of helpless innocence about him; clothed with rags and covered with chains; yet daring to raise his manacled hands to heaven, with a spirit soaring above the attributes of man; I looked on him and my blood curdled in my veins.

I will not shock the feelings of humanity, nor wound afresh the bosoms of the disconsolate sufferers in this unparalleled and inhuman massacre, by detailing the deeds of their fiend-like barbarity. There were two or three who were in the power of these wretches, had they known it, and who escaped in the most providential manner. There were two whom they thought they left dead on the field at Mr. Parker's, but who were only stunned by the blows of their guns, as they did not take time to re-load when they charged on them. The escape of a little girl who went to school at Mr. Waller's, and where the children were collecting for that purpose, excited general sympathy. As their teacher had not arrived, they were at play in the yard, and seeing the negroes approach, she ran up on a dirt chimney, (such as are common to log houses,) and remained there unnoticed during the massacre of the eleven that were killed at this place. She remained on her hiding place till just before the arrival of a party, who were in pursuit of the murderers, when she came down and fled to a swamp, where, a mere child as she was, with the horrors of the late scene before her, she lay concealed until the next day, when seeing a party go up to the house, she came up, and on being asked how she escaped, replied with the utmost simplicity, "The Lord helped her." She was taken up behind a gentleman of the party, and returned to the arms of her weeping mother. Miss Whitehead concealed herself between the bed and the mat that supported it, while they murdered her sister in the same room, without discovering her. She was afterwards carried off, and concealed for protection by a slave of the family, who gave evidence against several of them on their trial. Mrs. Nathaniel Francis, while concealed in a closet heard their blows, and the shrieks of the victims of these ruthless savages; they then entered the closet where she was concealed, and went out without discovering her. While in this hiding place, she heard two of her women in a quarrel about the division of her clothes. Mr. John T. Baron, discovering them approaching his house, told his wife to make her escape, and scorning to fly, fell fighting on his own threshold. After firing his rifle, he discharged his gun at them, and then broke it over the villain who first approached him, but he was overpowered, and slain. His bravery, however, saved from the hands of these monsters, his lovely and amiable wife, who will long lament a husband so deserving of her love. As directed by him, she attempted to escape through the garden, when she was caught and held by one of her servant girls, but another coming to her rescue, she fled to the woods, and concealed herself. Few indeed, were those who escaped their work of death. But fortunate for society, the hand of retributive justice has overtaken them; and not one that was known to be concerned has escaped.

The Commonwealth, } Charged with making insurrection,
     vs.   and plotting to take away the lives of
Nat Turner.   divers free white persons, &c.
                            on the 22d of August, 1831.

The court composed of ——, having met for the trial of Nat Turner, the prisoner was brought in and arraigned, and upon his arraignment pleaded *Not guilty;* saying to his counsel, that he did not feel so.

On the part of the Commonwealth, Levi Waller was introduced, who being sworn, deposed as follows: (*agreeably to Nat's own Confession.*) Col. Trezvant* was then introduced, who being sworn, numerated Nat's Confession to him, as

*The committing Magistrate.

follows: (*his Confession as given to Mr. Gray.*) The prisoner introduced no evidence, and the case was submitted without argument to the court, who having found him guilty, Jeremiah Cobb, Esq. Chairman, pronounced the sentence of the court, in the following words: "Nat Turner! Stand up. Have you any thing to say why sentence of death should not be pronounced against you?"

Ans. I have not. I have made a full confession to Mr. Gray, and I have nothing more to say.

Attend then to the sentence of the Court. You have been arraigned and tried before this court, and convicted of one of the highest crimes in our criminal code. You have been convicted of plotting in cold blood, the indiscriminate destruction of men, of helpless women, and of infant children. The evidence before us leaves not a shadow of doubt, but that your hands were often imbrued in the blood of the innocent; and your own confession tells us that they were stained with the blood of a master; in your own language, "too indulgent." Could I stop here, your crime would be sufficiently aggravated. But the original contriver of a plan, deep and deadly, one that never can be effected, you managed so far to put it into execution, as to deprive us of many of our most valuable citizens; and this was done when they were asleep, and defenceless; under circumstances shocking to humanity. And while upon this part of the subject, I cannot but call your attention to the poor misguided wretches who have gone before you. They are not few in number—they were your bosom associates; and the blood of all cries aloud, and calls upon you, as the author of their misfortune. Yes! You forced them unprepared, from Time to Eternity. Borne down by this load of guilt, your only justification is, that you were led away by fanaticism. If this be true, from my soul I pity you; and while you have my sympathies, I am, nevertheless called upon to pass the sentence of the court. The time between this and your execution, will necessarily be very short; and your only hope must be in another world. The judgment of the court is, that you be taken hence to the jail from whence you came, thence to the place of execution, and on Friday next, between the hours of 10 A. M. and 2 P. M. be hung by the neck until you are dead! dead! dead! and may the Lord have mercy upon your soul.

A list of persons murdered in the Insurrection, on the 21st and 22d of August, 1831.

Joseph Travers and wife and three children, Mrs. Elizabeth Turner, Hartwell Prebles, Sarah Newsome, Mrs. P. Reese and son William, Trajan Doyle, Henry Bryant and wife and child, and wife's mother, Mrs. Catharine Whitehead, son Richard and four daughters and grand-child, Salathiel Francis, Nathaniel Francis' overseer and two children, John T. Barrow, George Vaughan, Mrs. Levi Waller and ten children, William Williams, wife and two boys, Mrs. Caswell Worrell and child, Mrs. Rebecca Vaughan, Ann Eliza Vaughan, and son Arthur, Mrs. John K. Williams and child, Mrs. Jacob Williams and three children, and Edwin Drury—amounting to fifty-five.

A List of Negroes brought before the Court of Southampton, with their owners' names, and sentence.

Daniel, ...	Richard Porter,	Convicted.
Moses, ...	J. T. Barrow,	Do.
Tom, ...	Caty Whitehead,	Discharged.
Jack and Andrew, . . .	Caty Whitehead,	Con. and transported.
Jacob, ...	Geo. H. Charlton,	Disch'd without trial.
Isaac, ...	Ditto,	Convi. and transported.
Jack, ...	Everett Bryant,	Discharged.
Nathan, ...	Benj. Blunt's estate,	Convicted.
Nathan, Tom, and Davy, (boys,)	Nathaniel Francis,	Convicted and transported.
Davy, ...	Elizabeth Turner,	Convicted.
Curtis, ...	Thomas Ridley,	Do.
Stephen, ...	Do.	Do.
Hardy and Isham, . . .	Benjamin Edwards,	Convicted and transp'd.
Sam, ...	Nathaniel Francis,	Convicted.
Hark, ...	Joseph Travis' estate.	Do.
Moses, (a boy,)	Do.	Do. and transported
Davy, ...	Levi Waller,	Convicted.
Nelson, ...	Jacob Williams,	Do.
Nat, ...	Edm'd Turner's estate,	Do.
Jack, ...	Wm. Reese's estate,	Do.
Dred, ...	Nathaniel Francis,	Do.

Arnold, Artist, (free,) . . . . Discharged.
Sam, ... J. W. Parker, Acquitted.
Ferry and Archer, . . . J. W. Parker, Disch'd without trial.
Jim, ... William Vaughan, Acquitted.
Bob, ... Temperance Parker, Do.
Davy, ... Joseph Parker,
Daniel, ... Solomon D. Parker, Disch'd without trial.
Thomas Haithcock, (free,) . . . . Sent on for further trial.
Joe, ... John C. Turner, Convicted.
Lucy, ... John T. Barrow, Do.
Matt, ... Thomas Ridley, Acquitted.
Jim, ... Richard Porter, Do.
Exum Artes, (free,) . . . . Sent on for further trial.
Joe, ... Richard P. Briggs, Disch'd without trial.
Bury Newsome, (free,) . . . . Sent on for further trial.
Stephen, ... James Bell, Acquitted.
Jim and Isaac, ... Samuel Champion, Convicted and trans'd.
Preston, ... Hannah Williamson, Acquitted.
Frank, ... Solomon D. Parker, Convi'd and transp'd.
Jack and Shadrach, . . . Nathaniel Simmons, Acquitted.
Nelson, ... Benj. Blunt's estate, Do.
Sam, ... Peter Edwards, Convicted.
Archer, ... Arthur G. Reese, Acquitted.
Isham Turner, (free,) . . . . Sent on for further trial.
Nat Turner, ... Putnam Moore, dec'd, Convicted.

NARRATIVE

OF THE

LIFE

OF

FREDERICK DOUGLASS,

AN

AMERICAN SLAVE.

WRITTEN BY HIMSELF.

BOSTON:
PUBLISHED AT THE ANTI-SLAVERY OFFICE,
No. 25 CORNHILL
1845.

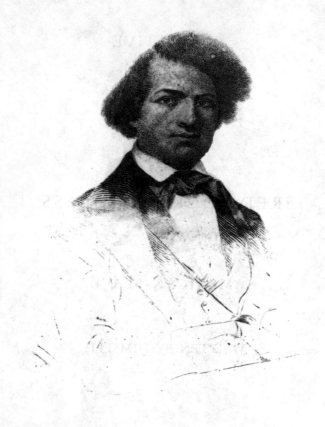

Frederick Douglass

PREFACE.

In the month of August, 1841, I attended an anti-slavery convention in Nantucket, at which it was my happiness to become acquainted with Frederick Douglass, the writer of the following Narrative. He was a stranger to nearly every member of that body; but, having recently made his escape from the southern prison-house of bondage, and feeling his curiosity excited to ascertain the principles and measures of the abolitionists,—of whom he had heard a somewhat vague description while he was a slave,—he was induced to give his attendance, on the occasion alluded to, though at that time a resident in New Bedford.

Fortunate, most fortunate occurrence!—fortunate for the millions of his manacled brethren, yet panting for deliverance from their awful thraldom!—fortunate for the cause of negro emancipation, and of universal liberty!—fortunate for the land of his birth, which he has already done so much to save and bless!—fortunate for a large circle of friends and acquaintances, whose sympathy and affection he has strongly secured by the many sufferings he has endured, by his virtuous traits of character, by his ever-abiding remembrance of those who are in bonds, as being bound with them!—fortunate for the multitudes, in various parts of our republic, whose minds he has enlightened on the subject of slavery, and who have been melted to tears by his pathos, or roused to virtuous indignation by his stirring eloquence against the enslavers of men!—fortunate for himself, as it at once brought him into the field of public usefulness, "gave the world assurance of a MAN," quickened the slumbering energies of his soul, and consecrated him to the great work of breaking the rod of the oppressor, and letting the oppressed go free!

I shall never forget his first speech at the convention—the extraordinary emotion it excited in my own mind—the powerful impression it created upon a crowded auditory, completely taken by surprise—the applause which followed from the beginning to the end of his felicitous remarks. I think I never hated slavery so intensely as at that moment; certainly, my perception of the enormous outrage which is inflicted by it, on the godlike nature of its victims, was rendered far more clear than ever. There stood one, in physical proportion and stature commanding and exact—in intellect richly endowed—in natural eloquence a prodigy—in soul manifestly "created but a little lower than the angels"—yet a slave, ay, a fugitive slave,—trembling for his safety, hardly daring to believe that on the American soil, a single white person could be found who would befriend him at all hazards, for the love of God and humanity! Capable of high attainments as an intellectual and moral being—needing nothing but a comparatively small amount of cultivation to make him an ornament to society and a blessing to his race—by the law of the land, by the voice of the people, by the terms of the slave code, he was only a piece of property, a beast of burden, a chattel personal, nevertheless!

A beloved friend from New Bedford prevailed on Mr. DOUGLASS to address the convention. He came forward to the platform with a hesitancy and embarrassment, necessarily the attendants of a sensitive mind in such a novel position. After apologizing for his ignorance, and reminding the audience that slavery was a poor school for the human intellect and heart, he proceeded to narrate some of the facts in his own history as a slave, and in the course of his speech gave utterance to many noble thoughts and thrilling reflections. As soon as he had taken his seat, filled with hope and admiration, I rose, and declared that PATRICK HENRY, of revolutionary fame, never made a speech more eloquent in the cause of liberty, than the one we had just listened to from the lips of that hunted fugitive. So I believed at that time—such is my belief now. I reminded the audience of the peril which surrounded this self-emancipated young man at the North,—even in Massachusetts, on the soil of the Pilgrim Fathers, among the descendants of revolutionary sires; and I appealed to them, whether they would ever allow him to be carried back into slavery,—law or no law, constitution or no constitution. The response was unanimous and in thunder-tones—"NO!" "Will you succor and protect him as a brother-man—a resident of the old Bay State?" "YES!" shouted the whole mass, with an energy so startling, that the ruthless tyrants south of Mason and Dixon's line might almost have heard the mighty burst of feeling, and recognized it as the pledge of an invincible determination, on the part of those who gave it, never to betray him that wanders, but to hide the outcast, and firmly to abide the consequences.

It was at once deeply impressed upon my mind, that, if Mr. DOUGLASS could be persuaded to consecrate his time and talents to the promotion of the anti-slavery enterprise, a powerful impetus would be given to it, and a stunning blow at the same time inflicted on northern prejudice against a colored complexion. I therefore endeavored to instil hope and courage into his mind, in order that he might dare to engage in a vocation so anomalous and responsible for a person in his situation; and I was seconded in this effort by warm-hearted friends, especially by the late General Agent of the Massachusetts Anti-Slavery Society, Mr. JOHN A. COLLINS, whose judgment in this instance entirely coincided with my own. At first, he could give no encouragement; with unfeigned diffidence, he expressed his conviction that he was not adequate to the performance of so great a task; the path marked out was wholly an untrodden one; he was sincerely apprehensive that he should do more harm than good. After much deliberation, however, he consented to make a trial; and ever since that period, he has acted as a lecturing agent, under the auspices either of the American or the Massachusetts Anti-Slavery Society. In labors he has been most abundant; and his success in combating prejudice, in gaining proselytes, in agitating the public mind, has far surpassed the most sanguine expectations that were raised at the commencement of his brilliant career. He has borne himself with gentleness and meekness, yet with true manliness of character. As a public speaker, he excels in pathos, wit, comparison, imitation, strength of reasoning, and fluency of language. There is in him that union of head and heart, which is indispensable to an enlightenment of the heads and a winning of the hearts of others. May his strength continue to be equal to his day! May he continue to "grow in grace, and in the knowledge of God," that he may be increasingly serviceable in the cause of bleeding humanity, whether at home or abroad!

It is certainly a very remarkable fact, that one of the most efficient advocates of the slave population, now before the public, is a fugitive slave, in the person of FREDERICK DOUG-LASS; and that the free colored population of the United States are as ably represented by one of their own number, in the person of CHARLES LENOX REMOND, whose eloquent appeals have extorted the highest applause of multitudes on both sides of the Atlantic. Let the calumniators of the colored race despise themselves for their baseness and illiberality of spirit, and henceforth cease to talk of the natural inferiority of those who require nothing but time and opportunity to attain to the highest point of human excellence.

It may, perhaps, be fairly questioned, whether any other portion of the population of the earth could have endured the privations, sufferings and horrors of slavery, without having become more degraded in the scale of humanity than the slaves of African descent. Nothing has been left undone to cripple their intellects, darken their minds, debase their moral nature, obliterate all traces of their relationship to mankind; and yet how wonderfully they have sustained the mighty load of a most frightful bondage, under which they have been groaning for centuries! To illustrate the effect of slavery on the white man,—to show that he has no powers of endurance, in such a condition, superior to those of his black brother,—DANIEL O'CONNELL, the distinguished advocate of universal emancipation, and the mightiest champion of prostrate but not conquered Ireland, relates the following anecdote in a speech delivered by him in the Conciliation Hall, Dublin, before the Loyal National Repeal Association, March 31, 1845. "No matter," said Mr. O'CONNELL, "under what specious term it may disguise itself, slavery is still hideous. *It has a natural, an inevitable tendency to brutalize every noble faculty of man.* An American sailor, who was cast away on the shore of Africa, where he was kept in slavery for three years, was, at the expiration of that period, found to be imbruted and stultified—he had lost all reasoning power; and having forgotten his native language, could only utter some savage gibberish between Arabic and English, which nobody could understand, and which even he himself found difficulty in pronouncing. So much for the humanizing influence of THE DOMESTIC INSTITUTION!" Admitting this to have been an extraordinary case of mental deterioration, it proves at least that the white slave can sink as low in the scale of humanity as the black one.

Mr. DOUGLASS has very properly chosen to write his own Narrative, in his own style, and according to the best of his ability, rather than to employ some one else. It is, therefore, entirely his own production; and, considering how long and dark was the career he had to run as a slave,—how few have been his opportunities to improve his mind since he broke his iron fetters,—it is, in my judgment, highly creditable to his head and heart. He who can peruse it without a tearful eye, a heaving breast, an afflicted spirit,—without being filled with an unutterable abhorrence of slavery and all its abettors, and animated with a determination to seek the immediate over-throw of that execrable system,—without trembling for the fate of this country in the hands of a righteous God, who is ever on the side of the oppressed, and whose arm is not short-ened that it cannot save,—must have a flinty heart, and be qualified to act the part of a trafficker "in slaves and the souls of men." I am confident that it is essentially true in all its statements; that nothing has been set down in malice, noth-ing exaggerated, nothing drawn from the imagination; that it comes short of the reality, rather than overstates a single fact in regard to SLAVERY AS IT IS. The experience of FREDERICK DOUGLASS, as a slave, was not a peculiar one; his lot was not especially a hard one; his case may be regarded as a very fair specimen of the treatment of slaves in Maryland, in which State it is conceded that they are better fed and less cruelly treated than in Georgia, Alabama, or Louisiana. Many have suffered incomparably more, while very few on the planta-tions have suffered less, than himself. Yet how deplorable was his situation! what terrible chastisements were inflicted upon his person! what still more shocking outrages were perpe-trated upon his mind! with all his noble powers and sublime aspirations, how like a brute was he treated, even by those professing to have the same mind in them that was in Christ Jesus! to what dreadful liabilities was he continually subjected! how destitute of friendly counsel and aid, even in his greatest extremities! how heavy was the midnight of woe which shrouded in blackness the last ray of hope, and filled the fu-ture with terror and gloom! what longings after freedom took possession of his breast, and how his misery augmented, in proportion as he grew reflective and intelligent,—thus demonstrating that a happy slave is an extinct man! how he thought, reasoned, felt, under the lash of the driver, with the chains upon his limbs! what perils he encountered in his endeavors to escape from his horrible doom! and how signal have been his deliverance and preservation in the midst of a nation of pitiless enemies!

This Narrative contains many affecting incidents, many passages of great eloquence and power; but I think the most thrilling one of them all is the description DOUGLASS gives of his feelings, as he stood soliloquizing respecting his fate, and the chances of his one day being a freeman, on the banks of the Chesapeake Bay—viewing the receding vessels as they flew with their white wings before the breeze, and apostrophizing them as animated by the living spirit of freedom. Who can read that passage, and be insensible to its pathos and sublimity? Compressed into it is a whole Alexandrian library of thought, feeling, and sentiment—all that can, all that need be urged, in the form of expostulation, entreaty, rebuke, against that crime of crimes,—making man the property of his fellow-man! O, how accursed is that system, which entombs the godlike mind of man, defaces the divine image, reduces those who by creation were crowned with glory and honor to a level with four-footed beasts, and exalts the dealer in human flesh above all that is called God! Why should its existence be prolonged one hour? Is it not evil, only evil, and that continually? What does its presence imply but the absence of all fear of God, all regard for man, on the part of the people of the United States? Heaven speed its eternal overthrow!

So profoundly ignorant of the nature of slavery are many persons, that they are stubbornly incredulous whenever they read or listen to any recital of the cruelties which are daily inflicted on its victims. They do not deny that the slaves are held as property; but that terrible fact seems to convey to their minds no idea of injustice, exposure to outrage, or savage barbarity. Tell them of cruel scourgings, of mutilations and brandings, of scenes of pollution and blood, of the banishment of all light and knowledge, and they affect to be greatly indignant at such enormous exaggerations, such wholesale misstatements, such abominable libels on the character of the southern planters! As if all these direful outrages were not the natural results of slavery! As if it were less cruel to reduce a human being to the condition of a thing, than to give him a severe flagellation, or to deprive him of necessary food and clothing! As if whips, chains, thumb-screws, paddles, bloodhounds, overseers, drivers, patrols, were not all indispensable to keep the slaves down, and to give protection to their ruthless oppressors! As if, when the marriage institution is abolished, concubinage, adultery, and incest, must not necessarily abound; when all the rights of humanity are annihilated, any barrier remains to protect the victim from the fury of the spoiler; when absolute power is assumed over life and liberty, it will not be wielded with destructive sway! Skeptics of this character abound in society. In some few instances, their incredulity arises from a want of reflection; but, generally, it indicates a hatred of the light, a desire to shield slavery from the assaults of its foes, a contempt of the colored race, whether bond or free. Such will try to discredit the shocking tales of slaveholding cruelty which are recorded in this truthful Narrative; but they will labor in vain. Mr. DOUGLASS has frankly disclosed the place of his birth, the names of those who claimed ownership in his body and soul, and the names also of those who committed the crimes which he has alleged against them. His statements, therefore, may easily be disproved, if they are untrue.

In the course of his Narrative, he relates two instances of murderous cruelty,—in one of which a planter deliberately shot a slave belonging to a neighboring plantation, who had unintentionally gotten within his lordly domain in quest of fish; and in the other, an overseer blew out the brains of a slave who had fled to a stream of water to escape a bloody scourging. Mr. DOUGLASS states that in neither of these instances was any thing done by way of legal arrest or judicial investigation. The Baltimore American, of March 17, 1845, relates a similar case of atrocity, perpetrated with similar impunity—as follows:—"*Shooting a Slave.*—We learn, upon the authority of a letter from Charles county, Maryland, received by a gentleman of this city, that a young man, named

Matthews, a nephew of General Matthews, and whose father, it is believed, holds an office at Washington, killed one of the slaves upon his father's farm by shooting him. The letter states that young Matthews had been left in charge of the farm; that he gave an order to the servant, which was disobeyed, when he proceeded to the house, *obtained a gun, and, returning, shot the servant.* He immediately, the letter continues, fled to his father's residence, where he still remains unmolested."—Let it never be forgotten, that no slaveholder or overseer can be convicted of any outrage perpetrated on the person of a slave, however diabolical it may be, on the testimony of colored witnesses, whether bond or free. By the slave code, they are adjudged to be as incompetent to testify against a white man, as though they were indeed a part of the brute creation. Hence, there is no legal protection in fact, whatever there may be in form, for the slave population; and any amount of cruelty may be inflicted on them with impunity. Is it possible for the human mind to conceive of a more horrible state of society?

The effect of a religious profession on the conduct of southern masters is vividly described in the following Narrative, and shown to be any thing but salutary. In the nature of the case, it must be in the highest degree pernicious. The testimony of Mr. DOUGLASS, on this point, is sustained by a cloud of witnesses, whose veracity is unimpeachable. "A slaveholder's profession of Christianity is a palpable imposture. He is a felon of the highest grade. He is a man-stealer. It is of no importance what you put in the other scale."

Reader! are you with the man-stealers in sympathy and purpose, or on the side of their down-trodden victims? If with the former, then are you the foe of God and man. If with the latter, what are you prepared to do and dare in their behalf? Be faithful, be vigilant, be untiring in your efforts to break every yoke, and let the oppressed go free. Come what may—cost what it may—inscribe on the banner which you unfurl to the breeze, as your religious and political motto—"No COMPROMISE WITH SLAVERY! NO UNION WITH SLAVEHOLDERS!"

WM. LLOYD GARRISON.

BOSTON, *May 1, 1845.*

LETTER
FROM WENDELL PHILLIPS, ESQ.

BOSTON, *April 22, 1845.*

My Dear Friend:

YOU remember the old fable of "The Man and the Lion," where the lion complained that he should not be so misrepresented "when the lions wrote history."

I am glad the time has come when the "lions write history." We have been left long enough to gather the character of slavery from the involuntary evidence of the masters. One might, indeed, rest sufficiently satisfied with what, it is evident, must be, in general, the results of such a relation, without seeking farther to find whether they have followed in every instance. Indeed, those who stare at the half-peck of corn a week, and love to count the lashes on the slave's back, are seldom the "stuff" out of which reformers and abolitionists are to be made. I remember that, in 1838, many were waiting for the results of the West India experiment, before they could come into our ranks. Those "results" have come long ago; but, alas! few of that number have come with them, as converts. A man must be disposed to judge of emancipation by other tests than whether it has increased the produce of sugar,—and to hate slavery for other reasons than because it starves men and whips women,—before he is ready to lay the first stone of his anti-slavery life.

I was glad to learn, in your story, how early the most neglected of God's children waken to a sense of their rights, and of the injustice done them. Experience is a keen teacher; and long before you had mastered your A B C, or knew where the "white sails" of the Chesapeake were bound, you began, I see, to gauge the wretchedness of the slave, not by his hunger and want, not by his lashes and toil, but by the cruel and blighting death which gathers over his soul.

In connection with this, there is one circumstance which makes your recollections peculiarly valuable, and renders your early insight the more remarkable. You come from that part of the country where we are told slavery appears with its fairest features. Let us hear, then, what it is at its best estate—gaze on its bright side, if it has one; and then imagination may task her powers to add dark lines to the picture, as she travels southward to that (for the colored man) Valley of the Shadow of Death, where the Mississippi sweeps along.

Again, we have known you long, and can put the most entire confidence in your truth, candor, and sincerity. Every one who has heard you speak has felt, and, I am confident, every one who reads your book will feel, persuaded that you give them a fair specimen of the whole truth. No one-sided portrait,—no wholesale complaints,—but strict justice done, whenever individual kindliness has neutralized, for a moment, the deadly system with which it was strangely allied. You have been with us, too, some years, and can fairly compare the twilight of rights, which your race enjoy at the North, with that "noon of night" under which they labor south of Mason and Dixon's line. Tell us whether, after all, the half-free colored man of Massachusetts is worse off than the pampered slave of the rice swamps!

In reading your life, no one can say that we have unfairly picked out some rare specimens of cruelty. We know that the bitter drops, which even you have drained from the cup, are no incidental aggravations, no individual ills, but such as must mingle always and necessarily in the lot of every slave. They are the essential ingredients, not the occasional results, of the system.

After all, I shall read your book with trembling for you. Some years ago, when you were beginning to tell me your real name and birthplace, you may remember I stopped you, and preferred to remain ignorant of all. With the exception of a vague description, so I continued, till the other day, when you read me your memoirs. I hardly knew, at the time, whether to thank you or not for the sight of them, when I reflected that it was still dangerous, in Massachusetts, for honest men to tell their names! They say the fathers, in 1776, signed the Declaration of Independence with the halter about their necks. You, too, publish your declaration of freedom with danger compassing you around. In all the broad lands which the Constitution of the United States overshadows, there is no single spot,—however narrow or desolate,—

where a fugitive slave can plant himself and say, "I am safe." The whole armory of Northern Law has no shield for you. I am free to say that, in your place, I should throw the MS. into the fire.

You, perhaps, may tell your story in safety, endeared as you are to so many warm hearts by rare gifts, and a still rarer devotion of them to the service of others. But it will be owing only to your labors, and the fearless efforts of those who, trampling the laws and Constitution of the country under their feet, are determined that they will "hide the outcast," and that their hearths shall be, spite of the law, an asylum for the oppressed, if, some time or other, the humblest may stand in our streets, and bear witness in safety against the cruelties of which he has been the victim.

Yet it is sad to think, that these very throbbing hearts which welcome your story, and form your best safeguard in telling it, are all beating contrary to the "statute in such case made and provided." Go on, my dear friend, till you, and those who, like you, have been saved, so as by fire, from the dark prison-house, shall stereotype these free, illegal pulses into statutes; and New England, cutting loose from a blood-stained Union, shall glory in being the house of refuge for the oppressed;—till we no longer merely "*hide* the outcast," or make a merit of standing idly by while he is hunted in our midst; but, consecrating anew the soil of the Pilgrims as an asylum for the oppressed, proclaim our *welcome* to the slave so loudly, that the tones shall reach every hut in the Carolinas, and make the broken-hearted bondman leap up at the thought of old Massachusetts.

God speed the day!

Till then, and ever,

Yours truly

WENDELL PHILLIPS.

FREDERICK DOUGLASS.

NARRATIVE

OF THE

LIFE OF FREDERICK DOUGLASS.

CHAPTER I.

I WAS born in Tuckahoe, near Hillsborough, and about twelve miles from Easton, in Talbot county, Maryland. I have no accurate knowledge of my age, never having seen any authentic record containing it. By far the larger part of the slaves know as little of their ages as horses know of theirs, and it is the wish of most masters within my knowledge to keep their slaves thus ignorant. I do not remember to have ever met a slave who could tell of his birthday. They seldom come nearer to it than planting-time, harvest-time, cherry-time, spring-time, or fall-time. A want of information concerning my own was a source of unhappiness to me even during childhood. The white children could tell their ages. I could not tell why I ought to be deprived of the same privilege. I was not allowed to make any inquiries of my master concerning it. He deemed all such inquiries on the part of a slave improper and impertinent, and evidence of a restless spirit. The nearest estimate I can give makes me now between twenty-seven and twenty-eight years of age. I come to this, from hearing my master say, some time during 1835, I was about seventeen years old.

My mother was named Harriet Bailey. She was the daughter of Isaac and Betsey Bailey, both colored, and quite dark. My mother was of a darker complexion than either my grandmother or grandfather.

My father was a white man. He was admitted to be such by all I ever heard speak of my parentage. The opinion was also whispered that my master was my father; but of the correctness of this opinion, I know nothing; the means of knowing was withheld from me. My mother and I were separated when I was but an infant—before I knew her as my mother. It is a common custom, in the part of Maryland from which I ran away, to part children from their mothers at a very early age. Frequently, before the child has reached its twelfth month, its mother is taken from it, and hired out on some farm a considerable distance off, and the child is placed under the care of an old woman, too old for field labor. For what this separation is done, I do not know, unless it be to hinder the development of the child's affection toward its mother, and to blunt and destroy the natural affection of the mother for the child. This is the inevitable result.

I never saw my mother, to know her as such, more than four or five times in my life; and each of these times was very short in duration, and at night. She was hired by a Mr. Stewart, who lived about twelve miles from my home. She made her journeys to see me in the night, travelling the whole distance on foot, after the performance of her day's work. She was a field hand, and a whipping is the penalty of not being in the field at sunrise, unless a slave has special permission from his or her master to the contrary—a permission which they seldom get, and one that gives to him that gives it the proud name of being a kind master. I do not recollect of ever seeing my mother by the light of day. She was with me in the night. She would lie down with me, and get me to sleep, but long before I waked she was gone. Very little communication ever took place between us. Death soon ended what little we could have while she lived, and with it her hardships and suffering. She died when I was about seven years old, on one of my master's farms, near Lee's Mill. I was not allowed to be present during her illness, at her death, or burial. She was gone long before I knew any thing about it. Never having enjoyed, to any considerable extent, her soothing presence, her tender and watchful care, I received the tidings of her death with much the same emotions I should have probably felt at the death of a stranger.

Called thus suddenly away, she left me without the slightest intimation of who my father was. The whisper that my master was my father, may or may not be true; and, true or false, it is of but little consequence to my purpose whilst the fact remains, in all its glaring odiousness, that slaveholders have ordained, and by law established, that the children of slave women shall in all cases follow the condition of their mothers; and this is done too obviously to administer to their own lusts, and make a gratification of their wicked desires profitable as well as pleasurable; for by this cunning arrangement, the slaveholder, in cases not a few, sustains to his slaves the double relation of master and father.

I know of such cases; and it is worthy of remark that such slaves invariably suffer greater hardships, and have more to contend with, than others. They are, in the first place, a constant offence to their mistress. She is ever disposed to find fault with them; they can seldom do any thing to please her; she is never better pleased than when she sees them under the lash, especially when she suspects her husband of showing to his mulatto children favors which he withholds from his black slaves. The master is frequently compelled to sell this class of his slaves, out of deference to the feelings of his white wife; and, cruel as the deed may strike any one to be, for a man to sell his own children to human flesh-mongers, it is often the dictate of humanity for him to do so; for, unless he does this, he must not only whip them himself, but must stand by and see one white son tie up his brother, of but few shades darker complexion than himself, and ply the gory lash to his naked back; and if he lisp one word of disapproval, it is set down to his parental partiality, and only makes a bad matter worse, both for himself and the slave whom he would protect and defend.

Every year brings with it multitudes of this class of slaves. It was doubtless in consequence of a knowledge of this fact, that one great statesman of the south predicted the downfall of slavery by the inevitable laws of population. Whether this prophecy is ever fulfilled or not, it is nevertheless plain that a very different-looking class of people are springing up at the south, and are now held in slavery, from those originally brought to this country from Africa; and if their increase will do no other good, it will do away the force of the argument, that God cursed Ham, and therefore American slavery is right. If the lineal descendants of Ham are alone to be scripturally enslaved, it is certain that slavery at the south must soon become unscriptural; for thousands are ushered into the world, annually, who, like myself, owe their existence to white fathers, and those fathers most frequently their own masters.

I have had two masters. My first master's name was Anthony. I do not remember his first name. He was generally called Captain Anthony—a title which, I presume, he acquired by sailing a craft on the Chesapeake Bay. He was not considered a rich slaveholder. He owned two or three farms, and about thirty slaves. His farms and slaves were under the care of an overseer. The overseer's name was Plummer. Mr. Plummer was a miserable drunkard, a profane swearer, and a savage monster. He always went armed with a cowskin and a heavy cudgel. I have known him to cut and slash the women's heads so horribly, that even master would be enraged at his cruelty, and would threaten to whip him if he did not mind himself. Master, however, was not a humane slaveholder. It required extraordinary barbarity on the part of an overseer to affect him. He was a cruel man, hardened by a long life of slaveholding. He would at times seem to take great pleasure in whipping a slave. I have often been awakened at the dawn of day by the most heart-rending shrieks of an own aunt of mine, whom he used to tie up to a joist, and whip upon her naked back till she was literally covered with blood. No words, no tears, no prayers, from his gory victim, seemed to move his iron heart from its bloody purpose. The louder she screamed, the harder he whipped; and where the blood ran fastest, there he whipped longest. He would whip her to make her scream, and whip her to make her hush; and not until overcome by fatigue, would he cease to swing the blood-clotted cowskin. I remember the first time I ever witnessed this horrible exhibition. I was quite a child, but I well remember it. I never shall forget it whilst I remember any thing. It was the first of a long series of such outrages, of which I was doomed to be a witness and a participant. It struck me with awful force. It was the blood-stained gate, the entrance to the hell of slavery, through which I was about to pass. It was a most terrible spectacle. I wish I could commit to paper the feelings with which I beheld it.

This occurrence took place very soon after I went to live with my old master, and under the following circumstances.

Aunt Hester went out one night,—where or for what I do not know,—and happened to be absent when my master desired her presence. He had ordered her not to go out evenings, and warned her that she must never let him catch her in company with a young man, who was paying attention to her, belonging to Colonel Lloyd. The young man's name was Ned Roberts, generally called Lloyd's Ned. Why master was so careful of her, may be safely left to conjecture. She was a woman of noble form, and of graceful proportions, having very few equals, and fewer superiors, in personal appearance, among the colored or white women of our neighborhood.

Aunt Hester had not only disobeyed his orders in going out, but had been found in company with Lloyd's Ned; which circumstance, I found, from what he said while whipping her, was the chief offence. Had he been a man of pure morals himself, he might have been thought interested in protecting the innocence of my aunt; but those who knew him will not suspect him of any such virtue. Before he commenced whipping Aunt Hester, he took her into the kitchen, and stripped her from neck to waist, leaving her neck, shoulders, and back, entirely naked. He then told her to cross her hands, calling her at the same time a d——d b——h. After crossing her hands, he tied them with a strong rope, and led her to a stool under a large hook in the joist, put in for the purpose. He made her get upon the stool, and tied her hands to the hook. She now stood fair for his infernal purpose. Her arms were stretched up at their full length, so that she stood upon the ends of her toes. He then said to her, "Now, you d——d b——h, I'll learn you how to disobey my orders!" and after rolling up his sleeves, he commenced to lay on the heavy cowskin, and soon the warm, red blood (amid heart-rending shrieks from her, and horrid oaths from him) came dripping to the floor. I was so terrified and horror-stricken at the sight, that I hid myself in a closet, and dared not venture out till long after the bloody transaction was over. I expected it would be my turn next. It was all new to me. I had never seen any thing like it before. I had always lived with my grandmother on the outskirts of the plantation, where she was put to raise the children of the younger women. I had therefore been, until now, out of the way of the bloody scenes that often occurred on the plantation.

CHAPTER II.

My master's family consisted of two sons, Andrew and Richard; one daughter, Lucretia, and her husband, Captain Thomas Auld. They lived in one house, upon the home plantation of Colonel Edward Lloyd. My master was Colonel Lloyd's clerk and superintendent. He was what might be called the overseer of the overseers. I spent two years of childhood on this plantation in my old master's family. It was here that I witnessed the bloody transaction recorded in the first chapter; and as I received my first impressions of slavery on this plantation, I will give some description of it, and of slavery as it there existed. The plantation is about twelve miles north of Easton, in Talbot county, and is situated on the border of Miles River. The principal products raised upon it were tobacco, corn, and wheat. These were raised in great abundance; so that, with the products of this and the other farms belonging to him, he was able to keep in almost constant employment a large sloop, in carrying them to market at Baltimore. This sloop was named Sally Lloyd, in honor of one of the colonel's daughters. My master's son-in-law, Captain Auld, was master of the vessel; she was otherwise manned by the colonel's own slaves. Their names were Peter, Isaac, Rich, and Jake. These were esteemed very highly by the other slaves, and looked upon as the privileged ones of the plantation; for it was no small affair, in the eyes of the slaves, to be allowed to see Baltimore.

Colonel Lloyd kept from three to four hundred slaves on his home plantation, and owned a large number more on the neighboring farms belonging to him. The names of the farms nearest to the home plantation were Wye Town and New Design. "Wye Town" was under the overseership of a man named Noah Willis. New Design was under the overseership of a Mr. Townsend. The overseers of these, and all the rest of the farms, numbering over twenty, received advice and direction from the managers of the home plantation. This was the great business place. It was the seat of government for the whole twenty farms. All disputes among the overseers were settled here. If a slave was convicted of any high misdemeanor, became unmanageable, or evinced a determination to run away, he was brought immediately here, severely whipped, put on board the sloop, carried to Baltimore, and sold to Austin Woolfolk, or some other slave-trader, as a warning to the slaves remaining.

Here, too, the slaves of all the other farms received their monthly allowance of food, and their yearly clothing. The men and women slaves received, as their monthly allowance of food, eight pounds of pork, or its equivalent in fish, and one bushel of corn meal. Their yearly clothing consisted of two coarse linen shirts, one pair of linen trousers, like the shirts, one jacket, one pair of trousers for winter, made of coarse negro cloth, one pair of stockings, and one pair of shoes; the whole of which could not have cost more than seven dollars. The allowance of the slave children was given to their mothers, or the old women having the care of them. The children unable to work in the field had neither shoes, stockings, jackets, nor trousers, given to them; their clothing consisted of two coarse linen shirts per year. When these failed them, they went naked until the next allowance-day. Children from seven to ten years old, of both sexes, almost naked, might be seen at all seasons of the year.

There were no beds given the slaves, unless one coarse blanket be considered such, and none but the men and women had these. This, however, is not considered a very great privation. They find less difficulty from the want of beds, than from the want of time to sleep; for when their day's work in the field is done, the most of them having their washing, mending, and cooking to do, and having few or none of the ordinary facilities for doing either of these, very many of their sleeping hours are consumed in preparing for the field the coming day; and when this is done, old and young, male and female, married and single, drop down side by side, on one common bed,—the cold, damp floor,—each covering himself or herself with their miserable blankets; and here they sleep till they are summoned to the field by the driver's horn. At the sound of this, all must rise, and be off to the field. There must be no halting; every one must be at his or her post; and woe betides them who hear not this morning summons to the field; for if they are not awakened by the sense of hearing, they are by the sense of feeling: no age nor sex finds any favor. Mr. Severe, the overseer, used to stand by the door of the quarter, armed with a large hickory stick and heavy cowskin, ready to whip any one who was so unfortunate as not to hear, or, from any other cause, was prevented from being ready to start for the field at the sound of the horn.

Mr. Severe was rightly named: he was a cruel man. I have seen him whip a woman, causing the blood to run half an hour at the time; and this, too, in the midst of her crying children, pleading for their mother's release. He seemed to take pleasure in manifesting his fiendish barbarity. Added to his cruelty, he was a profane swearer. It was enough to chill the blood and stiffen the hair of an ordinary man to hear him talk. Scarce a sentence escaped him but that was commenced or concluded by some horrid oath. The field was the place to witness his cruelty and profanity. His presence made it both the field of blood and of blasphemy. From the rising till the going down of the sun, he was cursing, raving, cutting, and slashing among the slaves of the field, in the most frightful manner. His career was short. He died very soon after I went to Colonel Lloyd's; and he died as he lived, uttering, with his dying groans, bitter curses and horrid oaths. His death was regarded by the slaves as the result of a merciful providence.

Mr. Severe's place was filled by a Mr. Hopkins. He was a very different man. He was less cruel, less profane, and made less noise, than Mr. Severe. His course was characterized by no extraordinary demonstrations of cruelty. He whipped, but seemed to take no pleasure in it. He was called by the slaves a good overseer.

The home plantation of Colonel Lloyd wore the appearance of a country village. All the mechanical operations for all the farms were performed here. The shoemaking and mending, the blacksmithing, cartwrighting, coopering, weaving, and grain-grinding, were all performed by the slaves on the home plantation. The whole place wore a business-like aspect very unlike the neighboring farms. The number of houses, too, conspired to give it advantage over the neighboring farms. It was called by the slaves the *Great House Farm*. Few privileges were esteemed higher, by the slaves of the out-farms, than that of being selected to do errands at the Great House Farm. It was associated in their minds with greatness. A representative could not be prouder of his election to a seat in the American Congress, than a slave on one of the out-farms would be of his election to do errands at the Great House Farm. They regarded it as evidence of great confidence reposed in them by their overseers; and it was on this account, as well as a constant desire to be out of the field from under the driver's lash, that they esteemed it a high privilege, one worth careful living for. He was called the smartest and most trusty fellow, who had this honor conferred upon him the most frequently. The competitors for this office sought as diligently to please their overseers, as the office-seekers in the political parties seek to please and deceive the people. The same traits of character might be seen in Colonel Lloyd's slaves, as are seen in the slaves of the political parties.

The slaves selected to go to the Great House Farm, for the monthly allowance for themselves and their fellow-slaves, were peculiarly enthusiastic. While on their way, they would make the dense old woods, for miles around, reverberate with their wild songs, revealing at once the highest joy and the deepest sadness. They would compose and sing as they went along, consulting neither time nor tune. The thought that came up, came out—if not in the word, in the sound;—and as frequently in the one as in the other. They would some-times sing the most pathetic sentiment in the most rapturous tone, and the most rapturous sentiment in the most pathetic tone. Into all of their songs they would manage to weave something of the Great House Farm. Especially would they do this, when leaving home. They would then sing most ex-ultingly the following words:—

> "I am going away to the Great House Farm!
> O, yea! O, yea! O!"

This they would sing, as a chorus, to words which to many would seem unmeaning jargon, but which, nevertheless, were full of meaning to themselves. I have sometimes thought that the mere hearing of those songs would do more to impress some minds with the horrible character of slavery, than the reading of whole volumes of philosophy on the subject could do.

I did not, when a slave, understand the deep meaning of those rude and apparently incoherent songs. I was myself within the circle; so that I neither saw nor heard as those without might see and hear. They told a tale of woe which was then altogether beyond my feeble comprehension; they were tones loud, long, and deep; they breathed the prayer and complaint of souls boiling over with the bitterest anguish. Every tone was a testimony against slavery, and a prayer to God for deliverance from chains. The hearing of those wild notes always depressed my spirit, and filled me with ineffable sadness. I have frequently found myself in tears while hearing them. The mere recurrence to those songs, even now, afflicts me; and while I am writing these lines, an expression of feeling has already found its way down my cheek. To those songs I trace my first glimmering conception of the dehumanizing character of slavery. I can never get rid of that conception. Those songs still follow me, to deepen my hatred of slavery, and quicken my sympathies for my brethren in bonds. If any one wishes to be impressed with the soul-killing effects of slavery, let him go to Colonel Lloyd's plantation, and, on allowance-day, place himself in the deep pine woods, and there let him, in silence, analyze the sounds that shall pass through the chambers of his soul,—and if he is not thus impressed, it will only be because "there is no flesh in his obdurate heart."

I have often been utterly astonished, since I came to the north, to find persons who could speak of the singing, among slaves, as evidence of their contentment and happiness. It is impossible to conceive of a greater mistake. Slaves sing most when they are most unhappy. The songs of the slave represent the sorrows of his heart; and he is relieved by them, only as an aching heart is relieved by its tears. At least, such is my experience. I have often sung to drown my sorrow, but seldom to express my happiness. Crying for joy, and singing for joy, were alike uncommon to me while in the jaws of slavery. The singing of a man cast away upon a desolate island might be as appropriately considered as evidence of contentment and happiness, as the singing of a slave; the songs of the one and of the other are prompted by the same emotion.

CHAPTER III.

COLONEL LLOYD kept a large and finely cultivated garden, which afforded almost constant employment for four men, besides the chief gardener, (Mr. M'Durmond.) This garden was probably the greatest attraction of the place. During the summer months, people came from far and near—from Baltimore, Easton, and Annapolis—to see it. It abounded in fruits of almost every description, from the hardy apple of the north to the delicate orange of the south. This garden was not the least source of trouble on the plantation. Its excellent fruit was quite a temptation to the hungry swarms of boys, as well as the older slaves, belonging to the colonel, few of whom had the virtue or the vice to resist it. Scarcely a day passed, during the summer, but that some slave had to take the lash for stealing fruit. The colonel had to resort to all kinds of stratagems to keep his slaves out of the garden. The last and most successful one was that of tarring his fence all around; after which, if a slave was caught with any tar upon his person, it was deemed sufficient proof that he had either been into the garden, or had tried to get in. In either case, he was severely whipped by the chief gardener. This plan worked well; the slaves became as fearful of tar as of the lash. They seemed to realize the impossibility of touching *tar* without being defiled.

The colonel also kept a splendid riding equipage. His stable and carriage-house presented the appearance of some of our large city livery establishments. His horses were of the finest form and noblest blood. His carriage-house contained three splendid coaches, three or four gigs, besides dearborns and barouches of the most fashionable style.

This establishment was under the care of two slaves—old Barney and young Barney—father and son. To attend to this establishment was their sole work. But it was by no means an easy employment; for in nothing was Colonel Lloyd more particular than in the management of his horses. The slightest inattention to these was unpardonable, and was visited upon those, under whose care they were placed, with the severest punishment; no excuse could shield them, if the colonel only suspected any want of attention to his horses—a supposition which he frequently indulged, and one which, of course, made the office of old and young Barney a very trying one. They never knew when they were safe from punishment. They were frequently whipped when least deserving, and escaped whipping when most deserving it. Every thing depended upon the looks of the horses, and the state of Colonel Lloyd's own mind when his horses were brought to him for use. If a horse did not move fast enough, or hold his head high enough, it was owing to some fault of his keepers. It was painful to stand near the stable-door, and hear the various complaints against the keepers when a horse was taken out for use. "This horse has not had proper attention. He has not been sufficiently rubbed and curried, or he has not been properly fed; his food was too wet or too dry; he got it too soon or too late; he was too hot or too cold; he had too much hay, and not enough of grain; or he had too much grain, and not enough of hay; instead of old Barney's attending to the horse, he had very improperly left it to his son." To all these complaints, no matter how unjust, the slave must answer never a word. Colonel Lloyd could not brook any contradiction from a slave. When he spoke, a slave must stand, listen, and tremble; and such was literally the case. I have seen Colonel Lloyd make old Barney, a man between fifty and sixty years of age, uncover his bald head, kneel down upon the cold, damp ground, and receive upon his naked and toil-worn shoulders more than thirty lashes at the time. Colonel Lloyd had three sons—Edward, Murray, and Daniel,—and three sons-in-law, Mr. Winder, Mr. Nicholson, and Mr. Lowndes. All of these lived at the Great House Farm, and enjoyed the luxury of whipping the servants when they pleased, from old Barney down to William Wilkes, the coach-driver. I have seen

Winder make one of the house-servants stand off from him a suitable distance to be touched with the end of his whip, and at every stroke raise great ridges upon his back.

To describe the wealth of Colonel Lloyd would be almost equal to describing the riches of Job. He kept from ten to fifteen house-servants. He was said to own a thousand slaves, and I think this estimate quite within the truth. Colonel Lloyd owned so many that he did not know them when he saw them; nor did all the slaves of the out-farms know him. It is reported of him, that, while riding along the road one day, he met a colored man, and addressed him in the usual manner of speaking to colored people on the public highways of the south: "Well, boy, whom do you belong to?" "To Colonel Lloyd," replied the slave. "Well, does the colonel treat you well?" "No, sir," was the ready reply. "What, does he work you too hard?" "Yes, sir." "Well, don't he give you enough to eat?" "Yes, sir, he gives me enough, such as it is."

The colonel, after ascertaining where the slave belonged, rode on; the man also went on about his business, not dreaming that he had been conversing with his master. He thought, said, and heard nothing more of the matter, until two or three weeks afterwards. The poor man was then informed by his overseer that, for having found fault with his master, he was now to be sold to a Georgia trader. He was immediately chained and handcuffed; and thus, without a moment's warning, he was snatched away, and forever sundered, from his family and friends, by a hand more unrelenting than death. This is the penalty of telling the truth, of telling the simple truth, in answer to a series of plain questions.

It is partly in consequence of such facts, that slaves, when inquired of as to their condition and the character of their masters, almost universally say they are contented, and that their masters are kind. The slaveholders have been known to send in spies among their slaves, to ascertain their views and feelings in regard to their condition. The frequency of this has had the effect to establish among the slaves the maxim, that a still tongue makes a wise head. They suppress the truth rather than take the consequences of telling it, and in so doing prove themselves a part of the human family. If they have any thing to say of their masters, it is generally in their masters' favor, especially when speaking to an untried man. I have been frequently asked, when a slave, if I had a kind master, and do not remember ever to have given a negative answer; nor did I, in pursuing this course, consider myself as uttering what was absolutely false; for I always measured the kindness of my master by the standard of kindness set up among slaveholders around us. Moreover, slaves are like other people, and imbibe prejudices quite common to others. They think their own better than that of others. Many, under the influence of this prejudice, think their own masters are better than the masters of other slaves; and this, too, in some cases, when the very reverse is true. Indeed, it is not uncommon for slaves even to fall out and quarrel among themselves about the relative goodness of their masters, each contending for the superior goodness of his own over that of the others. At the very same time, they mutually execrate their masters when viewed separately. It was so on our plantation. When Colonel Lloyd's slaves met the slaves of Jacob Jepson, they seldom parted without a quarrel about their masters; Colonel Lloyd's slaves contending that he was the richest, and Mr. Jepson's slaves that he was the smartest, and most of a man. Colonel Lloyd's slaves would boast his ability to buy and sell Jacob Jepson. Mr. Jepson's slaves would boast his ability to whip Colonel Lloyd. These quarrels would almost always end in a fight between the parties, and those that whipped were supposed to have gained the point at issue. They seemed to think that the greatness of their masters was transferable to themselves. It was considered as being bad enough to be a slave; but to be a poor man's slave was deemed a disgrace indeed!

CHAPTER IV.

MR. HOPKINS remained but a short time in the office of overseer. Why his career was so short, I do not know, but suppose he lacked the necessary severity to suit Colonel Lloyd. Mr. Hopkins was succeeded by Mr. Austin Gore, a man possessing, in an eminent degree, all those traits of character indispensable to what is called a first-rate overseer. Mr. Gore had served Colonel Lloyd, in the capacity of overseer, upon one of the out-farms, and had shown himself worthy of the high station of overseer upon the home or Great House Farm.

Mr. Gore was proud, ambitious, and persevering. He was artful, cruel, and obdurate. He was just the man for such a place, and it was just the place for such a man. It afforded scope for the full exercise of all his powers, and he seemed to be perfectly at home in it. He was one of those who could torture the slightest look, word, or gesture, on the part of the slave, into impudence, and would treat it accordingly. There must be no answering back to him; no explanation was allowed a slave, showing himself to have been wrongfully accused. Mr. Gore acted fully up to the maxim laid down by slaveholders,—"It is better that a dozen slaves suffer under the lash, than that the overseer should be convicted, in the presence of the slaves, of having been at fault." No matter how innocent a slave might be—it availed him nothing, when accused by Mr. Gore of any misdemeanor. To be accused was to be convicted, and to be convicted was to be punished; the one always following the other with immutable certainty. To escape punishment was to escape accusation; and few slaves had the fortune to do either, under the overseership of Mr. Gore. He was just proud enough to demand the most debasing homage of the slave, and quite servile enough to crouch, himself, at the feet of the master. He was ambitious enough to be contented with nothing short of the highest rank of overseers, and persevering enough to reach the height of his ambition. He was cruel enough to inflict the severest punishment, artful enough to descend to the lowest trickery, and obdurate enough to be insensible to the voice of a reproving conscience. He was, of all the overseers, the most dreaded by the slaves. His presence was painful; his eye flashed confusion; and seldom was his sharp, shrill voice heard, without producing horror and trembling in their ranks.

Mr. Gore was a grave man, and, though a young man, he indulged in no jokes, said no funny words, seldom smiled. His words were in perfect keeping with his looks, and his looks were in perfect keeping with his words. Overseers will sometimes indulge in a witty word, even with the slaves; not so with Mr. Gore. He spoke but to command, and commanded but to be obeyed; he dealt sparingly with his words, and bountifully with his whip, never using the former where the latter would answer as well. When he whipped, he seemed to do so from a sense of duty, and feared no consequences. He did nothing reluctantly, no matter how disagreeable; always at his post, never inconsistent. He never promised but to fulfil. He was, in a word, a man of the most inflexible firmness and stone-like coolness.

His savage barbarity was equalled only by the consummate coolness with which he committed the grossest and most savage deeds upon the slaves under his charge. Mr. Gore once undertook to whip one of Colonel Lloyd's slaves, by the name of Demby. He had given Demby but few stripes, when, to get rid of the scourging, he ran and plunged himself into a creek, and stood there at the depth of his shoulders, refusing to come out. Mr. Gore told him that he would give him three calls, and that, if he did not come out at the third call, he would shoot him. The first call was given. Demby made no response, but stood his ground. The second and third calls were given with the same result. Mr. Gore then, without consultation or deliberation with any one, not even giving Demby an additional call, raised his musket to his face, taking deadly aim at his standing victim, and in an instant poor Demby was no more. His mangled body sank out of sight, and blood and brains marked the water where he had stood.

A thrill of horror flashed through every soul upon the plantation, excepting Mr. Gore. He alone seemed cool and collected. He was asked by Colonel Lloyd and my old master, why he resorted to this extraordinary expedient. His reply was, (as well as I can remember,) that Demby had become unmanageable. He was setting a dangerous example to the other slaves,—one which, if suffered to pass without some such demonstration on his part, would finally lead to the total subversion of all rule and order upon the plantation. He argued that if one slave refused to be corrected, and escaped with his life, the other slaves would soon copy the example; the result of which would be, the freedom of the slaves, and the enslavement of the whites. Mr. Gore's defence was satisfactory. He was continued in his station as overseer upon the home plantation. His fame as an overseer went abroad. His horrid crime was not even submitted to judicial investigation. It was committed in the presence of slaves, and they of course could neither institute a suit, nor testify against him; and thus the guilty perpetrator of one of the bloodiest and most foul murders goes unwhipped of justice, and uncensured by the community in which he lives. Mr. Gore lived in St. Michael's, Talbot county, Maryland, when I left there; and if he is still alive, he very probably lives there now; and if so, he is now, as he was then, as highly esteemed and as much respected as though his guilty soul had not been stained with his brother's blood.

I speak advisedly when I say this,—that killing a slave, or any colored person, in Talbot county, Maryland, is not treated as a crime, either by the courts or the community. Mr. Thomas Lanman, of St. Michael's, killed two slaves, one of whom he killed with a hatchet, by knocking his brains out. He used to boast of the commission of the awful and bloody deed. I have heard him do so laughingly, saying, among other things, that he was the only benefactor of his country in the company, and that when others would do as much as he had done, we should be relieved of "the d——d niggers."

The wife of Mr. Giles Hick, living but a short distance from where I used to live, murdered my wife's cousin, a young girl between fifteen and sixteen years of age, mangling her person in the most horrible manner, breaking her nose and breastbone with a stick, so that the poor girl expired in a few hours afterward. She was immediately buried, but had not been in her untimely grave but a few hours before she was taken up and examined by the coroner, who decided that she had come to her death by severe beating. The offence for which this girl was thus murdered was this:—She had been set that night to mind Mrs. Hick's baby, and during the night she fell asleep, and the baby cried. She, having lost her rest for several nights previous, did not hear the crying. They were both in the room with Mrs. Hicks. Mrs. Hicks, finding the girl slow to move, jumped from her bed, seized an oak stick of wood by the fireplace, and with it broke the girl's nose and breastbone, and thus ended her life. I will not say that this most horrid murder produced no sensation in the community. It did produce sensation, but not enough to bring the murderess to punishment. There was a warrant issued for her arrest, but it was never served. Thus she escaped not only punishment, but even the pain of being arraigned before a court for her horrid crime.

Whilst I am detailing bloody deeds which took place during my stay on Colonel Lloyd's plantation, I will briefly narrate another, which occurred about the same time as the murder of Demby by Mr. Gore.

Colonel Lloyd's slaves were in the habit of spending a part of their nights and Sundays in fishing for oysters, and in this way made up the deficiency of their scanty allowance. An old man belonging to Colonel Lloyd, while thus engaged, happened to get beyond the limits of Colonel Lloyd's, and on the premises of Mr. Beal Bondly. At this trespass, Mr. Bondly took offence, and with his musket came down to the shore, and blew its deadly contents into the poor old man.

Mr. Bondly came over to see Colonel Lloyd the next day, whether to pay him for his property, or to justify himself in what he had done, I know not. At any rate, this whole fiendish transaction was soon hushed up. There was very little said about it at all, and nothing done. It was a common saying, even among little white boys, that it was worth a half-cent to kill a "nigger," and a half-cent to bury one.

CHAPTER V.

As to my own treatment while I lived on Colonel Lloyd's plantation, it was very similar to that of the other slave children. I was not old enough to work in the field, and there being little else than field work to do, I had a great deal of leisure time. The most I had to do was to drive up the cows at evening, keep the fowls out of the garden, keep the front yard clean, and run of errands for my old master's daughter, Mrs. Lucretia Auld. The most of my leisure time I spent in helping Master Daniel Lloyd in finding his birds, after he had shot them. My connection with Master Daniel was of some advantage to me. He became quite attached to me, and was a sort of protector of me. He would not allow the older boys to impose upon me, and would divide his cakes with me.

I was seldom whipped by my old master, and suffered little from any thing else than hunger and cold. I suffered much from hunger, but much more from cold. In hottest summer and coldest winter, I was kept almost naked—no shoes, no stockings, no jacket, no trousers, nothing on but a coarse tow linen shirt, reaching only to my knees. I had no bed. I must have perished with cold, but that, the coldest nights, I used to steal a bag which was used for carrying corn to the mill. I would crawl into this bag, and there sleep on the cold, damp, clay floor, with my head in and feet out. My feet have been so cracked with the frost, that the pen with which I am writing might be laid in the gashes.

We were not regularly allowanced. Our food was coarse corn meal boiled. This was called *mush*. It was put into a large wooden tray or trough, and set down upon the ground. The children were then called, like so many pigs, and like so many pigs they would come and devour the mush; some with oyster-shells, others with pieces of shingle, some with naked hands, and none with spoons. He that ate fastest got most; he that was strongest secured the best place; and few left the trough satisfied.

I was probably between seven and eight years old when I left Colonel Lloyd's plantation. I left it with joy. I shall never forget the ecstasy with which I received the intelligence that my old master (Anthony) had determined to let me go to Baltimore, to live with Mr. Hugh Auld, brother to my old master's son-in-law, Captain Thomas Auld. I received this information about three days before my departure. They were three of the happiest days I ever enjoyed. I spent the most part of all these three days in the creek, washing off the plantation scurf, and preparing myself for my departure.

The pride of appearance which this would indicate was not my own. I spent the time in washing, not so much because I wished to, but because Mrs. Lucretia had told me I must get all the dead skin off my feet and knees before I could go to Baltimore; for the people in Baltimore were very cleanly, and would laugh at me if I looked dirty. Besides, she was going to give me a pair of trousers, which I should not put on unless I got all the dirt off me. The thought of owning a pair of trousers was great indeed! It was almost a sufficient motive, not only to make me take off what would be called by pig-drovers the mange, but the skin itself. I went at it in good earnest, working for the first time with the hope of reward.

The ties that ordinarily bind children to their homes were all suspended in my case. I found no severe trial in my departure. My home was charmless; it was not home to me; on parting from it, I could not feel that I was leaving any thing which I could have enjoyed by staying. My mother was dead, my grandmother lived far off, so that I seldom saw her. I had two sisters and one brother, that lived in the same house with me; but the early separation of us from our mother had well nigh blotted the fact of our relationship from our memories. I looked for home elsewhere, and was confident of finding none which I should relish less than the one which I was leaving. If, however, I found in my new home hardship, hunger, whipping, and nakedness, I had the consolation that I should not have escaped any one of them by staying. Having already had more than a taste of them in the house of my old master, and having endured them there, I very naturally inferred my ability to endure them elsewhere, and especially at Baltimore; for I had something of the feeling about Baltimore that is expressed in the proverb, that "being hanged in England is preferable to dying a natural death in Ireland." I had the strongest desire to see Baltimore. Cousin Tom, though not fluent in speech, had inspired me with that desire by his eloquent description of the place. I could never point out any thing at the Great House, no matter how beautiful or powerful, but that he had seen something at Baltimore far exceeding, both in beauty and strength, the object which I pointed out to him. Even the Great House itself, with all its pictures, was far inferior to many buildings in Baltimore. So strong was my desire, that I thought a gratification of it would fully compensate for whatever loss of comforts I should sustain by the exchange. I left without a regret, and with the highest hopes of future happiness.

We sailed out of Miles River for Baltimore on a Saturday

morning. I remember only the day of the week, for at that time I had no knowledge of the days of the month, nor the months of the year. On setting sail, I walked aft, and gave to Colonel Lloyd's plantation what I hoped would be the last look. I then placed myself in the bows of the sloop, and there spent the remainder of the day in looking ahead, interesting myself in what was in the distance rather than in things near by or behind.

In the afternoon of that day, we reached Annapolis, the capital of the State. We stopped but a few moments, so that I had no time to go on shore. It was the first large town that I had ever seen, and though it would look small compared with some of our New England factory villages, I thought it a wonderful place for its size—more imposing even than the Great House Farm!

We arrived at Baltimore early on Sunday morning, landing at Smith's Wharf, not far from Bowley's Wharf. We had on board the sloop a large flock of sheep; and after aiding in driving them to the slaughter-house of Mr. Curtis on Louden Slater's Hill, I was conducted by Rich, one of the hands belonging on board of the sloop, to my new home in Alliciana Street, near Mr. Gardner's ship-yard, on Fells Point.

Mr. and Mrs. Auld were both at home, and met me at the door with their little son Thomas, to take care of whom I had been given. And here I saw what I had never seen before; it was a white face beaming with the most kindly emotions; it was the face of my new mistress, Sophia Auld. I wish I could describe the rapture that flashed through my soul as I beheld it. It was a new and strange sight to me, brightening up my pathway with the light of happiness. Little Thomas was told, there was his Freddy,—and I was told to take care of little Thomas; and thus I entered upon the duties of my new home with the most cheering prospect ahead.

I look upon my departure from Colonel Lloyd's plantation as one of the most interesting events of my life. It is possible, and even quite probable, that but for the mere circumstance of being removed from that plantation to Baltimore, I should have to-day, instead of being here seated by my own table, in the enjoyment of freedom and the happiness of home, writing this Narrative, been confined in the galling chains of slavery.

Going to live at Baltimore laid the foundation, and opened the gateway, to all my subsequent prosperity. I have ever regarded it as the first plain manifestation of that kind providence which has ever since attended me, and marked my life with so many favors. I regarded the selection of myself as being somewhat remarkable. There were a number of slave children that might have been sent from the plantation to Baltimore. There were those younger, those older, and those of the same age. I was chosen from among them all, and was the first, last, and only choice.

I may be deemed superstitious, and even egotistical, in regarding this event as a special interposition of divine Providence in my favor. But I should be false to the earliest sentiments of my soul, if I suppressed the opinion. I prefer to be true to myself, even at the hazard of incurring the ridicule of others, rather than to be false, and incur my own abhorrence. From my earliest recollection, I date the entertainment of a deep conviction that slavery would not always be able to hold me within its foul embrace; and in the darkest hours of my career in slavery, this living word of faith and spirit of hope departed not from me, but remained like ministering angels to cheer me through the gloom. This good spirit was from God, and to him I offer thanksgiving and praise.

CHAPTER VI.

My new mistress proved to be all she appeared when I first met her at the door,—a woman of the kindest heart and finest feelings. She had never had a slave under her control previously to myself, and prior to her marriage she had been dependent upon her own industry for a living. She was by trade a weaver; and by constant application to her business, she had been in a good degree preserved from the blighting and dehumanizing effects of slavery. I was utterly astonished at her goodness. I scarcely knew how to behave towards her. She was entirely unlike any other white woman I had ever seen. I could not approach her as I was accustomed to approach other white ladies. My early instruction was all out of place. The crouching servility, usually so acceptable a quality in a slave, did not answer when manifested toward her. Her favor was not gained by it; she seemed to be disturbed by it. She did not deem it impudent or unmannerly for a slave to look her in the face. The meanest slave was put fully at ease in her presence, and none left without feeling better for having seen her. Her face was made of heavenly smiles, and her voice of tranquil music.

But, alas! this kind heart had but a short time to remain such. The fatal poison of irresponsible power was already in her hands, and soon commenced its infernal work. That cheerful eye, under the influence of slavery, soon became red with rage; that voice, made all of sweet accord, changed to one of harsh and horrid discord; and that angelic face gave place to that of a demon.

Very soon after I went to live with Mr. and Mrs. Auld, she very kindly commenced to teach me the A, B, C. After I had learned this, she assisted me in learning to spell words of three or four letters. Just at this point of my progress, Mr. Auld found out what was going on, and at once forbade Mrs. Auld to instruct me further, telling her, among other things, that it was unlawful, as well as unsafe, to teach a slave to read. To use his own words, further, he said, "If you give a nigger an inch, he will take an ell. A nigger should know nothing but to obey his master—to do as he is told to do. Learning would *spoil* the best nigger in the world. Now," said he, "if you teach that nigger (speaking of myself) how to read, there would be no keeping him. It would forever unfit him to be a slave. He would at once become unmanageable, and of no value to his master. As to himself, it could do him no good, but a great deal of harm. It would make him discontented and unhappy." These words sank deep into my heart, stirred up sentiments within that lay slumbering, and called into existence an entirely new train of thought. It was a new and special revelation, explaining dark and mysterious things, with which my youthful understanding had struggled, but struggled in vain. I now understood what had been to me a most perplexing difficulty—to wit, the white man's power to enslave the black man. It was a grand achievement, and I prized it highly. From that moment, I understood the pathway from slavery to freedom. It was just what I wanted, and I got it at a time when I the least expected it. Whilst I was saddened by the thought of losing the aid of my kind mistress, I was gladdened by the invaluable instruction which, by the merest accident, I had gained from my master. Though conscious of the difficulty of learning without a teacher, I set out with high hope, and a fixed purpose, at whatever cost of trouble, to learn how to read. The very decided manner with which he spoke, and strove to impress his wife with the evil consequences of giving me instruction, served to convince me that he was deeply sensible of the truths he was uttering. It gave me the best assurance that I might rely with the utmost confidence on the results which, he said, would flow from teaching me to read. What he most dreaded, that I most desired. What he most loved, that I most hated. That which to him was a great evil, to be carefully shunned, was to me a great good, to be diligently sought; and the argument which he so warmly urged, against my learning to read, only served to inspire me with a desire and determination to learn. In learning to read, I owe almost as much to the bitter opposition of my master, as to the kindly aid of my mistress. I acknowledge the benefit of both.

I had resided but a short time in Baltimore before I observed a marked difference, in the treatment of slaves, from that which I had witnessed in the country. A city slave is almost a freeman, compared with a slave on the plantation. He is much better fed and clothed, and enjoys privileges altogether unknown to the slave on the plantation. There is a vestige of decency, a sense of shame, that does much to curb and check those outbreaks of atrocious cruelty so commonly enacted upon the plantation. He is a desperate slaveholder, who will shock the humanity of his non-slaveholding neighbors with the cries of his lacerated slave. Few are willing to incur the odium attaching to the reputation of being a cruel master; and above all things, they would not be known as not giving a slave enough to eat. Every city slaveholder is anxious to have it known of him, that he feeds his slaves well; and it is due to them to say, that most of them do give their slaves enough to eat. There are, however, some painful exceptions to this rule. Directly opposite to us, on Philpot Street, lived Mr. Thomas Hamilton. He owned two slaves. Their names were Henrietta and Mary. Henrietta was about twenty-two years of age, Mary was about fourteen; and of all the mangled and emaciated creatures I ever looked upon, these two were the most so. His heart must be harder than stone, that could look upon these unmoved. The head, neck, and shoulders of Mary were literally cut to pieces. I have frequently felt her head, and found it nearly covered with festering sores, caused by the lash of her cruel mistress. I do not know that her master ever whipped her, but I have been an eye-witness to the cruelty of Mrs. Hamilton. I used to be in Mr. Hamilton's house nearly every day. Mrs. Hamilton used to sit in a large chair in the middle of the room, with a heavy cowskin always by her side, and scarce an hour passed during the day but was marked by the blood of one of these slaves. The girls seldom passed her without her saying, "Move faster, you *black gip*!" at the same time giving them a blow with the cowskin over the head or shoulders, often drawing the blood. She would then say, "Take that, you *black gip*!"—continuing, "If you don't move faster, I'll move you!" Added to the cruel lashings to which these slaves were subjected, they were kept nearly half-starved. They seldom knew what it was to eat a full meal. I have seen Mary contending with the pigs for the offal thrown into the street. So much was Mary kicked and cut to pieces, that she was oftener called *"pecked"* than by her name.

CHAPTER VII.

I LIVED in Master Hugh's family about seven years. During this time, I succeeded in learning to read and write. In accomplishing this, I was compelled to resort to various stratagems. I had no regular teacher. My mistress, who had kindly commenced to instruct me, had, in compliance with the advice and direction of her husband, not only ceased to instruct, but had set her face against my being instructed by any one else. It is due, however, to my mistress to say of her, that she did not adopt this course of treatment immediately. She at first lacked the depravity indispensable to shutting me up in mental darkness. It was at least necessary for her to have some training in the exercise of irresponsible power, to make her equal to the task of treating me as though I were a brute.

My mistress was, as I have said, a kind and tender-hearted woman; and in the simplicity of her soul she commenced, when I first went to live with her, to treat me as she supposed one human being ought to treat another. In entering upon the duties of a slaveholder, she did not seem to perceive that I sustained to her the relation of a mere chattel, and that for her to treat me as a human being was not only wrong, but dangerously so. Slavery proved as injurious to her as it did to me. When I went there, she was a pious, warm, and tender-hearted woman. There was no sorrow or suffering for which she had not a tear. She had bread for the hungry, clothes for the naked, and comfort for every mourner that came within her reach. Slavery soon proved its ability to divest her of these heavenly qualities. Under its influence, the tender heart became stone, and the lamblike disposition gave way to one of tiger-like fierceness. The first step in her downward course was in her ceasing to instruct me. She now commenced to practise her husband's precepts. She finally became even more violent in her opposition than her husband himself. She was not satisfied with simply doing as well as he had commanded; she seemed anxious to do better. Nothing seemed to make her more angry than to see me with a newspaper. She seemed to think that here lay the danger. I have had her rush at me with a face made all up of fury, and snatch from me a newspaper, in a manner that fully revealed her apprehension. She was an apt woman; and a little experience soon demonstrated, to her satisfaction, that education and slavery were incompatible with each other.

From this time I was most narrowly watched. If I was in a separate room any considerable length of time, I was sure to be suspected of having a book, and was at once called to give an account of myself. All this, however, was too late. The first step had been taken. Mistress, in teaching me the alphabet, had given me the *inch*, and no precaution could prevent me from taking the *ell*.

The plan which I adopted, and the one by which I was most successful, was that of making friends of all the little white boys whom I met in the street. As many of these as I could, I converted into teachers. With their kindly aid, obtained at different times and in different places, I finally succeeded in learning to read. When I was sent of errands, I always took my book with me, and by going one part of my errand quickly, I found time to get a lesson before my return. I used also to carry bread with me, enough of which was always in the house, and to which I was always welcome; for I was much better off in this regard than many of the poor white children in our neighborhood. This bread I used to bestow upon the hungry little urchins, who, in return, would give me that more valuable bread of knowledge. I am strongly tempted to give the names of two or three of those little boys, as a testimonial of the gratitude and affection I bear them; but prudence forbids;—not that it would injure me, but it might embarrass them; for it is almost an unpardonable offence to teach slaves to read in this Christian country. It is enough to say of the dear little fellows, that they lived on Philpot Street, very near Durgin and Bailey's ship-yard. I used to talk this matter of slavery over with them. I would sometimes say to them, I wished I could be as free as they would be when they got to be men. "You will be free as soon as you are twenty-one, *but I am a slave for life!* Have not I as good a right to be free as you have?" These words used to trouble them; they would express for me the liveliest sympathy, and console me with the hope that something would occur by which I might be free.

I was now about twelve years old, and the thought of being *a slave for life* began to bear heavily upon my heart. Just about this time, I got hold of a book entitled "The Columbian Orator." Every opportunity I got, I used to read this book. Among much of other interesting matter, I found in it a dialogue between a master and his slave. The slave was represented as having run away from his master three times. The dialogue represented the conversation which took place between them, when the slave was retaken the third time. In this dialogue, the whole argument in behalf of slavery was brought forward by the master, all of which was disposed of by the slave. The slave was made to say some very smart as well as impressive things in reply to his master—things which had the desired though unexpected effect; for the conversation resulted in the voluntary emancipation of the slave on the part of the master.

In the same book, I met with one of Sheridan's mighty speeches on and in behalf of Catholic emancipation. These were choice documents to me. I read them over and over again with unabated interest. They gave tongue to interesting thoughts of my own soul, which had frequently flashed through my mind, and died away for want of utterance. The moral which I gained from the dialogue was the power of truth over the conscience of even a slaveholder. What I got from Sheridan was a bold denunciation of slavery, and a powerful vindication of human rights. The reading of these documents enabled me to utter my thoughts, and to meet the arguments brought forward to sustain slavery; but while they relieved me of one difficulty, they brought on another even more painful than the one of which I was relieved. The more I read, the more I was led to abhor and detest my enslavers. I could regard them in no other light than a band of successful robbers, who had left their homes, and gone to Africa, and stolen us from our homes, and in a strange land reduced us to slavery. I loathed them as being the meanest as well as the most wicked of men. As I read and contemplated the subject, behold! that very discontentment which Master Hugh had predicted would follow my learning to read had already come, to torment and sting my soul to unutterable anguish. As I writhed under it, I would at times feel that learning to read had been a curse rather than a blessing. It had given me a view of my wretched condition, without the remedy. It opened my eyes to the horrible pit, but to no ladder upon which to get out. In moments of agony, I envied my fellow-slaves for their stupidity. I have often wished myself a beast. I preferred the condition of the meanest reptile to my own. Any thing, no matter what, to get rid of thinking! It was this everlasting thinking of my condition that tormented me. There was no getting rid of it. It was pressed upon me by every object within sight or hearing, animate or inanimate. The silver trump of freedom had roused my soul to eternal wakefulness. Freedom now appeared, to disappear no more forever. It was heard in every sound, and seen in every thing. It was ever present to torment me with a sense of my wretched condition. I saw nothing without seeing it, I heard nothing without hearing it, and felt nothing without feeling it. It looked from every star, it smiled in every calm, breathed in every wind, and moved in every storm.

I often found myself regretting my own existence, and wishing myself dead; and but for the hope of being free, I have no doubt but that I should have killed myself, or done something for which I should have been killed. While in this state of mind, I was eager to hear any one speak of slavery. I was a ready listener. Every little while, I could hear something about the abolitionists. It was some time before I found what the word meant. It was always used in such connections as to make it an interesting word to me. If a slave ran away and succeeded in getting clear, or if a slave killed his master, set fire to a barn, or did any thing very wrong in the mind of a slaveholder, it was spoken of as the fruit of *abolition*. Hearing the word in this connection very often, I set about learning what it meant. The dictionary afforded me little or no help. I found it was "the act of abolishing;" but then I did not know what was to be abolished. Here I was perplexed. I did not dare to ask any one about its meaning, for I was satisfied that it was something they wanted me to know very little about. After a patient waiting, I got one of our city papers, containing an account of the number of petitions from the north, praying for the abolition of slavery in the District of Columbia, and of the slave trade between the States. From this time I understood the words *abolition* and *abolitionist*, and always drew near when that word was spoken, expecting to hear something of importance to myself and fellow-slaves. The light broke in upon me by degrees. I went one day down on the wharf of Mr. Waters; and seeing two Irishmen unloading a scow of stone, I went, unasked, and helped them. When we had finished, one of them came to me and asked me if I were a slave. I told him I was. He asked, "Are ye a slave for life?" I told him that I was. The good Irishman seemed to be deeply affected by the statement. He said to the other that it was a pity so fine a little fellow as myself should be a slave for life.

He said it was a shame to hold me. They both advised me to run away to the north; that I should find friends there, and that I should be free. I pretended not to be interested in what they said, and treated them as if I did not understand them; for I feared they might be treacherous. White men have been known to encourage slaves to escape, and then, to get the reward, catch them and return them to their masters. I was afraid that these seemingly good men might use me so; but I nevertheless remembered their advice, and from that time I resolved to run away. I looked forward to a time at which it would be safe for me to escape. I was too young to think of doing so immediately; besides, I wished to learn how to write, as I might have occasion to write my own pass. I consoled myself with the hope that I should one day find a good chance. Meanwhile, I would learn to write.

The idea as to how I might learn to write was suggested to me by being in Durgin and Bailey's ship-yard, and frequently seeing the ship carpenters, after hewing, and getting a piece of timber ready for use, write on the timber the name of that part of the ship for which it was intended. When a piece of timber was intended for the larboard side, it would be marked thus—"L." When a piece was for the starboard side, it would be marked thus—"S." A piece for the larboard side forward, would be marked thus—"L. F." When a piece was for starboard side forward, it would be marked thus—"S. F." For larboard aft, it would be marked thus—"L. A." For starboard aft, it would be marked thus—"S. A." I soon learned the names of these letters, and for what they were intended when placed upon a piece of timber in the ship-yard. I immediately commenced copying them, and in a short time was able to make the four letters named. After that, when I met with any boy who I knew could write, I would tell him I could write as well as he. The next word would be, "I don't believe you. Let me see you try it." I would then make the letters which I had been so fortunate as to learn, and ask him to beat that. In this way I got a good many lessons in writing, which it is quite possible I should never have gotten in any other way. During this time, my copy-book was the board fence, brick wall, and pavement; my pen and ink was a lump of chalk. With these, I learned mainly how to write. I then commenced and continued copying the Italics in Webster's Spelling Book, until I could make them all without looking on the book. By this time, my little Master Thomas had gone to school, and learned how to write, and had written over a number of copy-books. These had been brought home, and shown to some of our near neighbors, and then laid aside. My mistress used to go to class meeting at the Wilk Street meeting-house every Monday afternoon, and leave me to take care of the house. When left thus, I used to spend the time in writing in the spaces left in Master Thomas's copy-book, copying what he had written. I continued to do this until I could write a hand very similar to that of Master Thomas. Thus, after a long, tedious effort for years, I finally succeeded in learning how to write.

CHAPTER VIII.

In a very short time after I went to live at Baltimore, my old master's youngest son Richard died; and in about three years and six months after his death, my old master, Captain Anthony, died, leaving only his son, Andrew, and daughter, Lucretia, to share his estate. He died while on a visit to see his daughter at Hillsborough. Cut off thus unexpectedly, he left no will as to the disposal of his property. It was therefore necessary to have a valuation of the property, that it might be equally divided between Mrs. Lucretia and Master Andrew. I was immediately sent for, to be valued with the other property. Here again my feelings rose up in detestation of slavery. I had now a new conception of my degraded condition. Prior to this, I had become, if not insensible to my lot, at least partly so. I left Baltimore with a young heart overborne with sadness, and a soul full of apprehension. I took passage with Captain Rowe, in the schooner Wild Cat, and, after a sail of about twenty-four hours, I found myself near the place of my birth. I had now been absent from it almost, if not quite, five years. I, however, remembered the place very well. I was only about five years old when I left it, to go and live with my old master on Colonel Lloyd's plantation; so that I was now between ten and eleven years old.

We were all ranked together at the valuation. Men and women, old and young, married and single, were ranked with horses, sheep, and swine. There were horses and men, cattle and women, pigs and children, all holding the same rank in the scale of being, and were all subjected to the same narrow examination. Silvery-headed age and sprightly youth, maids and matrons, had to undergo the same indelicate inspection. At this moment, I saw more clearly than ever the brutalizing effects of slavery upon both slave and slaveholder.

After the valuation, then came the division. I have no language to express the high excitement and deep anxiety which were felt among us poor slaves during this time. Our fate for life was now to be decided. We had no more voice in that decision than the brutes among whom we were ranked. A single word from the white men was enough—against all our wishes, prayers, and entreaties—to sunder forever the dearest friends, dearest kindred, and strongest ties known to human beings. In addition to the pain of separation, there was the horrid dread of falling into the hands of Master Andrew. He was known to us all as being a most cruel wretch,—a common drunkard, who had, by his reckless mismanagement and profligate dissipation, already wasted a large portion of his father's property. We all felt that we might as well be sold at once to the Georgia traders, as to pass into his hands; for we knew that that would be our inevitable condition,—a condition held by us all in the utmost horror and dread.

I suffered more anxiety than most of my fellow-slaves. I had known what it was to be kindly treated; they had known nothing of the kind. They had seen little or nothing of the world. They were in very deed men and women of sorrow, and acquainted with grief. Their backs had been made familiar with the bloody lash, so that they had become callous; mine was yet tender; for while at Baltimore I got few whippings, and few slaves could boast of a kinder master and mistress than myself; and the thought of passing out of their hands into those of Master Andrew—a man who, but a few days before, to give me a sample of his bloody disposition, took my little brother by the throat, threw him on the ground, and with the heel of his boot stamped upon his head till the blood gushed from his nose and ears—was well calculated to make me anxious as to my fate. After he had committed this savage outrage upon my brother, he turned to me, and said that was the way he meant to serve me one of these days,—meaning, I suppose, when I came into his possession.

Thanks to a kind Providence, I fell to the portion of Mrs. Lucretia, and was sent immediately back to Baltimore, to live again in the family of Master Hugh. Their joy at my return equalled their sorrow at my departure. It was a glad day to me. I had escaped a worse than lion's jaws. I was absent from Baltimore, for the purpose of valuation and division, just about one month, and it seemed to have been six.

Very soon after my return to Baltimore, my mistress, Lucretia, died, leaving her husband and one child, Amanda; and in a very short time after her death, Master Andrew died. Now all the property of my old master, slaves included, was in the hands of strangers,—strangers who had had nothing to do with accumulating it. Not a slave was left free. All remained slaves, from the youngest to the oldest. If any one thing in my experience, more than another, served to deepen my conviction of the infernal character of slavery, and to fill me with unutterable loathing of slaveholders, it was their base ingratitude to my poor old grandmother. She had served my old master faithfully from youth to old age. She had been the source of all his wealth; she had peopled his plantation with slaves; she had become a great grandmother in his service. She had rocked him in infancy, attended him in childhood, served him through life, and at his death wiped from his icy brow the cold death-sweat, and closed his eyes forever. She was nevertheless left a slave—a slave for life—a slave in the hands of strangers; and in their hands she saw her children, her grandchildren, and her great-grandchildren, divided, like so many sheep, without being gratified with the small privilege of a single word, as to their or her own destiny. And, to cap the climax of their base ingratitude and fiendish barbarity, my grandmother, who was now very old, having outlived my old master and all his children, having seen the beginning and end of all of them, and her present owners finding she was of but little value, her frame already racked with the pains of old age, and complete helplessness fast stealing over her once active limbs, they took her to the woods, built her a little hut, put up a little mud-chimney, and then made her welcome to the privilege of supporting herself there in perfect loneliness; thus virtually turning her out to die! If my poor old grandmother now lives, she lives to suffer in utter lone-liness; she lives to remember and mourn over the loss of children, the loss of grandchildren, and the loss of great-grandchildren. They are, in the language of the slave's poet, Whittier,—

> "Gone, gone, sold and gone
>   To the rice swamp dank and lone,
>   Where the slave-whip ceaseless swings,
>   Where the noisome insect stings,
>   Where the fever-demon strews
>   Poison with the falling dews,
>   Where the sickly sunbeams glare
>   Through the hot and misty air:—
>   Gone, gone, sold and gone
>   To the rice swamp dank and lone,
>   From Virginia hills and waters—
>   Woe is me, my stolen daughters!"

The hearth is desolate. The children, the unconscious chil-dren, who once sang and danced in her presence, are gone. She gropes her way, in the darkness of age, for a drink of water. Instead of the voices of her children, she hears by day the moans of the dove, and by night the screams of the hid-eous owl. All is gloom. The grave is at the door. And now, when weighed down by the pains and aches of old age, when the head inclines to the feet, when the beginning and ending of human existence meet, and helpless infancy and painful old age combine together—at this time, this most needful time, the time for the exercise of that tenderness and affec-tion which children only can exercise towards a declining parent—my poor old grandmother, the devoted mother of twelve children, is left all alone, in yonder little hut, before a few dim embers. She stands—she sits—she staggers—she falls—she groans—she dies—and there are none of her children or grandchildren present, to wipe from her wrinkled brow the cold sweat of death, or to place beneath the sod her fallen remains. Will not a righteous God visit for these things?

In about two years after the death of Mrs. Lucretia, Master Thomas married his second wife. Her name was Rowena Hamilton. She was the eldest daughter of Mr. William Hamilton. Master now lived in St. Michael's. Not long after his marriage, a misunderstanding took place between himself and Master Hugh; and as a means of punishing his brother, he took me from him to live with himself at St. Michael's. Here I underwent another most painful separation. It, however, was not so severe as the one I dreaded at the division of property; for, during this interval, a great change had taken place in Master Hugh and his once kind and affectionate wife. The influence of brandy upon him, and of slavery upon her, had effected a disastrous change in the characters of both; so that, as far as they were concerned, I thought I had little to lose by the change. But it was not to them that I was attached. It was to those little Baltimore boys that I felt the strongest attachment. I had received many good lessons from them, and was still receiving them, and the thought of leaving them was painful indeed. I was leaving, too, without the hope of ever being allowed to return. Master Thomas had said he would never let me return again. The barrier betwixt himself and brother he considered impassable.

I then had to regret that I did not at least make the attempt to carry out my resolution to run away; for the chances of success are tenfold greater from the city than from the country.

I sailed from Baltimore for St. Michael's in the sloop Amanda, Captain Edward Dodson. On my passage, I paid particular attention to the direction which the steamboats took to go to Philadelphia. I found, instead of going down, on reaching North Point they went up the bay, in a north-easterly direction. I deemed this knowledge of the utmost importance.

My determination to run away was again revived. I resolved to wait only so long as the offering of a favorable opportunity. When that came, I was determined to be off.

CHAPTER IX.

I HAVE now reached a period of my life when I can give dates. I left Baltimore, and went to live with Master Thomas Auld, at St. Michael's, in March, 1832. It was now more than seven years since I lived with him in the family of my old master, on Colonel Lloyd's plantation. We of course were now almost entire strangers to each other. He was to me a new master, and I to him a new slave. I was ignorant of his temper and disposition; he was equally so of mine. A very short time, however, brought us into full acquaintance with each other. I was made acquainted with his wife not less than with himself. They were well matched, being equally mean and cruel. I was now, for the first time during a space of more than seven years, made to feel the painful gnawings of hunger—a something which I had not experienced before since I left Colonel Lloyd's plantation. It went hard enough with me then, when I could look back to no period at which I had enjoyed a sufficiency. It was tenfold harder after living in Master Hugh's family, where I had always had enough to eat, and of that which was good. I have said Master Thomas was a mean man. He was so. Not to give a slave enough to eat, is regarded as the most aggravated development of meanness even among slaveholders. The rule is, no matter how coarse the food, only let there be enough of it. This is the theory; and in the part of Maryland from which I came, it is the general practice,—though there are many exceptions. Master Thomas gave us enough of neither coarse nor fine food. There were four slaves of us in the kitchen—my sister Eliza, my aunt Priscilla, Henny, and myself; and we were allowed less than a half of a bushel of corn-meal per week, and very little else, either in the shape of meat or vegetables. It was not enough for us to subsist upon. We were therefore reduced to the wretched necessity of living at the expense of our neighbors. This we did by begging and stealing, whichever came handy in the time of need, the one being considered as legitimate as the other. A great many times have we poor creatures been nearly perishing with hunger, when food in abundance lay mouldering in the safe and smoke-house, and our pious mistress was aware of the fact; and yet that mistress and her husband would kneel every morning, and pray that God would bless them in basket and store!

Bad as all slaveholders are, we seldom meet one destitute of every element of character commanding respect. My master was one of this rare sort. I do not know of one single noble act ever performed by him. The leading trait in his character was meanness; and if there were any other element in his nature, it was made subject to this. He was mean; and, like most other mean men, he lacked the ability to conceal his meanness. Captain Auld was not born a slaveholder. He had been a poor man, master only of a Bay craft. He came into possession of all his slaves by marriage; and of all men, adopted slaveholders are the worst. He was cruel, but cowardly. He commanded without firmness. In the enforcement of his rules, he was at times rigid, and at times lax. At times, he spoke to his slaves with the firmness of Napoleon and the fury of a demon; at other times, he might well be mistaken for an inquirer who had lost his way. He did nothing of himself. He might have passed for a lion, but for his ears. In all things noble which he attempted, his own meanness shone most conspicuous. His airs, words, and actions, were the airs, words, and actions of born slaveholders, and, being assumed, were awkward enough. He was not even a good imitator. He possessed all the disposition to deceive, but wanted the power. Having no resources within himself, he was compelled to be the copyist of many, and being such, he was forever the victim of inconsistency; and of consequence he was an object of contempt, and was held as such even by his slaves. The luxury of having slaves of his own to wait upon him was something new and unprepared for. He was a slaveholder without the ability to hold slaves. He found himself incapable of managing his slaves either by force, fear, or fraud. We seldom called him "master;" we generally called him "Captain Auld," and were hardly disposed to title him at all. I doubt not that our conduct had much to do with making him appear awkward, and of consequence fretful. Our want of reverence for him must have perplexed him greatly. He wished to have us call him master, but lacked the firmness necessary to command us to do so. His wife used to insist upon our calling him so, but to no purpose. In August, 1832, my master attended a Methodist camp-meeting held in the Bay-side, Talbot county, and there experienced religion. I indulged a faint hope that his conversion would lead him to emancipate his slaves, and that, if he did not do this, it would, at any rate, make him more kind and humane. I was disappointed in both these respects. It neither made him to be humane to his slaves, nor to emancipate them. If it had any effect on his character, it made him more cruel and hateful in all his ways; for I believe him to have been a much worse man after his conversion than before. Prior to his conversion, he relied upon his own depravity to shield and sustain him in his savage barbarity; but after his conversion, he found religious sanction and support for his slaveholding cruelty. He made the greatest pretensions to piety. His house was the house of prayer. He prayed morning, noon, and night. He very soon distinguished himself among his brethren, and was soon made a class-leader and exhorter. His activity in revivals was great, and he proved himself an instrument in the hands of the church in converting many souls. His house was the preachers' home. They used to take great pleasure in coming there to put up; for while he starved us, he stuffed them. We have had three or four preachers there at a time. The names of those who used to come most frequently while I lived there, were Mr. Storks, Mr. Ewery, Mr. Humphry, and Mr. Hickey. I have also seen Mr. George Cookman at our house. We slaves loved Mr. Cookman. We believed him to be a good man. We thought him instrumental in getting Mr. Samuel Harrison, a very rich slaveholder, to emancipate his slaves; and by some means got the impression that he was laboring to effect the emancipation of all the slaves. When he was at our house, we were sure to be called in to prayers. When the others were there, we were sometimes called in and sometimes not. Mr. Cookman took more notice of us than either of the other ministers. He could not come among us without betraying his sympathy for us, and, stupid as we were, we had the sagacity to see it.

While I lived with my master in St. Michael's, there was a white young man, a Mr. Wilson, who proposed to keep a Sabbath school for the instruction of such slaves as might be disposed to learn to read the New Testament. We met but three times, when Mr. West and Mr. Fairbanks, both class-leaders, with many others, came upon us with sticks and other missiles, drove us off, and forbade us to meet again. Thus ended our little Sabbath school in the pious town of St. Michael's.

I have said my master found religious sanction for his cruelty. As an example, I will state one of many facts going to prove the charge. I have seen him tie up a lame young woman, and whip her with a heavy cowskin upon her naked shoulders, causing the warm red blood to drip; and, in justification of the bloody deed, he would quote this passage of Scripture— "He that knoweth his master's will, and doeth it not, shall be beaten with many stripes."

Master would keep this lacerated young woman tied up in this horrid situation four or five hours at a time. I have known him to tie her up early in the morning, and whip her before breakfast; leave her, go to his store, return at dinner, and whip her again, cutting her in the places already made raw with his cruel lash. The secret of master's cruelty toward "Henny" is found in the fact of her being almost helpless. When quite a child, she fell into the fire, and burned herself horribly. Her hands were so burnt that she never got the use of them. She could do very little but bear heavy burdens. She was to master a bill of expense; and as he was a mean man, she was a constant offence to him. He seemed desirous of getting the poor girl out of existence. He gave her away once to his sister; but, being a poor gift, she was not disposed to keep her. Finally, my benevolent master, to use his own words, "set her adrift to take care of herself." Here was a recently-converted man, holding on upon the mother, and at the same time turning out her helpless child, to starve and die! Master Thomas was one of the many pious slaveholders who hold slaves for the very charitable purpose of taking care of them.

My master and myself had quite a number of differences. He found me unsuitable to his purpose. My city life, he said, had

had a very pernicious effect upon me. It had almost ruined me for every good purpose, and fitted me for every thing which was bad. One of my greatest faults was that of letting his horse run away, and go down to his father-in-law's farm, which was about five miles from St. Michael's. I would then have to go after it. My reason for this kind of carelessness, or carefulness, was, that I could always get something to eat when I went there. Master William Hamilton, my master's father-in-law, always gave his slaves enough to eat. I never left there hungry, no matter how great the need of my speedy return. Master Thomas at length said he would stand it no longer. I had lived with him nine months, during which time he had given me a number of severe whippings, all to no good purpose. He resolved to put me out, as he said, to be broken; and, for this purpose, he let me for one year to a man named Edward Covey. Mr. Covey was a poor man, a farm-renter. He rented the place upon which he lived, as also the hands with which he tilled it. Mr. Covey had acquired a very high reputation for breaking young slaves, and this reputation was of immense value to him. It enabled him to get his farm tilled with much less expense to himself than he could have had it done without such a reputation. Some slaveholders thought it not much loss to allow Mr. Covey to have their slaves one year, for the sake of the training to which they were subjected, without any other compensation. He could hire young help with great ease, in consequence of this reputation. Added to the natural good qualities of Mr. Covey, he was a professor of religion—a pious soul—a member and a class-leader in the Methodist church. All of this added weight to his reputation as a "nigger-breaker." I was aware of all the facts, having been made acquainted with them by a young man who had lived there. I nevertheless made the change gladly; for I was sure of getting enough to eat, which is not the smallest consideration to a hungry man.

CHAPTER X.

I LEFT Master Thomas's house, and went to live with Mr. Covey, on the 1st of January, 1833. I was now, for the first time in my life, a field hand. In my new employment, I found myself even more awkward than a country boy appeared to be in a large city. I had been at my new home but one week before Mr. Covey gave me a very severe whipping, cutting my back, causing the blood to run, and raising ridges on my flesh as large as my little finger. The details of this affair are as follows: Mr. Covey sent me, very early in the morning of one of our coldest days in the month of January, to the woods, to get a load of wood. He gave me a team of unbroken oxen. He told me which was the in-hand ox, and which the off-hand one. He then tied the end of a large rope around the horns of the in-hand ox, and gave me the other end of it, and told me, if the oxen started to run, that I must hold on upon the rope. I had never driven oxen before, and of course I was very awkward. I, however, succeeded in getting to the edge of the woods with little difficulty; but I had got a very few rods into the woods, when the oxen took fright, and started full tilt, carrying the cart against trees, and over stumps, in the most frightful manner. I expected every moment that my brains would be dashed out against the trees. After running thus for a considerable distance, they finally upset the cart, dashing it with great force against a tree, and threw themselves into a dense thicket. How I escaped death, I do not know. There I was, entirely alone, in a thick wood, in a place new to me. My cart was upset and shattered, my oxen were entangled among the young trees, and there was none to help me. After a long spell of effort, I succeeded in getting my cart righted, my oxen disentangled, and again yoked to the cart. I now proceeded with my team to the place where I had, the day before, been chopping wood, and loaded my cart pretty heavily, thinking in this way to tame my oxen. I then proceeded on my way home. I had now consumed one half of the day. I got out of the woods safely, and now felt out of danger. I stopped my oxen to open the woods gate; and just as I did so, before I could get hold of my ox-rope, the oxen again started, rushed through the gate, catching it between the wheel and the body of the cart, tearing it to pieces, and coming within a few inches of crushing me against the gate-post. Thus twice, in one short day, I escaped death by the merest chance. On my return, I told Mr. Covey what had happened, and how it happened. He ordered me to return to the woods again immediately. I did so, and he followed on after me. Just as I got into the woods, he came up and told me to stop my cart, and that he would teach me how to trifle away my time, and break gates. He then went to a large gum-tree, and with his axe cut three large switches, and, after trimming them up neatly with his pocket-knife, he ordered me to take off my clothes. I made him no answer, but stood with my clothes on. He repeated his order. I still made him no answer, nor did I move to strip myself. Upon this he rushed at me with the fierceness of a tiger, tore off my clothes, and lashed me till he had worn out his switches, cutting me so savagely as to leave the marks visible for a long time after. This whipping was the first of a number just like it, and for similar offences.

I lived with Mr. Covey one year. During the first six months, of that year, scarce a week passed without his whipping me. I was seldom free from a sore back. My awkwardness was almost always his excuse for whipping me. We were worked fully up to the point of endurance. Long before day we were up, our horses fed, and by the first approach of day we were off to the field with our hoes and ploughing teams. Mr. Covey gave us enough to eat, but scarce time to eat it. We were often less than five minutes taking our meals. We were often in the field from the first approach of day till its last lingering ray had left us; and at saving-fodder time, midnight often caught us in the field binding blades.

Covey would be out with us. The way he used to stand it, was this. He would spend the most of his afternoons in bed. He would then come out fresh in the evening, ready to urge us on with his words, example, and frequently with the whip. Mr. Covey was one of the few slaveholders who could and did work with his hands. He was a hard-working man. He knew by himself just what a man or a boy could do. There was no deceiving him. His work went on in his absence almost as well as in his presence; and he had the faculty of making us feel that he was ever present with us. This he did by surprising us. He seldom approached the spot where we were at work openly, if he could do it secretly. He always aimed at taking us by surprise. Such was his cunning, that we used to call him, among ourselves, "the snake." When we were at work in the cornfield, he would sometimes crawl on his hands and knees to avoid detection, and all at once he would rise nearly in our midst, and scream out, "Ha, ha! Come, come! Dash on, dash on!" This being his mode of attack, it was never safe to stop a single minute. His comings were like a thief in the night. He appeared to us as being ever at hand. He was under every tree, behind every stump, in every bush, and at every window, on the plantation. He would sometimes mount his horse, as if bound to St. Michael's, a distance of seven miles, and in half an hour afterwards you would see him coiled up in the corner of the wood-fence, watching every motion of the slaves. He would, for this purpose, leave his horse tied up in the woods. Again, he would sometimes walk up to us, and give us orders as though he was upon the point of starting on a long journey, turn his back upon us, and make as though he was going to the house to get ready; and, before he would get half way thither, he would turn short and crawl into a fence-corner, or behind some tree, and there watch us till the going down of the sun.

Mr. Covey's *forte* consisted in his power to deceive. His life was devoted to planning and perpetrating the grossest deceptions. Every thing he possessed in the shape of learning or religion, he made conform to his disposition to deceive. He seemed to think himself equal to deceiving the Almighty. He would make a short prayer in the morning, and a long prayer at night; and, strange as it may seem, few men would at times appear more devotional than he. The exercises of his family devotions were always commenced with singing; and, as he was a very poor singer himself, the duty of raising the hymn generally came upon me. He would read his hymn, and nod at me to commence. I would at times do so; at others, I would not. My non-compliance would almost always produce much confusion. To show himself independent of me, he would start and stagger through with his hymn in the most discordant manner. In this state of mind, he prayed with more than ordinary spirit. Poor man! such was his disposition, and success at deceiving, I do verily believe that he sometimes deceived himself into the solemn belief, that he was a sincere worshipper of the most high God; and this, too, at a time when he may be said to have been guilty of compelling his woman slave to commit the sin of adultery. The facts in the case are these: Mr. Covey was a poor man; he was just commencing in life; he was only able to buy one slave; and, shocking as is the fact, he bought her, as he said, for *a breeder.* This woman was named Caroline. Mr. Covey bought her from Mr. Thomas Lowe, about six miles from St. Michael's. She was a large, able-bodied woman, about twenty years old. She had already given birth to one child, which proved her to be just what he wanted. After buying her, he hired a married man of Mr. Samuel Harrison, to live with him one year; and him he used to fasten up with her every night! The result was, that, at the end of the year, the miserable woman gave birth to twins. At this result Mr. Covey seemed to be highly pleased, both with the man and the wretched woman. Such was his joy, and that of his wife, that nothing they could do for Caroline during her confinement was too good, or too hard, to be done. The children were regarded as being quite an addition to his wealth.

If at any one time of my life more than another, I was made to drink the bitterest dregs of slavery, that time was during the first six months of my stay with Mr. Covey. We were worked in all weathers. It was never too hot or too cold; it could never rain, blow, hail, or snow, too hard for us to work in the field. Work, work, work, was scarcely more the order of the day than of the night. The longest days were too short for him, and the shortest nights too long for him. I was somewhat unmanageable when I first went there, but a few months of this discipline tamed me. Mr. Covey succeeded in breaking me. I was broken in body, soul, and spirit. My natural elasticity was crushed, my intellect languished, the disposition to read departed, the cheerful spark that lingered about my eye died; the dark night of slavery closed in upon me; and behold a man transformed into a brute!

Sunday was my only leisure time. I spent this in a sort of beast-like stupor, between sleep and wake, under some large tree. At times I would rise up, a flash of energetic freedom would dart through my soul, accompanied with a faint beam of hope, that flickered for a moment, and then vanished. I sank down again, mourning over my wretched condition. I was sometimes prompted to take my life, and that of Covey, but was prevented by a combination of hope and fear. My sufferings on this plantation seem now like a dream rather than a stern reality.

Our house stood within a few rods of the Chesapeake Bay, whose broad bosom was ever white with sails from every quarter of the habitable globe. Those beautiful vessels, robed in purest white, so delightful to the eye of freemen, were to me so many shrouded ghosts, to terrify and torment me with thoughts of my wretched condition. I have often, in the deep stillness of a summer's Sabbath, stood all alone upon the lofty banks of that noble bay, and traced, with saddened heart and tearful eye, the countless number of sails moving off to the mighty ocean. The sight of these always affected me powerfully. My thoughts would compel utterance; and there, with no audience but the Almighty, I would pour out my soul's complaint, in my rude way, with an apostrophe to the moving multitude of ships:—

"You are loosed from your moorings, and are free; I am fast in my chains, and am a slave! You move merrily before the gentle gale, and I sadly before the bloody whip! You are freedom's swift-winged angels, that fly round the world; I am confined in bands of iron! O that I were free! O, that I were on one of your gallant decks, and under your protecting wing! Alas! betwixt me and you, the turbid waters roll. Go on, go on. O that I could also go! Could I but swim! If I could fly! O, why was I born a man, of whom to make a brute! The glad ship is gone; she hides in the dim distance. I am left in the hottest hell of unending slavery. O God, save me! God, deliver me! Let me be free! Is there any God? Why am I a slave? I will run away. I will not stand it. Get caught, or get clear, I'll try it. I had as well die with ague as the fever. I have only one life to lose. I had as well be killed running as die standing. Only think of it; one hundred miles straight north, and I am free! Try it? Yes! God helping me, I will. It cannot be that I shall live and die a slave. I will take to the water. This very bay shall yet bear me into freedom. The steamboats steered in a north-east course from North Point. I will do the same; and when I get to the head of the bay, I will turn my canoe adrift, and walk straight through Delaware into Pennsylvania. When I get there, I shall not be required to have a pass; I can travel without being disturbed. Let but the first opportunity offer, and, come what will, I am off. Meanwhile, I will try to bear up under the yoke. I am not the only slave in the world. Why should I fret? I can bear as much as any of them. Besides, I am but a boy, and all boys are bound to some one. It may be that my misery in slavery will only increase my happiness when I get free. There is a better day coming."

Thus I used to think, and thus I used to speak to myself; goaded almost to madness at one moment, and at the next reconciling myself to my wretched lot.

I have already intimated that my condition was much worse, during the first six months of my stay at Mr. Covey's, than in the last six. The circumstances leading to the change in Mr. Covey's course toward me form an epoch in my humble history. You have seen how a man was made a slave; you shall see how a slave was made a man. On one of the hottest days of the month of August, 1833, Bill Smith, William Hughes, a slave named Eli, and myself, were engaged in fanning wheat. Hughes was clearing the fanned wheat from before the fan, Eli was turning, Smith was feeding, and I was carrying wheat to the fan. The work was simple, requiring strength rather than intellect; yet, to one entirely unused to such work, it came very hard. About three o'clock of that day, I broke down; my strength failed me; I was seized with a violent aching of the head, attended with extreme dizziness; I trembled in every limb. Finding what was coming, I nerved myself up, feeling it would never do to stop work. I stood as long as I could stagger to the hopper with grain. When I could stand no longer, I fell, and felt as if held down by an immense weight. The fan of course stopped; every one had his own work to do; and no one could do the work of the other, and have his own go on at the same time.

Mr. Covey was at the house, about one hundred yards from the treading-yard where we were fanning. On hearing the fan stop, he left immediately, and came to the spot where we were. He hastily inquired what the matter was. Bill answered that I was sick, and there was no one to bring wheat to the fan. I had by this time crawled away under the side of the post and rail-fence by which the yard was enclosed, hoping to find relief by getting out of the sun. He then asked where I was. He was told by one of the hands. He came to the spot, and, after looking at me awhile, asked me what was the matter. I told him as well as I could, for I scarce had strength to speak. He then gave me a savage kick in the side, and told me to get up. I tried to do so, but fell back in the attempt. He gave me another kick, and again told me to rise. I again tried, and succeeded in gaining my feet; but, stooping to get the tub with which I was feeding the fan, I again staggered and fell. While down in this situation, Mr. Covey took up the hickory slat with which Hughes had been striking off the half-bushel measure, and with it gave me a heavy blow upon the head, making a large wound, and the blood ran freely; and with this again told me to get up. I made no effort to comply, having now made up my mind to let him do his worst. In a short time after receiving this blow, my head grew better. Mr. Covey had now left me to my fate. At this moment I resolved, for the first time, to go to my master, enter a complaint, and ask his protection. In order to do this, I must that afternoon walk seven miles; and this, under the circumstances, was truly a severe undertaking. I was exceedingly feeble; made so as much by the kicks and blows which I received, as by the severe fit of sickness to which I had been subjected. I, however, watched my chance, while Covey was looking in an opposite direction, and started for St. Michael's. I succeeded in getting a considerable distance on my way to the woods, when Covey discovered me, and called after me to come back, threatening what he would do if I did not come. I disregarded both his calls and his threats, and made my way to the woods as fast as my feeble state would allow; and thinking I might be over-hauled by him if I kept the road, I walked through the woods, keeping far enough from the road to avoid detection, and near enough to prevent losing my way. I had not gone far before my little strength again failed me. I could go no farther. I fell down, and lay for a considerable time. The blood was yet oozing from the wound on my head. For a time I thought I should bleed to death; and think now that I should have done so, but that the blood so matted my hair as to stop the wound. After lying there about three quarters of an hour, I nerved myself up again, and started on my way, through bogs and briers, barefooted and bareheaded, tearing my feet sometimes at nearly every step; and after a journey of about seven miles, occupying some five hours to perform it, I arrived at master's store. I then presented an appearance enough to affect any but a heart of iron. From the crown of my head to my feet, I was covered with blood. My hair was all clotted with dust and blood; my shirt was stiff with blood. My legs and feet were torn in sundry places with briers and thorns, and were also covered with blood. I suppose I looked like a man who had escaped a den of wild beasts, and barely escaped them. In this state I appeared before my master, humbly entreating him to interpose his authority for my protection. I told him all the circumstances as well as I could, and it seemed, as I spoke, at times to affect him. He would then walk the floor, and seek to justify Covey by saying he expected I deserved it. He asked me what I wanted. I told him, to let me get a new home; that as sure as I lived with Mr. Covey again, I should live with but to die with him; that Covey would surely kill me; he was in a fair way for it. Master Thomas ridiculed the idea that there was any danger of Mr. Covey's killing me, and said that he knew Mr. Covey; that he was a good man, and that he could not think of taking me from him; that, should he do so, he would lose the whole year's wages; that I belonged to Mr. Covey for one year, and that I must go back to him, come what might; and that I must not trouble him with any more stories, or that he would himself *get hold of me*. After threatening me thus, he gave me a very large dose of salts, telling me that I might remain in St. Michael's that night, (it being quite late,) but that I must be off back to Mr. Covey's early in the morning; and that if I did not, he would *get hold of me*, which meant that he would whip me. I remained all night, and, according to his orders, I started off to Covey's in the morning, (Saturday morning,) wearied in body and broken in spirit. I got no supper that night, or breakfast that morning. I reached Covey's about nine o'clock; and just as I was getting over the fence that divided Mrs. Kemp's fields from ours, out ran Covey with his cowskin, to give me another whipping. Before he could reach me, I succeeded in getting to the cornfield; and as the corn was very high, it afforded me the means of hiding. He seemed very angry, and searched for me a long time. My behavior was altogether unaccountable. He finally gave up the chase, thinking, I suppose, that I must come home for something to eat; he would give himself no further trouble in looking for me. I spent that day mostly in the woods, having the alternative before me,—to go home and be whipped to death, or stay in the woods and be starved to death. That night, I fell in with Sandy Jenkins, a slave with whom I was somewhat acquainted. Sandy had a free wife, who lived about four miles from Mr. Covey's; and it being Saturday, he was on his way to see her. I told him my circumstances, and he very kindly invited me to go home with him. I went home with him, and talked this whole matter over, and got his advice as to what course it was best for me to pursue. I found Sandy an old adviser. He told me, with great solemnity, I must go back to Covey; but that before I went, I must go with him into another part of the woods, where there was a certain *root*, which, if I would take some of it with me, carrying it *always on my right side*, would render it impossible for Mr. Covey, or any other white man, to whip me. He said he had carried it for years; and since he had done so, he had never received a blow, and never expected to while he carried it. I at first rejected the idea, that the simple carrying of a root in my pocket would have any such effect as he had said, and was not disposed to take it; but Sandy impressed the necessity with much earnestness, telling me it could do no harm, if it did no good. To please him, I at length took the root, and, according to his direction, carried it upon my right side. This was Sunday morning. I immediately started for home; and upon entering the yard gate, out came Mr. Covey on his way to meeting. He spoke to me very kindly, bade me drive the pigs from a lot near by, and passed on towards the church. Now, this singular conduct of Mr. Covey really made me begin to think that there was something in the *root* which Sandy had given me; and had it been on any other day than Sunday, I could have attributed the conduct to no other cause than the influence of that root; and as it was, I was half inclined to think the *root* to be something more than I at first had taken it to be. All went well till Monday morning. On this morning, the virtue of the *root* was fully tested. Long before daylight, I was called to go and rub, curry, and feed, the horses. I obeyed, and was glad to obey. But whilst thus engaged, whilst in the act of throwing down some blades from the loft, Mr. Covey entered the stable with a long rope; and just as I was half out of the loft, he caught hold of my legs, and was about tying me. As soon as I found what he was up to, I gave a sudden spring, and as I did so, he holding to my legs, I was brought sprawling on the stable floor. Mr. Covey seemed now to think he had me, and could do what he pleased; but at this moment—from whence came the spirit I don't know—I resolved to fight; and, suiting my action to the resolution, I seized Covey hard by the throat; and as I did so, I rose. He held on to me, and I to him. My resistance was so entirely unexpected, that Covey seemed taken all aback. He trembled like a leaf. This gave me assurance, and I held him uneasy, causing the blood to run where I touched him with the ends of my fingers. Mr. Covey soon called out to Hughes for help. Hughes came, and, while Covey held me, attempted to tie my right hand. While he was in the act of doing so, I watched my chance, and gave him a heavy kick close under the ribs. This kick fairly sickened Hughes, so that he left me in the hands of Mr. Covey. This kick had the effect of not only weakening Hughes, but Covey also. When he saw Hughes bending over with pain, his courage quailed. He asked me if I meant to persist in my resistance. I told him I did, come what might; that he had used me like a brute for six months, and that I was determined to be used so no longer. With that, he strove to drag me to a stick that was lying just out of the stable door. He meant to knock me down. But just as he was leaning over to get the stick, I seized him with both hands by his collar, and brought him by a sudden snatch to the ground. By this time, Bill came. Covey called upon him for assistance. Bill wanted to know what he could do. Covey said, "Take hold of him, take hold of him!" Bill said his master hired him out to work, and not to help to whip me; so he left Covey and myself to fight our own battle out. We were at it for nearly two hours. Covey at length let me go, puffing and blowing at a great rate, saying that if I had not resisted, he would not have whipped me half so much. The truth was, that he had not whipped me at all. I considered him as getting entirely the worst end of the bargain; for he had drawn no blood from me, but I had from him. The whole six months afterwards, that I spent with Mr. Covey, he never laid the weight of his finger upon me in anger. He would occasionally say, he didn't want to get hold of me again. "No," thought I, "you need not; for you will come off worse than you did before."

This battle with Mr. Covey was the turning-point in my career as a slave. It rekindled the few expiring embers of freedom, and revived within me a sense of my own manhood. It recalled the departed self-confidence, and inspired me again with a determination to be free. The gratification afforded by the triumph was a full compensation for whatever else might follow, even death itself. He only can understand the deep satisfaction which I experienced, who has himself repelled by force the bloody arm of slavery. I felt as I never felt before. It was a glorious resurrection, from the tomb of slavery, to the heaven of freedom. My long-crushed spirit rose, cowardice departed, bold defiance took its place; and I now resolved that, however long I might remain a slave in form, the day had passed forever when I could be a slave in fact. I did not hesitate to let it be known of me, that the white man who expected to succeed in whipping, must also succeed in killing me.

From this time I was never again what might be called fairly whipped, though I remained a slave four years afterwards. I had several fights, but was never whipped.

It was for a long time a matter of surprise to me why Mr. Covey did not immediately have me taken by the constable to the whipping-post, and there regularly whipped for the crime of raising my hand against a white man in defence of myself. And the only explanation I can now think of does not entirely satisfy me; but such as it is, I will give it. Mr. Covey enjoyed the most unbounded reputation for being a first-rate overseer and negro-breaker. It was of considerable importance to him. That reputation was at stake; and had he sent me—a boy about sixteen years old—to the public whipping-post, his reputation would have been lost; so, to save his reputation, he suffered me to go unpunished.

My term of actual service to Mr. Edward Covey ended on Christmas day, 1833. The days between Christmas and New Year's day are allowed as holidays; and, accordingly, we were not required to perform any labor, more than to feed and take care of the stock. This time we regarded as our own, by the grace of our masters; and we therefore used or abused it nearly as we pleased. Those of us who had families at a distance, were generally allowed to spend the whole six days in their society. This time, however, was spent in various ways. The staid, sober, thinking and industrious ones of our number would employ themselves in making corn-brooms, mats, horse-collars, and baskets; and another class of us would spend the time in hunting opossums, hares, and coons. But by far the larger part engaged in such sports and merriments as playing ball, wrestling, running foot-races, fiddling, dancing, and drinking whisky; and this latter mode of spending the time was by far the most agreeable to the feelings of our masters. A slave who would work during the holidays was considered by our masters as scarcely deserving them. He was regarded as one who rejected the favor of his master. It was deemed a disgrace not to get drunk at Christmas; and he was regarded as lazy indeed, who had not provided himself with the necessary means, during the year, to get whisky enough to last him through Christmas.

From what I know of the effect of these holidays upon the slave, I believe them to be among the most effective means in the hands of the slaveholder in keeping down the spirit of insurrection. Were the slaveholders at once to abandon this practice, I have not the slightest doubt it would lead to an immediate insurrection among the slaves. These holidays serve as conductors, or safety-valves, to carry off the rebellious spirit of enslaved humanity. But for these, the slave would be forced up to the wildest desperation; and woe betide the slaveholder, the day he ventures to remove or hinder the operation of those conductors! I warn him that, in such an event, a spirit will go forth in their midst, more to be dreaded than the most appalling earthquake.

The holidays are part and parcel of the gross fraud, wrong,

and inhumanity of slavery. They are professedly a custom established by the benevolence of the slaveholders; but I undertake to say, it is the result of selfishness, and one of the grossest frauds committed upon the down-trodden slave. They do not give the slaves this time because they would not like to have their work during its continuance, but because they know it would be unsafe to deprive them of it. This will be seen by the fact, that the slaveholders like to have their slaves spend those days just in such a manner as to make them as glad of their ending as of their beginning. Their object seems to be, to disgust their slaves with freedom, by plunging them into the lowest depths of dissipation. For instance, the slaveholders not only like to see the slave drink of his own accord, but will adopt various plans to make him drunk. One plan is, to make bets on their slaves, as to who can drink the most whisky without getting drunk; and in this way they succeed in getting whole multitudes to drink to excess. Thus, when the slave asks for virtuous freedom, the cunning slaveholder, knowing his ignorance, cheats him with a dose of vicious dissipation, artfully labelled with the name of liberty. The most of us used to drink it down, and the result was just what might be supposed. many of us were led to think that there was little to choose between liberty and slavery. We felt, and very properly too, that we had almost as well be slaves to man as to rum. So, when the holidays ended, we staggered up from the filth of our wallowing, took a long breath, and marched to the field,—feeling, upon the whole, rather glad to go, from what our master had deceived us into a belief was freedom, back to the arms of slavery.

I have said that this mode of treatment is a part of the whole system of fraud and inhumanity of slavery. It is so. The mode here adopted to disgust the slave with freedom, by allowing him to see only the abuse of it, is carried out in other things. For instance, a slave loves molasses; he steals some. His master, in many cases, goes off to town, and buys a large quantity; he returns, takes his whip, and commands the slave to eat the molasses, until the poor fellow is made sick at the very mention of it. The same mode is sometimes adopted to make the slaves refrain from asking for more food than their regular allowance. A slave runs through his allowance, and applies for more. His master is enraged at him; but, not willing to send him off without food, gives him more than is necessary, and compels him to eat it within a given time. Then, if he complains that he cannot eat it, he is said to be satisfied neither full nor fasting, and is whipped for being hard to please! I have an abundance of such illustrations of the same principle, drawn from my own observation, but think the cases I have cited sufficient. The practice is a very common one.

On the first of January, 1834, I left Mr. Covey, and went to live with Mr. William Freeland, who lived about three miles from St. Michael's. I soon found Mr. Freeland a very different man from Mr. Covey. Though not rich, he was what would be called an educated southern gentleman. Mr. Covey, as I have shown, was a well-trained negro-breaker and slave-driver. The former (slaveholder though he was) seemed to possess some regard for honor, some reverence for justice, and some respect for humanity. The latter seemed totally insensible to all such sentiments. Mr. Freeland had many of the faults peculiar to slaveholders, such as being very passionate and fretful; but I must do him the justice to say, that he was exceedingly free from those degrading vices to which Mr. Covey was constantly addicted. The one was open and frank, and we always knew where to find him. The other was a most artful deceiver, and could be understood only by such as were skilful enough to detect his cunningly-devised frauds. Another advantage I gained in my new master was, he made no pretensions to, or profession of, religion; and this, in my opinion, was truly a great advantage. I assert most unhesitatingly, that the religion of the south is a mere covering for the most horrid crimes,—a justifier of the most appalling barbarity,—a sanctifier of the most hateful frauds,—and a dark shelter under, which the darkest, foulest, grossest, and most infernal deeds of slaveholders find the strongest protection. Were I to be again reduced to the chains of slavery, next to that enslavement, I should regard being the slave of a religious master the greatest calamity that could befall me. For of all slaveholders with whom I have ever met, religious slaveholders are the worst. I have ever found them the meanest and basest, the most cruel and cowardly, of all others. It was my unhappy lot not only to belong to a religious slaveholder, but to live in a community of such religionists. Very near Mr. Freeland lived the Rev. Daniel Weeden, and in the same neighborhood lived the Rev. Rigby Hopkins. These were members and ministers in the Reformed Methodist Church. Mr. Weeden owned, among others, a woman slave, whose name I have forgotten. This woman's back, for weeks, was kept literally raw, made so by the lash of this merciless, *religious* wretch. He used to hire hands. His maxim was, Behave well or behave ill, it is the duty of a master occasionally to whip a slave, to remind him of his master's authority. Such was his theory, and such his practice.

Mr. Hopkins was even worse than Mr. Weeden. His chief boast was his ability to manage slaves. The peculiar feature of his government was that of whipping slaves in advance of deserving it. He always managed to have one or more of his slaves to whip every Monday morning. He did this to alarm their fears, and strike terror into those who escaped. His plan was to whip for the smallest offences, to prevent the commission of large ones. Mr. Hopkins could always find some excuse for whipping a slave. It would astonish one, unaccustomed to a slaveholding life, to see with what wonderful ease a slaveholder can find things, of which to make occasion to whip a slave. A mere look, word, or motion,—a mistake, accident, or want of power,—are all matters for which a slave may be whipped at any time. Does a slave look dissatisfied? It is said, he has the devil in him, and it must be whipped out. Does he speak loudly when spoken to by his master? Then he is getting high-minded, and should be taken down a button-hole lower. Does he forget to pull off his hat at the approach of a white person? Then he is wanting in reverence, and should be whipped for it. Does he ever venture to vindicate his conduct, when censured for it? Then he is guilty of impudence,—one of the greatest crimes of which a slave can be guilty. Does he ever venture to suggest a different mode of doing things from that pointed out by his master? He is indeed presumptuous, and getting above himself; and nothing less than a flogging will do for him. Does he, while ploughing, break a plough,—or, while hoeing, break a hoe? It is owing to his carelessness, and for it a slave must always be whipped. Mr. Hopkins could always find something of this sort to justify the use of the lash, and he seldom failed to embrace such opportunities. There was not a man in the whole county, with whom the slaves who had the getting their own home, would not prefer to live, rather than with this Rev. Mr. Hopkins. And yet there was not a man any where round, who made higher professions of religion, or was more active in revivals,—more attentive to the class, love-feast, prayer and preaching meetings, or more devotional in his family,—that prayed earlier, later, louder, and longer,—than this same reverend slave-driver, Rigby Hopkins.

But to return to Mr. Freeland, and to my experience while in his employment. He, like Mr. Covey, gave us enough to eat; but, unlike Mr. Covey, he also gave us sufficient time to take our meals. He worked us hard, but always between sunrise and sunset. He required a good deal of work to be done, but gave us good tools with which to work. His farm was large, but he employed hands enough to work it, and with ease, compared with many of his neighbors. My treatment, while in his employment, was heavenly, compared with what I experienced at the hands of Mr. Edward Covey.

Mr. Freeland was himself the owner of but two slaves. Their names were Henry Harris and John Harris. The rest of his hands he hired. These consisted of myself, Sandy Jenkins,* and Handy Caldwell. Henry and John were quite intelligent, and in a very little while after I went there, I succeeded in creating in them a strong desire to learn how to read. This desire soon sprang up in the others also. They very soon mustered up some old spelling-books, and nothing would do but that I must keep a Sabbath school. I agreed to do so, and accordingly devoted my Sundays to teaching these my loved fellow-slaves how to read. Neither of them knew his letters when I went there. Some of the slaves of the

---

*This is the same man who gave me the roots to prevent my being whipped by Mr. Covey. He was "a clever soul." We used frequently to talk about the fight with Covey, and as often as we did so, he would claim my success as the result of the roots which he gave me. This superstition is very common among the more ignorant slaves. A slave seldom dies but that his death is attributed to trickery.

neighboring farms found what was going on, and also availed themselves of this little opportunity to learn to read. It was understood, among all who came, that there must be as little display about it as possible. It was necessary to keep our religious masters at St. Michael's unacquainted with the fact, that, instead of spending the Sabbath in wrestling, boxing, and drinking whisky, we were trying to learn how to read the will of God; for they had much rather see us engaged in those degrading sports, than to see us behaving like intellectual, moral, and accountable beings. My blood boils as I think of the bloody manner in which Messrs. Wright Fairbanks and Garrison West, both class-leaders, in connection with many others, rushed in upon us with sticks and stones, and broke up our virtuous little Sabbath school, at St. Michael's—all calling themselves Christians! humble followers of the Lord Jesus Christ! But I am again digressing.

I held my Sabbath school at the house of a free colored man, whose name I deem it imprudent to mention; for should it be known, it might embarrass him greatly, though the crime of holding the school was committed ten years ago. I had at one time over forty scholars, and those of the right sort, ardently desiring to learn. They were of all ages, though mostly men and women. I look back to those Sundays with an amount of pleasure not to be expressed. They were great days to my soul. The work of instructing my dear fellow-slaves was the sweetest engagement with which I was ever blessed. We loved each other, and to leave them at the close of the Sabbath was a severe cross indeed. When I think that these precious souls are to-day shut up in the prison-house of slavery, my feelings overcome me, and I am almost ready to ask, "Does a righteous God govern the universe? and for what does he hold the thunders in his right hand, if not to smite the oppressor, and deliver the spoiled out of the hand of the spoiler?" These dear souls came not to Sabbath school because it was popular to do so, nor did I teach them because it was reputable to be thus engaged. Every moment they spent in that school, they were liable to be taken up, and given thirty-nine lashes. They came because they wished to learn. Their minds had been starved by their cruel masters. They had been shut up in mental darkness. I taught them, because it was the delight of my soul to be doing something that looked like bettering the condition of my race. I kept up my school nearly the whole year I lived with Mr. Freeland; and, beside my Sabbath school, I devoted three evenings in the week, during the winter, to teaching the slaves at home. And I have the happiness to know, that several of those who came to Sabbath school learned how to read; and that one, at least, is now free through my agency.

The year passed off smoothly. It seemed only about half as long as the year which preceded it. I went through it without receiving a single blow. I will give Mr. Freeland the credit of being the best master I ever had, *till I became my own master.* For the ease with which I passed the year, I was, however, somewhat indebted to the society of my fellow-slaves. They were noble souls; they not only possessed loving hearts, but brave ones. We were linked and interlinked with each other. I loved them with a love stronger than any thing I have experienced since. It is sometimes said that we slaves do not love and confide in each other. In answer to this assertion, I can say, I never loved any or confided in any people more than my fellow-slaves, and especially those with whom I lived at Mr. Freeland's. I believe we would have died for each other. We never undertook to do any thing, of any importance, without a mutual consultation. We never moved separately. We were one; and as much so by our tempers and dispositions, as by the mutual hardships to which we were necessarily subjected by our condition as slaves.

At the close of the year 1834, Mr. Freeland again hired me of my master, for the year 1835. But, by this time, I began to want to live *upon free land* as well as *with Freeland*; and I was no longer content, therefore, to live with him or any other slaveholder. I began, with the commencement of the year, to prepare myself for a final struggle, which should decide my fate one way or the other. My tendency was upward. I was fast approaching manhood, and year after year had passed, and I was still a slave. These thoughts roused me—I must do something. I therefore resolved that 1835 should not pass without witnessing an attempt, on my part, to secure my liberty. But I was not willing to cherish this determination alone. My fellow-slaves were dear to me. I was anxious to have them participate with me in this, my life-giving determination. I therefore, though with great prudence, commenced early to ascertain their views and feelings in regard to their condition, and to imbue their minds with thoughts of freedom. I bent myself to devising ways and means for our escape, and meanwhile strove, on all fitting occasions, to impress them with the gross fraud and inhumanity of slavery. I went first to Henry, next to John, then to the others. I found, in them all, warm hearts and noble spirits. They were ready to hear, and ready to act when a feasible plan should be proposed. This was what I wanted. I talked to them of our want of manhood, if we submitted to our enslavement without at least one noble effort to be free. We met often, and consulted frequently, and told our hopes and fears, recounted the difficulties, real and imagined, which we should be called on to meet. At times we were almost disposed to give up, and try to content ourselves with our wretched lot; at others, we were firm and unbending in our determination to go. Whenever we suggested any plan, there was shrinking—the odds were fearful. Our path was beset with the greatest obstacles; and if we succeeded in gaining the end of it, our right to be free was yet questionable—we were yet liable to be returned to bondage. We could see no spot, this side of the ocean, where we could be free. We knew nothing about Canada. Our knowledge of the north did not extend farther than New York; and to go there, and be forever harassed with the frightful liability of being returned to slavery—with the certainty of being treated tenfold worse than before—the thought was truly a horrible one, and one which it was not easy to overcome. The case sometimes stood thus: At every gate through which we were to pass, we saw a watchman—at every ferry a guard—on every bridge a sentinel—and in every wood a patrol. We were hemmed in upon every side. Here were the difficulties, real or imagined—the good to be sought, and the evil to be shunned. On the one hand, there stood slavery, a stern reality, glaring frightfully upon us,—its robes already crimsoned with the blood of millions, and even now feasting itself greedily upon our own flesh. On the other hand, away back in the dim distance, under the flickering light of the north star, behind some craggy hill or snow-covered mountain, stood a doubtful freedom—half frozen—beckoning us to come and share its hospitality. This in itself was sometimes enough to stagger us; but when we permitted ourselves to survey the road, we were frequently appalled. Upon either side we saw grim death, assuming the most horrid shapes. Now it was starvation, causing us to eat our own flesh;—now we were contending with the waves, and were drowned;—now we were overtaken, and torn to pieces by the fangs of the terrible bloodhound. We were stung by scorpions, chased by wild beasts, bitten by snakes, and finally, after having nearly reached the desired spot,—after swimming rivers, encountering wild beasts, sleeping in the woods, suffering hunger and nakedness,—we were overtaken by our pursuers, and, in our resistance, we were shot dead upon the spot! I say, this picture sometimes appalled us, and made us

> "rather bear those ills we had,
> Than fly to others, that we knew not of."

In coming to a fixed determination to run away, we did more than Patrick Henry, when he resolved upon liberty or death. With us it was a doubtful liberty at most, and almost certain death if we failed. For my part, I should prefer death to hopeless bondage.

Sandy, one of our number, gave up the notion, but still encouraged us. Our company then consisted of Henry Harris, John Harris, Henry Bailey, Charles Roberts, and myself. Henry Bailey was my uncle, and belonged to my master. Charles married my aunt: he belonged to my master's father-in-law, Mr. William Hamilton.

The plan we finally concluded upon was, to get a large canoe belonging to Mr. Hamilton, and upon the Saturday night previous to Easter holidays, paddle directly up the Chesapeake Bay. On our arrival at the head of the bay, a distance of seventy or eighty miles from where we lived, it was our purpose to turn our canoe adrift, and follow the guidance of the north star till we got beyond the limits of Maryland. Our reason for taking the water route was, that we were less liable to be suspected as runaways; we hoped to be regarded as fishermen; whereas, if we should take the land route, we should be subjected to interruptions of almost every kind. Any one having a white face, and being so disposed, could stop us, and subject us to examination.

The week before our intended start, I wrote several protections, one for each of us. As well as I can remember, they were in the following words, to wit:—

"THIS is to certify that I, the undersigned, have given the bearer, my servant, full liberty to go to Baltimore, and spend the Easter holidays. Written with mine own hand, &c., 1835.

"WILLIAM HAMILTON,
"Near St. Michael's, in Talbot county, Maryland."

We were not going to Baltimore; but, in going up the bay, we went toward Baltimore, and these protections were only intended to protect us while on the bay.

As the time drew near for our departure, our anxiety became more and more intense. It was truly a matter of life and death with us. The strength of our determination was about to be fully tested. At this time, I was very active in explaining every difficulty, removing every doubt, dispelling every fear, and inspiring all with the firmness indispensable to success in our undertaking; assuring them that half was gained the instant we made the move; we had talked long enough; we were now ready to move; if not now, we never should be; and if we did not intend to move now, we had as well fold our arms, sit down, and acknowledge ourselves fit only to be slaves. This, none of us were prepared to acknowledge. Every man stood firm; and at our last meeting, we pledged ourselves afresh, in the most solemn manner, that, at the time appointed, we would certainly start in pursuit of freedom. This was in the middle of the week, at the end of which we were to be off. We went, as usual, to our several fields of labor, but with bosoms highly agitated with thoughts of our truly hazardous undertaking. We tried to conceal our feelings as much as possible; and I think we succeeded very well.

After a painful waiting, the Saturday morning, whose night was to witness our departure, came. I hailed it with joy, bring what of sadness it might. Friday night was a sleepless one for me. I probably felt more anxious than the rest, because I was, by common consent, at the head of the whole affair. The responsibility of success or failure lay heavily upon me. The glory of the one, and the confusion of the other, were alike mine. The first two hours of that morning were such as I never experienced before, and hope never to again. Early in the morning, we went, as usual, to the field. We were spreading manure; and all at once, while thus engaged, I was overwhelmed with an indescribable feeling, in the fulness of which I turned to Sandy, who was near by, and said, "We are betrayed!" "Well," said he, "that thought has this moment struck me." We said no more. I was never more certain of any thing.

The horn was blown as usual, and we went up from the field to the house for breakfast. I went for the form, more than for want of any thing to eat that morning. Just as I got to the house, in looking out at the lane gate, I saw four white men, with two colored men. The white men were on horseback, and the colored ones were walking behind, as if tied. I watched them a few moments till they got up to our lane gate. Here they halted, and tied the colored men to the gatepost. I was not yet certain as to what the matter was. In a few moments, in rode Mr. Hamilton, with a speed betokening great excitement. He came to the door, and inquired if Master William was in. He was told he was at the barn. Mr. Hamilton, without dismounting, rode up to the barn with extraordinary speed. In a few moments, he and Mr. Freeland returned to the house. By this time, the three constables rode up, and in great haste dismounted, tied their horses, and met Master William and Mr. Hamilton returning from the barn; and after talking awhile, they all walked up to the kitchen door. There was no one in the kitchen but myself and John. Henry and Sandy were up at the barn. Mr. Freeland put his head in at the door, and called me by name, saying, there were some gentlemen at the door who wished to see me. I stepped to the door, and inquired what they wanted. They at once seized me, and, without giving me any satisfaction, tied me—lashing my hands closely together. I insisted upon knowing what the matter was. They at length said, that they had learned I had been in a "scrape," and that I was to be examined before my master; and if their information proved false, I should not be hurt.

In a few moments, they succeeded in tying John. They then turned to Henry, who had by this time returned, and commanded him to cross his hands. "I won't!" said Henry, in a firm tone, indicating his readiness to meet the consequences of his refusal. "Won't you?" said Tom Graham, the constable. "No, I won't!" said Henry, in a still stronger tone. With this, two of the constables pulled out their shining pistols, and swore, by their Creator, that they would make him cross his hands or kill him. Each cocked his pistol, and, with fingers on the trigger, walked up to Henry, saying, at the same time, if he did not cross his hands, they would blow his damned heart out. "Shoot me, shoot me!" said Henry; "you can't kill me but once. Shoot, shoot,—and be damned! *I won't be tied!*" This he said in a tone of loud defiance; and at the same time, with a motion as quick as lightning, he with one single stroke dashed the pistols from the hand of each constable. As he did this, all hands fell upon him, and, after beating him some time, they finally overpowered him, and got him tied.

During the scuffle, I managed, I know not how, to get my pass out, and, without being discovered, put it into the fire. We were all now tied; and just as we were to leave for Easton jail, Betsy Freeland, mother of William Freeland, came to the door with her hands full of biscuits, and divided them between Henry and John. She then delivered herself of a speech, to the following effect:—addressing herself to me, she said, "*You devil! You yellow devil!* it was you that put it into the heads of Henry and John to run away. But for you, you long-legged mulatto devil! Henry nor John would never have thought of such a thing." I made no reply, and was immediately hurried off towards St. Michael's. Just a moment previous to the scuffle with Henry, Mr. Hamilton suggested the propriety of making a search for the protections which he had understood Frederick had written for himself and the rest. But, just at the moment he was about carrying his proposal into effect, his aid was needed in helping to tie Henry; and the excitement attending the scuffle caused them either to forget, or to deem it unsafe, under the circumstances, to search. So we were not yet convicted of the intention to run away.

When we got about half way to St. Michael's, while the constables having us in charge were looking ahead, Henry inquired of me what he should do with his pass. I told him to eat it with his biscuit, and own nothing; and we passed the word around, *"Own nothing;"* and *"Own nothing!"* said we all. Our confidence in each other was unshaken. We were resolved to succeed or fail together, after the calamity had befallen us as much as before. We were now prepared for any thing. We were to be dragged that morning fifteen miles behind horses, and then to be placed in the Easton jail. When we reached St. Michael's, we underwent a sort of examination. We all denied that we ever intended to run away. We did this more to bring out the evidence against us, than from any hope of getting clear of being sold; for, as I have said, we were ready for that. The fact was, we cared but little where we went, so we went together. Our greatest concern was about separation. We dreaded that more than any thing this side of death. We found the evidence against us to be the testimony of one person; our master would not tell who it was; but we came to a unanimous decision among ourselves as to who their informant was. We were sent off to the jail at Easton. When we got there, we were delivered up to the sheriff, Mr. Joseph Graham, and by him placed in jail. Henry, John, and myself, were placed in one room together—Charles, and Henry Bailey, in another. Their object in separating us was to hinder concert.

We had been in jail scarcely twenty minutes, when a swarm of slave traders, and agents for slave traders, flocked into jail to look at us, and to ascertain if we were for sale. Such a set of beings I never saw before! I felt myself surrounded by so many fiends from perdition. A band of pirates never looked more like their father, the devil. They laughed and grinned over us, saying, "Ah, my boys! we have got you, haven't we?" And after taunting us in various ways, they one by one went into an examination of us, with intent to ascertain our value. They would impudently ask us if we would not like to have them for our masters. We would make them no answer, and leave them to find out as best they could. Then they would curse and swear at us, telling us that they could take the devil out of us in a very little while, if we were only in their hands.

While in jail, we found ourselves in much more comfortable quarters than we expected when we went there. We did not get much to eat, nor that which was very good; but we had a good clean room, from the windows of which we could see what was going on in the street, which was very much better than though we had been placed in one of the dark, damp cells. Upon the whole, we got along very well, so far as the jail and its keeper were concerned. Immediately after the holidays were over, contrary to all our expectations, Mr. Hamilton and Mr. Freeland came up to Easton, and took Charles, the two Henrys, and John, out of jail, and carried them home, leaving me alone. I regarded this separation as a final one. It caused me more pain than any thing else in the whole transaction. I was ready for any thing rather than separation. I supposed that they had consulted together, and had decided that, as I was the whole cause of the intention of the others to run away, it was hard to make the innocent suffer with the guilty; and that they had, therefore, concluded to take the others home, and sell me, as a warning to the others that remained. It is due to the noble Henry to say, he seemed almost as reluctant at leaving the prison as at leaving home to come to the prison. But we knew we should, in all probability, be separated, if we were sold; and since he was in their hands, he concluded to go peaceably home.

I was now left to my fate. I was all alone, and within the walls of a stone prison. But a few days before, and I was full of hope. I expected to have been safe in a land of freedom; but now I was covered with gloom, sunk down to the utmost despair. I thought the possibility of freedom was gone. I was kept in this way about one week, at the end of which, Captain Auld, my master, to my surprise and utter astonishment, came up, and took me out, with the intention of sending me, with a gentleman of his acquaintance, into Alabama. But, from some cause or other, he did not send me to Alabama, but concluded to send me back to Baltimore, to live again with his brother Hugh, and to learn a trade.

Thus, after an absence of three years and one month, I was once more permitted to return to my old home at Baltimore. My master sent me away, because there existed against me a very great prejudice in the community, and he feared I might be killed.

In a few weeks after I went to Baltimore, Master Hugh hired me to Mr. William Gardner, an extensive ship-builder, on Fell's Point. I was put there to learn how to calk. It, however, proved a very unfavorable place for the accomplishment of this object. Mr. Gardner was engaged that spring in building two large man-of-war brigs, professedly for the Mexican government. The vessels were to be launched in the July of that year, and in failure thereof, Mr. Gardner was to lose a considerable sum; so that when I entered, all was hurry. There was no time to learn any thing. Every man had to do that which he knew how to do. In entering the ship-yard, my orders from Mr. Gardner were, to do whatever the carpenters commanded me to do. This was placing me at the beck and call of about seventy-five men. I was to regard all these as masters. Their word was to be my law. My situation was a most trying one. At times I needed a dozen pair of hands. I was called a dozen ways in the space of a single minute. Three or four voices would strike my ear at the same moment. It was—"Fred., come help me to cant this timber here."— "Fred., come carry this timber yonder."—"Fred., bring that roller here."—"Fred., go get a fresh can of water."—"Fred., come help saw off the end of this timber."—"Fred., go quick, and get the crowbar."—"Fred., hold on the end of this fall."—"Fred., go to the blacksmith's shop, and get a new punch."—"Hurra, Fred.! run and bring me a cold chisel."—"I say, Fred., bear a hand, and get up a fire as quick as lightning under that steam-box."—"Halloo, nigger! come, turn this grindstone."—"Come, come! move, move! and *bowse* this timber forward."—"I say, darky, blast your eyes, why don't you heat up some pitch?"—"Halloo! halloo! halloo!" (Three voices at the same time.) "Come here!—Go there!—Hold on where you are! Damn you, if you move, I'll knock your brains out!"

This was my school for eight months; and I might have remained there longer, but for a most horrid fight I had with four of the white apprentices, in which my left eye was nearly knocked out, and I was horribly mangled in other respects. The facts in the case were these: Until a very little while after I went there, white and black ship-carpenters worked side by side, and no one seemed to see any impropriety in it. All hands seemed to be very well satisfied. Many of the black carpenters were freemen. Things seemed to be going on very well. All at once, the white carpenters knocked off, and said they would not work with free colored workmen. Their reason for this, as alleged, was, that if free colored carpenters were encouraged, they would soon take the trade into their own hands, and poor white men would be thrown out of employment. They therefore felt called upon at once to put a stop to it. And, taking advantage of Mr. Gardner's necessities, they broke off, swearing they would work no longer, unless he would discharge his black carpenters. Now, though this did not extend to me in form, it did reach me in fact. My fellow-apprentices very soon began to feel it degrading to them to work with me. They began to put on airs, and talk about the "niggers" taking the country, saying we all ought to be killed; and, being encouraged by the journeymen, they commenced making my condition as hard as they could, by hectoring me around, and sometimes striking me. I, of course, kept the vow I made after the fight with Mr. Covey, and struck back again, regardless of consequences; and while I kept them from combining, I succeeded very well; for I could whip the whole of them, taking them separately. They, however, at length combined, and came upon me, armed with sticks, stones, and heavy handspikes. One came in front with a half brick. There was one at each side of me, and one behind me. While I was attending to those in front, and on either side, the one behind ran up with the handspike, and struck me a heavy blow upon the head. It stunned me. I fell, and with this they all ran upon me, and fell to beating me with their fists. I let them lay on for a while, gathering strength. In an instant, I gave a sudden surge, and rose to my hands and knees. Just as I did that, one of their number gave me, with his heavy boot, a powerful kick in the left eye. My eyeball seemed to have burst. When they saw my eye closed, and badly swollen, they left me. With this I seized the handspike, and for a time pursued them. But here the carpenters interfered, and I thought I might as well give it up. It was impossible to stand my hand against so many. All this took place in sight of not less than fifty white ship-carpenters, and not one interposed a friendly word; but some cried, "Kill the

damned nigger! Kill him! kill him! He struck a white person."
I found my only chance for life was in flight. I succeeded in
getting away without an additional blow, and barely so; for
to strike a white man is death by Lynch law,—and that was
the law in Mr. Gardner's ship-yard; nor is there much of any
other out of Mr. Gardner's ship-yard.

I went directly home, and told the story of my wrongs to
Master Hugh; and I am happy to say of him, irreligious as he
was, his conduct was heavenly, compared with that of his
brother Thomas under similar circumstances. He listened attentively to my narration of the circumstances leading to the
savage outrage, and gave many proofs of his strong indignation at it. The heart of my once overkind mistress was again
melted into pity. My puffed-out eye and blood-covered face
moved her to tears. She took a chair by me, washed the blood
from my face, and, with a mother's tenderness, bound up my
head, covering the wounded eye with a lean piece of fresh
beef. It was almost compensation for my suffering to witness,
once more, a manifestation of kindness from this, my once
affectionate old mistress. Master Hugh was very much enraged. He gave expression to his feelings by pouring out
curses upon the heads of those who did the deed. As soon as I
got a little the better of my bruises, he took me with him to
Esquire Watson's, on Bond Street, to see what could be done
about the matter. Mr. Watson inquired who saw the assault
committed. Master Hugh told him it was done in Mr. Gardner's ship-yard, at mid-day, where there were a large company of men at work. "As to that," he said, "the deed was
done, and there was no question as to who did it." His answer was, he could do nothing in the case, unless some white
man would come forward and testify. He could issue no warrant on my word. If I had been killed in the presence of a
thousand colored people, their testimony combined would
have been insufficient to have arrested one of the murderers.
Master Hugh, for once, was compelled to say this state of
things was too bad. Of course, it was impossible to get any
white man to volunteer his testimony in my behalf, and
against the white young men. Even those who may have sympathized with me were not prepared to do this. It required a

degree of courage unknown to them to do so; for just at that time, the slightest manifestation of humanity toward a colored person was denounced as abolitionism, and that name subjected its bearer to frightful liabilities. The watchwords of the bloody-minded in that region, and in those days, were, "Damn the abolitionists!" and "Damn the niggers!" There was nothing done, and probably nothing would have been done if I had been killed. Such was, and such remains, the state of things in the Christian city of Baltimore.

Master Hugh, finding he could get no redress, refused to let me go back again to Mr. Gardner. He kept me himself, and his wife dressed my wound till I was again restored to health. He then took me into the ship-yard of which he was foreman, in the employment of Mr. Walter Price. There I was immediately set to calking, and very soon learned the art of using my mallet and irons. In the course of one year from the time I left Mr. Gardner's, I was able to command the highest wages given to the most experienced calkers. I was now of some importance to my master. I was bringing him from six to seven dollars per week. I sometimes brought him nine dollars per week: my wages were a dollar and a half a day. After learning how to calk, I sought my own employment, made my own contracts, and collected the money which I earned. My pathway became much more smooth than before; my condition was now much more comfortable. When I could get no calking to do, I did nothing. During these leisure times, those old notions about freedom would steal over me again. When in Mr. Gardner's employment, I was kept in such a perpetual whirl of excitement, I could think of nothing, scarcely, but my life; and in thinking of my life, I almost forgot my liberty. I have observed this in my experience of slavery,—that whenever my condition was improved, instead of its increasing my contentment, it only increased my desire to be free, and set me to thinking of plans to gain my freedom. I have found that, to make a contented slave, it is necessary to make a thoughtless one. It is necessary to darken his moral and mental vision, and, as far as possible, to annihilate the power of reason. He must be able to detect no inconsistencies in slavery; he must be made to feel that slavery is right; and he can be brought to that only when he ceases to be a man.

I was now getting, as I have said, one dollar and fifty cents per day. I contracted for it; I earned it; it was paid to me; it was rightfully my own; yet, upon each returning Saturday night, I was compelled to deliver every cent of that money to Master Hugh. And why? Not because he earned it,—not because he had any hand in earning it,—not because I owed it to him,—nor because he possessed the slightest shadow of a right to it; but solely because he had the power to compel me to give it up. The right of the grim-visaged pirate upon the high seas is exactly the same.

CHAPTER XI.

I NOW come to that part of my life during which I planned, and finally succeeded in making, my escape from slavery. But before narrating any of the peculiar circumstances, I deem it proper to make known my intention not to state all the facts connected with the transaction. My reasons for pursuing this course may be understood from the following: First, were I to give a minute statement of all the facts, it is not only possible, but quite probable, that others would thereby be involved in the most embarrassing difficulties. Secondly, such a statement would most undoubtedly induce greater vigilance on the part of slaveholders than has existed heretofore among them; which would, of course, be the means of guarding a door whereby some dear brother bondman might escape his galling chains. I deeply regret the necessity that impels me to suppress any thing of importance connected with my experience in slavery. It would afford me great pleasure indeed, as well as materially add to the interest of my narrative, were I at liberty to gratify a curiosity, which I know exists in the minds of many, by an accurate statement of all the facts pertaining to my most fortunate escape. But I must deprive myself of this pleasure, and the curious of the gratification which such a statement would afford. I would allow myself to suffer under the greatest imputations which evil-minded men might suggest, rather than exculpate myself, and thereby run the hazard of closing the slightest avenue by which a brother slave might clear himself of the chains and fetters of slavery.

I have never approved of the very public manner in which some of our western friends have conducted what they call the *underground railroad*, but which, I think, by their open declarations, has been made most emphatically the *upperground railroad*. I honor those good men and women for their noble daring, and applaud them for willingly subjecting themselves to bloody persecution, by openly avowing their participation in the escape of slaves. I, however, can see very little good resulting from such a course, either to themselves or the slaves escaping; while, upon the other hand, I see and feel assured that those open declarations are a positive evil to the slaves remaining, who are seeking to escape. They do nothing towards enlightening the slave, whilst they do much towards enlightening the master. They stimulate him to greater watchfulness, and enhance his power to capture his slave. We owe something to the slaves south of the line as well as to those north of it; and in aiding the latter on their way to freedom, we should be careful to do nothing which would be likely to hinder the former from escaping from slavery. I would keep the merciless slaveholder profoundly ignorant of the means of flight adopted by the slave. I would leave him to imagine himself surrounded by myriads of invisible tormentors, ever ready to snatch from his infernal grasp his trembling prey. Let him be left to feel his way in the dark; let darkness commensurate with his crime hover over him; and let him feel that at every step he takes, in pursuit of the flying bondman, he is running the frightful risk of having his hot brains dashed out by an invisible agency. Let us render the tyrant no aid; let us not hold the light by which he can trace the footprints of our flying brother. But enough of this. I will now proceed to the statement of those facts, connected with my escape, for which I am alone responsible, and for which no one can be made to suffer but myself.

In the early part of the year 1838, I became quite restless. I could see no reason why I should, at the end of each week, pour the reward of my toil into the purse of my master.

When I carried to him my weekly wages, he would, after counting the money, look me in the face with a robber-like fierceness, and ask, "Is this all?" He was satisfied with nothing less than the last cent. He would, however, when I made him six dollars, sometimes give me six cents, to encourage me. It had the opposite effect. I regarded it as a sort of admission of my right to the whole. The fact that he gave me any part of my wages was proof, to my mind, that he believed me entitled to the whole of them. I always felt worse for having received any thing; for I feared that the giving me a few cents would ease his conscience, and make him feel himself to be a pretty honorable sort of robber. My discontent grew upon me. I was ever on the look-out for means of escape; and, finding no direct means, I determined to try to hire my time, with a view of getting money with which to make my escape. In the spring of 1838, when Master Thomas came to Baltimore to purchase his spring goods, I got an opportunity, and applied to him to allow me to hire my time. He unhesitatingly refused my request, and told me this was another stratagem by which to escape. He told me I could go nowhere but that he could get me; and that, in the event of my running away, he should spare no pains in his efforts to catch me. He exhorted me to content myself, and be obedient. He told me, if I would be happy, I must lay out no plans for the future. He said, if I behaved myself properly, he would take care of me. Indeed, he advised me to complete thoughtlessness of the future, and taught me to depend solely upon him for happiness. He seemed to see fully the pressing necessity of setting aside my intellectual nature, in order to contentment in slavery. But in spite of him, and even in spite of myself, I continued to think, and to think about the injustice of my enslavement, and the means of escape.

About two months after this, I applied to Master Hugh for the privilege of hiring my time. He was not acquainted with the fact that I had applied to Master Thomas, and had been refused. He too, at first, seemed disposed to refuse; but, after some reflection, he granted me the privilege, and proposed the following terms: I was to be allowed all my time, make all contracts with those for whom I worked, and find my own employment; and, in return for this liberty, I was to pay him three dollars at the end of each week; find myself in calking tools, and in board and clothing. My board was two dollars and a half per week. This, with the wear and tear of clothing and calking tools, made my regular expenses about six dollars per week. This amount I was compelled to make up, or relinquish the privilege of hiring my time. Rain or shine, work or no work, at the end of each week the money must be forthcoming, or I must give up my privilege. This arrangement, it will be perceived, was decidedly in my master's favor. It relieved him of all need of looking after me. His money was sure. He received all the benefits of slaveholding without its evils; while I endured all the evils of a slave, and suffered all the care and anxiety of a freeman. I found it a hard bargain. But, hard as it was, I thought it better than the old mode of getting along. It was a step towards freedom to be allowed to bear the responsibilities of a freeman, and I was determined to hold on upon it. I bent myself to the work of making money. I was ready to work at night as well as day, and by the most untiring perseverance and industry, I made enough to meet my expenses, and lay up a little money every week. I went on thus from May till August. Master Hugh then refused to allow me to hire my time longer. The ground for his refusal was a failure on my part, one Saturday night, to pay him for my week's time. This failure was occasioned by my attending a camp meeting about ten miles from Baltimore. During the week, I had entered into an engagement with a number of young friends to start from Baltimore to the camp ground early Saturday evening; and being detained by my employer, I was unable to get down to Master Hugh's without disappointing the company. I knew that Master Hugh was in no special need of the money that night. I therefore decided to go to camp meeting, and upon my return pay him the three dollars. I staid at the camp meeting one day longer than I intended when I left. But as soon as I returned, I called upon him to pay him what he considered his due. I found him very angry; he could scarce restrain his wrath. He said he had a great mind to give me a severe whipping. He wished to know how I dared go out of the city without asking his permission. I told him I hired my time, and while I paid him the price which he asked for it, I did not know that I was bound to ask him when and where I should go. This reply troubled him; and, after reflecting a few moments, he turned to me, and said I should hire my time no longer; that the next thing he should know of, I would be running away. Upon the same plea, he told me to bring my tools and clothing home forthwith. I did so; but instead of seeking work, as I had been accustomed to do previously to hiring my time, I spent the whole week without the performance of a single stroke of work. I did this in retaliation. Saturday night, he called upon me as usual for my week's wages. I told him I had no wages; I had done no work that week. Here we were upon the point of coming to blows. He raved, and swore his determination to get hold of me. I did not allow myself a single word; but was resolved, if he laid the weight of his hand upon me, it should be blow for blow. He did not strike me, but told me that he would find me in constant employment in future. I thought the matter over during the next day, Sunday, and finally resolved upon the third day of September, as the day upon which I would make a second attempt to secure my freedom. I now had three weeks during which to prepare for my journey. Early on Monday morning, before Master Hugh had time to make any engagement for me, I went out and got employment of Mr. Butler, at his ship-yard near the drawbridge, upon what is called the City Block, thus making it unnecessary for him to seek employment for me. At the end of the week, I brought him between eight and nine dollars. He seemed very well pleased, and asked me why I did not do the same the week before. He little knew what my plans were. My object in working steadily was to remove any suspicion he might entertain of my intent to run away; and in this I succeeded admirably. I suppose he thought I was never better satisfied with my condition than at the very time during which I was planning my escape. The second week passed, and again I carried him my full wages; and so well pleased was he, that he gave me twenty-five cents, (quite a large sum for a slaveholder to give a slave,) and bade me to make a good use of it. I told him I would.

Things went on without very smoothly indeed, but within there was trouble. It is impossible for me to describe my feelings as the time of my contemplated start drew near. I had a number of warm-hearted friends in Baltimore,—friends that I loved almost as I did my life,—and the thought of being separated from them forever was painful beyond expression. It is my opinion that thousands would escape from slavery, who now remain, but for the strong cords of affection that bind them to their friends. The thought of leaving my friends was decidedly the most painful thought with which I had to contend. The love of them was my tender point, and shook my decision more than all things else. Besides the pain of separation, the dread and apprehension of a failure exceeded what I had experienced at my first attempt. The appalling defeat I then sustained returned to torment me. I felt assured that, if I failed in this attempt, my case would be a hopeless one—it would seal my fate as a slave forever. I could not hope to get off with any thing less than the severest punishment, and being placed beyond the means of escape. It required no very vivid imagination to depict the most frightful scenes through which I should have to pass, in case I failed. The wretchedness of slavery, and the blessedness of freedom, were perpetually before me. It was life and death with me. But I remained firm, and, according to my resolution, on the third day of September, 1838, I left my chains, and succeeded in reaching New York without the slightest interruption of any kind. How I did so,—what means I adopted,—what direction I travelled, and by what mode of conveyance,—I must leave unexplained, for the reasons before mentioned.

I have been frequently asked how I felt when I found myself in a free State. I have never been able to answer the question with any satisfaction to myself. It was a moment of the highest excitement I ever experienced. I suppose I felt as one may imagine the unarmed mariner to feel when he is rescued by a friendly man-of-war from the pursuit of a pirate. In writing to a dear friend, immediately after my arrival at New York, I said I felt like one who had escaped a den of hungry lions. This state of mind, however, very soon subsided; and I was again seized with a feeling of great insecurity and loneliness. I was yet liable to be taken back, and subjected to all the tortures of slavery. This in itself was enough to damp the ardor of my enthusiasm. But the loneliness overcame me. There I was in the midst of thousands, and yet a perfect stranger; without home and without friends, in the midst of thousands of my own brethren—children of a common Father, and yet I dared not to unfold to any one of them my sad condition. I was afraid to speak to any one for fear of speaking to the wrong one, and thereby falling into the hands of money-loving kidnappers, whose business it was to lie in wait for the panting fugitive, as the ferocious beasts of the forest lie in wait for their prey. The motto which I adopted when I started from slavery was this—"Trust no man!" I saw in every white man an enemy, and in almost every colored man cause for distrust. It was a most painful situation; and, to understand it, one must needs experience it, or imagine himself in similar circumstances. Let him be a fugitive slave in a strange land—a land given up to be the hunting-ground for slave-holders—whose inhabitants are legalized kidnappers—where he is every moment subjected to the terrible liability of being seized upon by his fellow-men, as the hideous crocodile seizes upon his prey!—I say, let him place himself in my situation—without home or friends—without money or credit—wanting shelter, and no one to give it—wanting bread, and no money to buy it,—and at the same time let him feel that he is pursued by merciless men-hunters, and in total darkness as to what to do, where to go, or where to stay,—perfectly helpless both as to the means of defence and means of escape,—in the midst of plenty, yet suffering the terrible gnawings of hunger,—in the midst of houses, yet having no home,—among fellow-men, yet feeling as if in the midst of wild beasts, whose greediness to swallow up the trembling and half-famished fugitive is only equalled by that with which the monsters of the deep swallow up the helpless fish upon which they subsist,—I say, let him be placed in this most trying situation,—the situation in which I was placed,—then, and not till then, will he fully appreciate the hardships of, and know how to sympathize with, the toil-worn and whip-scarred fugitive slave.

Thank Heaven, I remained but a short time in this distressed situation. I was relieved from it by the humane hand of Mr. DAVID RUGGLES, whose vigilance, kindness, and perseverance, I shall never forget. I am glad of an opportunity to express, as far as words can, the love and gratitude I bear him.

Mr. Ruggles is now afflicted with blindness, and is himself in need of the same kind offices which he was once so forward in the performance of toward others. I had been in New York but a few days, when Mr. Ruggles sought me out, and very kindly took me to his boarding-house at the corner of Church and Lespenard Streets. Mr. Ruggles was then very deeply engaged in the memorable *Darg* case, as well as attending to a number of other fugitive slaves, devising ways and means for their successful escape; and, though watched and hemmed in on almost every side, he seemed to be more than a match for his enemies.

Very soon after I went to Mr. Ruggles, he wished to know of me where I wanted to go; as he deemed it unsafe for me to remain in New York. I told him I was a calker, and should like to go where I could get work. I thought of going to Canada; but he decided against it, and in favor of my going to New Bedford, thinking I should be able to get work there at my trade. At this time, Anna,* my intended wife, came on; for I wrote to her immediately after my arrival at New York, (notwithstanding my homeless, houseless, and helpless condition,) informing her of my successful flight, and wishing her to come on forthwith. In a few days after her arrival, Mr. Ruggles called in the Rev. J. W. C. Pennington, who, in the presence of Mr. Ruggles, Mrs. Michaels, and two or three others, performed the marriage ceremony, and gave us a certificate, of which the following is an exact copy:—

> "THIS may certify, that I joined together in holy matrimony Frederick Johnson† and Anna Murray, as man and wife, in the presence of Mr. David Ruggles and Mrs. Michaels.
>
> "JAMES W. C. PENNINGTON.
> "*New York, Sept. 15, 1838.*"

Upon receiving this certificate, and a five-dollar bill from Mr. Ruggles, I shouldered one part of our baggage, and Anna took up the other, and we set out forthwith to take passage on board of the steamboat John W. Richmond for Newport, on our way to New Bedford. Mr. Ruggles gave me

*She was free.
†I had changed my name from Frederick *Bailey* to that of *Johnson*.

a letter to a Mr. Shaw in Newport, and told me, in case my money did not serve me to New Bedford, to stop in Newport and obtain further assistance; but upon our arrival at Newport, we were so anxious to get to a place of safety, that, notwithstanding we lacked the necessary money to pay our fare, we decided to take seats in the stage, and promise to pay when we got to New Bedford. We were encouraged to do this by two excellent gentlemen, residents of New Bedford, whose names I afterward ascertained to be Joseph Ricketson and William C. Taber. They seemed at once to understand our circumstances, and gave us such assurance of their friendliness as put us fully at ease in their presence. It was good indeed to meet with such friends, at such a time. Upon reaching New Bedford, we were directed to the house of Mr. Nathan Johnson, by whom we were kindly received, and hospitably provided for. Both Mr. and Mrs. Johnson took a deep and lively interest in our welfare. They proved themselves quite worthy of the name of abolitionists. When the stage-driver found us unable to pay our fare, he held on upon our baggage as security for the debt. I had but to mention the fact to Mr. Johnson, and he forthwith advanced the money.

We now began to feel a degree of safety, and to prepare ourselves for the duties and responsibilities of a life of freedom. On the morning after our arrival at New Bedford, while at the breakfast-table, the question arose as to what name I should be called by. The name given me by my mother was, "Frederick Augustus Washington Bailey." I, however, had dispensed with the two middle names long before I left Maryland, so that I was generally known by the name of "Frederick Bailey." I started from Baltimore bearing the name of "Stanley." When I got to New York, I again changed my name to "Frederick Johnson," and thought that would be the last change. But when I got to New Bedford, I found it necessary again to change my name. The reason of this necessity was, that there were so many Johnsons in New Bedford, it was already quite difficult to distinguish between them. I gave Mr. Johnson the privilege of choosing me a name, but told him he must not take from me the name of "Frederick." I must hold on to that, to preserve a sense of my identity. Mr. Johnson had just been reading the "Lady of the Lake," and at once suggested that my name be "Douglass." From that time until now I have been called "Frederick Douglass;" and as I am more widely known by that name than by either of the others, I shall continue to use it as my own.

I was quite disappointed at the general appearance of things in New Bedford. The impression which I had received respecting the character and condition of the people of the north, I found to be singularly erroneous. I had very strangely supposed, while in slavery, that few of the comforts, and scarcely any of the luxuries, of life were enjoyed at the north, compared with what were enjoyed by the slaveholders of the south. I probably came to this conclusion from the fact that northern people owned no slaves. I supposed that they were about upon a level with the non-slaveholding population of the south. I knew *they* were exceedingly poor, and I had been accustomed to regard their poverty as the necessary consequence of their being non-slaveholders. I had somehow imbibed the opinion that, in the absence of slaves, there could be no wealth, and very little refinement. And upon coming to the north, I expected to meet with a rough, hard-handed, and uncultivated population, living in the most Spartan-like simplicity, knowing nothing of the ease, luxury, pomp, and grandeur of southern slaveholders. Such being my conjectures, any one acquainted with the appearance of New Bedford may very readily infer how palpably I must have seen my mistake.

In the afternoon of the day when I reached New Bedford, I visited the wharves, to take a view of the shipping. Here I found myself surrounded with the strongest proofs of wealth. Lying at the wharves, and riding in the stream, I saw many ships of the finest model, in the best order, and of the largest size. Upon the right and left, I was walled in by granite warehouses of the widest dimensions, stowed to their utmost capacity with the necessaries and comforts of life. Added to this, almost every body seemed to be at work, but noiselessly so, compared with what I had been accustomed to in Baltimore. There were no loud songs heard from those engaged in loading and unloading ships. I heard no deep oaths or horrid curses on the laborer. I saw no whipping of men; but all seemed to go smoothly on. Every man appeared to understand his work, and went at it with a sober, yet cheerful earnestness, which betokened the deep interest which he felt in what he was doing, as well as a sense of his own dignity as a man. To me this looked exceedingly strange. From the wharves I strolled around and over the town, gazing with wonder and admiration at the splendid churches, beautiful dwellings, and finely-cultivated gardens; evincing an amount of wealth, comfort, taste, and refinement, such as I had never seen in any part of slaveholding Maryland.

Every thing looked clean, new, and beautiful. I saw few or no dilapidated houses, with poverty-stricken inmates; no half-naked children and barefooted women, such as I had been accustomed to see in Hillsborough, Easton, St. Michael's, and Baltimore. The people looked more able, stronger, healthier, and happier, than those of Maryland. I was for once made glad by a view of extreme wealth, without being saddened by seeing extreme poverty. But the most astonishing as well as the most interesting thing to me was the condition of the colored people, a great many of whom, like myself, had escaped thither as a refuge from the hunters of men. I found many, who had not been seven years out of their chains, living in finer houses, and evidently enjoying more of the comforts of life, than the average of slaveholders in Maryland. I will venture to assert that my friend Mr. Nathan Johnson (of whom I can say with a grateful heart, "I was hungry, and he gave me meat; I was thirsty, and he gave me drink; I was a stranger, and he took me in") lived in a neater house; dined at a better table; took, paid for, and read, more newspapers; better understood the moral, religious, and political character of the nation,—than nine tenths of the slaveholders in Talbot county, Maryland. Yet Mr. Johnson was a working man. His hands were hardened by toil, and not his alone, but those also of Mrs. Johnson. I found the colored people much more spirited than I had supposed they would be. I found among them a determination to protect each other from the blood-thirsty kidnapper, at all hazards. Soon after my arrival, I was told of a circumstance which illustrated their spirit. A colored man and a fugitive slave were on unfriendly terms. The former was heard to threaten the latter with informing his master of his whereabouts. Straightway a meeting was called among the colored people, under the stereotyped notice, "Business of importance!" The betrayer was invited to attend. The people came at the appointed hour, and organized the meeting by appointing a very religious old gentleman as president, who, I believe, made a prayer, after which he addressed the meeting as follows: *"Friends, we have got him here, and I would recommend that you young men just take him outside the door, and kill him!"* With this, a number of them bolted at him; but they were intercepted by some more timid than themselves, and the betrayer escaped their vengeance, and has not been seen in New Bedford since. I believe there have been no more such threats, and should there be hereafter, I doubt not that death would be the consequence.

I found employment, the third day after my arrival, in stowing a sloop with a load of oil. It was new, dirty, and hard work for me; but I went at it with a glad heart and a willing hand. I was now my own master. It was a happy moment, the rapture of which can be understood only by those who have been slaves. It was the first work, the reward of which was to be entirely my own. There was no Master Hugh standing ready, the moment I earned the money, to rob me of it. I worked that day with a pleasure I had never before experienced. I was at work for myself and newly-married wife. It was to me the starting-point of a new existence. When I got through with that job, I went in pursuit of a job of calking; but such was the strength of prejudice against color, among the white calkers, that they refused to work with me, and of course I could get no employment.* Finding my trade of no immediate benefit, I threw off my calking habiliments, and prepared myself to do any kind of work I could get to do. Mr. Johnson kindly let me have his wood-horse and saw, and I very soon found myself a plenty of work. There was no work too hard—none too dirty. I was ready to saw wood, shovel coal, carry the hod, sweep the chimney, or roll oil casks,—all of which I did for nearly three years in New Bedford, before I became known to the anti-slavery world.

In about four months after I went to New Bedford, there came a young man to me, and inquired if I did not wish to

---

*I am told that colored persons can now get employment at calking in New Bedford—a result of anti-slavery effort.

take the "Liberator." I told him I did; but, just having made my escape from slavery, I remarked that I was unable to pay for it then. I, however, finally became a subscriber to it. The paper came, and I read it from week to week with such feelings as it would be quite idle for me to attempt to describe. The paper became my meat and my drink. My soul was set all on fire. Its sympathy for my brethren in bonds—its scathing denunciations of slaveholders—its faithful exposures of slavery—and its powerful attacks upon the upholders of the institution—sent a thrill of joy through my soul, such as I had never felt before!

I had not long been a reader of the "Liberator," before I got a pretty correct idea of the principles, measures and spirit of the anti-slavery reform. I took right hold of the cause. I could do but little; but what I could, I did with a joyful heart, and never felt happier than when in an anti-slavery meeting. I seldom had much to say at the meetings, because what I wanted to say was said so much better by others. But, while attending an anti-slavery convention at Nantucket, on the 11th of August, 1841, I felt strongly moved to speak, and was at the same time much urged to do so by Mr. William C. Coffin, a gentleman who had heard me speak in the colored people's meeting at New Bedford. It was a severe cross, and I took it up reluctantly. The truth was, I felt myself a slave, and the idea of speaking to white people weighed me down. I spoke but a few moments, when I felt a degree of freedom, and said what I desired with considerable ease. From that time until now, I have been engaged in pleading the cause of my brethren—with what success, and with what devotion, I leave those acquainted with my labors to decide.

APPENDIX.

I find, since reading over the foregoing Narrative, that I have, in several instances, spoken in such a tone and manner, respecting religion, as may possibly lead those unacquainted with my religious views to suppose me an opponent of all religion. To remove the liability of such misapprehension, I deem it proper to append the following brief explanation. What I have said respecting and against religion, I mean strictly to apply to the *slaveholding religion* of this land, and with no possible reference to Christianity proper; for, between the Christianity of this land, and the Christianity of Christ, I recognize the widest possible difference—so wide, that to receive the one as good, pure, and holy, is of necessity to reject the other as bad, corrupt, and wicked. To be the friend of the one, is of necessity to be the enemy of the other. I love the pure, peaceable, and impartial Christianity of Christ: I therefore hate the corrupt, slaveholding, women-whipping, cradle-plundering, partial and hypocritical Christianity of this land. Indeed, I can see no reason, but the most deceitful one, for calling the religion of this land Christianity. I look upon it as the climax of all misnomers, the boldest of all frauds, and the grossest of all libels. Never was there a clearer case of "stealing the livery of the court of heaven to serve the devil in." I am filled with unutterable loathing when I contemplate the religious pomp and show, together with the horrible inconsistencies, which every where surround me. We have men-stealers for ministers, women-whippers for missionaries, and cradle-plunderers for church members. The man who wields the blood-clotted cowskin during the week fills the pulpit on Sunday, and claims to be a minister of the meek and lowly Jesus. The man who robs me of my earnings at the end of each week meets me as a class-leader on Sunday morning, to show me the way of life, and the path of salvation. He who sells my sister, for purposes of prostitution, stands forth as the pious advocate of purity. He who proclaims it a religious duty to read the Bible denies me the right of learning to read the name of the God who made me. He who is the religious advocate of marriage robs whole millions of its sacred influence, and leaves them to the ravages of wholesale pollution. The warm defender of the sacredness of the family relation is the same that scatters whole families,—sundering husbands and wives, parents and children, sisters and brothers,—leaving the hut vacant, and the hearth desolate. We see the thief preaching against theft, and the adulterer against adultery. We have men sold to build churches, women sold to support the gospel, and babes sold to purchase Bibles for the *poor heathen! all for the glory of God and the good of souls!* The slave auctioneer's bell and the church-going bell chime in with each other, and the bitter cries of the heart-broken slave are drowned in the religious shouts of his pious master. Revivals of religion and revivals in the slave-trade go hand in hand together. The slave prison and the church stand near each other. The clanking of fetters and the rattling of chains in the prison, and the pious psalm and solemn prayer in the church, may be heard at the same time. The dealers in the bodies and souls of men erect their stand in the presence of the pulpit, and they mutually help each other. The dealer gives his blood-stained gold to support the pulpit, and the pulpit, in return, covers his infernal business with the garb of Christianity. Here we have religion and robbery the allies of each other—devils dressed in angels' robes, and hell presenting the semblance of paradise.

> "Just God! and these are they,
>   Who minister at thine altar, God of right!
>   Men who their hands, with prayer and blessing, lay
>   On Israel's ark of light.
>
> "What! preach, and kidnap men?
>   Give thanks, and rob thy own afflicted poor?
>   Talk of thy glorious liberty, and then
>   Bolt hard the captive's door?
>
> "What! servants of thy own
>   Merciful Son, who came to seek and save
>   The homeless and the outcast, fettering down
>   The tasked and plundered slave!

"Pilate and Herod friends!
Chief priests and rulers, as of old, combine!
Just God and holy! is that church which lends
Strength to the spoiler thine?"

The Christianity of America is a Christianity, of whose votaries it may be as truly said, as it was of the ancient scribes and Pharisees, "They bind heavy burdens, and grievous to be borne, and lay them on men's shoulders, but they themselves will not move them with one of their fingers. All their works they do for to be seen of men.——They love the uppermost rooms at feasts, and the chief seats in the synagogues, ... and to be called of men, Rabbi, Rabbi.——But woe unto you, scribes and Pharisees, hypocrites! for ye shut up the kingdom of heaven against men; for ye neither go in yourselves, neither suffer ye them that are entering to go in. Ye devour widows' houses, and for a pretence make long prayers; therefore ye shall receive the greater damnation. Ye compass sea and land to make one proselyte, and when he is made, ye make him twofold more the child of hell than yourselves. ——Woe unto you, scribes and Pharisees, hypocrites! for ye pay tithe of mint, and anise, and cumin, and have omitted the weightier matters of the law, judgment, mercy, and faith; these ought ye to have done, and not to leave the other undone. Ye blind guides! which strain at a gnat, and swallow a camel. Woe unto you, scribes and Pharisees, hypocrites! for ye make clean the outside of the cup and of the platter; but within, they are full of extortion and excess.——Woe unto you, scribes and Pharisees, hypocrites! for ye are like unto whited sepulchres, which indeed appear beautiful outward, but are within full of dead men's bones, and of all uncleanness. Even so ye also outwardly appear righteous unto men, but within ye are full of hypocrisy and iniquity."

Dark and terrible as is this picture, I hold it to be strictly true of the overwhelming mass of professed Christians in America. They strain at a gnat, and swallow a camel. Could any thing be more true of our churches? They would be shocked at the proposition of fellowshipping a *sheep*-stealer; and at the same time they hug to their communion a *man-*

stealer, and brand me with being an infidel, if I find fault with them for it. They attend with Pharisaical strictness to the outward forms of religion, and at the same time neglect the weightier matters of the law, judgment, mercy, and faith. They are always ready to sacrifice, but seldom to show mercy. They are they who are represented as professing to love God whom they have not seen, whilst they hate their brother whom they have seen. They love the heathen on the other side of the globe. They can pray for him, pay money to have the Bible put into his hand, and missionaries to instruct him; while they despise and totally neglect the heathen at their own doors.

Such is, very briefly, my view of the religion of this land; and to avoid any misunderstanding, growing out of the use of general terms, I mean, by the religion of this land, that which is revealed in the words, deeds, and actions, of those bodies, north and south, calling themselves Christian churches, and yet in union with slaveholders. It is against religion, as presented by these bodies, that I have felt it my duty to testify.

I conclude these remarks by copying the following portrait of the religion of the south, (which is, by communion and fellowship, the religion of the north,) which I soberly affirm is "true to the life," and without caricature or the slightest exaggeration. It is said to have been drawn, several years before the present anti-slavery agitation began, by a northern Methodist preacher, who, while residing at the south, had an opportunity to see slaveholding morals, manners, and piety, with his own eyes. "Shall I not visit for these things? saith the Lord. Shall not my soul be avenged on such a nation as this?"

"A PARODY.

"Come, saints and sinners, hear me tell
How pious priests whip Jack and Nell,
And women buy and children sell,
And preach all sinners down to hell,
And sing of heavenly union.

"They'll bleat and baa, dona like goats,
 Gorge down black sheep, and strain at motes,
 Array their backs in fine black coats,
 Then seize their negroes by their throats,
     And choke, for heavenly union.

"They'll church you if you sip a dram,
 And damn you if you steal a lamb;
 Yet rob old Tony, Doll, and Sam,
 Of human rights, and bread and ham;
     Kidnapper's heavenly union.

"They'll loudly talk of Christ's reward,
 And bind his image with a cord,
 And scold, and swing the lash abhorred,
 And sell their brother in the Lord
     To handcuffed heavenly union.

"They'll read and sing a sacred song,
 And make a prayer both loud and long,
 And teach the right and do the wrong,
 Hailing the brother, sister throng,
     With words of heavenly union.

"We wonder how such saints can sing,
 Or praise the Lord upon the wing,
 Who roar, and scold, and whip, and sting,
 And to their slaves and mammon cling,
     In guilty conscience union.

"They'll raise tobacco, corn, and rye,
 And drive, and thieve, and cheat, and lie,
 And lay up treasures in the sky,
 By making switch and cowskin fly,
     In hope of heavenly union.

"They'll crack old Tony on the skull,
 And preach and roar like Bashan bull,
 Or braying ass, of mischief full,
 Then seize old Jacob by the wool,
     And pull for heavenly union.

"A roaring, ranting, sleek man-thief,
 Who lived on mutton, veal, and beef,
 Yet never would afford relief
 To needy, sable sons of grief,
     Was big with heavenly union.

" 'Love not the world,' the preacher said,
 And winked his eye, and shook his head;
 He seized on Tom, and Dick, and Ned,
 Cut short their meat, and clothes, and bread,
     Yet still loved heavenly union.

"Another preacher whining spoke
 Of One whose heart for sinners broke:
 He tied old Nanny to an oak,
 And drew the blood at every stroke,
     And prayed for heavenly union.

"Two others oped their iron jaws,
 And waved their children-stealing paws;
 There sat their children in gewgaws;
 By stinting negroes' backs and maws,
     They kept up heavenly union.

"All good from Jack another takes,
 And entertains their flirts and rakes,
 Who dress as sleek as glossy snakes,
 And cram their mouths with sweetened cakes;
     And this goes down for union."

Sincerely and earnestly hoping that this little book may do something toward throwing light on the American slave system, and hastening the glad day of deliverance to the millions of my brethren in bonds—faithfully relying upon the power of truth, love, and justice, for success in my humble efforts—and solemnly pledging myself anew to the sacred cause,—I subscribe myself,

FREDERICK DOUGLASS.

Lynn, *Mass., April 28, 1845.*

NARRATIVE

OF

WILLIAM W. BROWN,

A

FUGITIVE SLAVE.

WRITTEN BY HIMSELF.

————Is there not some chosen curse,
Some hidden thunder in the stores of heaven,
Red with uncommon wrath, to blast the man
Who gains his fortune from the blood of souls?
COWPER.

BOSTON:
PUBLISHED AT THE ANTI-SLAVERY OFFICE,
No. 25 CORNHILL.
1847.

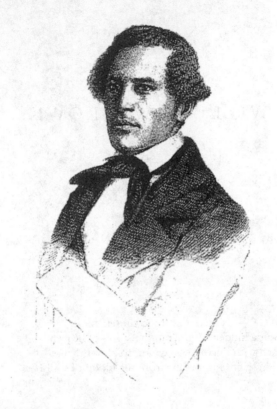

Wm. W. Brown.

TO WELLS BROWN, OF OHIO.

THIRTEEN years ago, I came to your door, a weary fugitive from chains and stripes. I was a stranger, and you took me in. I was hungry, and you fed me. Naked was I, and you clothed me. Even a name by which to be known among men, slavery had denied me. You bestowed upon me your own. Base indeed should I be, if I ever forget what I owe to you, or do anything to disgrace that honored name!

As a slight testimony of my gratitude to my earliest benefactor, I take the liberty to inscribe to you this little Narrative of the sufferings from which I was fleeing when you had compassion upon me. In the multitude that you have succored, it is very possible that you may not remember me; but until I forget God and myself, I can never forget you.

Your grateful friend,
WILLIAM WELLS BROWN.

LETTER FROM
EDMUND QUINCY, ESQ.

DEDHAM, JULY 1, 1847.

TO WILLIAM W. BROWN.

MY DEAR FRIEND:—I heartily thank you for the privilege of reading the manuscript of your Narrative. I have read it with deep interest and strong emotion. I am much mistaken if it be not greatly successful and eminently useful. It presents a different phase of the infernal slave-system from that portrayed in the admirable story of Mr. Douglass, and gives us a glimpse of its hideous cruelties in other portions of its domain.

Your opportunities of observing the workings of this accursed system have been singularly great. Your experiences in the Field, in the House, and especially on the River in the service of the slave-trader, Walker, have been such as few individuals have had;—no one, certainly, who has been competent to describe them. What I have admired, and marvelled at, in your Narrative, is the simplicity and calmness with which you describe scenes and actions which might well "move the very stones to rise and mutiny" against the National Institution which makes them possible.

You will perceive that I have made very sparing use of your flattering permission to alter what you had written. To correct a few errors, which appeared to be merely clerical ones, committed in the hurry of composition, under unfavorable circumstances, and to suggest a few curtailments, is all that I have ventured to do. I should be a bold man, as well as a vain one, if I should attempt to improve your descriptions of what you have seen and suffered. Some of the scenes are not unworthy of De Foe himself.

I trust and believe that your Narrative will have a wide circulation. I am sure it deserves it. At least, a man must be differently constituted from me, who can rise from the perusal of your Narrative without feeling that he understands slavery better, and hates it worse, than he ever did before.

I am, very faithfully and respectfully,

Your friend,

EDMUND QUINCY.

PREFACE.

THE FRIENDS of freedom may well congratulate each other on the appearance of the following Narrative. It adds another volume to the rapidly increasing anti-slavery literature of the age. It has been remarked by a close observer of human nature, "Let me make the songs of a nation, and I care not who makes its laws;" and it may with equal truth be said, that, among a reading people like our own, their books will at least give character to their laws. It is an influence which goes forth noiselessly upon its mission, but fails not to find its way to many a warm heart, to kindle on the altar thereof the fires of freedom, which will one day break forth in a living flame to consume oppression.

This little book is a voice from the prison-house, unfolding the deeds of darkness which are there perpetrated. Our cause has received efficient aid from this source. The names of those who have come from thence, and battled manfully for the right, need not to be recorded here. The works of some of them are an enduring monument of praise, and their perpetual record shall be found in the grateful hearts of the redeemed bondman.

Few persons have had greater facilities for becoming acquainted with slavery, in all its horrible aspects, than WILLIAM W. BROWN. He has been behind the curtain. He has visited its secret chambers. Its iron has entered his own soul. The dearest ties of nature have been riven in his own person. A mother has been cruelly scourged before his own eyes. A father,—alas! slaves have no father. A brother has been made the subject of its tender mercies. A sister has been given up to the irresponsible control of the pale-faced oppressor. This nation looks on approvingly. The American Union sanctions the deed. The Constitution shields the criminals. American religion sanctifies the crime. But the tide is turning. Already, a mighty under-current is sweeping onward. The voice of warning, of remonstrance, of rebuke, of entreaty, has gone forth. Hand is linked in hand, and heart mingles with heart, in this great work of the slave's deliverance.

The convulsive throes of the monster, even now, give evidence of deep wounds.

The writer of this Narrative was hired by his master to a "*soul-driver*," and has witnessed all the horrors of the traffic, from the buying up of human cattle in the slave-breeding States, which produced a constant scene of separating the victims from all those whom they loved, to their final sale in the southern market, to be worked up in seven years, or given over to minister to the lust of southern *Christians*.

Many harrowing scenes are graphically portrayed; and yet with that simplicity and ingenuousness which carries with it a conviction of the truthfulness of the picture.

This book will do much to unmask those who have "clothed themselves in the livery of the court of heaven" to cover up the enormity of their deeds.

During the past three years, the author has devoted his entire energies to the anti-slavery cause. Laboring under all the disabilities and disadvantages growing out of his education in slavery—subjected, as he had been from his birth, to all the wrongs and deprivations incident to his condition—he yet went forth, impelled to the work by a love of liberty—stimulated by the remembrance of his own sufferings—urged on by the consideration that a mother, brothers, and sister, were still grinding in the prison-house of bondage, in common with three millions of our Father's children—sustained by an unfaltering faith in the omnipotence of truth and the final triumph of justice—to plead the cause of the slave, and by the eloquence of earnestness carried conviction to many minds, and enlisted the sympathy and secured the co-operation of many to the cause.

His labors have been chiefly confined to Western New York, where he has secured many warm friends, by his untiring zeal, persevering energy, continued fidelity, and universal kindness.

Reader, are you an Abolitionist? What have you done for the slave? What are you doing in his behalf? What do you purpose to do? There is a great work before us! Who will be an idler now? This is the great humanity movement of the age, swallowing up, for the time being, all other questions, com-

paratively speaking. The course of human events, in obedience to the unchangeable laws of our being, is fast hastening
the final crisis, and

> "Have ye chosen, O my people, on whose party ye shall
>   stand,
>   Ere the Doom from its worn sandal shakes the dust
>   against our land?"

Are you a Christian? This is the carrying out of practical
Christianity; and there is no other. Christianity is *practical* in
its very nature and essence. It is a life, springing out of a soul
imbued with its spirit. Are you a friend of the missionary
cause? This is the greatest missionary enterprize of the day.
Three millions of *Christian*, law-manufactured heathen are
longing for the glad tidings of the Gospel of freedom. Are
you a friend of the Bible? Come, then, and help us to restore
to these millions, whose eyes have been bored out by slavery,
their sight, that they may see to read the Bible. Do you love
God whom you have not seen? Then manifest that love, by
restoring to your brother whom you have seen, his rightful
inheritance, of which he has been so long and so cruelly deprived.

It is not for a single generation alone, numbering three millions—sublime as would be that effort—that we are working.
It is for HUMANITY, the wide world over, not only now, but
for all coming time, and all future generations:—

> "For he who settles Freedom's principles,
>   Writes the death-warrant of all tyranny."

It is a vast work—a glorious enterprize—worthy the un-
swerving devotion of the entire life-time of the great and the
good.

Slaveholding and slaveholders must be rendered disrep-
utable and odious. They must be stripped of their respectability and Christian reputation. They must be treated as
"MEN-STEALERS—guilty of the highest kind of theft, and sinners of the first rank." Their more guilty accomplices in the
persons of *northern apologists*, both in Church and State, must
be placed in the same category. Honest men must be made to

look upon their crimes with the same abhorrence and loathing, with which they regard the less guilty robber and assassin, until

> "The common damned shun their society,
> And look upon themselves as fiends less foul."

When a just estimate is placed upon the crime of slaveholding, the work will have been accomplished, and the glorious day ushered in—

> "When man nor woman in all our wide domain,
> Shall buy, or sell, or hold, or be a slave."

J. C. HATHAWAY.

—Farmington, N. Y., 1847.

NARRATIVE.

CHAPTER I.

I was born in Lexington, Ky. The man who stole me as soon as I was born, recorded the births of all the infants which he claimed to be born his property, in a book which he kept for that purpose. My mother's name was Elizabeth. She had seven children, viz: Solomon, Leander, Benjamin, Joseph, Millford, Elizabeth, and myself. No two of us were children of the same father. My father's name, as I learned from my mother, was George Higgins. He was a white man, a relative of my master, and connected with some of the first families in Kentucky.

My master owned about forty slaves, twenty-five of whom were field hands. He removed from Kentucky to Missouri, when I was quite young, and settled thirty or forty miles above St. Charles, on the Missouri, where, in addition to his practice as a physician, he carried on milling, merchandizing and farming. He had a large farm, the principal productions of which were tobacco and hemp. The slave cabins were situated on the back part of the farm, with the house of the overseer, whose name was Grove Cook, in their midst. He had the entire charge of the farm, and having no family, was allowed a woman to keep house for him, whose business it was to deal out the provisions for the hands.

A woman was also kept at the quarters to do the cooking for the field hands, who were summoned to their unrequited toil every morning at four o'clock, by the ringing of a bell, hung on a post near the house of the overseer. They were allowed half an hour to eat their breakfast, and get to the field. At half past four, a horn was blown by the overseer, which was the signal to commence work; and every one that was not on the spot at the time, had to receive ten lashes from the negro-whip, with which the overseer always went armed. The handle was about three feet long, with the butt-end filled with lead, and the lash six or seven feet in length, made of cowhide, with platted wire on the end of it. This whip was put in requisition very frequently and freely, and a small offence on the part of a slave furnished an occasion for its use. During the time that Mr. Cook was overseer, I was a house servant—a situation preferable to that of a field hand, as I was better fed, better clothed, and not obliged to rise at the ringing of the bell, but about half an hour after. I have often laid and heard the crack of the whip, and the screams of the slave. My mother was a field hand, and one morning was ten or fifteen minutes behind the others in getting into the field. As soon as she reached the spot where they were at work, the overseer commenced whipping her. She cried, "Oh! pray—Oh! pray—Oh! pray"—these are generally the words of slaves, when imploring mercy at the hands of their oppressors. I heard her voice, and knew it, and jumped out of my bunk, and went to the door. Though the field was some distance from the house, I could hear every crack of the whip, and every groan and cry of my poor mother. I remained at the door, not daring to venture any farther. The cold chills ran over me, and I wept aloud. After giving her ten lashes, the sound of the whip ceased, and I returned to my bed, and found no consolation but in my tears. It was not yet daylight.

CHAPTER II.

MY master being a political demagogue, soon found those who were ready to put him into office, for the favors he could render them; and a few years after his arrival in Missouri, he was elected to a seat in the Legislature. In his absence from home, everything was left in charge of Mr. Cook, the overseer, and he soon became more tyrannical and cruel. Among the slaves on the plantation, was one by the name of Randall. He was a man about six feet high, and well-proportioned, and known as a man of great strength and power. He was considered the most valuable and able-bodied slave on the plantation; but no matter how good or useful a slave may be, he seldom escapes the lash. But it was not so with Randall. He had been on the plantation since my earliest recollection, and

I had never known of his being flogged. No thanks were due to the master or overseer for this. I have often heard him declare, that no white man should ever whip him—that he would die first.

Cook, from the time that he came upon the plantation, had frequently declared, that he could and would flog any nigger that was put into the field to work under him. My master had repeatedly told him not to attempt to whip Randall, but he was determined to try it. As soon as he was left sole dictator, he thought the time had come to put his threats into execution. He soon began to find fault with Randall, and threatened to whip him, if he did not do better. One day he gave him a very hard task,—more than he could possibly do; and at night, the task not being performed, he told Randall that he should remember him the next morning. On the following morning, after the hands had taken breakfast, Cook called out to Randall, and told him that he intended to whip him, and ordered him to cross his hands and be tied. Randall asked why he wished to whip him. He answered, because he had not finished his task the day before. Randall said that the task was too great, or he should have done it. Cook said it made no difference,—he should whip him. Randall stood silent for a moment, and then said, "Mr. Cook, I have always tried to please you since you have been on the plantation, and I find you are determined not to be satisfied with my work, let me do as well as I may. No man has laid hands on me, to whip me, for the last ten years, and I have long since come to the conclusion not to be whipped by any man living." Cook, finding by Randall's determined look and gestures, that he would resist, called three of the hands from their work, and commanded them to seize Randall, and tie him. The hands stood still;—they knew Randall—and they also knew him to be a powerful man, and were afraid to grapple with him. As soon as Cook had ordered the men to seize him, Randall turned to them, and said—"Boys, you all know me; you know that I can handle any three of you, and the man that lays hands on me shall die. This white man can't whip me himself, and therefore he has called you to help him." The overseer was unable to prevail upon them to seize and secure Randall, and finally ordered them all to go to their work together.

Nothing was said to Randall by the overseer, for more than a week. One morning, however, while the hands were at work in the field, he came into it, accompanied by three friends of his, Thompson, Woodbridge and Jones. They came up to where Randall was at work, and Cook ordered him to leave his work, and go with them to the barn. He refused to go; whereupon he was attacked by the overseer and his companions, when he turned upon them, and laid them, one after another, prostrate on the ground. Woodbridge drew out his pistol, and fired at him, and brought him to the ground by a pistol ball. The others rushed upon him with their clubs, and beat him over the head and face, until they succeeded in tying him. He was then taken to the barn, and tied to a beam. Cook gave him over one hundred lashes with a heavy cowhide, had him washed with salt and water, and left him tied during the day. The next day he was untied, and taken to a blacksmith's shop, and had a ball and chain attached to his leg. He was compelled to labor in the field, and perform the same amount of work that the other hands did. When his master returned home, he was much pleased to find that Randall had been subdued in his absence.

CHAPTER III.

SOON afterwards, my master removed to the city of St. Louis, and purchased a farm four miles from there, which he placed under the charge of an overseer by the name of Friend Haskell. He was a regular Yankee from New England. The Yankees are noted for making the most cruel overseers.

My mother was hired out in the city, and I was also hired out there to Major Freeland, who kept a public house. He was formerly from Virginia, and was a horse-racer, cock-fighter, gambler, and withal an inveterate drunkard. There were ten or twelve servants in the house, and when he was present, it was cut and slash—knock down and drag out. In his fits of anger, he would take up a chair, and throw it at a servant; and in his more rational moments, when he wished to chastise one, he would tie them up in the smoke-house, and whip them; after which, he would cause a fire to be made of tobacco stems, and smoke them. This he called "*Virginia play.*"

I complained to my master of the treatment which I received from Major Freeland; but it made no difference. He cared nothing about it, so long as he received the money for my labor. After living with Major Freeland five or six months, I ran away, and went into the woods back of the city; and when night came on, I made my way to my master's farm, but was afraid to be seen, knowing that if Mr. Haskell, the overseer, should discover me, I should be again carried back to Major Freeland; so I kept in the woods. One day, while in the woods, I heard the barking and howling of dogs, and in a short time they came so near, that I knew them to be the bloodhounds of Major Benjamin O'Fallon. He kept five or six, to hunt runaway slaves with.

As soon as I was convinced that it was them, I knew there was no chance of escape. I took refuge in the top of a tree, and the hounds were soon at its base, and there remained until the hunters came up in a half or three quarters of an hour afterwards. There were two men with the dogs, who, as soon as they came up, ordered me to descend. I came down, was tied, and taken to St. Louis jail. Major Freeland soon made his appearance, and took me out, and ordered me to follow him, which I did. After we returned home, I was tied up in the smoke-house, and was very severely whipped. After the Major had flogged me to his satisfaction, he sent out his son Robert, a young man eighteen or twenty years of age, to see that I was well smoked. He made a fire of tobacco stems, which soon set me to coughing and sneezing. This, Robert told me, was the way his father used to do to his slaves in Virginia. After giving me what they conceived to be a decent smoking, I was untied and again set to work.

Robert Freeland was a "chip of the old block." Though quite young, it was not unfrequently that he came home in a state of intoxication. He is now, I believe, a popular commander of a steamboat on the Mississippi river. Major Freeland soon after failed in business, and I was put on board the steamboat Missouri, which plied between St. Louis and Galena. The commander of the boat was William B. Culver. I remained on her during the sailing season, which was the most pleasant time for me that I had ever experienced. At the close of navigation, I was hired to Mr. John Colburn, keeper of the Missouri Hotel. He was from one of the Free States; but a more inveterate hater of the negro, I do not believe ever walked on God's green earth. This hotel was at that time one of the largest in the city, and there were employed in it twenty or thirty servants, mostly slaves.

Mr. Colburn was very abusive, not only to the servants, but to his wife also, who was an excellent woman, and one from whom I never knew a servant to receive a harsh word; but never did I know a kind one to a servant from her husband. Among the slaves employed in the hotel, was one by the name of Aaron, who belonged to Mr. John F. Darby, a lawyer. Aaron was the knife-cleaner. One day, one of the knives was put on the table, not as clean as it might have been. Mr. Colburn, for this offence, tied Aaron up in the wood-house, and gave him over fifty lashes on the bare back with a cowhide, after which, he made me wash him down with rum. This seemed to put him into more agony than the whipping. After being untied, he went home to his master, and complained of the treatment which he had received. Mr. Darby would give no heed to anything he had to say, but sent him directly back. Colburn, learning that he had been to his master with complaints, tied him up again, and gave him a more severe whipping than before. The poor fellow's back was literally cut to pieces; so much so, that he was not able to work for ten or twelve days.

There was also, among the servants, a girl whose master resided in the country. Her name was Patsey. Mr. Colburn tied her up one evening, and whipped her until several of the boarders came out and begged him to desist. The reason for whipping her was this. She was engaged to be married to a man belonging to Major William Christy, who resided four or five miles north of the city. Mr. Colburn had forbid her to see John Christy. The reason of this was said to be the regard which he himself had for Patsey. She went to meeting that evening, and John returned home with her. Mr. Colburn had intended to flog John, if he came within the inclosure; but John knew too well the temper of his rival, and kept at a safe distance;—so he took vengeance on the poor girl. If all the slave-drivers had been called together, I do not think a more cruel man than John Colburn,—and he too a northern man,—could have been found among them.

While living at the Missouri Hotel, a circumstance occurred which caused me great unhappiness. My master sold my mother, and all her children, except myself. They were sold to different persons in the city of St. Louis.

CHAPTER IV.

I WAS soon after taken from Mr. Colburn's, and hired to Elijah P. Lovejoy, who was at that time publisher and editor of the "St. Louis Times." My work, while with him, was mainly in the printing office, waiting on the hands, working the press, &c. Mr. Lovejoy was a very good man, and decidedly the best master that I had ever had. I am chiefly indebted to him, and to my employment in the printing office, for what little learning I obtained while in slavery.

Though slavery is thought, by some, to be mild in Missouri, when compared with the cotton, sugar and rice growing States, yet no part of our slave-holding country, is more noted for the barbarity of its inhabitants, than St. Louis. It was here that Col. Harney, a United States officer, whipped a slave woman to death. It was here that Francis McIntosh, a free colored man from Pittsburgh, was taken from the steamboat Flora, and burned at the stake. During a residence of eight years in this city, numerous cases of extreme cruelty came under my own observation;—to record them all, would occupy more space than could possibly be allowed in this little volume. I shall, therefore, give but a few more, in addition to what I have already related.

Capt. J. B. Brunt, who resided near my master, had a slave named John. He was his body servant, carriage driver, &c. On one occasion, while driving his master through the city,— the streets being very muddy, and the horses going at a rapid rate,— some mud spattered upon a gentleman by the name of Robert More. More was determined to be revenged. Some three or four months after this occurrence, he purchased John, for the express purpose, as he said, "to tame the d——d nigger." After the purchase, he took him to a blacksmith's shop, and had a ball and chain fastened to his leg, and then put him to driving a yoke of oxen, and kept him at hard labor, until the iron around his leg was so worn into the flesh, that it was thought mortification would ensue. In addition to this, John told me that his master whipped him regularly three times a week for the first two months:—and all this to "*tame him.*" A more noble looking man than he, was not to be found in all St. Louis, before he fell into the hands of More; and a more degraded and spirit-crushed looking being was never seen on a southern plantation, after he had been subjected to this "*taming*" process for three months. The last time that I saw him, he had nearly lost the entire use of his limbs.

While living with Mr. Lovejoy, I was often sent on errands to the office of the "Missouri Republican," published by Mr. Edward Charles. Once, while returning to the office with type, I was attacked by several large boys, sons of slave-holders, who pelted me with snow-balls. Having the heavy form of type in my hands, I could not make my escape by running; so I laid down the type and gave them battle. They gathered around me, pelting me with stones and sticks, until they overpowered me, and would have captured me, if I had not resorted to my heels. Upon my retreat, they took possession of the type; and what to do to regain it I could not devise. Knowing Mr. Lovejoy to be a very humane man, I went to the office, and laid the case before him. He told me to remain in the office. He took one of the apprentices with him, and went after the type, and soon returned with it; but on his return informed me that Samuel McKinney had told him that he would whip me, because I had hurt his boy. Soon after, McKinney was seen making his way to the office by one of the printers, who informed me of the fact, and I made my escape through the back door.

McKinney not being able to find me on his arrival, left the office in a great rage, swearing that he would whip me to death. A few days after, as I was walking along Main Street, he seized me by the collar, and struck me over the head five or six times with a large cane, which caused the blood to gush from my nose and ears in such a manner that my clothes were completely saturated with blood. After beating me to his satisfaction, he let me go, and I returned to the office so weak from the loss of blood, that Mr. Lovejoy sent me home to my master. It was five weeks before I was able to walk again. During this time, it was necessary to have some one to supply my place at the office, and I lost the situation.

After my recovery, I was hired to Capt. Otis Reynolds, as a waiter on board the steamboat Enterprize, owned by Messrs. John and Edward Walsh, commission merchants at St. Louis. This boat was then running on the upper Mississippi. My employment on board was to wait on gentlemen, and the captain being a good man, the situation was a pleasant one to me;— but in passing from place to place, and seeing new faces every day, and knowing that they could go where they pleased, I soon became unhappy, and several times thought of leaving the boat at some landing place, and trying to make my escape to Canada, which I had heard much about as a place where the slave might live, be free, and be protected.

But whenever such thoughts would come into my mind, my resolution would soon be shaken by the remembrance that my dear mother was a slave in St. Louis, and I could not bear the idea of leaving her in that condition. She had often taken me upon her knee, and told me how she had carried me upon her back to the field when I was an infant—how often she had been whipped for leaving her work to nurse me—and how happy I would appear when she would take me into her arms. When these thoughts came over me, I would resolve never to leave the land of slavery without my mother. I thought that to leave her in slavery, after she had undergone and suffered so much for me, would be proving recreant to the duty which I owed to her. Besides this, I had three brothers and a sister there,—two of my brothers having died.

My mother, my brothers Joseph and Millford, and my sister Elizabeth, belonged to Mr. Isaac Mansfield, formerly from one of the Free States, (Massachusetts, I believe.) He was a tinner by trade, and carried on a large manufacturing establishment. Of all my relatives, mother was first, and sister next. One evening, while visiting them, I made some allusion to a proposed journey to Canada, and sister took her seat by my side, and taking my hand in hers, said, with tears in her eyes,—

"Brother, you are not going to leave mother and your dear sister here without a friend, are you?"

I looked into her face, as the tears coursed swiftly down her cheeks, and bursting into tears myself, said—

"No, I will never desert you and mother."

She clasped my hand in hers, and said—

"Brother, you have often declared that you would not end your days in slavery. I see no possible way in which you can escape with us; and now, brother, you are on a steamboat where there is some chance for you to escape to a land of liberty. I beseech you not to let us hinder you. If we cannot get our liberty, we do not wish to be the means of keeping you from a land of freedom."

I could restrain my feelings no longer, and an outburst of my own feelings, caused her to cease speaking upon that subject. In opposition to their wishes, I pledged myself not to leave them in the hand of the oppressor. I took leave of them, and returned to the boat, and laid down in my bunk; but "sleep departed from my eyes, and slumber from my eyelids."

A few weeks after, on our downward passage, the boat took on board, at Hannibal, a drove of slaves, bound for the New Orleans market. They numbered from fifty to sixty, consisting of men and women from eighteen to forty years of age. A drove of slaves on a southern steamboat, bound for the cotton or sugar regions, is an occurrence so common, that no one, not even the passengers, appear to notice it, though they clank their chains at every step. There was, however, one in this gang that attracted the attention of the passengers and crew. It was a beautiful girl, apparently about twenty years of age, perfectly white, with straight light hair and blue eyes. But it was not the whiteness of her skin that created such a sensation among those who gazed upon her—it was her almost unparalleled beauty. She had been on the boat but a short time, before the attention of all the passengers, including the ladies, had been called to her, and the common topic of conversation was about the beautiful slave-girl. She was not in chains. The man who claimed this article of human merchandize was a

Mr. Walker,—a well known slave-trader, residing in St. Louis. There was a general anxiety among the passengers and crew to learn the history of the girl. Her master kept close by her side, and it would have been considered impudent for any of the passengers to have spoken to her, and the crew were not allowed to have any conversation with them. When we reached St. Louis, the slaves were removed to a boat bound for New Orleans, and the history of the beautiful slave-girl remained a mystery.

I remained on the boat during the season, and it was not an unfrequent occurrence to have on board gangs of slaves on their way to the cotton, sugar and rice plantations of the South.

Toward the latter part of the summer, Captain Reynolds left the boat, and I was sent home. I was then placed on the farm under Mr. Haskell, the overseer. As I had been some time out of the field, and not accustomed to work in the burning sun, it was very hard; but I was compelled to keep up with the best of the hands.

I found a great difference between the work in a steamboat cabin and that in a corn-field.

My master, who was then living in the city, soon after removed to the farm, when I was taken out of the field to work in the house as a waiter. Though his wife was very peevish, and hard to please, I much preferred to be under her control than the overseer's. They brought with them Mr. Sloane, a Presbyterian minister; Miss Martha Tulley, a neice of theirs from Kentucky; and their nephew William. The latter had been in the family a number of years, but the others were all new-comers.

Mr. Sloane was a young minister, who had been at the South but a short time, and it seemed as if his whole aim was to please the slaveholders, especially my master and mistress. He was intending to make a visit during the winter, and he not only tried to please them, but I think he succeeded admirably. When they wanted singing, he sung; when they wanted praying, he prayed; when they wanted a story told, he told a story. Instead of his teaching my master theology, my master taught theology to him. While I was with Captain Reynolds, my master "got religion," and new laws were made on the plantation. Formerly, we had the privilege of hunting, fishing, making splint brooms, baskets, &c. on Sunday; but this was all stopped. Every Sunday, we were all compelled to attend meeting. Master was so religious, that he induced some others to join him in hiring a preacher to preach to the slaves.

CHAPTER V.

My master had family worship, night and morning. At night, the slaves were called in to attend; but in the mornings, they had to be at their work, and master did all the praying. My master and mistress were great lovers of mint julep, and every morning, a pitcher-full was made, of which they all partook freely, not excepting little master William. After drinking freely all round, they would have family worship, and then breakfast. I cannot say but I loved the julep as well as any of them, and during prayer was always careful to seat myself close to the table where it stood, so as to help myself when they were all busily engaged in their devotions. By the time prayer was over, I was about as happy as any of them. A sad accident happened one morning. In helping myself, and at the same time keeping an eye on my old mistress, I accidentally let the pitcher fall upon the floor, breaking it in pieces, and spilling the contents. This was a bad affair for me; for as soon as prayer was over, I was taken and severely chastised.

My master's family consisted of himself, his wife, and their nephew, William Moore. He was taken into the family, when only a few weeks of age. His name being that of my own, mine was changed, for the purpose of giving precedence to his, though I was his senior by ten or twelve years. The plantation being four miles from the city, I had to drive the family to church. I always dreaded the approach of the Sabbath; for, during service, I was obliged to stand by the horses in the hot broiling sun, or in the rain, just as it happened.

One Sabbath, as we were driving past the house of D. D. Page, a gentleman who owned a large baking establishment, as I was sitting upon the box of the carriage, which was very much elevated, I saw Mr. Page pursuing a slave around the yard, with a long whip, cutting him at every jump. The man soon escaped from the yard, and was followed by Mr. Page. They came running past us, and the slave perceiving that he would be overtaken, stopped suddenly, and Page stumbled over him, and falling on the stone pavement, fractured one of his legs, which crippled him for life. The same gentleman, but a short time previous, tied up a woman of his, by the name of Delphia, and whipped her nearly to death; yet he was a deacon in the Baptist church, in good and regular standing. Poor Delphia! I was well acquainted with her, and called to see her while upon her sick bed; and I shall never forget her appearance. She was a member of the same church with her master.

Soon after this, I was hired out to Mr. Walker; the same man whom I have mentioned as having carried a gang of slaves down the river, on the steamboat Enterprize. Seeing me in the capacity of steward on the boat, and thinking that I would make a good hand to take care of slaves, he determined to have me for that purpose; and finding that my master would not sell me, he hired me for the term of one year.

When I learned the fact of my having been hired to a negro speculator, or a "soul-driver" as they are generally called among slaves, no one can tell my emotions. Mr. Walker had offered a high price for me, as I afterwards learned, but I suppose my master was restrained from selling me by the fact that I was a near relative of his. On entering the service of Mr. Walker, I found that my opportunity of getting to a land of liberty was gone, at least for the time being. He had a gang of slaves in readiness to start for New Orleans, and in a few days we were on our journey. I am at a loss for language to express my feelings on that occasion. Although my master had told me that he had not sold me, and Mr. Walker had told me that he had not purchased me, I did not believe them; and not until I had been to New Orleans, and was on my return, did I believe that I was not sold.

There was on the boat a large room on the lower deck, in which the slaves were kept, men and women, promiscuously—all chained two and two, and a strict watch kept that they did not get loose; for cases have occurred in which slaves have got off their chains, and made their escape at landing-places, while the boats were taking in wood;—and with all our care, we lost one woman who had been taken from her husband and children, and having no desire to live without them, in the agony of her soul jumped overboard, and drowned herself. She was not chained.

It was almost impossible to keep that part of the boat clean.

On landing at Natchez, the slaves were all carried to the slave-pen, and there kept one week, during which time, several of them were sold. Mr. Walker fed his slaves well. We took on board, at St. Louis, several hundred pounds of bacon (smoked meat) and corn-meal, and his slaves were better fed than slaves generally were in Natchez, so far as my observation extended.

At the end of a week, we left for New Orleans, the place of our final destination, which we reached in two days. Here the slaves were placed in a negro-pen, where those who wished to purchase could call and examine them. The negro-pen is a small yard, surrounded by buildings, from fifteen to twenty feet wide, with the exception of a large gate with iron bars. The slaves are kept in the buildings during the night, and turned out into the yard during the day. After the best of the stock was sold at private sale at the pen, the balance were taken to the Exchange Coffee House Auction Rooms, kept by Isaac L. McCoy, and sold at public auction. After the sale of this lot of slaves, we left New Orleans for St. Louis.

CHAPTER VI.

On our arrival at St. Louis, I went to Dr. Young, and told him that I did not wish to live with Mr. Walker any longer. I was heart-sick at seeing my fellow-creatures bought and sold. But the Dr. had hired me for the year, and stay I must. Mr. Walker again commenced purchasing another gang of slaves. He bought a man of Colonel John O'Fallon, who resided in the suburbs of the city. This man had a wife and three children. As soon as the purchase was made, he was put in jail for safe keeping, until we should be ready to start for New Orleans. His wife visited him while there, several times, and several times when she went for that purpose was refused admittance.

In the course of eight or nine weeks Mr. Walker had his cargo of human flesh made up. There was in this lot a number of old men and women, some of them with gray locks. We left St. Louis in the steamboat Carlton, Captain Swan, bound for New Orleans. On our way down, and before we reached Rodney, the place where we made our first stop, I had to prepare the old slaves for market. I was ordered to have the old men's whiskers shaved off, and the grey hairs plucked out, where they were not too numerous, in which case he had a preparation of blacking to color it, and with a blacking-brush we would put it on. This was new business to me, and was performed in a room where the passengers could not see us. These slaves were also taught how old they were by Mr. Walker, and after going through the blacking process, they looked ten or fifteen years younger; and I am sure that some of those who purchased slaves of Mr. Walker, were dreadfully cheated, especially in the ages of the slaves which they bought.

We landed at Rodney, and the slaves were driven to the pen in the back part of the village. Several were sold at this place, during our stay of four or five days, when we proceeded to Natchez. There we landed at night, and the gang were put in the warehouse until morning, when they were driven to the pen. As soon as the slaves are put in these pens, swarms of planters may be seen in and about them. They knew when Walker was expected, as he always had the time advertised beforehand when he would be in Rodney, Natchez, and New Orleans. These were the principal places where he offered his slaves for sale.

When at Natchez the second time, I saw a slave very cruelly whipped. He belonged to a Mr. Broadwell, a merchant who kept a store on the wharf. The slave's name was Lewis. I had known him several years, as he was formerly from St. Louis. We were expecting a steamboat down the river, in which we were to take passage for New Orleans. Mr. Walker sent me to the landing to watch for the boat, ordering me to inform him on its arrival. While there, I went into the store to see Lewis. I saw a slave in the store, and asked him where Lewis was. Said he, "They have got Lewis hanging between the heavens and the earth." I asked him what he meant by that. He told me to go into the warehouse and see. I went in, and found Lewis there. He was tied up to a beam, with his toes just touching the floor. As there was no one in the warehouse but himself, I inquired the reason of his being in that situation. He said Mr. Broadwell had sold his wife to a planter six miles from the city, and that he had been to visit her,— that he went in the night, expecting to return before daylight, and went without his master's permission. The patrol had taken him up before he reached his wife. He was put in jail, and his master had to pay for his catching and keeping, and that was what he was tied up for.

Just as he finished his story, Mr. Broadwell came in, and inquired what I was doing there. I knew not what to say, and while I was thinking what reply to make, he struck me over the head with the cowhide, the end of which struck me over my right eye, sinking deep into the flesh, leaving a scar which I carry to this day. Before I visited Lewis, he had received fifty lashes. Mr. Broadwell gave him fifty lashes more after I came out, as I was afterwards informed by Lewis himself.

The next day we proceeded to New Orleans, and put the gang in the same negro-pen which we occupied before. In a short time, the planters came flocking to the pen to purchase slaves. Before the slaves were exhibited for sale, they were dressed and driven out into the yard. Some were set to dancing, some to jumping, some to singing, and some to playing cards. This was done to make them appear cheerful and happy. My business was to see that they were placed in those situations before the arrival of the purchasers, and I have often set them to dancing when their cheeks were wet with tears. As slaves were in good demand at that time, they were all soon disposed of, and we again set out for St. Louis.

On our arrival, Mr. Walker purchased a farm five or six miles from the city. He had no family, but made a housekeeper of one of his female slaves. Poor Cynthia! I knew her well. She was a quadroon, and one of the most beautiful women I ever saw. She was a native of St. Louis, and bore an irreproachable character for virtue and propriety of conduct. Mr. Walker bought her for the New Orleans market, and took her down with him on one of the trips that I made with him. Never shall I forget the circumstances of that voyage! On the first night that we were on board the steamboat, he directed me to put her into a state-room he had provided for her, apart from the other slaves. I had seen too much of the workings of slavery, not to know what this meant. I accordingly watched him into the state-room, and listened to hear what passed between them. I heard him make his base offers, and her reject them. He told her that if she would accept his vile proposals, he would take her back with him to St. Louis, and establish her as his housekeeper at his farm. But if she persisted in rejecting them, he would sell her as a field hand on the worst plantation on the river. Neither threats nor bribes prevailed, however, and he retired, disappointed of his prey.

The next morning, poor Cynthia told me what had past, and bewailed her sad fate with floods of tears. I comforted and encouraged her all I could; but I foresaw but too well what the result must be. Without entering into any farther particulars, suffice it to say that Walker performed his part of the contract, at that time. He took her back to St. Louis, established her as his mistress and housekeeper at his farm, and before I left, he had two children by her. But, mark the end! Since I have been at the North, I have been credibly informed that Walker has been married, and, as a previous measure, sold poor Cynthia and her four children (she having had two more since I came away) into hopeless bondage!

He soon commenced purchasing to make up the third gang. We took steamboat, and went to Jefferson City, a town on the Missouri river. Here we landed, and took stage for the interior of the State. He bought a number of slaves as he passed the different farms and villages. After getting twenty-two or twenty-three men and women, we arrived at St. Charles, a village on the banks of the Missouri. Here he purchased a woman who had a child in her arms, appearing to be four or five weeks old.

We had been travelling by land for some days, and were in hopes to have found a boat at this place for St. Louis, but were disappointed. As no boat was expected for some days, we started for St. Louis by land. Mr. Walker had purchased two horses. He rode one, and I the other. The slaves were chained together, and we took up our line of march, Mr. Walker taking the lead, and I bringing up the rear. Though the distance was not more than twenty miles, we did not reach it the first day. The road was worse than any that I have ever travelled.

Soon after we left St. Charles, the young child grew very cross, and kept up a noise during the greater part of the day. Mr. Walker complained of its crying several times, and told the mother to stop the child's d——d noise, or he would. The woman tried to keep the child from crying, but could not. We put up at night with an acquaintance of Mr. Walker, and in the morning, just as we were about to start, the child again commenced crying. Walker stepped up to her, and told her to give the child to him. The mother tremblingly obeyed. He took the child by one arm, as you would a cat by the leg, walked into the house, and said to the lady,

"Madam, I will make you a present of this little nigger; it keeps such a noise that I can't bear it."

"Thank you, sir," said the lady.

The mother, as soon as she saw that her child was to be left, ran up to Mr. Walker, and falling upon her knees begged him to let her have her child; she clung around his legs, and cried, "Oh, my child! my child! master, do let me have my child! oh, do, do, do. I will stop its crying, if you will only let me have it again." When I saw this woman crying for her child so piteously, a shudder,—a feeling akin to horror, shot through my frame. I have often since in imagination heard her crying for her child:—

> "O, master, let me stay to catch
>   My baby's sobbing breath,
> His little glassy eye to watch,
>   And smooth his limbs in death,
>
> And cover him with grass and leaf,
>   Beneath the large oak tree:
> It is not sullenness, but grief,—
>   O, master, pity me!
>
> The morn was chill—I spoke no word,
>   But feared my babe might die,
> And heard all day, or thought I heard,
>   My little baby cry.

At noon, oh, how I ran and took
  My baby to my breast!
I lingered—and the long lash broke
  My sleeping infant's rest.

I worked till night—till darkest night,
  In torture and disgrace;
Went home and watched till morning light,
  To see my baby's face.

Then give me but one little hour—
  O! do not lash me so!
One little hour—one little hour—
  And gratefully I'll go."

Mr. Walker commanded her to return into the ranks with the other slaves. Women who had children were not chained, but those that had none were. As soon as her child was disposed of, she was chained in the gang.

The following song I have often heard the slaves sing, when about to be carried to the far south. It is said to have been composed by a slave.

"See these poor souls from Africa
  Transported to America;
We are stolen, and sold to Georgia,
  Will you go along with me?
We are stolen, and sold to Georgia,
  Come sound the jubilee!

See wives and husbands sold apart,
  Their children's screams will break my heart;—
There's a better day a coming,
  Will you go along with me?
There's a better day a coming,
  Go sound the jubilee!

O, gracious Lord! when shall it be,
  That we poor souls shall all be free;
Lord, break them slavery powers—
  Will you go along with me?
Lord break them slavery powers,
  Go sound the jubilee!

Dear Lord, dear Lord, when slavery'll cease,
Then we poor souls will have our peace;—
There's a better day a coming,
Will you go along with me?
There's a better day a coming,
Go sound the jubilee!"

We finally arrived at Mr. Walker's farm. He had a house built during our absence to put slaves in. It was a kind of domestic jail. The slaves were put in the jail at night, and worked on the farm during the day. They were kept here until the gang was completed, when we again started for New Orleans, on board the steamboat North America, Capt. Alexander Scott. We had a large number of slaves in this gang. One, by the name of Joe, Mr. Walker was training up to take my place, as my time was nearly out, and glad was I. We made our first stop at Vicksburg, where we remained one week and sold several slaves.

Mr. Walker, though not a good master, had not flogged a slave since I had been with him, though he had threatened me. The slaves were kept in the pen, and he always put up at the best hotel, and kept his wines in his room, for the accommodation of those who called to negotiate with him for the purchase of slaves. One day while we were at Vicksburg, several gentlemen came to see him for this purpose, and as usual the wine was called for. I took the tray and started around with it, and having accidentally filled some of the glasses too full, the gentlemen spilled the wine on their clothes as they went to drink. Mr. Walker apologized to them for my carelessness, but looked at me as though he would see me again on this subject.

After the gentlemen had left the room, he asked me what I meant by my carelessness, and said that he would attend to me. The next morning, he gave me a note to carry to the jailer, and a dollar in money to give to him. I suspected that all was not right, so I went down near the landing where I met with a sailor, and walking up to him, asked him if he would be so kind as to read the note for me. He read it over, and then looked at me. I asked him to tell me what was in it. Said he,

"They are going to give you hell."

"Why?" said I.

He said, "This is a note to have you whipped, and says that you have a dollar to pay for it."

He handed me back the note, and off I started. I knew not what to do, but was determined not to be whipped. I went up to the jail—took a look at it, and walked off again. As Mr. Walker was acquainted with the jailer, I feared that I should be found out if I did not go, and be treated in consequence of it still worse.

While I was meditating on the subject, I saw a colored man about my size walk up, and the thought struck me in a moment to send him with my note. I walked up to him, and asked him who he belonged to. He said he was a free man, and had been in the city but a short time. I told him I had a note to go into the jail, and get a trunk to carry to one of the steamboats; but was so busily engaged that I could not do it, although I had a dollar to pay for it. He asked me if I would not give him the job. I handed him the note and the dollar, and off he started for the jail.

I watched to see that he went in, and as soon as I saw the door close behind him, I walked around the corner, and took my station, intending to see how my friend looked when he came out. I had been there but a short time, when a colored man came around the corner, and said to another colored man with whom he was acquainted—

"They are giving a nigger scissors in the jail."

"What for?" said the other. The man continued,

"A nigger came into the jail, and asked for the jailer. The jailer came out, and he handed him a note, and said he wanted to get a trunk. The jailer told him to go with him, and he would give him the trunk. So he took him into the room, and told the nigger to give up the dollar. He said a man had given him the dollar to pay for getting the trunk. But that lie would not answer. So they made him strip himself, and then they tied him down, and are now whipping him."

I stood by all the while listening to their talk, and soon found out that the person alluded to was my customer. I went into the street opposite the jail, and concealed myself in such a manner that I could not be seen by any one coming out. I had been there but a short time, when the young man made his appearance, and looked around for me. I, unobserved, came forth from my hiding-place, behind a pile of brick, and he pretty soon saw me and came up to me complaining bitterly, saying that I had played a trick upon him. I denied any knowledge of what the note contained, and asked him what they had done to him. He told me in substance what I heard the man tell who had come out of the jail.

"Yes," said he, "they whipped me and took my dollar, and gave me this note."

He showed me the note which the jailer had given him, telling him to give it to his master. I told him I would give him fifty cents for it,—that being all the money I had. He gave it to me, and took his money. He had received twenty lashes on his bare back, with the negro-whip.

I took the note and started for the hotel where I had left Mr. Walker. Upon reaching the hotel, I handed it to a stranger whom I had not seen before, and requested him to read it to me. As near as I can recollect, it was as follows:—

> "DEAR SIR:—By your direction, I have given your boy twenty lashes. He is a very saucy boy, and tried to make me believe that he did not belong to you, and I put it on to him well for lying to me.
>   I remain,
>   Your obedient servant."

It is true that in most of the slave-holding cities, when a gentleman wishes his servants whipped, he can send him to the jail and have it done. Before I went in where Mr. Walker was, I wet my cheeks a little, as though I had been crying. He looked at me, and inquired what was the matter. I told him that I had never had such a whipping in my life, and handed him the note. He looked at it and laughed;—"and so you told him that you did not belong to me." "Yes, sir," said I. "I did not know that there was any harm in that." He told me I must behave myself, if I did not want to be whipped again.

This incident shows how it is that slavery makes its victims lying and mean; for which vices it afterwards reproaches them, and uses them as arguments to prove that they deserve no better fate. I have often, since my escape, deeply regretted the deception I practised upon this poor fellow; and I heartily desire that it may be, at some time or other, in my power to make him amends for his vicarious sufferings in my behalf.

CHAPTER VII.

In a few days we reached New Orleans, and arriving there in the night, remained on board until morning. While at New Orleans this time, I saw a slave killed; an account of which has been published by Theodore D. Weld, in his book entitled, "Slavery as it is." The circumstances were as follows. In the evening, between seven and eight o'clock, a slave came running down the levee, followed by several men and boys. The whites were crying out, "Stop that nigger; stop that nigger;" while the poor panting slave, in almost breathless accents, was repeating, "I did not steal the meat—I did not steal the meat." The poor man at last took refuge in the river. The whites who were in pursuit of him, run on board of one of the boats to see if they could discover him. They finally espied him under the bow of the steamboat Trenton. They got a pike-pole, and tried to drive him from his hiding place. When they would strike at him, he would dive under the water. The water was so cold, that it soon became evident that he must come out or be drowned.

While they were trying to drive him from under the bow of the boat or drown him, he would in broken and imploring accents say, "I did not steal the meat; I did not steal the meat. My master lives up the river. I want to see my master. I did not steal the meat. Do let me go home to master." After punching him, and striking him over the head for some time, he at last sunk in the water, to rise no more alive.

On the end of the pike-pole with which they were striking him was a hook which caught in his clothing, and they hauled him up on the bow of the boat. Some said he was dead, others said he was "*playing possum*," while others kicked him to make him get up, but it was of no use—he was dead.

As soon as they became satisfied of this, they commenced leaving, one after another. One of the hands on the boat informed the captain that they had killed the man, and that the dead body was lying on the deck. The captain came on deck, and said to those who were remaining, "You have killed this nigger; now take him off of my boat." The captain's name was Hart. The dead body was dragged on shore and left there. I went on board of the boat where our gang of slaves were, and during the whole night my mind was occupied with what I had seen. Early in the morning, I went on shore to see if the dead body remained there. I found it in the same position that it was left the night before. I watched to see what they would do with it. It was left there until between eight and nine o'clock, when a cart, which takes up the trash out of the streets, came along, and the body was thrown in, and in a few minutes more was covered over with dirt which they were removing from the streets. During the whole time, I did not see more than six or seven persons around it, who, from their manner, evidently regarded it as no uncommon occurrence.

During our stay in the city, I met with a young white man with whom I was well acquainted in St. Louis. He had been sold into slavery, under the following circumstances. His father was a drunkard, and very poor, with a family of five or six children. The father died, and left the mother to take care of and provide for the children as best she might. The eldest was a boy, named Burrill, about thirteen years of age, who did chores in a store kept by Mr. Riley, to assist his mother in procuring a living for the family. After working with him two years, Mr. Riley took him to New Orleans to wait on him while in that city on a visit, and when he returned to St. Louis, he told the mother of the boy that he had died with the yellow fever. Nothing more was heard from him, no one supposing him to be alive. I was much astonished when Burrill told me his story. Though I sympathized with him, I could not assist him. We were both slaves. He was poor, uneducated, and without friends; and if living, is, I presume, still held as a slave.

After selling out this cargo of human flesh, we returned to St. Louis, and my time was up with Mr. Walker. I had served him one year, and it was the longest year I ever lived.

CHAPTER VIII.

I WAS sent home, and was glad enough to leave the service of one who was tearing the husband from the wife, the child from the mother, and the sister from the brother,—but a trial more severe and heart-rending than any which I had yet met with awaited me. My dear sister had been sold to a man who was going to Natchez, and was lying in jail awaiting the hour of his departure. She had expressed her determination to die, rather than go to the far south, and she was put in jail for safe keeping. I went to the jail the same day that I arrived, but as the jailor was not in, I could not see her.

I went home to my master, in the country, and the first day after my return, he came where I was at work, and spoke to me very politely. I knew from his appearance that something was the matter. After talking about my several journeys to New Orleans with Mr. Walker, he told me that he was hard pressed for money, and as he had sold my mother and all her children except me, he thought it would be better to sell me than any other one, and that as I had been used to living in the city, he thought it probable that I would prefer it to a country life. I raised up my head, and looked him full in the face. When my eyes caught his, he immediately looked to the ground. After a short pause, I said,

"Master, mother has often told me that you are a near relative of mine, and I have often heard you admit the fact; and after you have hired me out, and received, as I once heard you say, nine hundred dollars for my services,—after receiving this large sum, will you sell me to be carried to New Orleans or some other place?"

"No," said he, "I do not intend to sell you to a negro trader. If I had wished to have done that, I might have sold you to Mr. Walker for a large sum, but I would not sell you to a negro trader. You may go to the city, and find you a good master."

"But," said I, "I cannot find a good master in the whole city of St. Louis."

"Why?" said he.

"Because there are no good masters in the State."

"Do you not call me a good master?"

"If you were, you would not sell me."

"Now I will give you one week to find a master in, and surely you can do it in that time."

The price set by my evangelical master upon my soul and body was the trifling sum of five hundred dollars. I tried to enter into some arrangement by which I might purchase my freedom; but he would enter into no such arrangement.

I set out for the city with the understanding that I was to return in a week with some one to become my new master. Soon after reaching the city, I went to the jail, to learn if I could once more see my sister; but could not gain admission. I then went to mother, and learned from her that the owner of my sister intended to start for Natchez in a few days.

I went to the jail again the next day, and Mr. Simonds, the keeper, allowed me to see my sister for the last time. I cannot give a just description of the scene at that parting interview. Never, never can be erased from my heart the occurrences of that day! When I entered the room where she was, she was seated in one corner, alone. There were four other women in the same room, belonging to the same man. He had purchased them, he said, for his own use. She was seated with her face towards the door where I entered, yet she did not look up until I walked up to her. As soon as she observed me, she sprung up, threw her arms around my neck, leaned her head upon my breast, and, without uttering a word, burst into tears. As soon as she recovered herself sufficiently to speak, she advised me to take mother, and try to get out of slavery. She said there was no hope for herself,— that she must live and die a slave. After giving her some advice, and taking from my finger a ring and placing it upon hers, I bade her farewell forever, and returned to my mother, and then and there made up my mind to leave for Canada as soon as possible.

I had been in the city nearly two days, and as I was to be absent only a week, I thought best to get on my journey as soon as possible. In conversing with mother, I found her unwilling to make the attempt to reach a land of liberty, but she counselled me to get my liberty if I could. She said, as all her children were in slavery, she did not wish to leave them. I could not bear the idea of leaving her among those pirates, when there was a prospect of being able to get away from them. After much persuasion, I succeeded in inducing her to make the attempt to get away.

The time fixed for our departure was the next night. I had with me a little money that I had received, from time to time, from gentlemen for whom I had done errands. I took my scanty means and purchased some dried beef, crackers and cheese, which I carried to mother, who had provided herself with a bag to carry it in. I occasionally thought of my old master, and of my mission to the city to find a new one. I waited with the most intense anxiety for the appointed time to leave the land of slavery, in search of a land of liberty.

The time at length arrived, and we left the city just as the clock struck nine. We proceeded to the upper part of the city, where I had been two or three times during the day, and selected a skiff to carry us across the river. The boat was not mine, nor did I know to whom it did belong; neither did I care. The boat was fastened with a small pole, which, with the aid of a rail, I soon loosened from its moorings. After hunting round and finding a board to use as an oar, I turned to the city, and bidding it a long farewell, pushed off my boat. The current running very swift, we had not reached the middle of the stream before we were directly opposite the city.

We were soon upon the Illinois shore, and, leaping from the boat, turned it adrift, and the last I saw of it, it was going down the river at good speed. We took the main road to Alton, and passed through just at daylight, when we made for the woods, where we remained during the day. Our reason for going into the woods was, that we expected that Mr. Mansfield (the man who owned my mother) would start in pursuit of her as soon as he discovered that she was missing. He also knew that I had been in the city looking for a new master, and we thought probably he would go out to my master's to see if he could find my mother, and in so doing, Dr. Young might be led to suspect that I had gone to Canada to find a purchaser.

We remained in the woods during the day, and as soon as darkness overshadowed the earth, we started again on our gloomy way, having no guide but the NORTH STAR. We continued to travel by night, and secrete ourselves in woods by day; and every night, before emerging from our hiding-place, we would anxiously look for our friend and leader,—the NORTH STAR.

CHAPTER IX.

As we travelled towards a land of liberty, my heart would at times leap for joy. At other times, being, as I was, almost constantly on my feet, I felt as though I could travel no further. But when I thought of slavery with its Democratic whips—its Republican chains—its evangelical blood-hounds, and its religious slave-holders—when I thought of all this paraphernalia of American Democracy and Religion behind me, and the prospect of liberty before me, I was encouraged to press forward, my heart was strengthened, and I forgot that I was tired or hungry.

On the eighth day of our journey, we had a very heavy rain, and in a few hours after it commenced, we had not a dry thread upon our bodies. This made our journey still more unpleasant. On the tenth day, we found ourselves entirely destitute of provisions, and how to obtain any we could not tell. We finally resolved to stop at some farmhouse, and try to get something to eat. We had no sooner determined to do this, than we went to a house, and asked them for some food. We were treated with great kindness, and they not only gave us something to eat, but gave us provisions to carry with us. They advised us to travel by day, and lye by at night. Finding ourselves about one hundred and fifty miles from St. Louis, we concluded that it would be safe to travel by daylight, and did not leave the house until the next morning. We travelled on that day through a thickly settled country, and through one small village. Though we were fleeing from a land of oppression, our hearts were still there. My dear sister and two beloved brothers were behind us, and the idea of giving them up, and leaving them forever, made us feel sad. But with all this depression of heart, the thought that I should one day be free, and call my body my own, buoyed me up, and made my heart leap for joy. I had just been telling mother how I should try to get employment as soon as we reached Canada, and how I intended to purchase us a little farm, and how I would earn money enough to buy sister and brothers, and how happy we would be in our own FREE HOME,—when three men came up on horseback, and ordered us to stop.

I turned to the one who appeared to be the principal man, and asked him what he wanted. He said he had a warrant to take us up. The three immediately dismounted, and one took from his pocket a handbill, advertising us as runaways, and offering a reward of two hundred dollars for our apprehension, and delivery in the city of St. Louis. The advertisement had been put out by Isaac Mansfield and John Young.

While they were reading the advertisement, mother looked me in the face, and burst into tears. A cold chill ran over me, and such a sensation I never experienced before, and I hope never to again. They took out a rope and tied me, and we were taken back about six miles, to the house of the individual who appeared to be the leader. We reached there about seven o'clock in the evening, had supper, and were separated for the night. Two men remained in the room during the night. Before the family retired to rest, they were all called together to attend prayers. The man who but a few hours before had bound my hands together with a strong cord, read a chapter from the Bible, and then offered up prayer, just as though God sanctioned the act he had just committed upon a poor panting, fugitive slave.

The next morning, a blacksmith came in, and put a pair of handcuffs on me, and we started on our journey back to the land of whips, chains and Bibles. Mother was not tied, but was closely watched at night. We were carried back in a wagon, and after four days travel, we came in sight of St. Louis. I cannot describe my feelings upon approaching the city.

As we were crossing the ferry, Mr. Wiggins, the owner of the ferry, came up to me, and inquired what I had been doing that I was in chains. He had not heard that I had run away. In a few minutes, we were on the Missouri side, and were taken directly to the jail. On the way thither, I saw several of my friends, who gave me a nod of recognition as I passed them. After reaching the jail, we were locked up in different apartments.

CHAPTER X.

I HAD been in jail but a short time when I heard that my master was sick, and nothing brought more joy to my heart than that intelligence. I prayed fervently for him—not for his recovery, but for his death. I knew he would be exasperated at having to pay for my apprehension, and knowing his cruelty, I feared him. While in jail, I learned that my sister Elizabeth, who was in prison when we left the city, had been carried off four days before our arrival.

I had been in jail but a few hours when three negro-traders, learning that I was secured thus for running away, came to my prison-house and looked at me, expecting that I would be offered for sale. Mr. Mansfield, the man who owned mother, came into the jail as soon as Mr. Jones, the man who arrested us, informed him that he had brought her back. He told her that he would not whip her, but would sell her to a negro-trader, or take her to New Orleans himself. After being in jail about one week, master sent a man to take me out of jail, and send me home. I was taken out and carried home, and the old man was well enough to sit up. He had me brought into the room where he was, and as I entered, he asked me where I had been? I told I had acted according to his orders. He had told me to look for a master, and I had been to look for one. He answered that he did not tell me to go to Canada to look for a master. I told him that as I had served him faithfully, and had been the means of putting a number of hundreds of dollars into his pocket, I thought I had a right to my liberty. He said he had promised my father that I should not be sold to supply the New Orleans market, or he would sell me to a negro-trader.

I was ordered to go into the field to work, and was closely watched by the overseer during the day, and locked up at night. The overseer gave me a severe whipping on the second day that I was in the field. I had been at home but a short time, when master was able to ride to the city; and on his return, he informed me that he had sold me to Samuel Willi, a merchant tailor. I knew Mr. Willi. I had lived with him three or four months some years before, when he hired me of my master.

Mr. Willi was not considered by his servants as a very bad man, nor was he the best of masters. I went to my new home, and found my new mistress very glad to see me. Mr. Willi owned two servants before he purchased me,—Robert and Charlotte. Robert was an excellent white-washer, and hired his time from his master, paying him one dollar per day, besides taking care of himself. He was known in the city by the name of Bob Music. Charlotte was an old woman, who attended to the cooking, washing, &c. Mr. Willi was not a wealthy man, and did not feel able to keep many servants around his house; so he soon decided to hire me out, and as I had been accustomed to service in steamboats, he gave me the privilege of finding such employment.

I soon secured a situation on board the steamer Otto, Capt. J. B. Hill, which sailed from St. Louis to Independence, Missouri. My former master, Dr. Young, did not let Mr. Willi know that I had run away, or he would not have permitted me to go on board a steamboat. The boat was not quite ready to commence running, and therefore I had to remain with Mr. Willi. But during this time, I had to undergo a trial, for which I was entirely unprepared. My mother, who had been in jail since her return until the present time, was now about being carried to New Orleans, to die on a cotton, sugar, or rice plantation!

I had been several times to the jail, but could obtain no interview with her. I ascertained, however, the time the boat in which she was to embark would sail, and as I had not seen mother since her being thrown into prison, I felt anxious for the hour of sailing to come. At last, the day arrived when I was to see her for the first time after our painful separation, and, for aught that I knew, for the last time in this world!

At about ten o'clock in the morning I went on board of the boat, and found her there in company with fifty or sixty other slaves. She was chained to another woman. On seeing me, she immediately dropped her head upon her heaving bosom. She moved not, neither did she weep. Her emotions were too deep for tears. I approached, threw my arms around her neck, kissed her, and fell upon my knees, begging her forgiveness, for I thought myself to blame for her sad condition; for if I had not persuaded her to accompany me, she would not then have been in chains.

She finally raised her head, looked me in the face, (and such a look none but an angel can give!) and said, *"My dear son, you are not to blame for my being here. You have done nothing more nor less than your duty. Do not, I pray you, weep for me. I cannot last long upon a cotton plantation. I feel that my heavenly master will soon call me home, and then I shall be out of the hands of the slave-holders!"*

I could bear no more—my heart struggled to free itself from the human form. In a moment she saw Mr. Mansfield coming toward that part of the boat, and she whispered into my ear, *"My child, we must soon part to meet no more this side of the grave. You have ever said that you would not die a slave; that you would be a freeman. Now try to get your liberty! You will soon have no one to look after but yourself!"* and just as she whispered the last sentence into my ear, Mansfield came up to me, and with an oath, said, "Leave here this instant; you have been the means of my losing one hundred dollars to get this wench back,"—at the same time kicking me with a heavy pair of boots. As I left her, she gave one shriek, saying, "God be with you!" It was the last time that I saw her, and the last word I heard her utter.

I walked on shore. The bell was tolling. The boat was about to start. I stood with a heavy heart, waiting to see her leave the wharf. As I thought of my mother, I could but feel that I had lost

> "———the glory of my life,
> My blessing and my pride!
> I half forgot the name of slave,
> When she was by my side."

CHAPTER XI.

THE love of liberty that had been burning in my bosom, had well nigh gone out. I felt as though I was ready to die. The boat moved gently from the wharf, and while she glided down the river, I realized that my mother was indeed

"Gone,—gone,—sold and gone,
To the rice swamp dank and lone!"

After the boat was out of sight, I returned home; but my thoughts were so absorbed in what I had witnessed, that I knew not what I was about half of the time. Night came, but it brought no sleep to my eyes.

In a few days, the boat upon which I was to work being ready, I went on board to commence. This employment suited me better than living in the city, and I remained until the close of navigation; though it proved anything but pleasant. The captain was a drunken, profligate, hard-hearted creature, not knowing how to treat himself, or any other person.

The boat, on its second trip, brought down Mr. Walker, the man of whom I have spoken in a previous chapter, as hiring my time. He had between one and two hundred slaves, chained and manacled. Among them was a man that formerly belonged to my old master's brother, Aaron Young. His name was Solomon. He was a preacher, and belonged to the same church with his master. I was glad to see the old man. He wept like a child when he told me how he had been sold from his wife and children.

The boat carried down, while I remained on board, four or five gangs of slaves. Missouri, though a comparatively new State, is very much engaged in raising slaves to supply the southern market. In a former chapter, I have mentioned that I was once in the employ of a slave-trader, or driver, as he is called at the south. For fear that some may think that I have misrepresented a slave-driver, I will here give an extract from a paper published in a slaveholding State, Tennessee, called the "Millennial Trumpeter."

"Droves of negroes, chained together in dozens and scores, and hand-cuffed, have been driven through our country in numbers far surpassing any previous year, and these vile slave-drivers and dealers are swarming like buzzards around a carrion. Through this county, you cannot pass a few miles in the great roads without having every feeling of humanity insulted and lacerated by this spectacle, nor can you go into any county or any neighborhood, scarcely, without seeing or hearing of some of these despicable creatures, called negro-drivers.

"Who is a negro-driver? One whose eyes dwell with delight on lacerated bodies of helpless men, women and children; whose soul feels diabolical raptures at the chains, and hand-cuffs, and cart-whips, for inflicting tortures on weeping mothers torn from helpless babes, and on husbands and wives torn asunder forever!"

Dark and revolting as is the picture here drawn, it is from the pen of one living in the midst of slavery. But though these men may cant about negro-drivers, and tell what despicable creatures they are, who is it, I ask, that supplies them with the human beings that they are tearing asunder? I answer, as far as I have any knowledge of the State where I came from, that those who raise slaves for the market are to be found among all classes, from Thomas H. Benton down to the lowest political demagogue, who may be able to purchase a woman for the purpose of raising stock, and from the Doctor of Divinity down to the most humble lay member in the church.

It was not uncommon in St. Louis to pass by an auction-stand, and behold a woman upon the auction-block, and hear the seller crying out, *"How much is offered for this woman? She is a good cook, good washer, a good obedient servant. She has got religion!"* Why should this man tell the purchasers that she has religion? I answer, because in Missouri, and as far as I have any knowledge of slavery in the other States, the religious teaching consists in teaching the slave that he must never strike a white man; that God made him for a slave; and that, when whipped, he must not find fault,—for the Bible says, "He that knoweth his master's will, and doeth it not, shall be beaten with many stripes!" And slaveholders find such religion very profitable to them.

After leaving the steamer Otto, I resided at home, in Mr. Willi's family, and again began to lay my plans for making my escape from slavery. The anxiety to be a freeman would not let me rest day or night. I would think of the northern cities that I had heard so much about;—of Canada, where so many of my acquaintances had found refuge. I would dream at night that I was in Canada, a freeman, and on waking in the morning, weep to find myself so sadly mistaken.

"I would think of Victoria's domain,
    And in a moment I seemed to be there!
But the fear of being taken again,
    Soon hurried me back to despair."

Mr. Willi treated me better than Dr. Young ever had; but instead of making me contented and happy, it only rendered me the more miserable, for it enabled me better to appreciate liberty. Mr. Willi was a man who loved money as most men do, and without looking for an opportunity to sell me, he found one in the offer of Captain Enoch Price, a steamboat owner and commission merchant, living in the city of St. Louis. Captain Price tendered seven hundred dollars, which was two hundred more than Mr. Willi had paid. He therefore thought best to accept the offer. I was wanted for a carriage driver, and Mrs. Price was very much pleased with the captain's bargain. His family consisted besides of one child. He had three servants besides myself—one man and two women.

Mrs. Price was very proud of her servants, always keeping them well dressed, and as soon as I had been purchased, she resolved to have a new carriage. And soon one was procured, and all preparations were made for a turn-out in grand style, I being the driver.

One of the female servants was a girl some eighteen or twenty years of age, named Maria. Mrs. Price was very soon determined to have us united, if she could so arrange matters. She would often urge upon me the necessity of having a wife, saying that it would be so pleasant for me to take one in the same family! But getting married, while in slavery, was the last of my thoughts; and had I been ever so inclined, I should not have married Maria, as my love had already gone in another quarter. Mrs. Price soon found out that her efforts at this match-making between Maria and myself would not prove successful. She also discovered (or thought she had) that I was rather partial to a girl named Eliza, who was owned by Dr. Mills. This induced her at once to endeavor the purchase of Eliza, so great was her desire to get me a wife!

Before making the attempt, however, she deemed it best to talk to me a little upon the subject of love, courtship, and marriage. Accordingly one afternoon she called me into her room—telling me to take a chair and sit down. I did so, thinking it rather strange, for servants are not very often asked thus to sit down in the same room with the master or mistress. She said that she had found out that I did not care enough about Maria to marry her. I told her that was true. She then asked me if there was not a girl in the city that I loved. Well, now, this was coming into too close quarters with me! People, generally, don't like to tell their love stories to everybody that may think fit to ask about them, and it was so with me. But, after blushing awhile and recovering myself, I told her that I did not want a wife. She then asked me, if I did not think something of Eliza. I told her that I did. She then said that if I wished to marry Eliza, she would purchase her if she could.

I gave but little encouragement to this proposition, as I was determined to make another trial to get my liberty, and I knew that if I should have a wife, I should not be willing to leave her behind; and if I should attempt to bring her with me, the chances would be difficult for success. However, Eliza was purchased, and brought into the family.

CHAPTER XII.

But the more I thought of the trap laid by Mrs. Price to make me satisfied with my new home, by getting me a wife, the more I determined never to marry any woman on earth until I should get my liberty. But this secret I was compelled to keep to myself, which placed me in a very critical position. I must keep upon good terms with Mrs. Price and Eliza. I therefore promised Mrs. Price that I would marry Eliza; but said that I was not then ready. And I had to keep upon good terms with Eliza, for fear that Mrs. Price would find out that I did not intend to get married.

I have here spoken of marriage, and it is very common among slaves themselves to talk of it. And it is common for slaves to be married; or at least have the marriage ceremony performed. But there is no such thing as slaves being lawfully married. There has never yet a case occurred where a slave has been tried for bigamy. The man may have as many women as he wishes, and the women as many men; and the law takes no cognizance of such acts among slaves. And in fact some masters, when they have sold the husband from the wife, compel her to take another.

There lived opposite Captain Price's, Doctor Farrar, well known in St. Louis. He sold a man named Ben, to one of the traders. He also owned Ben's wife, and in a few days he compelled Sally (that was her name) to marry Peter, another man belonging to him. I asked Sally "why she married Peter so soon after Ben was sold." She said, "because master made her do it."

Mr. John Calvert, who resided near our place, had a woman named Lavinia. She was quite young, and a man to whom she was about to be married was sold, and carried into the country near St. Charles, about twenty miles from St. Louis. Mr. Calvert wanted her to get a husband; but she had resolved not to marry any other man, and she refused. Mr. Calvert whipped her in such a manner that it was thought she would die. Some of the citizens had him arrested, but it was soon hushed up. And that was the last of it. The woman did not die, but it would have been the same if she had.

Captain Price purchased me in the month of October, and I remained with him until December, when the family made a voyage to New Orleans, in a boat owned by himself, and named the "Chester." I served on board, as one of the stewards. On arriving at New Orleans, about the middle of the month, the boat took in freight for Cincinnati; and it was decided that the family should go up the river in her, and what was of more interest to me, I was to accompany them.

The long looked for opportunity to make my escape from slavery was near at hand.

Captain Price had some fears as to the propriety of taking me near a free State, or a place where it was likely I could run away, with a prospect of liberty. He asked me if I had ever been in a free State. "Oh yes," said I, "I have been in Ohio; my master carried me into that State once, but I never liked a free State."

It was soon decided that it would be safe to take me with

them, and what made it more safe, Eliza was on the boat with us, and Mrs. Price, to try me, asked if I thought as much as ever of Eliza. I told her that Eliza was very dear to me indeed, and that nothing but death should part us. It was the same as if we were married. This had the desired effect. The boat left New Orleans, and proceeded up the river.

I had at different times obtained little sums of money, which I had reserved for a "rainy day." I procured some cotton cloth, and made me a bag to carry provisions in. The trials of the past were all lost in hopes for the future. The love of liberty, that had been burning in my bosom for years, and had been well nigh extinguished, was now resuscitated. At night, when all around was peaceful, I would walk the decks, meditating upon my happy prospects.

I should have stated, that before leaving St. Louis, I went to an old man named Frank, a slave, owned by a Mr. Sarpee. This old man was very distinguished (not only among the slave population, but also the whites) as a fortune-teller. He was about seventy years of age, something over six feet high, and very slender. Indeed, he was so small around his body that it looked as though it was not strong enough to hold up his head.

Uncle Frank was a very great favorite with the young ladies, who would go to him in great numbers to get their fortunes told. And it was generally believed that he could really penetrate into the mysteries of futurity. Whether true or not, he had the *name*, and that is about half of what one needs in this gullible age. I found Uncle Frank seated in the chimney corner, about ten o'clock at night. As soon as I entered, the old man left his seat. I watched his movement as well as I could by the dim light of the fire. He soon lit a lamp, and coming up, looked me full in the face, saying, "Well, my son, you have come to get uncle to tell your fortune, have you?" "Yes," said I. But how the old man should know what I had come for, I could not tell. However, I paid the fee of twenty-five cents, and he commenced by looking into a gourd, filled with water. Whether the old man was a prophet, or the son of a prophet, I cannot say; but there is one thing certain, many of his predictions were verified.

I am no believer in soothsaying; yet I am sometimes at a

loss to know how Uncle Frank could tell so accurately what would occur in the future. Among the many things he told was one which was enough to pay me for all the trouble of hunting him up. It was that *I should be free!* He further said, that in trying to get my liberty, I would meet with many severe trials. I thought to myself, any fool could tell me that!

The first place in which we landed in a free State was Cairo, a small village at the mouth of the Ohio river. We remained here but a few hours, when we proceeded to Louisville. After unloading some of the cargo, the boat started on her upward trip. The next day was the first of January. I had looked forward to New Year's day as the commencement of a new era in the history of my life. I had decided upon leaving the peculiar institution that day.

During the last night that I served in slavery, I did not close my eyes a single moment. When not thinking of the future, my mind dwelt on the past. The love of a dear mother, a dear sister, and three dear brothers, yet living, caused me to shed many tears. If I could only have been assured of their being dead, I should have felt satisfied; but I imagined I saw my dear mother in the cotton-field, followed by a merciless taskmaster, and no one to speak a consoling word to her! I beheld my dear sister in the hands of a slave-driver, and compelled to submit to his cruelty! None but one placed in such a situation can for a moment imagine the intense agony to which these reflections subjected me.

CHAPTER XIII.

At last the time for action arrived. The boat landed at a point which appeared to me the place of all others to start from. I found that it would be impossible to carry anything with me, but what was upon my person. I had some provisions, and a single suit of clothes, about half worn. When the boat was discharging her cargo, and the passengers engaged carrying their baggage on and off shore, I improved the opportunity to convey myself with my little effects on land. Taking up a trunk, I went up the wharf, and was soon out of the crowd. I made directly for the woods, where I remained until night, knowing well that I could not travel, even in the State of Ohio, during the day, without danger of being arrested.

I had long since made up my mind that I would not trust myself in the hands of any man, white or colored. The slave is brought up to look upon every white man as an enemy to him and his race; and twenty-one years in slavery had taught me that there were traitors, even among colored people. After dark, I emerged from the woods into a narrow path, which led me into the main travelled road. But I knew not which way to go. I did not know North from South, East from West. I looked in vain for the North Star; a heavy cloud hid it from my view. I walked up and down the road until near midnight, when the clouds disappeared, and I welcomed the sight of my friend,—truly the slave's friend,—the North Star!

As soon as I saw it, I knew my course, and before daylight I travelled twenty or twenty-five miles. It being in the winter, I suffered intensely from the cold; being without an overcoat, and my other clothes rather thin for the season. I was provided with a tinder-box, so that I could make up a fire when necessary. And but for this, I should certainly have frozen to death; for I was determined not to go to any house for shelter. I knew of a man belonging to Gen. Ashly, of St. Louis, who had run away near Cincinnati, on the way to Washington, but had been caught and carried back into slavery; and I felt that a similar fate awaited me, should I be seen by any one. I travelled at night, and lay by during the day.

On the fourth day, my provisions gave out, and then what to do I could not tell. Have something to eat, I must; but how to get it was the question! On the first night after my food was gone, I went to a barn on the road-side, and there found some ears of corn. I took ten or twelve of them, and kept on my journey. During the next day, while in the woods, I roasted my corn and feasted upon it, thanking God that I was so well provided for.

My escape to a land of freedom now appeared certain, and the prospects of the future occupied a great part of my thoughts. What should be my occupation, was a subject of much anxiety to me; and the next thing what should be my name? I have before stated that my old master, Dr. Young, had no children of his own, but had with him a nephew, the son of his brother, Benjamin Young. When this boy was brought to Doctor Young, his name being William, the same as mine, my mother was ordered to change mine to something else. This, at the time, I thought to be one of the most cruel acts that could be committed upon my rights; and I received several very severe whippings for telling people that my name was William, after orders were given to change it. Though young, I was old enough to place a high appreciation upon my name. It was decided, however, to call me "Sandford," and this name I was known by, not only upon my master's plantation, but up to the time that I made my escape. I was sold under the name of Sandford.

But as soon as the subject came to my mind, I resolved on adopting my old name of William, and let Sandford go by the board, for I always hated it. Not because there was anything peculiar in the name; but because it had been forced upon me. It is sometimes common at the south, for slaves to take the name of their masters. Some have a legitimate right to do so. But I always detested the idea of being called by the name of either of my masters. And as for my father, I would rather have adopted the name of "Friday," and been known as the servant of some Robinson Crusoe, than to have taken his name. So I was not only hunting for my liberty, but also hunting for a name; though I regarded the latter as of little consequence, if I could but gain the former. Travelling along the road, I would sometimes speak to myself, sounding my name over, by way of getting used to it, before I should arrive among civilized human beings. On the fifth or sixth day, it rained very fast, and it froze about as fast as it fell, so that my clothes were one glare of ice. I travelled on at night until I became so chilled and benumbed—the wind blowing into my face—that I found it impossible to go any further, and accordingly took shelter in a barn, where I was obliged to walk about to keep from freezing.

I have ever looked upon that night as the most eventful part of my escape from slavery. Nothing but the providence of God, and that old barn, saved me from freezing to death. I received a very severe cold, which settled upon my lungs, and from time to time my feet had been frost-bitten, so that it was with difficulty I could walk. In this situation I travelled two days, when I found that I must seek shelter somewhere, or die.

The thought of death was nothing frightful to me, compared with that of being caught, and again carried back into slavery. Nothing but the prospect of enjoying liberty could have induced me to undergo such trials, for

> "Behind I left the whips and chains,
>   Before me were sweet Freedom's plains!"

This, and this alone, cheered me onward. But I at last resolved to seek protection from the inclemency of the weather, and therefore I secured myself behind some logs and brush, intending to wait there until some one should pass by; for I thought it probable that I might see some colored person, or, if not, some one who was not a slaveholder; for I had an idea that I should know a slaveholder as far as I could see him.

CHAPTER XIV.

THE first person that passed was a man in a buggy-wagon. He looked too genteel for me to hail him. Very soon, another passed by on horseback. I attempted speaking to him, but fear made my voice fail me. As he passed, I left my hiding-place, and was approaching the road, when I observed an old man walking towards me, leading a white horse. He had on a broad-brimmed hat and a very long coat, and was evidently walking for exercise. As soon as I saw him, and observed his dress, I thought to myself, "You are the man that I have been looking for!" Nor was I mistaken. He was the very man!

On approaching me, he asked me, "if I was not a slave." I looked at him some time, and then asked him "if he knew of any one who would help me, as I was sick." He answered that he would; but again asked, if I was not a slave. I told him I was. He then said that I was in a very pro-slavery neighborhood, and if I would wait until he went home, he would get a covered wagon for me. I promised to remain. He mounted his horse, and was soon out of sight.

After he was gone, I meditated whether to wait or not; being apprehensive that he had gone for some one to arrest me. But I finally concluded to remain until he should return; removing some few rods to watch his movements. After a suspense of an hour and a half or more, he returned with a two horse covered-wagon, such as are usually seen under the shed of a Quaker meeting-house on Sundays and Thursdays; for the old man proved to be a Quaker of the George Fox stamp.

He took me to his house, but it was some time before I could be induced to enter it; not until the old lady came out, did I venture into the house. I thought I saw something in the old lady's cap that told me I was not only safe, but welcome, in her house. I was not, however, prepared to receive their hospitalities. The only fault I found with them was their being too kind. I had never had a white man to treat me as an equal, and the idea of a white lady waiting on me at the table was still worse! Though the table was loaded with the good things of this life, I could not eat. I thought if I could only be allowed the privilege of eating in the kitchen, I should be more than satisfied!

Finding that I could not eat, the old lady, who was a "Thompsonian," made me a cup of "composition," or "number six;" but it was so strong and hot, that I called it "*number seven*!" However, I soon found myself at home in this family. On different occasions, when telling these facts, I have been asked how I felt upon finding myself regarded as a man by a white family; especially just having run away from one. I cannot say that I have ever answered the question yet.

The fact that I was in all probability a freeman, sounded in my ears like a charm. I am satisfied that none but a slave could place such an appreciation upon liberty as I did at that time. I wanted to see mother and sister, that I might tell them "I was free!" I wanted to see my fellow slaves in St. Louis, and let them know that the chains were no longer upon my limbs. I wanted to see Captain Price, and let him learn from my own lips that I was no more a chattel, but a man! I was anxious, too, thus to inform Mrs. Price that she must get another coachman. And I wanted to see Eliza more than I did either Mr. or Mrs. Price!

The fact that I was a freeman—could walk, talk, eat and sleep as a man, and no one to stand over me with the blood-clotted cowhide—all this made me feel that I was not myself.

The kind friend that had taken me in was named Wells Brown. He was a devoted friend of the slave; but was very old, and not in the enjoyment of good health. After being by the fire awhile, I found that my feet had been very much frozen. I was seized with a fever which threatened to confine me to my bed. But my Thompsonian friends soon raised me, treating me as kindly as if I had been one of their own children. I remained with them twelve or fifteen days, during which time they made me some clothing, and the old gentleman purchased me a pair of boots.

I found that I was about fifty or sixty miles from Dayton, in the State of Ohio, and between one and two hundred miles from Cleaveland, on lake Erie, a place I was desirous of reaching on my way to Canada. This I know will sound strangely to the ears of people in foreign lands, but it is nevertheless true. An American citizen was fleeing from a Democratic, Republican, Christian government, to receive protection under the monarchy of Great Britain. While the people of the United States boast of their freedom, they at the same time keep three millions of their own citizens in chains; and while I am seated here in sight of Bunker Hill Monument, writing this narrative, I am a slave, and no law, not even in Massachusetts, can protect me from the hands of the slaveholder!

Before leaving this good Quaker friend, he inquired what my name was besides William. I told him that I had no other name. "Well," said he, "thee must have another name. Since thee has got out of slavery, thee has become a man, and men always have two names."

I told him that he was the first man to extend the hand of friendship to me, and I would give him the privilege of naming me.

"If I name thee," said he, "I shall call thee Wells Brown, after myself."

"But," said I, "I am not willing to lose my name of William. As it was taken from me once against my will, I am not willing to part with it again upon any terms."

"Then," said he, "I will call thee William Wells Brown."

"So be it," said I; and I have been known by that name ever since I left the house of my first white friend, Wells Brown.

After giving me some little change, I again started for Canada. In four days I reached a public house, and went in to warm myself. I there learned that some fugitive slaves had just passed through the place. The men in the bar-room were talking about it, and I thought that it must have been myself they referred to, and I was therefore afraid to start, fearing they would seize me; but I finally mustered courage enough, and took my leave. As soon as I was out of sight, I went into the woods, and remained there until night, when I again regained the road, and travelled on until the next day.

Not having had any food for nearly two days, I was faint with hunger, and was in a dilemma what to do, as the little cash supplied me by my adopted father, and which had contributed to my comfort, was now all gone. I however concluded to go to a farm-house, and ask for something to eat. On approaching the door of the first one presenting itself, I knocked, and was soon met by a man who asked me what I wanted. I told him that I would like something to eat. He asked where I was from, and where I was going. I replied that I had come some way, and was going to Cleaveland.

After hesitating a moment or two, he told me that he could give me nothing to eat, adding, "that if I would work, I could get something to eat."

I felt bad, being thus refused something to sustain nature, but did not dare tell him that I was a slave.

Just as I was leaving the door, with a heavy heart, a woman, who proved to be the wife of this gentleman, came to the door, and asked her husband what I wanted? He did not seem inclined to inform her. She therefore asked me herself. I told her that I had asked for something to eat. After a few other questions, she told me to come in, and that she would give me something to eat.

I walked up to the door, but the husband remained in the passage, as if unwilling to let me enter.

She asked him two or three times to get out of the way, and let me in. But as he did not move, she pushed him on one side, bidding me walk in! I was never before so glad to see a woman push a man aside! Ever since that act, I have been in favor of "woman's rights!"

After giving me as much food as I could eat, she presented me with ten cents, all the money then at her disposal, accompanied with a note to a friend, a few miles further on the road. Thanking this angel of mercy from an overflowing heart, I pushed on my way, and in three days arrived at Cleaveland, Ohio.

Being an entire stranger in this place, it was difficult for me to find where to stop. I had no money, and the lake being frozen, I saw that I must remain until the opening of navigation, or go to Canada by way of Buffalo. But believing myself to be somewhat out of danger, I secured an engagement at the Mansion House, as a table waiter, in payment for my board. The proprietor, however, whose name was E. M. Segur, in a short time, hired me for twelve dollars per month; on which terms I remained until spring, when I found good employment on board a lake steamboat.

I purchased some books, and at leisure moments perused them with considerable advantage to myself. While at Cleaveland, I saw, for the first time, an anti-slavery newspaper. It was the "*Genius of Universal Emancipation*," published by Benjamin Lundy, and though I had no home, I subscribed for the paper. It was my great desire, being out of slavery myself, to do what I could for the emancipation of my brethren yet in chains, and while on Lake Erie, I found many opportunities of "helping their cause along."

It is well known, that a great number of fugitives make their escape to Canada, by way of Cleaveland; and while on the lake, I always made arrangement to carry them on the boat to Buffalo or Detroit, and thus effect their escape to the "promised land." The friends of the slave, knowing that I would transport them without charge, never failed to have a delegation when the boat arrived at Cleaveland. I have sometimes had four or five on board, at one time.

In the year 1842, I conveyed, from the first of May to the first of December, sixty-nine fugitives over Lake Erie to Canada. In 1843, I visited Malden, in Upper Canada, and counted seventeen, in that small village, who owed their escape to my humble efforts.

Soon after coming North, I subscribed for the Liberator, edited by that champion of freedom, William Lloyd Garrison. I labored a season to promote the temperance cause among the colored people, but for the last three years, have been pleading for the victims of American slavery.

WILLIAM WELLS BROWN.

Boston, Mass., June, 1847.

NARRATIVE

OF THE

LIFE AND ADVENTURES

OF

HENRY BIBB,

AN AMERICAN SLAVE,

WRITTEN BY HIMSELF.

WITH

AN INTRODUCTION

BY LUCIUS C. MATLACK.

NEW YORK:
PUBLISHED BY THE AUTHOR; 5 SPRUCE STREET.
1849.

INTRODUCTION.

From the most obnoxious substances we often see spring forth, beautiful and fragrant, flowers of every hue, to regale the eye, and perfume the air. Thus, frequently, are results originated which are wholly unlike the cause that gave them birth. An illustration of this truth is afforded by the history of American Slavery.

Naturally and necessarily, the enemy of literature, it has become the prolific theme of much that is profound in argument, sublime in poetry, and thrilling in narrative. From the soil of slavery itself have sprung forth some of the most brilliant productions, whose logical levers will ultimately upheave and overthrow the system. Gushing fountains of poetic thought, have started from beneath the rod of violence, that will long continue to slake the feverish thirst of humanity outraged, until swelling to a flood it shall rush with wasting violence over the ill-gotten heritage of the oppressor. Startling incidents authenticated, far excelling fiction in their touching pathos, from the pen of self-emancipated slaves, do now exhibit slavery in such revolting aspects, as to secure the execrations of all good men, and become a monument more enduring than marble, in testimony strong as sacred writ against it.

Of the class last named, is the narrative of the life of Henry Bibb, which is equally distinguished as a revolting portrait of the hideous slave system, a thrilling narrative of individual suffering, and a triumphant vindication of the slave's manhood and mental dignity. And all this is associated with unmistakable traces of originality and truthfulness.

To many, the elevated style, purity of diction, and easy flow of language, frequently exhibited, will appear unaccountable and contradictory, in view of his want of early mental culture. But to the thousands who have listened with delight to his speeches on anniversary and other occasions, these same traits will be noted as unequivocal evidence of originality. Very few men present in their written composition, so perfect a transcript of their style as is exhibited by Mr. Bibb.

Moreover, the writer of this introduction is well acquainted with his handwriting and style. The entire manuscript I have examined and prepared for the press. Many of the closing pages of it were written by Mr. Bibb in my office. And the whole is preserved for inspection now. An examination of it will show that no alteration of sentiment, language or style, was necessary to make it what it now is, in the hands of the reader. The work of preparation for the press was that of orthography and punctuation merely, an arrangement of the chapters, and a table of contents—little more than falls to the lot of publishers generally.

The fidelity of the narrative is sustained by the most satisfactory and ample testimony. Time has proved its claims to truth. Thorough investigation has sifted and analysed every essential fact alleged, and demonstrated clearly that this thrilling and eloquent narrative, though stranger than fiction, is undoubtedly true.

It is only necessary to present the following documents to the reader, to sustain this declaration. For convenience of reference, and that they may be more easily understood, the letters will be inserted consecutively, with explanations following the last.

The best preface to these letters, is the report of a committee appointed to investigate the truth of Mr. Bibb's narrative as he has delivered it in public for years past.

REPORT

OF THE UNDERSIGNED, COMMITTEE APPOINTED BY THE DETROIT LIBERTY ASSOCIATION TO INVESTIGATE THE TRUTH OF THE NARRATIVE OF HENRY BIBB, A FUGITIVE FROM SLAVERY, AND REPORT THEREON:

Mr. Bibb has addressed several assemblies in Michigan, and his narrative is generally known. Some of his hearers, among whom were Liberty men, felt doubt as to the truth of his statements. Respect for their scruples and the obligation of duty to the public induced the formation of the present Committee.

The Committee entered on the duty confided to them, resolved on a searching scrutiny, and an unreserved publication of its result. Mr. Bibb acquiesced in the inquiry with a praiseworthy spirit. He attended before the Committee and gave willing aid to its object. He was subjected to a rigorous examination. Facts—dates—persons—and localities were demanded and cheerfully furnished. Proper inquiry—either by letter, or personally, or through the medium of friends was then made from *every* person, and in *every* quarter likely to elucidate the truth. In fact no test for its ascertainment, known to the sense or experience of the Committee, was omitted. The result was the collection of a large body of testimony from very diversified quarters. Slave owners, slave dealers, fugitives from slavery, political friends and political foes contributed to a mass of testimony, every part of which pointed to a common conclusion—the undoubted truth of Mr. Bibb's statements.

In the Committee's opinion no individual can substantiate the events of his life by testimony more conclusive and harmonious than is now before them in confirmation of Mr. Bibb. The main facts of his narrative, and many of the minor ones are corroborated beyond all question. No inconsistency has been disclosed nor anything revealed to create suspicion. The Committee have no hesitation in declaring their conviction that Mr. Bibb is amply sustained, and is entitled to public confidence and high esteem.

The bulk of testimony precludes its publication, but it is in the Committee's hands for the inspection of any applicant.

A. L. PORTER,
C. H. STEWART,
SILAS M. HOLMES.

DETROIT, *April 22, 1845.* Committee.

————

From the bulk of testimony obtained, a part only is here introduced. The remainder fully corroborates and strengthens that.

[No. 1. An Extract] DAWN MILLS, FEB. 19th, 1845.
CHARLES H. STEWART, ESQ.
MY DEAR BROTHER:
Your kind communication of the 13th came to hand yesterday. I have made inquiries respecting Henry Bibb which may

be of service to you. Mr. Wm. Harrison, to whom you allude in your letter, is here. He is a respectable and worthy man—a man of piety. I have just had an interview with him this evening. He testifies, that he was well acquainted with Henry Bibb in Trimble County, Ky., and that he sent a letter to him by Thomas Henson, and got one in return from him. He says that Bibb came out to Canada some three years ago, and went back to get his wife up, but was betrayed at Cincinnati by a colored man—that he was taken to Louisville but got away—was taken again and lodged in jail, and sold off to New Orleans, or he, (Harrison,) understood that he was taken to New Orleans. He testifies that Bibb is a Methodist man, and says that two persons who came on with him last Summer, knew Bibb. One of these, Simpson Young, is now at Malden.

*   *   *

Very respectfully, thy friend,

HIRAM WILSON.

———

[No. 2.]   BEDFORD, TRIMBLE CO., KENTUCKY.
                                            March 4, 1845.

SIR:—Your letter under date of the 13th ult., is now before me, making some inquiry about a person supposed to be a fugitive from the South, "who is lecturing to your religious community on Slavery and the South."

I am pleased to inform you that I have it in my power to give you the information you desire. The person spoken of by you I have no doubt is Walton, a yellow man, who once belonged to my father, William Gatewood. He was purchased by him from John Sibly, and by John Sibly of his brother Albert G. Sibly, and Albert G. Sibly became possessed of him by his marriage with Judge David White's daughter, he being born Judge White's slave.

The boy Walton at the time he belonged to John Sibly, married a slave of my father's, a mulatto girl, and sometime afterwards solicited him to buy him; the old man after much importuning from Walton, consented to do so, and accordingly paid Sibly eight hundred and fifty dollars. He did not buy him because he needed him, but from the fact that he had a wife there, and Walton on his part promising every thing that my father could desire.

It was not long, however, before Walton became indolent and neglectful of his duty; and in addition to this, he was guilty, as the old man thought, of worse offences. He watched his conduct more strictly, and found he was guilty of disposing of articles from the farm for his own use, and pocketing the money.

He actually caught him one day stealing wheat—he had conveyed one sack full to a neighbor and whilst he was delivering the other my father caught him in the very act.

He confessed his guilt and promised to do better for the future—and on his making promises of this kind my father was disposed to keep him still, not wishing to part him from his wife, for whom he professed to entertain the strongest affection. When the Christmas Holidays came on, the old man, as is usual in this country, gave his negroes a week Holiday. Walton, instead of regaling himself by going about visiting his colored friends, took up his line of march for her Britanic Majesty's dominions.

He was gone about two years I think, when I heard of him in Cincinnati; I repaired thither, with some few friends to aid me, and succeeded in securing him.

He was taken to Louisville, and on the next morning after our arrival there, he escaped, almost from before our face, while we were on the street before the Tavern. He succeeded in eluding our pursuit, and again reached Canada in safety.

Nothing daunted he returned, after a lapse of some twelve or eighteen months, with the intention, as I have since learned, of conducting off his wife and eight or ten more slaves to Canada.

I got news of his whereabouts, and succeeded in recapturing him. I took him to Louisville and together with his wife and child, (she going along with him at her owner's request,) sold him. He was taken from thence to New Orleans—and from hence to Red River, Arkansas—and the next news I had of him he was again wending his way to Canada, and I suppose now is at or near Detroit.

In relation to his character, it was the general opinion here that he was a notorious liar, and a rogue. These things I can procure any number of respectable witnesses to prove.

In proof of it, he says his mother belonged to James Bibb, which is a lie, there not having been such a man about here, much less brother of Secretary Bibb. He says that Bibb's daughter married A. G. Sibly, when the fact is Sibly married Judge David White's daughter, and his mother belonged to White also and is now here, free.

So you will perceive he is guilty of lying for no effect, and what might it not be supposed he would do where he could effect anything by it.

I have been more tedious than I should have been, but being anxious to give you his rascally conduct in full, must be my apology. You are at liberty to publish this letter, or make any use you see proper of it. If you do publish it, let me have a paper containing the publication—at any rate let me hear from you again.

Respectfully yours, &c.,
SILAS GATEWOOD.

To C. H. STEWART, ESQ.

———

[No. 3. An Extract.]   CINCINNATI, *March 10, 1845*.

MY DEAR SIR:—Mrs. Path, Nickens and Woodson did not see Bibb on his first visit, in 1837, when he staid with Job Dundy, but were subsequently told of it by Bibb. They first saw him in May, 1838. Mrs. Path remembers this date because it was the month in which she removed from Broadway to Harrison street, and Bibb assisted her to remove. Mrs. Path's garden adjoined Dundy's back yard. While engaged in digging up flowers, she was addressed by Bibb, who was staying with Dundy, and who offered to dig them up for her. She hired him to do it. Mrs. Dundy shortly after called over and told Mrs. Path that he was a slave. After that Mrs. Path took him into her house and concealed him. While concealed, he astonished his good protectress by his ingenuity in bottoming chairs with cane. When the furniture was removed, Bibb insisted on helping, and was, after some remonstrances, permitted. At the house on Harrison street, he was employed for several days in digging a cellar, and was so employed when seized on Saturday afternoon by the constables. He held frequent conversations with Mrs. Path and others, in which he gave them the same account which he has given you.

On Saturday afternoon, two noted slave-catching constables, E. V. Brooks and O'Neil, surprised Bibb as he was digging in the cellar. Bibb sprang for the fence and gained the top of it, where he was seized and dragged back. They took him immediately before William Doty, a Justice of infamous notoriety as an accomplice of kidnappers, proved property, paid charges and took him away.

His distressed friends were surprised by his re-appearance in a few days after, the Wednesday following, as they think. He reached the house of Dr. Woods, (a colored man since deceased,) before day-break, and staid until dusk. Mrs. Path, John Woodson and others made up about twelve dollars for him. Woodson accompanied him out of town a mile and bid him "God speed." He has never been here since. Woodson and Clark saw him at Detroit two years ago.

Yours truly,
WILLIAM BIRNEY.

———

[No. 4.] LOUISVILLE, *March 14, 1845.*

MR. STEWART.—Yours of the 1st came to hand on the 13th inst. You wished me to inform you what became of a boy that was in the work-house in the fall of '39. The boy you allude to went by the name of Walton; he had ran away from Kentucky some time before, and returned for his wife—was caught and sold to Garrison; he was taken to Louisiana, I think—he was sold on Red River to a planter. As Garrison is absent in the City of New Orleans at this time, I cannot inform you who he was sold to. Garrison will be in Louisville some time this Spring; if you wish me, I will inquire of Garrison and inform you to whom he was sold, and where his master lives at this time.

Yours,
W. PORTER.

———

[No. 5.]   BEDFORD, TRIMBLE COUNTY, KY.
C. H. STEWART, ESQ.,

SIR.—I received your note on the 16th inst., and in accordance with it I write you these lines. You stated that you would wish to know something about Walton H. Bibb, and whether he had a wife and child, and whether they were sold to New Orleans. Sir, before I answer these inquiries, I should like to know who Charles H. Stewart is, and why you should make these inquiries of me, and how you knew who I was, as you are a stranger to me and I must be to you. In your next if you will tell me the intention of your inquiries, I will give you a full history of the whole case.

I have a boy in your county by the name of King, a large man and very black; if you are acquainted with him, give him my compliments, and tell him I am well, and all of his friends. W. H. Bibb is acquainted with him.

I wait your answer.

                                    Your most obedient,
March 17, 1845.   W. H. GATEWOOD.

————

[No. 6.]   BEDFORD, KENTUCKY, *April 6th, 1845.*
   MR. CHARLES H. STEWART.

SIR:—Yours of the 1st March is before me, inquiring if one Walton Bibb, a colored man, escaped from me at Louisville, Ky., in the Spring of 1839. To that inquiry I answer, he did. The particulars are these: He ran off from William Gatewood some time in 1838 I think, and was heard of in Cincinnati. Myself and some others went there and took him, and took him to Louisville for sale, by the directions of his master. While there he made his escape and was gone some time, I think about one year or longer. He came back it was said, to get his wife and child, so report says. He was again taken by his owner; he together with his wife and child was taken to Louisville and sold to a man who traded in negroes, and was taken by him to New Orleans and sold with his wife and child to some man up Red River, so I was informed by the man who sold him. He then ran off and left his wife and child and got back, it seems, to your country. I can say for Gatewood he was a good master, and treated him well. Gatewood bought him from a Mr. Sibly, who was going to send him down the river. Walton, to my knowledge, influenced Gatewood to buy him, and promised if he would, never to disobey him or run off. Who he belongs to now, I do not know. I know Gatewood sold his wife and child at a great sacrifice, to satisfy him. If any other information is necessary I will give it, if required. You will please write me again what he is trying to do in your country, or what he wishes the inquiry from me for.

Yours, truly,
DANIEL S. LANE.

These letters need little comment. Their testimony combined is most harmonious and conclusive. Look at the points established.

1. Hiram Wilson gives the testimony of reputable men now in Canada, who knew Henry Bibb as a slave in Kentucky.

2. Silas Gatewood, with a peculiar relish, fills three pages of foolscap, "being anxious to give his rascally conduct in full," as he says. But he vaults over the saddle and lands on the other side. His testimony is invaluable as an endorsement of Mr. Bibb's truthfulness. He illustrates all the essential facts of this narrative. He also labors to prove him deceitful and a liar.

Deceit in a slave, is only a slight reflex of the stupendous fraud practised by his master. And its indulgence has far more logic in its favor, than the ablest plea ever written for slave holding, under ever such peculiar circumstances. The attempt to prove Mr. Bibb in the lie, is a signal failure, as he never affirmed what Gatewood denies. With this offset, the letter under notice is a triumphant vindication of one, whom he thought there by to injure sadly. As Mr. Bibb has most happily acknowledged the wheat, (see page 556,) I pass the charge of stealing by referring to the logic there used, which will be deemed convincing.

3. William Birney, Esq., attests the facts of Mr. Bibb's arrest in Cincinnati, and the subsequent escape, as narrated by him, from the declaration of eye witnesses.

4. W. Porter, Jailor, states that Bibb was in the work-house at Louisville, held and sold afterwards to the persons and at the places named in this volume.

5. W. H. Gatewood, with much Southern dignity, will answer no questions, but shows his relation to these matters by naming "King"—saying, "W. H. Bibb is acquainted with him," and promising "a full history of the case."

6. Daniel S. Lane, with remarkable straight-forwardness and stupidity, tells all he knows, and then wants to know what they ask him for. The writer will answer that question. He wanted to prove by two or more witnesses, the truth of his own statements; which has most surely been accomplished.

Having thus presented an array of testimony sustaining the facts alleged in this narrative, the introduction will be concluded by introducing a letter signed by respectable men of Detroit, and endorsed by Judge Wilkins, showing the high esteem in which Mr. Bibb is held by those who know him well where he makes his home. Their testimony expresses their present regard as well as an opinion of his past character. It is introduced here with the greatest satisfaction, as the writer is assured, from an intimate acquaintance with Henry Bibb, that all who know him hereafter will entertain the same sentiments toward him:

———

DETROIT, *March 10, 1845.*

The undersigned have pleasure in recommending Henry Bibb to the kindness and confidence of Anti-slavery friends in every State. He has resided among us for some years. His deportment, his conduct, and his christian course have won our esteem and affection. The narrative of his sufferings and more early life has been thoroughly investigated by a Committee appointed for the purpose. They sought evidence respecting it in every proper quarter, and their report attested its undoubted truth. In this conclusion we all cordially unite.

H. Bibb has for some years publicly made this narrative to assemblies, whose number cannot be told; it has commanded public attention in this State, and provoked inquiry. Occasionally too we see persons from the South, who knew him in early years, yet not a word or fact worthy of impairing its truth has reached us; but on the contrary, every thing tended to its corroboration.

Mr. Bibb's Anti-slavery efforts in this State have produced

incalculable benefit. The Lord has blessed him into an instrument of great power. He has labored much, and for very inadequate compensation. Lucrative offers for other quarters did not tempt him to a more profitable field. His sincerity and disinterestedness are therefore beyond suspicion.

We bid him "God-speed," on his route. We bespeak for him every kind consideration.   *   *   *   *

H. HALLOCK,
President of the Detroit Lib. Association.
CULLEN BROWN, *Vice-President.*
S. M. HOLMES, *Secretary.*
J. D. BALDWIN,
CHARLES H. STEWART,
MARTIN WILSON,
WILLIAM BARNUM.

DETROIT, Nov. 11, 1845.

The undersigned, cheerfully concurs with Mr. Hallock and others in their friendly recommendation of Mr. Henry Bibb. The undersigned has known him for many months in the Sabbath School in this City, partly under his charge, and can certify to his correct deportment, and commend him to the sympathies of Christian benevolence.

ROSS WILKINS.

———

The task now performed, in preparing for the press and introducing to the public the narrative of Henry Bibb, has been one of the most pleasant ever required at my hands. And I conclude it with an expression of the hope that it may afford interest to the reader, support to the author in his efforts against slavery, and be instrumental in advancing the great work of emancipation in this country.

LUCIUS C. MATLACK.

NEW YORK CITY, *July 1st, 1849.*

AUTHOR'S PREFACE.

THIS work has been written during irregular intervals, while I have been travelling and laboring for the emancipation of my enslaved countrymen. The reader will remember that I make no pretension to literature; for I can truly say, that I have been educated in the school of adversity, whips, and chains. Experience and observation have been my principal teachers, with the exception of three weeks schooling which I have had the good fortune to receive since my escape from the "grave yard of the mind," or the dark prison of human bondage. And nothing but untiring perseverance has enabled me to prepare this volume for the public eye; and I trust by the aid of Divine Providence to be able to make it intelligible and instructive. I thank God for the blessings of Liberty—the contrast is truly great between freedom and slavery. To be changed from a chattel to a human being, is no light matter, though the process with myself practically was very simple. And if I could reach the ears of every slave to-day, throughout the whole continent of America, I would teach the same lesson, I would sound it in the ears of every hereditary bondman, "break your chains and fly for freedom!"

It may be asked why I have written this work, when there has been so much already written and published of the same character from other fugitives? And, why publish it after having told it publicly all through New England and the Western States to multiplied thousands?

My answer is, that in no place have I given orally the detail of my narrative; and some of the most interesting events of my life have never reached the public ear. Moreover, it was at the request of many friends of down-trodden humanity, that I have undertaken to write the following sketch, that light and truth might be spread on the sin and evils of slavery as far as possible. I also wanted to leave my humble testimony on record against this man-destroying system, to be read by succeeding generations when my body shall lie mouldering in the dust.

But I would not attempt by any sophistry to misrepresent

slavery in order to prove its dreadful wickedness. For, I presume there are none who may read this narrative through,
whether Christians or slaveholders, males or females, but what
will admit it to be a system of the most high-handed oppression and tyranny that ever was tolerated by an enlightened
nation.

HENRY BIBB

NARRATIVE

OF THE

LIFE OF HENRY BIBB.

CHAPTER I.

Sketch of my Parentage.—Early separation from my Mother.—
Hard Fare.—First Experiments at running away.—Earnest
longing for Freedom.—Abhorrent nature of Slavery.

I WAS born May 1815, of a slave mother, in Shelby County,
Kentucky, and was claimed as the property of David White
Esq. He came into possession of my mother long before I was
born. I was brought up in the Counties of Shelby, Henry,
Oldham, and Trimble. Or, more correctly speaking, in the
above counties, I may safely say, I was *flogged up;* for where I
should have received moral, mental, and religious instruction,
I received stripes without number, the object of which was to
degrade and keep me in subordination. I can truly say, that I
drank deeply of the bitter cup of suffering and woe. I have
been dragged down to the lowest depths of human degradation and wretchedness, by Slaveholders.

My mother was known by the name of Milldred Jackson.
She is the mother of seven slaves only, all being sons, of
whom I am the eldest. She was also so fortunate or unfortunate, as to have some of what is called the slaveholding blood
flowing in her veins. I know not how much; but not enough
to prevent her children though fathered by slaveholders, from
being bought and sold in the slave markets of the South. It is
almost impossible for slaves to give a correct account of their
male parentage. All that I know about it is, that my mother
informed me that my fathers name was JAMES BIBB. He was
doubtless one of the present Bibb family of Kentucky; but I
have no personal knowledge of him at all, for he died before
my recollection.

The first time I was separated from my mother, I was
young and small. I knew nothing of my condition then as a
slave. I was living with Mr. White, whose wife died and left

him a widower with one little girl, who was said to be the legitimate owner of my mother, and all her children. This girl was also my playmate when we were children.

I was taken away from my mother, and hired out to labor for various persons, eight or ten years in succession; and all my wages were expended for the education of Harriet White, my playmate. It was then my sorrows and sufferings commenced. It was then I first commenced seeing and feeling that I was a wretched slave, compelled to work under the lash without wages, and often without clothes enough to hide my nakedness. I have often worked without half enough to eat, both late and early, by day and by night. I have often laid my wearied limbs down at night to rest upon a dirt floor, or a bench, without any covering at all, because I had no where else to rest my wearied body, after having worked hard all the day. I have also been compelled in early life, to go at the bidding of a tyrant, through all kinds of weather, hot or cold, wet or dry, and without shoes frequently, until the month of December, with my bare feet on the cold frosty ground, cracked open and bleeding as I walked. Reader, believe me when I say, that no tongue, nor pen ever has or can express the horrors of American Slavery. Consequently I despair in finding language to express adequately the deep feeling of my soul, as I contemplate the past history of my life. But although I have suffered much from the lash, and for want of food and raiment; I confess that it was no disadvantage to be passed through the hands of so many families, as the only source of information that I had to enlighten my mind, consisted in what I could see and hear from others. Slaves were not allowed books, pen, ink, nor paper, to improve their minds. But it seems to me now, that I was particularly observing, and apt to retain what came under my observation. But more especially, all that I heard about liberty and freedom to the slaves, I never forgot. Among other good trades I learned the art of running away to perfection. I made a regular business of it, and never gave it up, until I had broken the bands of slavery, and landed myself safely in Canada, where I was regarded as a man, and not as a thing.

The first time in my life that I ran away, was for ill treatment, in 1835. I was living with a Mr. Vires, in the village of

Newcastle. His wife was a very cross woman. She was every day flogging me, boxing, pulling my ears, and scolding, so that I dreaded to enter the room where she was. This first started me to running away from them. I was often gone several days before I was caught. They would abuse me for going off, but it did no good. The next time they flogged me, I was off again; but after awhile they got sick of their bargain, and returned me back into the hands of my owners. By this time Mr. White had married his second wife. She was what I call a tyrant. I lived with her several months, but she kept me almost half of my time in the woods, running from under the bloody lash. While I was at home she kept me all the time rubbing furniture, washing, scrubbing the floors; and when I was not doing this, she would often seat herself in a large rocking chair, with two pillows about her, and would make me rock her, and keep off the flies. She was too lazy to scratch her own head, and would often make me scratch and comb it for her. She would at other times lie on her bed, in warm weather, and make me fan her while she slept, scratch and rub her feet; but after awhile she got sick of me, and preferred a maiden servant to do such business. I was then hired out again; but by this time I had become much better skilled in running away, and would make calculation to avoid detection, by taking with me a bridle. If any body should see me in the woods, as they have, and asked "what are you doing here sir! you are a runaway!"—I said, "no, sir, I am looking for our old mare;" at other times, "looking for our cows." For such excuses I was let pass. In fact, the only weapon of self defence that I could use successfully, was that of deception. It is useless for a poor helpless slave, to resist a white man in a slave-holding State. Public opinion and the law is against him; and resistance in many cases is death to the slave, while the law declares, that he shall submit or die.

The circumstances in which I was then placed, gave me a longing desire to be free. It kindled a fire of liberty within my breast which has never yet been quenched. This seemed to be a part of my nature; it was first revealed to me by the inevitable laws of nature's God. I could see that the All-wise Creator, had made man a free, moral, intelligent and accountable being; capable of knowing good and evil. And I believed then, as I believe now, that every man has a right to wages for his labor; a right to his own wife and children; a right to liberty and the pursuit of happiness; and a right to worship God according to the dictates of his own conscience. But here, in the light of these truths, I was a slave, a prisoner for life; I could possess nothing, nor acquire anything but what must belong to my keeper. No one can imagine my feelings in my reflecting moments, but he who has himself been a slave. Oh! I have often wept over my condition, while sauntering through the forest, to escape cruel punishment.

> "No arm to protect me from tyrants aggression;
>   No parents to cheer me when laden with grief.
>   Man may picture the bounds of the rocks and the rivers,
>   The hills and the valleys, the lakes and the ocean,
>   But the horrors of slavery, he never can trace."

The term slave to this day sounds with terror to my soul,— a word too obnoxious to speak—a system too intolerable to be endured. I know this from long and sad experience. I now feel as if I had just been aroused from sleep, and looking back with quickened perception at the state of torment from whence I fled. I was there held and claimed as a slave; as such I was subjected to the will and power of my keeper, in all respects whatsoever. That the slave is a human being, no one can deny. It is his lot to be exposed in common with other men, to the calamities of sickness, death, and the misfortunes incident to life. But unlike other men, he is denied the consolation of struggling against external difficulties, such as destroy the life, liberty, and happiness of himself and family. A slave may be bought and sold in the market like an ox. He is liable to be sold off to a distant land from his family. He is bound in chains hand and foot; and his sufferings are aggravated a hundred fold, by the terrible thought, that he is not allowed to struggle against misfortune, corporeal punishment, insults, and outrages committed upon himself and family; and he is not allowed to help himself, to resist or escape the blow, which he sees impending over him.

This idea of utter helplessness, in perpetual bondage, is the more distressing, as there is no period even with the remotest generation when it shall terminate.

CHAPTER II.

*A fruitless effort for education.—The Sabbath among Slaves.—
Degrading amusements.—Why religion is rejected.—Condi-
tion of poor white people.—Superstition among slaves.—
Education forbidden.*

In 1833, I had some very serious religious impressions, and
there was quite a number of slaves in that neighborhood, who
felt very desirous to be taught to read the Bible. There was a
Miss Davis, a poor white girl, who offered to teach a Sabbath
School for the slaves, notwithstanding public opinion and the
law was opposed to it. Books were furnished and she commenced the school; but the news soon got to our owners that
she was teaching us to read. This caused quite an excitement
in the neighborhood. Patrols* were appointed to go and
break it up the next Sabbath. They were determined that we
should not have a Sabbath School in operation. For slaves this
was called an incendiary movement.

The Sabbath is not regarded by a large number of the slaves
as a day of rest. They have no schools to go to; no moral nor
religious instruction at all in many localities where there are
hundreds of slaves. Hence they resort to some kind of amusement. Those who make no profession of religion, resort to
the woods in large numbers on that day to gamble, fight, get
drunk, and break the Sabbath. This is often encouraged by
slaveholders. When they wish to have a little sport of that
kind, they go among the slaves and give them whiskey, to see
them dance, "pat juber," sing and play on the banjo. Then
get them to wrestling, fighting, jumping, running foot races,
and butting each other like sheep. This is urged on by giving
them whiskey; making bets on them; laying chips on one
slave's head, and daring another to tip it off with his hand;
and if he tipped it off, it would be called an insult, and cause
a fight. Before fighting, the parties choose their seconds to
stand by them while fighting; a ring or a circle is formed to
fight in, and no one is allowed to enter the ring while they are
fighting, but their seconds, and the white gentlemen. They

*Police peculiar to the South.

are not allowed to fight a duel, nor to use weapons of any kind. The blows are made by kicking, knocking, and butting with their heads; they grab each other by their ears, and jam their heads together like sheep. If they are likely to hurt each other very bad, their masters would rap them with their walking canes, and make them stop. After fighting, they make friends, shake hands, and take a dram together, and there is no more of it.

But this is all principally for want of moral instruction. This is where they have no Sabbath Schools; no one to read the Bible to them; no one to preach the gospel who is competent to expound the Scriptures, except slaveholders. And the slaves, with but few exceptions, have no confidence at all in their preaching, because they preach a pro-slavery doctrine. They say, "Servants be obedient to your masters;—and he that knoweth his master's will and doeth it not, shall be beaten with many stripes;—" means that God will send them to hell, if they disobey their masters. This kind of preaching has driven thousands into infidelity. They view themselves as suffering unjustly under the lash, without friends, without protection of law or gospel, and the green eyed monster tyranny staring them in the face. They know that they are destined to die in that wretched condition, unless they are delivered by the arm of Omnipotence. And they cannot believe or trust in such a religion, as above named.

The poor and loafering class of whites, are about on a par in point of morals with the slaves at the South. They are generally ignorant, intemperate, licentious, and profane. They associate much with the slaves; are often found gambling together on the Sabbath; encouraging slaves to steal from their owners, and sell to them, corn, wheat, sheep, chickens, or any thing of the kind which they can well conceal. For such offences there is no law to reach a slave but lynch law. But if both parties are caught in the act by a white person, the slave is punished with the lash, while the white man is often punished with both lynch and common law. But there is another class of poor white people in the South, who, I think would be glad to see slavery abolished in self defence; they despise the institution because it is impoverishing and degrading to them and their children.

The slave holders are generally rich, aristocratic, overbearing; and they look with utter contempt upon a poor laboring man, who earns his bread by the "sweat of his brow," whether he be moral or immoral, honest or dishonest. No matter whether he is white or black; if he performs manual labor for a livelihood, he is looked upon as being inferior to a slaveholder, and but little better off than the slave, who toils without wages under the lash. It is true, that the slaveholder, and non-slaveholder, are living under the same laws in the same State. But the one is rich, the other is poor; one is educated, the other is uneducated; one has houses, land and influence, the other has none. This being the case, that class of the non-slaveholders would be glad to see slavery abolished, but they dare not speak it aloud.

There is much superstition among the slaves. Many of them believe in what they call "conjuration," tricking, and witchcraft; and some of them pretend to understand the art, and say that by it they can prevent their masters from exercising their will over their slaves. Such are often applied to by others, to give them power to prevent their masters from flogging them. The remedy is most generally some kind of bitter root; they are directed to chew it and spit towards their masters when they are angry with their slaves. At other times they prepare certain kinds of powders, to sprinkle about their masters dwellings. This is all done for the purpose of defending themselves in some peaceable manner, although I am satisfied that there is no virtue at all in it. I have tried it to perfection when I was a slave at the South. I was then a young man, full of life and vigor, and was very fond of visiting our neighbors slaves, but had no time to visit only Sundays, when I could get a permit to go, or after night, when I could slip off without being seen. If it was found out, the next morning I was called up to give an account of myself for going off without permission; and would very often get a flogging for it.

I got myself into a scrape at a certain time, by going off in this way, and I expected to be severely punished for it. I had a strong notion of running off, to escape being flogged, but was advised by a friend to go to one of those conjurers, who could prevent me from being flogged. I went and informed him of the difficulty. He said if I would pay him a small sum, he would prevent my being flogged. After I had paid him, he mixed up some alum, salt and other stuff into a powder, and said I must sprinkle it about my master, if he should offer to strike me; this would prevent him. He also gave me some kind of bitter root to chew, and spit towards him, which would certainly prevent my being flogged. According to order I used his remedy, and for some cause I was let pass without being flogged that time.

I had then great faith in conjuration and witchcraft. I was led to believe that I could do almost as I pleased, without being flogged. So on the next Sabbath my conjuration was fully tested by my going off, and staying away until Monday morning, without permission. When I returned home, my master declared that he would punish me for going off; but I did not believe that he could do it while I had this root and dust; and as he approached me, I commenced talking saucy to him. But he soon convinced me that there was no virtue in them. He became so enraged at me for saucing him, that he grasped a handful of switches and punished me severely, in spite of all my roots and powders.

But there was another old slave in that neighborhood, who professed to understand all about conjuration, and I thought I would try his skill. He told me that the first one was only a quack, and if I would only pay him a certain amount in cash, that he would tell me how to prevent any person from striking me. After I had paid him his charge, he told me to go to the cow-pen after night, and get some fresh cow manure, and mix it with red pepper and white people's hair, all to be put into a pot over the fire, and scorched until it could be ground into snuff. I was then to sprinkle it about my master's bedroom, in his hat and boots, and it would prevent him from ever abusing me in any way. After I got it all ready prepared, the smallest pinch of it scattered over a room, was enough to make a horse sneeze from the strength of it; but it did no good. I tried it to my satisfaction. It was my business to make fires in my master's chamber, night and morning. Whenever I could get a chance, I sprinkled a little of this dust about the linen of the bed, where they would breathe it on retiring. This was to act upon them as what is called a kind of love powder, to change their sentiments of anger, to those of love, towards me, but this all proved to be vain imagination. The old man had my money, and I was treated no better for it.

One night when I went in to make a fire, I availed myself of the opportunity of sprinkling a very heavy charge of this powder about my master's bed. Soon after their going to bed, they began to cough and sneeze. Being close around the house, watching and listening, to know what the effect would be, I heard them ask each other what in the world it could be, that made them cough and sneeze so. All the while, I was trembling with fear, expecting every moment I should be called and asked if I knew any thing about it. After this, for fear they might find me out in my dangerous experiments upon them, I had to give them up, for the time being. I was then convinced that running away was the most effectual way by which a slave could escape cruel punishment.

As all the instrumentalities which I as a slave, could bring to bear upon the system, had utterly failed to palliate my sufferings, all hope and consolation fled. I must be a slave for life, and suffer under the lash or die. The influence which this had only tended to make me more unhappy. I resolved that I would be free if running away could make me so. I had heard that Canada was a land of liberty, somewhere in the North; and every wave of trouble that rolled across my breast, caused me to think more and more about Canada, and liberty. But more especially after having been flogged, I have fled to the highest hills of the forest, pressing my way to the North for refuge; but the river Ohio was my limit. To me it was an impassable gulf. I had no rod wherewith to smite the stream, and thereby divide the waters. I had no Moses to go before me and lead the way from bondage to a promised land. Yet I was in a far worse state than Egyptian bondage; for they had houses and land; I had none; they had oxen and sheep; I had none; they had a wise counsel, to tell them what to do, and where to go, and even to go with them; I had none. I was surrounded by opposition on every hand. My friends were few and far between. I have often felt when running away as if I had scarcely a friend on earth.

Sometimes standing on the Ohio River bluff, looking over on a free State, and as far north as my eyes could see, I have eagerly gazed upon the blue sky of the free North, which at times constrained me to cry out from the depths of my soul, Oh! Canada, sweet land of rest—Oh! when shall I get there! Oh, that I had the wings of a dove, that I might soar away to where there is no slavery; no clanking of chains, no captives, no lacerating of backs, no parting of husbands and wives; and where man ceases to be the property of his fellow man. These thoughts have revolved in my mind a thousand times. I have stood upon the lofty banks of the river Ohio, gazing upon the splendid steamboats, wafted with all their magnificence up and down the river, and I thought of the fishes of the water, the fowls of the air, the wild beasts of the forest, all appeared to be free, to go just where they pleased, and I was an unhappy slave!

But my attention was gradually turned in a measure from this subject, by being introduced into the society of young women. This for the time being took my attention from running away, as waiting on the girls appeared to be perfectly congenial to my nature. I wanted to be well thought of by them, and would go to great lengths to gain their affection. I had been taught by the old superstitious slaves, to believe in conjuration, and it was hard for me to give up the notion, for all I had been deceived by them. One of these conjurers, for a small sum agreed to teach me to make any girl love me that I wished. After I had paid him, he told me to get a bull frog, and take a certain bone out of the frog, dry it, and when I got a chance I must step up to any girl whom I wished to make love me, and scratch her somewhere on her naked skin with this bone, and she would be certain to love me, and would follow me in spite of herself; no matter who she might be engaged to, nor who she might be walking with.

So I got me a bone for a certain girl, whom I knew to be under the influence of another young man. I happened to meet her in the company of her lover, one Sunday evening, walking out; so when I got a chance, I fetched her a tremendous rasp across her neck with this bone, which made her jump. But in place of making her love me, it only made her angry with me. She felt more like running after me to retaliate on me for thus abusing her, than she felt like loving me. After I found there was no virtue in the bone of a frog, I thought I would try some other way to carry out my object.

I then sought another counsellor among the old superstitious influential slaves; one who professed to be a great friend of mine, told me to get a lock of hair from the head of any girl, and wear it in my shoes: this would cause her to love me above all other persons. As there was another girl whose affections I was anxious to gain, but could not succeed, I thought, without trying the experiment of this hair. I slipped off one night to see the girl, and asked her for a lock of her hair; but she refused to give it. Believing that my success depended greatly upon this bunch of hair, I was bent on having a lock before I left that night let it cost what it might. As it was time for me to start home in order to get any sleep that night, I grasped hold of a lock of her hair, which caused her to screech, but I never let go until I had pulled it out. This of course made the girl mad with me, and I accomplished nothing but gained her displeasure.

Such are the superstitious notions of the great masses of southern slaves. It is given to them by tradition, and can never be erased, while the doors of education are bolted and barred against them. But there is a prohibition by law, of mental and religious instruction. The state of Georgia, by an act of 1770, declared "that it shall not be lawful for any number of free negroes, molattoes or mestinos, or even slaves in company with white persons, to meet together for the purpose of mental instruction, either before the rising of the sun or after the going down of the same." 2d Brevard's Digest, 254–5. Similar laws exist in most of the slave States, and patrols are sent out after night and on the Sabbath day to enforce them. They go through their respective towns to prevent slaves from meeting for religious worship or mental instruction.

This is the regulation and law of American Slavery, as sanctioned by the Government of the United States, and without which it could not exist. And almost the whole moral, political, and religious power of the nation are in favor of slavery and aggression, and against liberty and justice. I only judge by their actions, which speak louder than words. Slaveholders are put into the highest offices in the gift of the people in both Church and State, thereby making slaveholding popular and reputable.

CHAPTER III.

My Courtship and Marriage.—Change of owner.—My first born.—Its sufferings.—My wife abused.—My own anguish.

THE circumstances of my courtship and marriage, I consider to be among the most remarkable events of my life while a slave. To think that after I had determined to carry out the great idea which is so universally and practically acknowledged among all the civilized nations of the earth, that I would be free or die, I suffered myself to be turned aside by the fascinating charms of a female, who gradually won my attention from an object so high as that of liberty; and an object which I held paramount to all others.

But when I had arrived at the age of eighteen, which was in the year of 1833, it was my lot to be introduced to the favor of a mulatto slave girl named Malinda, who lived in Oldham County, Kentucky, about four miles from the residence of my owner. Malinda was a medium sized girl, graceful in her walk, of an extraordinary make, and active in business. Her skin was of a smooth texture, red cheeks, with dark and penetrating eyes. She moved in the highest circle* of slaves, and free people of color. She was also one of the best singers I ever heard, and was much esteemed by all who knew her, for her benevolence, talent and industry. In fact, I considered Malinda to be equalled by few, and surpassed by none, for the above qualities, all things considered.

It is truly marvellous to see how sudden a man's mind can be changed by the charms and influence of a female. The first two or three visits that I paid this dear girl, I had no intention of courting or marrying her, for I was aware that such a step would greatly obstruct my way to the land of liberty. I only visited Malinda because I liked her company, as a highly interesting girl. But in spite of myself, before I was aware of it, I was deeply in love; and what made this passion so effectual

---

*The distinction among slaves is as marked, as the classes of society are in any aristocratic community. Some refusing to associate with others whom they deem beneath them in point of character, color, condition, or the superior importance of their respective masters.

and almost irresistable, I became satisfied that it was recipro-cal. There was a union of feeling, and every visit made the impression stronger and stronger. One or two other young men were paying attention to Malinda, at the same time; one of whom her mother was anxious to have her marry. This of course gave me a fair opportunity of testing Malinda's sincer-ity. I had just about opposition enough to make the subject interesting. That Malinda loved me above all others on earth, no one could deny. I could read it by the warm reception with which the dear girl always met me, and treated me in her mother's house. I could read it by the warm and affectionate shake of the hand, and gentle smile upon her lovely cheek. I could read it by her always giving me the preference of her company; by her pressing invitations to visit even in opposi-tion to her mother's will. I could read it in the language of her bright and sparkling eye, penciled by the unchangable fin-ger of nature, that spake but could not lie. These strong temptations gradually diverted my attention from my actual condition and from liberty, though not entirely.

But oh! that I had only then been enabled to have seen as I do now, or to have read the following slave code, which is but a stereotyped law of American slavery. It would have saved me I think from having to lament that I was a husband and am the father of slaves who are still left to linger out their days in hopeless bondage. The laws of Kentucky, my native State, with Maryland and Virginia, which are said to be the mildest slave States in the Union, noted for their humanity, Christianity and democracy, declare that "Any slave, for ram-bling in the night, or riding horseback without leave, or run-ning away, may be punished by whipping, cropping and branding in the cheek, or otherwise, not rendering him unfit for labor." "Any slave convicted of petty larceny, murder, or wilfully burning of dwelling houses, may be sentenced to have his right hand cut off; to be hanged in the usual manner, or the head severed from the body, the body divided into four quarters, and head and quarters stuck up in the most public place in the county, where such act was committed."

At the time I joined my wife in holy wedlock, I was igno-rant of these ungodly laws; I knew not that I was propo-gating victims for this kind of torture and cruelty. Malinda's mother was free, and lived in Bedford, about a quarter of a mile from her daughter; and we often met and passed off the time pleasantly. Agreeable to promise, on one Saturday evening, I called to see Malinda, at her mother's residence, with an intention of letting her know my mind upon the subject of marriage. It was a very bright moonlight night; the dear girl was standing in the door, anxiously waiting my arrival. As I approached the door she caught my hand with an affectionate smile, and bid me welcome to her mother's fireside. After having broached the subject of marriage, I informed her of the difficulties which I conceived to be in the way of our marriage, and that I could never engage myself to marry any girl only on certain conditions; near as I can recollect the substance of our conversation upon the subject, it was, that I was religiously inclined; that I intended to try to comply with the requisitions of the gospel, both theoretically and practically through life. Also that I was decided on becoming a freeman before I died; and that I expected to get free by running away, and going to Canada, under the British Government. Agreement on those two cardinal questions I made my test for marriage.

I said, "I never will give my heart nor hand to any girl in marriage, until I first know her sentiments upon the all-important subjects of Religion and Liberty. No matter how well I might love her nor how great the sacrifice in carrying out these God-given principles. And I here pledge myself from this course never to be shaken while a single pulsation of my heart shall continue to throb for Liberty." With this idea Malinda appeared to be well pleased, and with a smile she looked me in the face and said, "I have long entertained the same views, and this has been one of the greatest reasons why I have not felt inclined to enter the married state while a slave; I have always felt a desire to be free; I have long cherished a hope that I should yet be free, either by purchase or running away. In regard to the subject of Religion, I have always felt that it was a good thing, and something that I would seek for at some future period." After I found that Malinda was right upon these all important questions, and that she truly loved me well enough to make me an affectionate wife, I made proposals for marriage. She very modestly declined answering the question then, considering it to be one of a grave character, and upon which our future destiny greatly depended. And notwithstanding she confessed that I had her entire affections, she must have some time to consider the matter. To this I of course consented, and was to meet her on the next Saturday night to decide the question. But for some cause I failed to come, and the next week she sent for me, and on the Sunday evening following I called on her again; she welcomed me with all the kindness of an affectionate lover, and seated me by her side. We soon broached the old subject of marriage, and entered upon a conditional contract of matrimony, viz: that we would marry if our minds should not change within one year; that after marriage we would change our former course and live a pious life; and that we would embrace the earliest opportunity of running away to Canada for our liberty. Clasping each other by the hand, pledging our sacred honor that we would be true, we called on high heaven to witness the rectitude of our purpose. There was nothing that could be more binding upon us as slaves than this; for marriage among American slaves, is disregarded by the laws of this country. It is counted a mere temporary matter; it is a union which may be continued or broken off, with or without the consent of a slaveholder, whether he is a priest or a libertine.

There is no legal marriage among the slaves of the South; I never saw nor heard of such a thing in my life, and I have been through seven of the slave states. A slave marrying according to law, is a thing unknown in the history of American Slavery. And be it known to the disgrace of our country that every slaveholder, who is the keeper of a number of slaves of both sexes, is also the keeper of a house or houses of ill-fame. Licentious white men, can and do, enter at night or day the lodging places of slaves; break up the bonds of affection in families; destroy all their domestic and social union for life; and the laws of the country afford them no protection. Will any man count, if they can be counted, the churches of Maryland, Kentucky, and Virginia, which have slaves connected with them, living in an open state of adultery, never having been married according to the laws of the State, and yet regular members of these various denominations, but more especially the Baptist and Methodist churches? And I hazard nothing in saying, that this state of things exists to a very wide extent in the above states.

I am happy to state that many fugitive slaves, who have been enabled by the aid of an over-ruling providence to escape to the free North with those whom they claim as their wives, notwithstanding all their ignorance and superstition, are not at all disposed to live together like brutes, as they have been compelled to do in slaveholding Churches. But as soon as they get free from slavery they go before some anti-slavery clergyman, and have the solemn ceremony of marriage performed according to the laws of the country. And if they profess religion, and have been baptized by a slaveholding minister, they repudiate it after becoming free, and are re-baptized by a man who is worthy of doing it according to the gospel rule.

The time and place of my marriage, I consider one of the most trying of my life. I was opposed by friends and foes; my mother opposed me because she thought I was too young, and marrying she thought would involve me in trouble and difficulty. My mother-in-law opposed me, because she wanted her daughter to marry a slave who belonged to a very rich man living near by, and who was well known to be the son of his master. She thought no doubt that his master or father might chance to set him free before he died, which would enable him to do a better part by her daughter than I could! and there was no prospect then of my ever being free. But his master has neither died nor yet set his son free, who is now about forty years of age, toiling under the lash, waiting and hoping that his master may die and will him to be free.

The young men were opposed to our marriage for the same reason that Paddy opposed a match when the clergyman was about to pronounce the marriage ceremony of a young couple. He said "if there be any present who have any objections to this couple being joined together in holy wedlock, let them speak now, or hold their peace henceforth." At this time Paddy sprang to his feet and said, "Sir, I object to this." Every eye was fixed upon him. "What is your objection?" said the clergyman. "Faith," replied Paddy, "Sir I want her myself."

The man to whom I belonged was opposed, because he

feared my taking off from his farm some of the fruits of my own labor for Malinda to eat, in the shape of pigs, chickens, or turkeys, and would count it not robbery. So we formed a resolution, that if we were prevented from joining in wedlock, that we would run away, and strike for Canada, let the consequences be what they might. But we had one consolation; Malinda's master was very much in favor of the match, but entirely upon selfish principles. When I went to ask his permission to marry Malinda, his answer was in the affirmative with but one condition which I consider to be too vulgar to be written in this book. Our marriage took place one night during the Christmas holydays; at which time we had quite a festival given us. All appeared to be wide awake, and we had quite a jolly time at my wedding party. And notwithstanding our marriage was without license or sanction of law, we believed it to be honorable before God, and the bed undefiled. Our Christmas holydays were spent in matrimonial visiting among our friends, while it should have been spent in running away to Canada, for our liberty. But freedom was little thought of by us, for several months after marriage. I often look back to that period even now as one of the most happy seasons of my life; notwithstanding all the contaminating and heart-rendering features with which the horrid system of slavery is marked, and must carry with it to its final grave, yet I still look back to that season with sweet remembrance and pleasure, that yet hath power to charm and drive back dull cares which have been accumulated by a thousand painful recollections of slavery. Malinda was to me an affectionate wife. She was with me in the darkest hours of adversity. She was with me in sorrow, and joy, in fasting and feasting, in trial and persecution, in sickness and health, in sunshine and in shade.

Some months after our marriage, the unfeeling master to whom I belonged, sold his farm with the view of moving his slaves to the State of Missouri, regardless of the separation of husbands and wives forever; but for fear of my resuming my old practice of running away, if he should have forced me to leave my wife, by my repeated requests, he was constrained to sell me to his brother, who lived within seven miles of Wm. Gatewood, who then held Malinda as his property. I was permitted to visit her only on Saturday nights, after my work was done, and I had to be at home before sunrise on Monday mornings or take a flogging. He proved to be so oppressive, and so unreasonable in punishing his victims, that I soon found that I should have to run away in self-defence. But he soon began to take the hint, and sold me to Wm. Gatewood the owner of Malinda. With my new residence I confess that I was much dissatisfied. Not that Gatewood was a more cruel master than my former owner—not that I was opposed to living with Malinda, who was then the centre and object of my affections—but to live where I must be eye witness to her insults, scourgings and abuses, such as are common to be inflicted upon slaves, was more than I could bear. If my wife must be exposed to the insults and licentious passions of wicked slavedrivers and overseers; if she must bear the stripes of the lash laid on by an unmerciful tyrant; if this is to be done with impunity, which is frequently done by slaveholders and their abettors, Heaven forbid that I should be compelled to witness the sight.

Not many months after I took up my residence on Wm. Gatewood's plantation, Malinda made me a father. The dear little daughter was called Mary Frances. She was nurtured and caressed by her mother and father, until she was large enough to creep over the floor after her parents, and climb up by a chair before I felt it to be my duty to leave my family and go into a foreign country for a season. Malinda's business was to labor out in the field the greater part of her time, and there was no one to take care of poor little Frances, while her mother was toiling in the field. She was left at the house to creep under the feet of an unmerciful old mistress, whom I have known to slap with her hand the face of little Frances, for crying after her mother, until her little face was left black and blue. I recollect that Malinda and myself came from the field one summer's day at noon, and poor little Frances came creeping to her mother smiling, but with large tear drops standing in her dear little eyes, sobbing and trying to tell her mother that she had been abused, but was not able to utter a word. Her little face was bruised black with the whole print of Mrs. Gatewood's hand. This print was plainly to be seen for eight days after it was done. But oh! this darling child was a slave; born of a slave mother. Who can imagine what could be the feelings of a father and mother, when looking upon their infant child whipped and tortured with impunity, and they placed in a situation where they could afford it no protection. But we were all claimed and held as property; the father and mother were slaves!

On this same plantation I was compelled to stand and see my wife shamefully scourged and abused by her master; and the manner in which this was done, was so violently and inhumanly committed upon the person of a female, that I despair in finding decent language to describe the bloody act of cruelty. My happiness or pleasure was then all blasted; for it was sometimes a pleasure to be with my little family even in slavery. I loved them as my wife and child. Little Frances was a pretty child; she was quiet, playful, bright, and interesting. She had a keen black eye, and the very image of her mother was stamped upon her cheek; but I could never look upon the dear child without being filled with sorrow and fearful apprehensions, of being separated by slaveholders, because she was a slave, regarded as property. And unfortunately for me, I am the father of a slave, a word too obnoxious to be spoken by a fugitive slave. It calls fresh to my mind the separation of husband and wife; of stripping, tying up and flogging; of tearing children from their parents, and selling them on the auction block. It calls to mind female virtue trampled under foot with impunity. But oh! when I remember that my daughter, my only child, is still there, destined to share the fate of all these calamities, it is too much to bear. If ever there was any one act of my life while a slave, that I have to lament over, it is that of being a father and a husband of slaves. I have the satisfaction of knowing that I am only the father of one slave. She is bone of my bone, and flesh of my flesh; poor unfortunate child. She was the first and shall be the last slave that ever I will father, for chains and slavery on this earth.

CHAPTER IV.

My first adventure for liberty.—Parting Scene.—Journey up the river.—Safe arrival in Cincinnati.—Journey to Canada.— Suffering from cold and hunger.—Denied food and shelter by some.—One noble exception.—Subsequent success.—Arrival at Perrysburgh.—I obtained employment through the winter.—My return to Kentucky to get my family.

In the fall or winter of 1837 I formed a resolution that I would escape, if possible, to Canada, for my Liberty. I commenced from that hour making preparations for the dangerous experiment of breaking the chains that bound me as a slave. My preparation for this voyage consisted in the accumulation of a little money, perhaps not exceeding two dollars and fifty cents, and a suit which I had never been seen or known to wear before; this last was to avoid detection.

On the twenty-fifth of December, 1837, my long anticipated time had arrived when I was to put into operation my former resolution, which was to bolt for Liberty or consent to die a Slave. I acted upon the former, although I confess it to be one of the most self-denying acts of my whole life, to take leave of an affectionate wife, who stood before me on my departure, with dear little Frances in her arms, and with tears of sorrow in her eyes as she bid me a long farewell. It required all the moral courage that I was master of to suppress my feelings while taking leave of my little family.

Had Malinda known my intention at that time, it would not have been possible for me to have got away, and I might have this day been a slave. Notwithstanding every inducement was held out to me to run away if I would be free, and the voice of liberty was thundering in my very soul, "Be free, oh, man! be free," I was struggling against a thousand obstacles which had clustered around my mind to bind my wounded spirit still in the dark prison of mental degradation. My strong attachments to friends and relatives, with all the love of home and birth-place which is so natural among the human family, twined about my heart and were hard to break away from. And withal, the fear of being pursued with guns and bloodhounds, and of being killed, or captured and taken to the extreme South, to linger out my days in hopeless bondage on some cotton or sugar plantation, all combined to deter me. But I had counted the cost, and was fully prepared to make the sacrifice. The time for fulfilling my pledge was then at hand. I must forsake friends and neighbors, wife and child, or consent to live and die a slave.

By the permission of my keeper, I started out to work for myself on Christmas. I went to the Ohio River, which was but a short distance from Bedford. My excuse for wanting to go there was to get work. High wages were offered for hands to work in a slaughter-house. But in place of my going to work there, according to promise, when I arrived at the river I managed to find a conveyance to cross over into a free state. I was landed in the village of Madison, Indiana, where steamboats were landing every day and night, passing up and down the river, which afforded me a good opportunity of getting a boat passage to Cincinnati. My anticipation being worked up to the highest pitch, no sooner was the curtain of night dropped over the village, than I secreted myself where no one could see me, and changed my suit ready for the passage. Soon I heard the welcome sound of a Steamboat coming up the river Ohio, which was soon to waft me beyond the limits of the human slave markets of Kentucky. When the boat had landed at Madison, notwithstanding my strong desire to get off, my heart trembled within me in view of the great danger to which I was exposed in taking passage on board of a Southern Steamboat; hence before I took passage, I kneeled down before the Great I Am, and prayed for his aid and protection, which He bountifully bestowed even beyond my expectation; for I felt myself to be unworthy. I then stept boldly on the deck of this splendid swift-running Steamer, bound for the city of Cincinnati. This being the first voyage that I had ever taken on board of a Steamboat, I was filled with fear and excitement, knowing that I was surrounded by the vilest enemies of God and man, liable to be seized and bound hand and foot, by any white man, and taken back into captivity. But I crowded myself back from the light among the deck passengers, where it would be difficult to distinguish me from a white man. Every time during the night that the mate came round with a light after the hands, I was afraid he would see I was a colored man, and take me up; hence I kept from the light as much as possible. Some men love darkness rather than light, because their deeds are evil; but this was not the case with myself; it was to avoid detection in doing right. This was one of the instances of my adventures that my affinity with the Anglo-Saxon race, and even slaveholders, worked well for my escape. But no thanks to them for it. While in their midst they have not only robbed me of my labor and liberty, but they have almost entirely robbed me of my dark complexion. Being so near the color of a slaveholder, they could not, or did not find me out that night among the white passengers. There was one of the deck hands on board called out on his watch, whose hammock was swinging up near by me. I asked him if he would let me lie in it. He said if I would pay him twenty-five cents that I might lie in it until day. I readily paid him the price and got into the hammock. No one could see my face to know whether I was white or colored, while I was in the hammock; but I never closed my eyes for sleep that night. I had often heard of explosions on board of Steamboats; and every time the boat landed, and blowed off steam, I was afraid the boilers had bursted and we should all be killed; but I lived through the night amid the many dangers to which I was exposed. I still maintained my position in the hammock, until the next morning about 8 o'clock, when I heard the passengers saying the boat was near Cincinnati; and by this time I supposed that the attention of the people would be turned to the city, and I might pass off unnoticed.

There were no questions asked me while on board the boat. The boat landed about 9 o'clock in the morning in Cincinnati, and I waited until after most of the passengers had gone off of the boat; I then walked as gracefully up street as if I was not running away, until I had got pretty well up Broadway. My object was to go to Canada, but having no knowledge of the road, it was necessary for me to make some inquiry before I left the city. I was afraid to ask a white person, and I could see no colored person to ask. But fortunately for me I found a company of little boys at play in the street, and through these little boys, by asking them indirect questions, I found the residence of a colored man.

"Boys, can you tell me where that old colored man lives who saws wood, and works at jobs around the streets?"

"What is his name?" said one of the boys.

"I forget."

"Is it old Job Dundy?"

"Is Dundy a colored man?"

"Yes, sir."

"That is the very man I am looking for; will you show me where he lives?"

"Yes," said the little boy, and pointed me out the house.

Mr. D. invited me in, and I found him to be a true friend. He asked me if I was a slave from Kentucky, and if I ever intended to go back into slavery? Not knowing yet whether he was truly in favor of slaves running away, I told him that I had just come over to spend my christmas holydays, and that I was going back. His reply was, "my son, I would never go back if I was in your place; you have a right to your liberty." I then asked him how I should get my freedom? He referred me to Canada, over which waved freedom's flag, defended by the British Government, upon whose soil there cannot be the foot print of a slave.

He then commenced telling me of the facilities for my escape to Canada; of the Abolitionists; of the Abolition Societies, and of their fidelity to the cause of suffering humanity. This was the first time in my life that ever I had heard of such people being in existence as the Abolitionists. I supposed that they were a different race of people. He conducted me to the house of one of these warm-hearted friends of God and the slave. I found him willing to aid a poor fugitive on his way to Canada, even to the dividing of the last cent, or morsel of bread if necessary.

These kind friends gave me something to eat and started me on my way to Canada, with a recommendation to a friend on my way. This was the commencement of what was called the under ground rail road to Canada. I walked with bold courage, trusting in the arm of Omnipotence; guided by the unchangable North Star by night, and inspired by an elevated thought that I was fleeing from a land of slavery and oppression, bidding farewell to handcuffs, whips, thumb-screws and chains.

I travelled on until I had arrived at the place where I was directed to call on an Abolitionist, but I made no stop: so great were my fears of being pursued by the pro-slavery hunting dogs of the South. I prosecuted my journey vigorously for nearly forty-eight hours without food or rest, struggling against external difficulties such as no one can imagine who has never experienced the same: not knowing what moment I might be captured while travelling among strangers, through cold and fear, breasting the north winds, being thinly clad, pelted by the snow storms through the dark hours of the night and not a house in which I could enter to shelter me from the storm.

The second night from Cincinnati, about midnight, I thought that I should freeze; my shoes were worn through, and my feet were exposed to the bare ground. I approached a house on the road-side, knocked at the door, and asked admission to their fire, but was refused. I went to the next house, and was refused the privilege of their fire-side, to prevent my freezing. This I thought was hard treatment among the human family. But—

"Behind a frowning Providence there was a smiling face,"

which soon shed beams of light upon unworthy me.

The next morning I was still found struggling on my way faint, hungry, lame, and rest-broken. I could see people taking breakfast from the road-side, but I did not dare to enter their houses to get my breakfast, for neither love nor money. In passing a low cottage, I saw the breakfast table spread with all its bounties, and I could see no male person about the house; the temptation for food was greater than I could resist.

I saw a lady about the table, and I thought that if she was ever so much disposed to take me up, that she would have to catch and hold me, and that would have been impossible. I stepped up to the door with my hat off, and asked her if she would be good enough to sell me a sixpence worth of bread and meat. She cut off a piece and brought it to me; I thanked her for it, and handed her the pay, but instead of receiving it, she burst into tears, and said "never mind the money," but gently turned away bidding me go on my journey. This was altogether unexpected to me: I had found a friend in the time of need among strangers, and nothing could be more cheering in the day of trouble than this. When I left that place I started with bolder courage. The next night I put up at a tavern, and continued stopping at public houses until my means were about gone. When I got to the Black Swamp in the county of Wood, Ohio, I stopped one night at a hotel, after travelling all day through mud and snow; but I soon found that I should not be able to pay my bill. This was about the time that the "wild-cat banks" were in a flourishing state, and "shin plasters"* in abundance; they would charge a dollar for one night's lodging.

After I had found out this, I slipped out of the bar room into the kitchen where the landlady was getting supper; as she had quite a number of travellers to cook for that night, I told her if she would accept my services, I would assist her in getting supper; that I was a cook. She very readily accepted the offer, and I went to work.

She was very much pleased with my work, and the next morning I helped her to get breakfast. She then wanted to hire me for all winter, but I refused for fear I might be pursued. My excuse to her was that I had a brother living in Detroit, whom I was going to see on some important business, and after I got that business attended to, I would come back and work for them all winter.

When I started the second morning they paid me fifty cents beside my board, with the understanding that I was to return; but I have not gone back yet.

I arrived the next morning in the village of Perrysburgh, where I found quite a settlement of colored people, many of whom were fugitive slaves. I made my case known to them and they sympathized with me. I was a stranger, and they took me in and persuaded me to spend the winter in Perrysburgh, where I could get employment and go to Canada the next spring, in a steamboat which run from Perrysburgh, if I thought it proper so to do.

I got a job of chopping wood during that winter which enabled me to purchase myself a suit, and after paying my board

---

*Nickname for temporary paper money.

the next spring, I had saved fifteen dollars in cash. My intention was to go back to Kentucky after my wife.

When I got ready to start, which was about the first of May, my friends all persuaded me not to go, but to get some other person to go, for fear I might be caught and sold off from my family into slavery forever. But I could not refrain from going back myself, believing that I could accomplish it better than a stranger.

The money that I had would not pass in the South, and for the purpose of getting it off to a good advantage, I took a steamboat passage to Detroit, Michigan, and there I spent all my money for dry goods, to peddle out on my way back through the State of Ohio. I also purchased myself a pair of false whiskers to put on when I got back to Kentucky, to prevent any one from knowing me after night, should they see me. I then started back after my little family.

CHAPTER V.

My safe arrival at Kentucky.—Surprise and delight to find my family.—Plan for their escape projected.—Return to Cincinnati.—My betrayal by traitors.—Imprisonment in Covington, Kentucky.—Return to slavery.—Infamous proposal of the slave catchers.—My reply.

I SUCCEEDED very well in selling out my goods, and when I arrived in Cincinnati, I called on some of my friends who had aided me on my first escape. They also opposed me in going back only for my own good. But it has ever been characteristic of me to persevere in what I undertake.

I took a Steamboat passage which would bring me to where I should want to land about dark, so as to give me a chance to find my family during the night if possible. The boat landed me at the proper place, and at the proper time accordingly. This landing was about six miles from Bedford, where my mother and wife lived, but with different families. My mother was the cook at a tavern, in Bedford. When I approached the house where mother was living, I remembered where she slept in the kitchen; her bed was near the window.

It was a bright moonlight night, and in looking through the kitchen window, I saw a person lying in bed about where my mother had formerly slept. I rapped on the glass which awakened the person, in whom I recognised my dear mother, but she knew me not, as I was dressed in disguise with my false whiskers on; but she came to the window and asked who I was and what I wanted. But when I took off my false whiskers, and spoke to her, she knew my voice, and quickly sprang to the door, clasping my hand, exclaiming, "Oh! is this my son," drawing me into the room, where I was so fortunate as to find Malinda, and little Frances, my wife and child, whom I had left to find the fair climes of liberty, and whom I was then seeking to rescue from perpetual slavery.

They never expected to see me again in this life. I am entirely unable to describe what my feelings were at that time. It was almost like the return of the prodigal son. There was weeping and rejoicing. They were filled with surprise and fear;

with sadness and joy. The sensation of joy at that moment flashed like lightning over my afflicted mind, mingled with a thousand dreadful apprehensions, that none but a heart wounded slave father and husband like myself can possibly imagine. After talking the matter over, we decided it was not best to start with my family that night, as it was very uncertain whether we should get a boat passage immediately. And in case of failure, if Malinda should get back even before daylight the next morning, it would have excited suspicion against her, as it was not customary for slaves to leave home at that stage of the week without permission. Hence we thought it would be the most effectual way for her to escape, to start on Saturday night; this being a night on which the slaves of Kentucky are permitted to visit around among their friends, and are often allowed to stay until the afternoon on Sabbath day.

I gave Malinda money to pay her passage on board of a Steamboat to Cincinnati, as it was not safe for me to wait for her until Saturday night; but she was to meet me in Cincinnati, if possible, the next Sunday. Her father was to go with her to the Ohio River on Saturday night, and if a boat passed up during the night she was to get on board at Madison, and come to Cincinnati. If she should fail in getting off that night, she was to try it the next Saturday night. This was the understanding when we separated. This we thought was the best plan for her escape, as there had been so much excitement caused by my running away.

The owners of my wife were very much afraid that she would follow me; and to prevent her they had told her and other slaves that I had been persuaded off by the Abolitionists, who had promised to set me free, but had sold me off to New Orleans. They told the slaves to beware of the abolitionists, that their object was to decoy off slaves and then sell them off in New Orleans. Some of them believed this, and others believed it not; and the owners of my wife were more watchful over her than they had ever been before as she was unbelieving.

This was in the month of June, 1838. I left Malinda on a bright but lonesome Wednesday night. When I arrived at the river Ohio, I found a small craft chained to a tree, in which I ferried myself across the stream.

I succeeded in getting a Steamboat passage back to Cincinnati, where I put up with one of my abolition friends who knew that I had gone after my family, and who appeared to be much surprised to see me again. I was soon visited by several friends who knew of my having gone back after my family. They wished to know why I had not brought my family with me; but after they understood the plan, and that my family was expected to be in Cincinnati within a few days, they thought it the best and safest plan for us to take a stage passage out to Lake Erie. But being short of money, I was not able to pay my passage in the stage, even if it would have prevented me from being caught by the slave hunters of Cincinnati, or save me from being taken back into bondage for life.

These friends proposed helping me by subscription; I accepted their kind offer, but in going among friends to solicit aid for me, they happened to get among traitors, and kidnappers, both white and colored men, who made their living by that kind of business. Several persons called on me and made me small donations, and among them two white men came in professing to be my friends. They told me not to be afraid of them, they were abolitionists. They asked me a great many questions. They wanted to know if I needed any help? and they wanted to know if it could be possible that a man so near white as myself could be a slave? Could it be possible that men would make slaves of their own children? They expressed great sympathy for me, and gave me fifty cents each; by this they gained my confidence. They asked my master's name; where he lived, &c. After which they left the room, bidding me God speed. These traitors, or land pirates, took passage on board of the first Steamboat down the river, in search of my owners. When they found them, they got a reward of three hundred dollars offered for the re-capture of this "stray" which they had so long and faithfully been hunting, by day and by night, by land and by water, with dogs and with guns, but all without success. This being the last and only chance for dragging me back into hopeless bondage, time and money was no object when they saw a prospect of my being re-taken.

Mr. Gatewood got two of his slaveholding neighbors to go with him to Cincinnati, for the purpose of swearing to anything which might be necessary to change me back into property. They came on to Cincinnati, and with but little effort they soon rallied a mob of ruffians who were willing to become the watch-dogs of slaveholders, for a dram, in connection with a few slavehunting petty constables.

While I was waiting the arrival of my family, I got a job of digging a cellar for the good lady where I was stopping, and while I was digging under the house, all at once I heard a man enter the house; another stept up to the cellar door to where I was at work; he looked in and saw me with my coat off at work. He then rapped over the cellar door on the house side, to notify the one who had entered the house to look for me that I was in the cellar. This strange conduct soon excited suspicion so strong in me, that I could not stay in the cellar and started to come out, but the man who stood by the door, rapped again on the house side, for the other to come to his aid, and told me to stop. I attempted to pass out by him, and he caught hold of me, and drew a pistol, swearing if I did not stop he would shoot me down. By this time I knew that I was betrayed.

I asked him what crime I had committed that I should be murdered.

"I will let you know, very soon," said he.

By this time there were others coming to his aid, and I could see no way by which I could possibly escape the jaws of that hell upon earth.

All my flattering prospects of enjoying my own fire-side, with my little family, were then blasted and gone; and I must bid farewell to friends and freedom forever.

In vain did I look to the infamous laws of the Commonwealth of Ohio, for that protection against violence and outrage, that even the vilest criminal with a white skin might enjoy. But oh! the dreadful thought, that after all my sacrifice and struggling to rescue my family from the hands of the oppressor; that I should be dragged back into cruel bondage to suffer the penalty of a tyrant's law, to endure stripes and imprisonment, and to be shut out from all moral as well as intellectual improvement, and linger out almost a living death.

When I saw a crowd of blood-thirsty, unprincipled slave hunters rushing upon me armed with weapons of death, it was no use for me to undertake to fight my way through against such fearful odds.

But I broke away from the man who stood by with his pistol drawn to shoot me if I should resist, and reached the fence and attempted to jump over it before I was overtaken; but the fence being very high I was caught by my legs before I got over.

I kicked and struggled with all my might to get away, but without success. I kicked a new cloth coat off of his back, while he was holding on to my leg. I kicked another in his eye; but they never let me go until they got more help. By this time, there was a crowd on the out side of the fence with clubs to beat me back. Finally, they succeeded in dragging me from the fence and overpowered me by numbers and choked me almost to death.

These ruffians dragged me through the streets of Cincinnati, to what was called a justice office. But it was more like an office of injustice.

When I entered the room I was introduced to three slaveholders, one of whom was a son of Wm. Gatewood, who claimed me as his property. They pretended to be very glad to see me.

They asked me if I did not want to see my wife and child; but I made no reply to any thing that was said until I was delivered up as a slave. After they were asked a few questions by the court, the old pro-slavery squire very gravely pronounced me to be the property of Mr. Gatewood.

The office being crowded with spectators, many of whom were colored persons, Mr. G. was afraid to keep me in Cincinnati, two or three hours even, until a steamboat got ready to leave for the South. So they took me across the river, and locked me up in Covington jail, for safe keeping. This was the first time in my life that I had been put into a jail. It was truly distressing to my feelings to be locked up in a cold dungeon for no crime. The jailor not being at home, his wife had to act in his place. After my owners had gone back to Cincinnati, the jailor's wife, in company with another female, came into the jail and talked with me very friendly.

I told them all about my situation, and these ladies said they hoped that I might get away again, and went so far as to tell me if I should be kept in the jail that night, there was a hole under the wall of the jail where a prisoner had got out. It was only filled up with loose dirt, they said, and I might scratch it out and clear myself.

This I thought was a kind word from an unexpected friend: I had power to have taken the key from those ladies, in spite of them, and have cleared myself; but knowing that they would have to suffer perhaps for letting me get away, I thought I would wait until after dark, at which time I should try to make my escape, if they should not take me out before that time. But within two or three hours, they came after me, and conducted me on board of a boat, on which we all took passage down to Louisville. I was not confined in any way, but was well guarded by five men, three of whom were slave-holders, and the two young men from Cincinnati, who had betrayed me.

After the boat had got fairly under way, with these vile men standing around me on the upper deck of the boat, and she under full speed carrying me back into a land of torment, I could see no possible way of escape. Yet, while I was permitted to gaze on the beauties of nature, on free soil, as I passed down the river, things looked to me uncommonly pleasant: The green trees and wild flowers of the forest; the ripening harvest fields waving with the gentle breezes of Heaven; and the honest farmers tilling their soil and living by their own toil. These things seem to light upon my vision with a peculiar charm. I was conscious of what must be my fate; a wretched victim for Slavery without limit; to be sold like an ox, into hopeless bondage, and to be worked under the flesh devouring lash during life, without wages.

This was to me an awful thought; every time the boat run near the shore, I was tempted to leap from the deck down into the water, with a hope of making my escape. Such was then my feeling.

But on a moment's reflection, reason with her warning

voice overcame this passion by pointing out the dreadful consequences of one's committing suicide. And this I thought
would have a very striking resemblance to the act, and I declined putting into practice this dangerous experiment,
though the temptation was great.

These kidnapping gentlemen, seeing that I was much dissatisfied, commenced talking to me, by saying that I must not
be cast down; they were going to take me back home to live
with my family, if I would promise not to run away again.

To this I agreed, and told them that this was all that I could
ask, and more than I had expected.

But they were not satisfied with having recaptured me, because they had lost other slaves and supposed that I knew
their whereabouts; and truly I did. They wanted me to tell
them; but before telling I wanted them to tell who it was that
had betrayed me into their hands. They said that I was betrayed by two colored men in Cincinnati, whose names they
were backward in telling, because their business in connection
with themselves was to betray and catch fugitive slaves for the
reward offered. They undertook to justify the act by saying if
they had not betrayed me, that somebody else would, and if
I would tell them where they could catch a number of other
runaway slaves, they would pay for me and set me free, and
would then take me in as one of the Club. They said I would
soon make money enough to buy my wife and child out of
slavery.

But I replied, "No, gentlemen, I cannot commit or do an
act of that kind, even if it were in my power so to do. I know
that I am now in the power of a master who can sell me from
my family for life, or punish me for the crime of running
away, just as he pleases: I know that I am a prisoner for life,
and have no way of extricating myself; and I also know that I
have been deceived and betrayed by men who professed to be
my best friends; but can all this justify me in becoming a traitor to others? Can I do that which I complain of others for
doing unto me? Never, I trust, while a single pulsation of my
heart continues to beat, can I consent to betray a fellow man
like myself back into bondage, who has escaped. Dear as I
love my wife and little child, and as much as I should like to

enjoy freedom and happiness with them, I am unwilling to bring this about by betraying and destroying the liberty and happiness of others who have never offended me!"

I then asked them again if they would do me the kindness to tell me who it was betrayed me into their hands at Cincinnati? They agreed to tell me with the understanding that I was to tell where there was living, a family of slaves at the North, who had run away from Mr. King of Kentucky. I should not have agreed to this, but I knew the slaves were in Canada, where it was not possible for them to be captured. After they had told me the names of the persons who betrayed me, and how it was done, then I told them their slaves were in Canada, doing well. The two white men were Constables, who claimed the right of taking up any strange colored person as a slave; while the two colored kidnappers, under the pretext of being abolitionists, would find out all the fugitives they could, and inform these Constables for which they got a part of the reward, after they had found out where the slaves were from, the name of his master, &c. By the agency of these colored men, they were seized by a band of white ruffians, locked up in jail, and their master sent for. These colored kidnappers, with the Constables, were getting rich by betraying fugitive slaves. This was told to me by one of the Constables, while they were all standing around trying to induce me to engage in the same business for the sake of regaining my own liberty, and that of my wife and child. But my answer even there, under the most trying circumstances, surrounded by the strongest enemies of God and man, was most emphatically in the negative. "Let my punishment be what it may, either with the lash or by selling me away from my friends and home; let my destiny be what you please, I can never engage in this business for the sake of getting free."

They said I should not be sold nor punished with the lash for what I had done, but I should be carried back to Bedford, to live with my wife. Yet when the boat got to where we should have landed, she wafted by without making any stop. I felt awful in view of never seeing my family again; they asked what was the matter? what made me look so cast down? I informed them that I knew I was to be sold in the Louisville slave market, or in New Orleans, and I never expected to see my family again. But they tried to pacify me by promising not to sell me to a slave trader who would take me off to New Orleans; cautioning me at the same time not to let it be known that I had been a runaway. This would very much lessen the value of me in market. They would not punish me by putting irons on my limbs, but would give me a good name, and sell me to some gentleman in Louisville for a house servant. They thought I would soon make money enough to buy myself, and would not part with me if they could get along without. But I had cost them so much in advertising and looking for me, that they were involved by it. In the first place they paid eight hundred and fifty dollars for me; and when I first run away, they paid one hundred for advertising and looking after me; and now they had to pay about forty dollars, expenses travelling to and from Cincinnati, in addition to the three hundred dollars reward; and they were not able to pay the reward without selling me.

I knew then the only alternative left for me to extricate myself was to use deception, which is the most effectual defence a slave can use. I pretended to be satisfied for the purpose of getting an opportunity of giving them the slip.

But oh, the distress of mind, the lamentable thought that I should never again see the face nor hear the gentle voice of my nearest and dearest friends in this life. I could imagine what must be my fate from my peculiar situation. To be sold to the highest bidder, and then wear the chains of slavery down to the grave. The day star of liberty which had once cheered and gladdened my heart in freedom's land, had then hidden itself from my vision, and the dark and dismal frown of slavery had obscured the sunshine of freedom from me, as they supposed for all time to come.

But the understanding between us was, I was not to be tied, chained, nor flogged; for if they should take me into the city handcuffed and guarded by five men the question might be asked what crime I had committed? And if it should be known that I had been a runaway to Canada, it would lessen the value of me at least one hundred dollars.

CHAPTER VI.

Arrival at Louisville, Ky.—Efforts to sell me.—Fortunate escape from the man-stealers in the public street.—I return to Bedford, Ky.—The rescue of my family again attempted.—I started alone expecting them to follow.—After waiting some months I resolve to go back again to Kentucky.

WHEN the boat arrived at Louisville, the day being too far spent for them to dispose of me, they had to put up at a Hotel. When we left the boat, they were afraid of my bolting from them in the street, and to prevent this they took hold of my arms, one on each side of me, gallanting me up to the hotel with as much propriety as if I had been a white lady. This was to deceive the people, and prevent my getting away from them.

They called for a bed-room to which I was conducted and locked within. That night three of them lodged in the same room to guard me. They locked the door and put the key under the head of their bed. I could see no possible way for my escape without jumping out of a high three story house window.

It was almost impossible for me to sleep that night in my peculiar situation. I passed the night in prayer to our Heavenly Father, asking that He would open to me even the smallest chance for escape.

The next morning after they had taken breakfast, four of them left me in the care of Dan Lane. He was what might be called one of the watch dogs of Kentucky. There was nothing too mean for him to do. He never blushed to rob a slave mother of her children, no matter how young or small. He was also celebrated for slave selling, kidnapping, and negro hunting. He was well known in that region by the slaves as well as the slaveholders, to have all the qualifications necessary for his business. He was a drunkard, a gambler, a profligate, and a slaveholder.

While the other four were looking around through the city for a purchaser, Dan was guarding me with his bowie knife and pistols. After a while the others came in with two persons

476

to buy me, but on seeing me they remarked that they thought I would run away, and asked me if I had ever run away. Dan sprang to his feet and answered the question for me, by telling one of the most palpable falsehoods that ever came from the lips of a slaveholder. He declared that I had never run away in my life!

Fortunately for me, Dan, while the others were away, became unwell; and from taking salts, or from some other cause, was compelled to leave his room. Off he started to the horse stable which was located on one of the most public streets of Louisville, and of course I had to accompany him. He gallanted me into the stable by the arm, and placed himself back in one of the horses stalls and ordered me to stand by until he was ready to come out.

At this time a thousand thoughts were flashing through my mind with regard to the propriety of trying the springs of my heels, which nature had so well adapted for taking the body out of danger, even in the most extraordinary emergencies. I thought in the attempt to get away by running, if I should not succeed, it could make my condition no worse, for they could but sell me and this they were then trying to do These thoughts impelled me to keep edging towards the door, though very cautiously. Dan kept looking around after me as if he was not satisfied at my getting so near to the door. But the last I saw of him in the stable was just as he turned his eyes from me; I nerved myself with all the moral courage I could command and bolted for the door, perhaps with the fleetness of a much frightened deer, who never looks behind in time of peril. Dan was left in the stable to make ready for the race, or jump out into the street half dressed, and thereby disgrace himself before the public eye.

It would be impossible for me to set forth the speed with which I run to avoid my adversary; I succeeded in turning a corner before Dan got sight of me, and by fast running, turning corners, and jumping high fences, I was enabled to effect my escape.

In running so swiftly through the public streets, I thought it would be a safer course to leave the public way, and as quick as thought I spied a high board fence by the way and attempted to leap over it. The top board broke and down I came into a hen-coop which stood by the fence. The dogs barked, and the hens flew and cackled so, that I feared it would lead to my detection before I could get out of the yard.

The reader can only imagine how great must have been the excited state of my mind while exposed to such extraordinary peril and danger on every side. In danger of being seized by a savage dog, which sprang at me when I fell into the hen-coop; in danger of being apprehended by the tenants of the lot; in danger of being shot or wounded by any one who might have attempted to stop me, a runaway slave; and in danger on the other hand of being overtaken and getting in conflict with my adversary. With these fearful apprehensions, caution dictated me not to proceed far by day-light in this slaveholding city.

At this moment every nerve and muscle of my whole system was in full stretch; and every facility of the mind brought into action striving to save myself from being re-captured. I dared not go to the forest, knowing that I might be tracked by blood-hounds, and overtaken. I was so fortunate as to find a hiding place in the city which seemed to be pointed out by the finger of Providence. After running across lots, turning corners, and shunning my fellow men, as if they were wild ferocious beasts. I found a hiding place in a pile of boards or scantling, where I kept concealed during that day.

No tongue nor pen can describe the dreadful apprehensions under which I labored for the space of ten or twelve hours. My hiding place happened to be between two work-shops, where there were men at work within six or eight feet of me. I could imagine that I heard them talking about me, and at other times thought I heard the footsteps of Daniel Lane in close pursuit. But I retained my position there until 9 or 10 o'clock at night, without being discovered; after which I attempted to find my way out, which was exceedingly difficult. The night being very dark, in a strange city, among slaveholders and slave hunters, to me it was like a person entering a wilderness among wolves and vipers, blindfolded. I was compelled from necessity to enter this place for refuge under the most extraordinary state of excitement, without regard to its geographical position. I found myself surrounded with a large block of buildings, which comprised a whole square, built up mostly on three sides, so that I could see no way to pass out without exposing myself perhaps to the gaze of patrols, or slave catchers.

In wandering around through the dark, I happened to find a calf in a back yard, which was bawling after the cow; the cow was also lowing in another direction, as if they were trying to find each other. A thought struck me that there must be an outlet somewhere about, where the cow and calf were trying to meet. I started in the direction where I heard the lowing of the cow, and I found an arch or tunnel extending between two large brick buildings, where I could see nothing of the cow but her eyes, shining like balls of fire through the dark tunnel, between the walls, through which I passed to where she stood. When I entered the streets I found them well lighted up. My heart was gladdened to know there was another chance for my escape. No bird ever let out of a cage felt more like flying, than I felt like running.

Before I left the city, I chanced to find by the way, an old man of color. Supposing him to be a friend, I ventured to make known my situation, and asked him if he would get me a bite to eat. The old man most cheerfully complied with my request. I was then about forty miles from the residence of Wm. Gatewood, where my wife, whom I sought to rescue from slavery, was living. This was also in the direction it was necessary for me to travel in order to get back to the free North. Knowing that the slave catchers would most likely be watching the public highway for me, to avoid them I made my way over the rocky hills, woods and plantations, back to Bedford.

I travelled all that night, guided on my way by the shining stars of heaven alone. The next morning just before the break of day, I came right to a large plantation, about which I secreted myself, until the darkness of the next night began to disappear. The morning larks commenced to chirp and sing merrily—pretty soon I heard the whip crack, and the voice of the ploughman driving in the corn field. About breakfast time, I heard the sound of a horn; saw a number of slaves in the field with a white man, who I supposed to be their overseer. He started to the house before the slaves, which gave me an opportunity to get the attention of one of the slaves, whom I met at the fence, before he started to his breakfast, and made known to him my wants and distresses. I also requested him to bring me a piece of bread if he could when he came back to the field.

The hospitable slave complied with my request. He came back to the field before his fellow laborers, and brought me something to eat, and as an equivolent for his kindness, I instructed him with regard to liberty, Canada, the way of escape, and the facilities by the way. He pledged his word that himself and others would be in Canada, in less than six months from that day. This closed our interview, and we separated. I concealed myself in the forest until about sunset, before I pursued my journey; and the second night from Louisville, I arrived again in the neighborhood of Bedford, where my little family were held in bondage, whom I so earnestly strove to rescue.

I concealed myself by the aid of a friend in that neighborhood, intending again to make my escape with my family. This confidential friend then carried a message to Malinda, requesting her to meet me on one side of the village.

We met under the most fearful apprehensions, for my pursuers had returned from Louisville, with the lamentable story that I was gone, and yet they were compelled to pay three hundred dollars to the Cincinnati slave catchers for re-capturing me there.

Daniel Lane's account of my escape from him, looked so unreasonable to slaveholders, that many of them charged him with selling me and keeping the money; while others believed that I had got away from him, and was then in the neighborhood, trying to take off my wife and child, which was true. Lane declared that in less than five minutes after I run out of the stable in Louisville, he had over twenty men running and looking in every direction after me; but all without success. They could hear nothing of me. They had turned over several tons of hay in a large loft, in search, and I was not to be found there. Dan imputed my escape to my godliness! He said that I must have gone up in a chariot of fire, for I went off by flying; and that he should never again have any thing to do with a praying negro.

Great excitement prevailed in Bedford, and many were out watching for me at the time Malinda was relating to me these facts. The excitement was then so great among the slaveholders—who were anxious to have me re-captured as a means of discouraging other slaves from running away—that time and money were no object while there was the least prospect of their success. I therefore declined making an effort just at that time to escape with my little family. Malinda managed to get me into the house of a friend that night, in the village, where I kept concealed several days seeking an opportunity to escape with Malinda and Frances to Canada.

But for some time Malinda was watched so very closely by white and by colored persons, both day and night, that it was not possible for us to escape together. They well knew that my little family was the only object of attraction that ever had or ever would induce me to come back and risk my liberty over the threshold of slavery—therefore this point was well guarded by the watch dogs of slavery, and I was compelled again to forsake my wife for a season, or surrender, which was suicidal to the cause of freedom, in my judgment.

The next day after my arrival in Bedford, Daniel Lane came to the very house wherein I was concealed and talked in my hearing to the family about my escape from him out of the stable in Louisville. He was near enough for me to have laid my hands on his head while in that house—and the intimidation which this produced on me was more than I could bear. I was also aware of the great temptation of the reward offered to white or colored persons for my apprehension; I was exposed to other calamities which rendered it altogether unsafe for me to stay longer under that roof.

One morning about 2 o'clock, I took leave of my little family and started for Canada. This was almost like tearing off the limbs from my body. When we were about to separate, Malinda clasped my hand exclaiming, "oh my soul! my heart is almost broken at the thought of this dangerous separation. This may be the last time we shall ever see each other's faces in this life, which will destroy all my future prospects of life and happiness forever." At this time the poor unhappy woman burst into tears and wept loudly; and my eyes were not dry. We separated with the understanding that she was to wait until the excitement was all over; after which she was to meet me at a certain place in the State of Ohio; which would not be longer than two months from that time.

I succeeded that night in getting a steamboat conveyance back to Cincinnati, or within ten miles of the city. I was apprehensive that there were slave-hunters in Cincinnati, watching the arrival of every boat up the river, expecting to catch me; and the boat landing to take in wood ten miles below the city, I got off and walked into Cincinnati, to avoid detection.

On my arrival at the house of a friend, I heard that the two young men who betrayed me for the three hundred dollars had returned and were watching for me. One of my friends in whom they had great confidence, called on the traitors, after he had talked with me, and asked them what they had done with me. Their reply was that I had given them the slip, and that they were glad of it, because they believed that I was a good man, and if they could see me on my way to Canada, they would give me money to aid me on my escape. My friend assured them that if they would give any thing to aid me on my way, much or little, if they would put the same into his hands, he would give it to me that night, or return it to them the next morning.

They then wanted to know where I was and whether I was in the city; but he would not tell them, but one of them gave him one dollar for me, promising that if I was in the city, and he would let him know the next morning, he would give me ten dollars.

But I never waited for the ten dollars. I received one dollar of the amount which they got for betraying me, and started that night for the north. Their excuse for betraying me, was, that catching runaways was their business, and if they had not done it somebody else would, but since they had got the reward they were glad that I had made my escape.

Having travelled the road several times from Cincinnati to Lake Erie, I travelled through without much fear or difficulty. My friends in Perrysburgh, who knew that I had gone back into the very jaws of slavery after my family, were much surprised at my return, for they had heard that I was re-captured.

After I had waited three months for the arrival of Malinda, and she came not, it caused me to be one of the most unhappy fugitives that ever left the South. I had waited eight or nine months without hearing from my family. I felt it to be my duty, as a husband and father, to make one more effort. I felt as if I could not give them up to be sacrificed on the "bloody altar of slavery." I felt as if love, duty, humanity and justice, required that I should go back, putting my trust in the God of Liberty for success.

CHAPTER VII.

My safe return to Kentucky.—The perils I encountered there.—
Again betrayed, and taken by a mob; ironed and impris-
oned.—Narrow escape from death.—Life in a slave prison.

I PREPARED myself for the journey before named, and started
back in the month of July, 1839.

My intention was, to let no person know my business until
I returned back to the North. I went to Cincinnati, and got a
passage down on board of a boat just as I did the first time,
without any misfortune or delay. I called on my mother, and
the raising of a dead body from the grave could not have been
more surprising to any one than my arrival was to her, on that
sad summer's night. She was not able to suppress her feelings.
When I entered the room, there was but one other person in
the house with my mother, and this was a little slave girl who
was asleep when I entered. The impulsive feeling which is
ever ready to act itself out at the return of a long absent
friend, was more than my bereaved mother could suppress.
And unfortunately for me, the loud shouts of joy at that late
hour of the night, awakened the little slave girl, who afterwards betrayed me. She kept perfectly still, and never let either of us know that she was awake, in order that she might
hear our conversation and report it. Mother informed me
where my family was living, and that she would see them the
next day, and would make arrangements for us to meet the
next night at that house after the people in the village had
gone to bed. I then went off and concealed myself during the
next day, and according to promise came back the next night
about eleven o'clock.

When I got near the house, moving very cautiously, filled
with fearful apprehensions, I saw several men walking around
the house as if they were looking for some person. I went
back and waited about one hour, before I returned, and the
number of men had increased. They were still to be seen lurking about this house, with dogs following them. This strange
movement frightened me off again, and I never returned until

after midnight, at which time I slipped up to the window, and rapped for my mother, who sprang to it and informed me that I was betrayed by the girl who overheard our conversation the night before. She thought that if I could keep out of the way for a few days, the white people would think that this girl was mistaken, or had lied. She had told her old mistress that I was there that night, and had made a plot with my mother to get my wife and child there the next night, and that I was going to take them off to Canada.

I went off to a friend of mine, who rendered me all the aid that one slave could render another, under the circumstances. Thank God he is now free from slavery, and is doing well. He was a messenger for me to my wife and mother, until at the suggestion of my mother, I changed an old friend for a new one, who betrayed me for the sum of five dollars.

We had set the time when we were to start for Canada, which was to be on the next Saturday night. My mother had an old friend whom she thought was true, and she got him to conceal me in a barn, not over two miles from the village. This man brought provisions to me, sent by my mother, and would tell me the news which was in circulation about me, among the citizens. But the poor fellow was not able to withstand the temptation of money.

My owners had about given me up, and thought the report of the slave girl was false; but they had offered a little reward among the slaves for my apprehension. The night before I was betrayed, I met with my mother and wife, and we had set up nearly all night plotting to start on the next Saturday night. I hid myself away in the flax in the barn, and being much rest broken I slept until the next morning about 9 o'clock. Then I was awakened by a mob of blood thirsty slaveholders, who had come armed with all the implements of death, with a determination to reduce me again to a life of slavery, or murder me on the spot.

When I looked up and saw that I was surrounded, they were exclaiming at the top of their voices, "shoot him down! shoot him down!" "If he offers to run, or to resist, kill him!"

I saw it was no use then for me to make any resistance, as I should be murdered. I felt confident that I had been betrayed by a slave, and all my flattering prospects of rescuing my family were gone for ever, and the grim monster slavery with all its horrors was staring me in the face.

I surrendered myself to this hostile mob at once. The first thing done, after they had laid violent hands on me, was to bind my hands behind me with a cord, and rob me of all I possessed.

In searching my pockets, they found my certificate from the Methodist E. Church, which had been given me by my classleader, testifying to my worthiness as a member of that church. And what made the matter look more disgraceful to me, many of this mob were members of the M. E. Church, and they were the persons who took away my church ticket, and then robbed me also of fourteen dollars in cash, a silver watch for which I paid ten dollars, a pocket knife for which I paid seventy-five cents, and a Bible for which I paid sixty-two and one half cents. All this they tyrannically robbed me of, and yet my owner, Wm. Gatewood, was a regular member of the same church to which I belonged.

He then had me taken to a blacksmith's shop, and most wickedly had my limbs bound with heavy irons, and then had my body locked within the cold dungeon walls of the Bedford jail, to be sold to a Southern slave trader.

My heart was filled with grief—my eyes were filled with tears. I could see no way of escape. I could hear no voice of consolation. Slaveholders were coming to the dungeon window in great numbers to ask me questions. Some were rejoicing—some swearing, and others saying that I ought to be hung; while others were in favor of sending both me and my wife to New Orleans. They supposed that I had informed her all about the facilities for slaves to escape to Canada, and that she would tell other slaves after I was gone; hence we must all be sent off to where we could neither escape ourselves, nor instruct others the way.

In the afternoon of the same day Malinda was permitted to visit the prison wherein I was locked, but was not permitted to enter the door. When she looked through the dungeon grates and saw my sad situation, which was caused by my repeated adventures to rescue her and my little daughter from the grasp of slavery, it was more than she could bear without bursting in tears. She plead for admission into the cold dungeon where I was confined, but without success. With manacled limbs; with wounded spirit; with sympathising tears and with bleeding heart, I intreated Malinda to weep not for me, for it only added to my grief, which was greater than I could bear.

I have often suffered from the sting of the cruel slave driver's lash on my quivering flesh—I have suffered from corporeal punishment in its various forms—I have mingled my sorrows with those that were bereaved by the ungodly soul drivers—and I also know what it is to shed the sympathetic tear at the grave of a departed friend; but all this is but a mere trifle compared with my sufferings from then to the end of six months subsequent.

The second night while I was in jail, two slaves came to the dungeon grates about the dead hour of night, and called me to the grates to have some conversation about Canada, and the facilities for getting there. They knew that I had travelled over the road, and they were determined to run away and go where they could be free. I of course took great pleasure in giving them directions how and where to go, and they started in less than a week from that time and got clear to Canada. I have seen them both since I came back to the north myself. They were known by the names of King and Jack.

The third day I was brought out of the prison to be carried off with my little family to the Louisville slave market. My hands were fastened together with heavy irons, and two men to guard me with loaded rifles, one of whom led the horse upon which I rode. My wife and child were set upon another nag. After we were all ready to start my old master thought I was not quite safe enough, and ordered one of the boys to bring him a bed cord from the store. He then tied my feet together under the horse, declaring that if I flew off this time, I should fly off with the horse.

Many tears were shed on that occasion by our friends and relatives, who saw us dragged off in irons to be sold in the human flesh market. No tongue could express the deep anguish of my soul when I saw the silent tear drops streaming down the sable cheeks of an aged slave mother, at my departure; and that too, caused by a black hearted traitor who was himself a slave:

"I love the man with a feeling soul.
  Whose passions are deep and strong;
  Whose cords, when touched with a kindred power,
  Will vibrate loud and long:

"The man whose word is bond and law—
  Who ne'er for gold or power,
  Would kiss the hand that would stab the heart
  In adversity's trying hour."

"I love the man who delights to help
  The panting, struggling poor:
  The man that will open his heart,
  Nor close against the fugitive at his door.

"Oh give me a heart that will firmly stand,
  When the storm of affliction shall lower—
  A hand that will never shrink, if grasped,
  In misfortune's darkest hour."

As we approached the city of Louisville, we attracted much attention, my being tied and handcuffed, and a person leading the horse upon which I rode. The horse appeared to be much frightened at the appearance of things in the city, being young and skittish. A carriage passing by jammed against the nag, which caused him to break from the man who was leading him, and in his fright throw me off backwards. My hands being confined with irons, and my feet tied under the horse with a rope, I had no power to help myself. I fell back off of the horse and could not extricate myself from this dreadful condition; the horse kicked with all his might while I was tied so close to his rump that he could only strike me with his legs by kicking.

The breath was kicked out of my body, but my bones were not broken. No one who saw my situation would have given five dollars for me. It was thought by all that I was dead and would never come to life again. When the horse was caught the cords were cut from my limbs, and I was rubbed with whiskey, camphor, &c., which brought me to life again.

Many bystanders expressed sympathy for me in my deplorable condition, and contempt for the tyrant who tied me to the young horse.

I was then driven through the streets of the city with my little family on foot, to jail, wherein I was locked with handcuffs yet on. A physician was then sent for, who doctored me several days before I was well enough to be sold in market.

The jail was one of the most disagreeable places I ever was confined in. It was not only disagreeable on account of the filth and dirt of the most disagreeable kind; but there were bed-bugs, fleas, lice and musquitoes in abundance, to contend with. At night we had to lie down on the floor in this filth. Our food was very scanty, and of the most inferior quality. No gentleman's dog would eat what we were compelled to eat or starve.

I had not been in this prison many days before Madison Garrison, the soul driver, bought me and my family to sell again in the New Orleans slave market. He was buying up slaves to take to New Orleans. So he took me and my little family to the work-house, to be kept under lock and key at work until he had bought up as many as he wished to take off to the South.

The work-house of Louisville was a very large brick building, built on the plan of a jail or State's prison, with many apartments to it, divided off into cells wherein prisoners were locked up after night. The upper apartments were occupied by females, principally. This prison was enclosed by a high stone wall, upon which stood watchmen with loaded guns to guard the prisoners from breaking out, and on either side there were large iron gates.

When Garrison conducted me with my family to the prison in which we were to be confined until he was ready to take us to New Orleans, I was shocked at the horrid sight of the prisoners on entering the yard. When the large iron gate or door was thrown open to receive us, it was astonishing to see so many whites as well as colored men loaded down with irons, at hard labor, under the supervision of overseers.

Some were sawing stone, some cutting stone, and others breaking stone. The first impression which was made on my mind when I entered this place of punishment, made me think of hell, with all its terrors of torment; such as "weeping, wailing, and gnashing of teeth," which was then the idea that I had of the infernal regions from oral instruction. And I doubt whether there can be a better picture of it drawn, than may be sketched from an American slave prison.

In this prison almost every prisoner had a heavy log chain riveted about his leg. It would indeed be astonishing to a christian man to stand in that prison one half hour and hear and see the contaminating influences of Southern slavery on the body and mind of man—you may there find almost every variety of character to look on. Some singing, some crying, some praying, and others swearing. The people of color who were in there were slaves, there without crime, but for safe keeping, while the whites were some of the most abandoned characters living. The keeper took me up to the anvil block and fastened a chain about my leg, which I had to drag after me both day and night during three months. My labor was sawing stone; my food was coarse corn bread and beef shanks and cows heads with pot liquor, and a very scanty allowance of that.

I have often seen the meat spoiled when brought to us, covered with flies and fly blows, and even worms crawling over it, when we were compelled to eat it, or go without any at all. It was all spread out on a long table in separate plates; and at the sound of a bell, every one would take his plate, asking no questions. After hastily eating, we were hurried back to our work, each man dragging a heavy log chain after him to his work.

About a half hour before night they were commanded to stop work, take a bite to eat, and then be locked up in a small cell until the next morning after sunrise. The prisoners were locked in, two together. My bed was a cold stone floor with but little bedding! My visitors were bed-bugs and musquitoes.

CHAPTER VIII.

Character of my prison companions.—Jail breaking contemplated.—Defeat of our plan.—My wife and child removed.—Disgraceful proposal to her, and cruel punishment.—Our departure in a coffle for New Orleans.—Events of our journey.

MOST of the inmates of this prison I have described, were white men who had been sentenced there by the law, for depredations committed by them. There was in that prison, gamblers, drunkards, thieves, robbers, adulterers, and even murderers. There were also in the female department, harlots, pick-pockets, and adulteresses. In such company, and under such influences, where there was constant swearing, lying, cheating, and stealing, it was almost impossible for a virtuous person to avoid pollution, or to maintain their virtue. No place or places in this country can be better calculated to inculcate vice of every kind than a Southern work house or house of correction.

After a profligate, thief, or a robber, has learned all that they can out of the prison, they might go in one of those prisons and learn something more—they might properly be called robber colleges; and if slaveholders understood this they would never let their slaves enter them. No man would give much for a slave who had been kept long in one of these prisons.

I have often heard them telling each other how they robbed houses, and persons on the high way, by knocking them down, and would rob them, pick their pockets, and leave them half dead. Others would tell of stealing horses, cattle, sheep, and slaves; and when they would be sometimes apprehended, by the aid of their friends, they would break jail. But they could most generally find enough to swear them clear of any kind of villany. They seemed to take great delight in telling of their exploits in robbery. There was a regular combination of them who had determined to resist law, wherever they went, to carry out their purposes.

In conversing with myself, they learned that I was notorious for running away, and professed sympathy for me. They thought that I might yet get to Canada, and be free, and suggested a plan by which I might accomplish it; and one way was, to learn to read and write, so that I might write myself a pass ticket, to go just where I pleased, when I was taken out of the prison; and they taught me secretly all they could while in the prison.

But there was another plan which they suggested to me to get away from slavery; that was to break out of the prison and leave my family. I consented to engage in this plot, but not to leave my family.

By my conduct in the prison, after having been there several weeks, I had gained the confidence of the keeper, and the turnkey. So much so, that when I wanted water or anything of the kind, they would open my door and hand it in to me. One of the turnkeys was an old colored man, who swept and cleaned up the cells, supplied the prisoners with water, &c.

On Sundays in the afternoon, the watchmen of the prison were most generally off, and this old slave, whose name was Stephen, had the prisoners to attend to. The white prisoners formed a plot to break out on Sunday in the afternoon, by making me the agent to get the prison keys from old Stephen.

I was to prepare a stone that would weigh about one pound, tie it up in a rag, and keep it in my pocket to strike poor old Stephen with, when he should open my cell door. But this I would not consent to do, without he should undertake to betray me.

I gave old Stephen one shilling to buy me a water melon, which he was to bring to me in the afternoon. All the prisoners were to be ready to strike, just as soon as I opened their doors. When Stephen opened my door to hand me the melon, I was to grasp him by the collar, raise the stone over his head, and say to him, that if he made any alarm that I should knock him down with the stone. But if he would be quiet he should not be hurt. I was then to take all the keys from him, and lock him up in the cell—take a chisel and cut the chain from my own leg, then unlock all the cells below, and let out the other prisoners, who were all to cut off their chains. We were then to go and let out old Stephen, and make him go off with us. We were to form a line and march to the front gate of the prison with a sledge hammer, and break it open, and if we should be discovered, and there should be any out-cry, we were all to run and raise the alarm of fire, so as to avoid detection. But while we were all listening for Stephen to open the door with the melon, he came and reported that he could not get one, and handed me back the money through the window. All were disappointed, and nothing done. I looked upon it as being a fortunate thing for me, for it was certainly a very dangerous experiment for a slave, and they could never get me to consent to be the leader in that matter again.

A few days after, another plot was concocted to to break prison, but it was betrayed by one of the party, which resulted in the most cruel punishment to the prisoners concerned in it; and I felt thankful that my name was not connected with it. They were not only flogged, but they were kept on bread and water alone, for many days. A few days after we were put in this prison, Garrison came and took my wife and child out, I knew not for what purpose, nor to what place, but after the absence of several days I supposed that he had sold them. But one morning, the outside door was thrown open, and Malinda thrust in by the ruthless hand of Garrison, whose voice was pouring forth the most bitter oaths and abusive language that could be dealt out to a female; while her heart-rending shrieks and sobbing, was truly melting to the soul of a father and husband.

The language of Malinda was, "Oh! my dear little child is gone? What shall I do? my child is gone." This most distressing sound struck a sympathetic chord through all the prison among the prisoners. I was not permitted to go to my wife and inquire what had become of little Frances. I never expected to see her again, for I supposed that she was sold.

That night, however, I had a short interview with my much abused wife, who told me the secret. She said that Garrison had taken her to a private house where he kept female slaves for the basest purposes. It was a resort for slave trading profligates and soul drivers, who were interested in the same business.

Soon after she arrived at this place, Garrison gave her to understand what he brought her there for, and made a most disgraceful assault on her virtue, which she promptly repeled;

and for which Garrison punished her with the lash, threatening her that if she did not submit that he would sell her child. The next day he made the same attempt, which she resisted, declaring that she would not submit to it; and again he tied her up and flogged her until her garments were stained with blood.

He then sent our child off to another part of the city, and said he meant to sell it, and that she should never see it again. He then drove Malinda before him to the work-house, swearing by his Maker that she should submit to him or die. I have already described her entrance in the prison.

Two days after this he came again and took Malinda out of the prison. It was several weeks before I saw her again, and learned that he had not sold her or the child. At the same time he was buying up other slaves to take to New Orleans. At the expiration of three months he was ready to start with us for the New Orleans slave market, but we never knew when we were to go, until the hour had arrived for our departure.

One Sabbath morning Garrison entered the prison and commanded that our limbs should be made ready for the coffles. They called us up to an anvill block, and the heavy log chains which we had been wearing on our legs during three months, were cut off. I had been in the prison over three months; but he had other slaves who had not been there so long. The hand-cuffs were then put on to our wrists. We were coupled together two and two—the right hand of one to the left hand of another, and a long chain to connect us together.

The other prisoners appeared to be sorry to see us start off in this way. We marched off to the river Ohio, to take passage on board of the steamboat Water Witch. But this was at a very low time of water, in the fall of 1839. The boat got aground, and did not get off that night; and Garrison had to watch us all night to keep any from getting away. He also had a very large savage dog, which was trained up to catch runaway slaves.

We were more than six weeks getting to the city of New Orleans, in consequence of low water. We were shifted on to several boats before we arrived at the mouth of the river Ohio. But we got but very little rest at night. As all were chained together night and day, it was impossible to sleep, being annoyed by the bustle and crowd of the passengers on board; by the terrible thought that we were destined to be sold in market as sheep or oxen; and annoyed by the galling chains that cramped our wearied limbs on the tedious voyage. But I had several opportunities to have run away from Garrison before we got to the mouth of the Ohio river. While they were shifting us from one boat to another, my hands were some times loosed, until they got us all on board—and I know that I should have broke away had it not been for the sake of my wife and child who was with me. I could see no chance to get them off, and I could not leave them in that condition—and Garrison was not so much afraid of my running away from him while he held on to my family, for he knew from the great sacrifices which I had made to rescue them from slavery, that my attachment was too strong to run off and leave them in his hands, while there was the least hope of ever getting them away with me.

CHAPTER IX.

Our arrival and examination at Vicksburg.—An account of slave sales.—Cruel punishment with the paddle.—Attempts to sell myself by Garrison's direction.—Amusing interview with a slave buyer.—Deacon Whitfield's examination.—He purchases the family.—Character of the Deacon.

WHEN we arrived at the city of Vicksburg, he intended to sell a portion of his slaves there, and stopped for three weeks trying to sell. But he met with very poor success.

We had there to pass through an examination or inspection by a city officer, whose business it was to inspect slave property that was brought to that market for sale. He examined our backs to see if we had been much scarred by the lash. He examined our limbs, to see whether we were inferior.

As it is hard to tell the ages of slaves, they look in their mouths at their teeth, and prick up the skin on the back of their hands, and if the person is very far advanced in life, when the skin is pricked up, the pucker will stand so many seconds on the back of the hand.

But the most rigorous examinations of slaves by those slave inspectors, is on the mental capacity. If they are found to be very intelligent, this is pronounced the most objectionable of all other qualities connected with the life of a slave. In fact, it undermines the whole fabric of his chattelhood; it prepares for what slaveholders are pleased to pronounce the unpardonable sin when committed by a slave. It lays the foundation for running away, and going to Canada. They also see in it a love for freedom, patriotism, insurrection, bloodshed, and exterminating war against American slavery.

Hence they are very careful to inquire whether a slave who is for sale can read or write. This question has been asked me often by slave traders, and cotton planters, while I was there for market. After conversing with me, they have sworn by their Maker, that they would not have me among their negroes; and that they saw the devil in my eye; I would run away, &c.

I have frequently been asked also, if I had ever run away;

but Garrison would generally answer this question for me in the negative. He could have sold my little family without any trouble, for the sum of one thousand dollars. But for fear he might not get me off at so great an advantage, as the people did not like my appearance, he could do better by selling us all together. They all wanted my wife, while but very few wanted me. He asked for me and my family twenty-five hundred dollars, but was not able to get us off at that price.

He tried to speculate on my Christian character. He tried to make it appear that I was so pious and honest that I would not runaway for ill treatment; which was a gross mistake, for I never had religion enough to keep me from running away from slavery in my life.

But we were taken from Vicksburgh, to the city of New Orleans, were we were to be sold at any rate. We were taken to a trader's yard or a slave prison on the corner of St. Joseph street. This was a common resort for slave traders, and planters who wanted to buy slaves; and all classes of slaves were kept there for sale, to be sold in private or public— young or old, males or females, children or parents, husbands or wives.

Every day at 10 o'clock they were exposed for sale. They had to be in trim for showing themselves to the public for sale. Every one's head had to be combed, and their faces washed, and those who were inclined to look dark and rough, were compelled to wash in greasy dish water, in order to make them look slick and lively.

When spectators would come in the yard, the slaves were ordered out to form a line. They were made to stand up straight, and look as sprightly as they could; and when they were asked a question, they had to answer it as promptly as they could, and try to induce the spectators to buy them. If they failed to do this, they were severely paddled after the spectators were gone. The object for using the paddle in the place of a lash was, to conceal the marks which would be made by the flogging. And the object for flogging under such circumstances, is to make the slaves anxious to be sold.

The paddle is made of a piece of hickory timber, about one inch thick, three inches in width, and about eighteen inches in length. The part which is applied to the flesh is bored full of quarter inch auger holes; and every time this is applied to the flesh of the victim, the blood gushes through the holes of the paddle, or a blister makes its appearance. The persons who are thus flogged, are always stripped naked, and their hands tied together. They are then bent over double, their knees are forced between their elbows, and a stick is put through between the elbows and the bend of the legs, in order to hold the victim in that position, while the paddle is applied to those parts of the body which would not be so likely to be seen by those who wanted to buy slaves.

I was kept in this prison for several months, and no one would buy me for fear I would run away. One day while I was in this prison, Garrison got mad with my wife, and took her off in one of the rooms, with his paddle in hand, swearing that he would paddle her; and I could afford her no protection at all, while the strong arm of the law, public opinion and custom, were all against me. I have often heard Garrison say, that he had rather paddle a female, than eat when he was hungry—that it was music for him to hear them scream, and to see their blood run.

After the lapse of several months, he found that he could not dispose of my person to a good advantage, while he kept me in that prison confined among the other slaves. I do not speak with vanity when I say the contrast was so great between myself and ordinary slaves, from the fact that I had enjoyed superior advantages, to which I have already referred. They have their slaves classed off and numbered.

Garrison came to me one day and informed me that I might go out through the city and find myself a master. I was to go to the Hotels, boarding houses, &c.—tell them that my wife was a good cook, wash-woman, &c.,—and that I was a good dining room servant, carriage driver, or porter—and in this way I might find some gentleman who would buy us both; and that this was the only hope of our being sold together.

But before starting me out, he dressed me up in a suit of his old clothes, so as to make me look respectable, and I was so much better dressed than usual that I felt quite gay. He would not allow my wife to go out with me however, for fear we might get away. I was out every day for several weeks, three or four hours in each day, trying to find a new master, but without success.

Many of the old French inhabitants have taken slaves for their wives, in this city, and their own children for their servants. Such commonly are called Creoles. They are better treated than other slaves, and I resembled this class in appearance so much that the French did not want me. Many of them set their mulatto children free, and make slaveholders of them.

At length one day I heard that there was a gentleman in the city from the State of Tennessee, to buy slaves. He had brought down two rafts of lumber for market, and I thought if I could get him to buy me with my family, and take us to Tennessee, from there, I would stand a better opportunity to run away again and get to Canada, than I would from the extreme South.

So I brushed up myself and walked down to the river's bank, where the man was pointed out to me standing on board of his raft, I approached him, and after passing the usual compliments I said:

"Sir, I understand that you wish to purchase a lot of servants and I have called to know if it is so."

He smiled and appeared to be much pleased at my visit on such laudable business, supposing me to be a slave trader. He commenced rubbing his hands together, and replied by saying: "Yes sir, I am glad to see you. It is a part of my business here to buy slaves, and if I could get you to take my lumber in part pay I should like to buy four or five of your slaves at any rate. What kind of slaves have you, sir?"

After I found that he took me to be a slave trader I knew that it would be of no use for me to tell him that I was myself a slave looking for a master, for he would have doubtless brought up the same objection that others had brought up,— that I was too white; and that they were afraid that I could read and write; and would never serve as a slave, but run away. My reply to the question respecting the quality of my slaves was, that I did not think his lumber would suit me— that I must have the cash for my negroes, and turned on my heel and left him!

I returned to the prison and informed my wife of the fact

that I had been taken to be a slaveholder. She thought that in addition to my light complexion my being dressed up in Garrison's old slave trading clothes might have caused the man to think that I was a slave trader, and she was afraid that we should yet be separated if I should not succeed in finding some body to buy us.

Every day to us was a day of trouble, and every night brought new and fearful apprehensions that the golden link which binds together husband and wife might be broken by the heartless tyrant before the light of another day.

Deep has been the anguish of my soul when looking over my little family during the silent hours of the night, knowing the great danger of our being sold off at auction the next day and parted forever. That this might not come to pass, many have been the tears and prayers which I have offered up to the God of Israel that we might be preserved.

While waiting here to be disposed of, I heard of one Francis Whitfield, a cotton planter, who wanted to buy slaves. He was represented to be a very pious soul, being a deacon of a Baptist church. As the regulations, as well as public opinion generally, were against slaves meeting for religious worship, I thought it would give me a better opportunity to attend to my religious duties should I fall into the hands of this deacon.

So I called on him and tried to show to the best advantage, for the purpose of inducing him to buy me and my family. When I approached him, I felt much pleased at his external appearance—I addressed him in the following words as well as I can remember:

"Sir, I understand you are desirous of purchasing slaves?"

With a very pleasant smile, he replied, "Yes, I do want to buy some, are you for sale?"

"Yes sir, with my wife and one child."

Garrison had given me a note to show wherever I went, that I was for sale, speaking of my wife and child, giving us a very good character of course—and I handed him the note.

After reading it over he remarked, "I have a few questions to ask you, and if you will tell me the truth like a good boy, perhaps I may buy you with your family. In the first place, my boy, you are a little too near white. I want you to tell me now whether you can read or write?"

My reply was in the negative.

"Now I want you to tell me whether you have run away? Don't tell me no stories now, like a good fellow, and perhaps I may buy you."

But as I was not under oath to tell him the whole truth, I only gave him a part of it, by telling him that I had run away once.

He appeared to be pleased at that, but cautioned me to tell him the truth, and asked me how long I stayed away, when I run off?

I told him that I was gone a month.

He assented to this by a bow of his head, and making a long grunt saying, "That's right, tell me the truth like a good boy."

The whole truth was that I had been off in the state of Ohio, and other free states, and even to Canada; besides this I was notorious for running away, from my boyhood.

I never told him that I had been a runaway longer than one month—neither did I tell him that I had not run away more than once in my life; for these questions he never asked me.

I afterwards found him to be one of the basest hypocrites that I ever saw. He looked like a saint—talked like the best of slave holding Christians, and acted at home like the devil.

When he saw my wife and child, he concluded to buy us. He paid for me twelve hundred dollars, and one thousand for my wife and child. He also bought several other slaves at the same time, and took home with him. His residence was in the parish of Claiborn, fifty miles up from the mouth of Red River.

When we arrived there, we found his slaves poor, ragged, stupid, and half-starved. The food he allowed them per week, was one peck of corn for each grown person, one pound of pork, and sometimes a quart of molasses. This was all that they were allowed, and if they got more they stole it.

He had one of the most cruel overseers to be found in that section of country. He weighed and measured out to them, their week's allowance of food every Sabbath morning. The overseer's horn was sounded two hours before daylight for them in the morning, in order that they should be ready for work before daylight. They were worked from daylight until after dark, without stopping but one half hour to eat or rest, which was at noon. And at the busy season of the year, they were compelled to work just as hard on the Sabbath, as on any other day.

CHAPTER X.

Cruel treatment on Whitfield's farm—Exposure of the chil-
dren—Mode of extorting extra labor—Neglect of the sick—
Strange medicine used—Death of our second child.

My first impressions when I arrived on the Deacon's farm, were that he was far more like what the people call the devil, than he was like a deacon. Not many days after my arrival there, I heard the Deacon tell one of the slave girls, that he had bought her for a wife for his boy Stephen, which office he compelled her fully to perform against her will. This he enforced by a threat. At first the poor girl neglected to do this, having no sort of affection for the man—but she was finally forced to it by an application of the driver's lash, as threatened by the Deacon.

The next thing I observed was that he made the slave driver strip his own wife, and flog her for not doing just as her master had ordered. He had a white overseer, and a colored man for a driver, whose business it was to watch and drive the slaves in the field, and do the flogging according to the orders of the overseer.

Next a mulatto girl who waited about the house, on her mistress, displeased her, for which the Deacon stripped and tied her up. He then handed me the lash and ordered me to put it on—but I told him I never had done the like, and hoped he would not compel me to do it. He then informed me that I was to be his overseer, and that he had bought me for that purpose. He was paying a man eight hundred dollars a year to oversee, and he believed I was competent to do the same business, and if I would do it up right he would put nothing harder on me to do; and if I knew not how to flog a slave, he would set me an example by which I might be governed. He then commenced on this poor girl, and gave her two hundred lashes before he had her untied.

After giving her fifty lashes, he stopped and lectured her a while, asking her if she thought that she could obey her mistress, &c. She promised to do all in her power to please him and her mistress, if he would have mercy on her. But this plea was all vain. He commenced on her again; and this flogging was carried on in the most inhuman manner until she had received two hundred stripes on her naked quivering flesh, tied up and exposed to the public gaze of all. And this was the example that I was to copy after.

He then compelled me to wash her back off with strong salt brine, before she was untied, which was so revolting to my feelings, that I could not refrain from shedding tears.

For some cause he never called on me again to flog a slave. I presume he saw that I was not savage enough. The above were about the first items of the Deacon's conduct which struck me with peculiar disgust.

After having enjoyed the blessings of civil and religious liberty for a season, to be dragged into that horrible place with my family, to linger out my existence without the aid of religious societies, or the light of revelation, was more than I could endure. I really felt as if I had got into one of the darkest corners of the earth. I thought I was almost out of humanity's reach, and should never again have the pleasure of hearing the gospel sound, as I could see no way by which I could extricate myself; yet I never omitted to pray for deliverance. I had faith to believe that the Lord could see our wrongs and hear our cries.

I was not used quite as bad as the regular field hands, as the greater part of my time was spent working about the house; and my wife was the cook.

This country was full of pine timber, and every slave had to prepare a light wood torch, over night, made of pine knots, to meet the overseer with, before daylight in the morning. Each person had to have his torch lit, and come with it in his hand to the gin house, before the overseer and driver, so as to be ready to go to the cotton field by the time they could see to pick out cotton. These lights looked beautiful at a distance.

The object of blowing the horn for them two hours before day, was, that they should get their bite to eat, before they went to the field, that they need not stop to eat but once during the day. Another object was, to do up their flogging which had been omitted over night. I have often heard the sound of the slave driver's lash on the backs, of the slaves and their heart-rending shrieks, which were enough to melt the heart of humanity, even among the most barbarous nations of the earth.

But the Deacon would keep no overseer on his plantation, who neglected to perform this every morning. I have heard him say that he was no better pleased than when he could hear the overseer's loud complaining voice, long before daylight in the morning, and the sound of the driver's lash among the toiling slaves.

This was a very warm climate, abounding with musquitoes, galinippers and other insects which were exceedingly annoying to the poor slaves by night and day, at their quarters and in the field. But more especially to their helpless little children, which they had to carry with them to the cotton fields, where they had to set on the damp ground alone from morning till night, exposed to the scorching rays of the sun, liable to be bitten by poisonous rattle snakes which are plenty in that section of the country, or to be devoured by large alligators, which are often seen creeping through the cotton fields going from swamp to swamp seeking their prey.

The cotton planters generally, never allow a slave mother time to go to the house, or quarter during the day to nurse her child; hence they have to carry them to the cotton fields and tie them in the shade of a tree, or in clusters of high weeds about in the fields, where they can go to them at noon, when they are allowed to stop work for one half hour. This is the reason why so very few slave children are raised on these cotton plantations, the mothers have no time to take care of them—and they are often found dead in the field and in the quarter for want of the care of their mothers. But I never was eye witness to a case of this kind but have heard many narrated by my slave brothers and sisters, some of which occurred on the deacon's plantation.

Their plan of getting large quantities of cotton picked is not only to extort it from them by the lash, but hold out an inducement and deceive them by giving small prizes. For example; the overseer will offer something worth one or two dollars to any slave who will pick out the most cotton in one day, dividing the hands off in three classes and offering a prize to the one who will pick out the most cotton in each of the classes. By this means they are all interested in trying to get the prize.

After making them try it over several times and weighing what cotton they pick every night, the overseer can tell just how much every hand can pick. He then gives the present to those that pick the most cotton, and then if they do not pick just as much afterward they are flogged.

I have known the slaves to be so much fatigued from labor that they could scarcely get to their lodging places from the field at night. And then they would have to prepare something to eat before they could lie down to rest. Their corn they had to grind on a hand mill for bread stuff, or pound it in a mortar; and by the time they would get their suppers it would be midnight; then they would herd down all together and take but two or three hours rest, before the overseer's horn called them up again to prepare for the field.

At the time of sickness among slaves they had but very little attention. The master was to be the judge of their sickness, but never had studied the medical profession. He always pronounced a slave who said he was sick, a liar and a hypocrite; said there was nothing the matter, and he only wanted to keep from work.

His remedy was most generally strong red pepper tea, boiled till it was red. He would make them drink a pint cup full of it at one dose. If he should not get better very soon after it, the dose was repeated. If that should not accomplish the object for which it was given, or have the desired effect, a pot or kettle was then put over the fire with a large quantity of chimney soot, which was boiled down until it was as strong as the juice of tobacco, and the poor sick slave was compelled to drink a quart of it.

This would operate on the system like salts, or castor oil. But if the slave should not be very ill, he would rather work as long as he could stand up, than to take this dreadful medicine.

If it should be a very valuable slave, sometimes a physician was sent for and something done to save him. But no special aid is afforded the suffering slave even in the last trying hour, when he is called to grapple with the grim monster death. He has no Bible, no family altar, no minister to address to him the consolations of the gospel, before he launches into the spirit world. As to the burial of slaves, but very little more care is taken of their dead bodies than if they were dumb beasts.

My wife was very sick while we were both living with the Deacon. We expected every day would be her last. While she was sick, we lost our second child, and I was compelled to dig my own child's grave and bury it myself without even a box to put it in.

CHAPTER XI.

I attend a prayer meeting.—Punishment therefor threatened.—
I attempt to escape alone.—My return to take my family.—
Our sufferings.—Dreadful attack of wolves.—Our recapture.

SOME months after Malinda had recovered from her sickness, I got permission from the Deacon, on one Sabbath day, to attend a prayer meeting, on a neighboring plantation, with a few old superannuated slaves, although this was contrary to the custom of the country—for slaves were not allowed to assemble for religious worship. Being more numerous than the whites there was fear of rebellion, and the overpowering of their oppressors in order to obtain freedom.

But this gentleman on whose plantation I attended the meeting was not a Deacon nor a professor of religion. He was not afraid of a few old Christian slaves rising up to kill their master because he allowed them to worship God on the Sabbath day.

We had a very good meeting, although our exercises were not conducted in accordance with an enlightened Christianity; for we had no Bible—no intelligent leader—but a conscience, prompted by our own reason, constrained us to worship God the Creator of all things.

When I returned home from meeting I told the other slaves what a good time we had at our meeting, and requested them to go with me to meeting there on the next Sabbath. As no slave was allowed to go from the plantation on a visit without a written pass from his master, on the next Sabbath several of us went to the Deacon, to get permission to attend that prayer meeting; but he refused to let any go. I thought I would slip off and attend the meeting and get back before he would miss me, and would not know that I had been to the meeting.

When I returned home from the meeting as I approached the house I saw Malinda, standing out at the fence looking in the direction in which I was expected to return. She hailed my approach, not with joy, but with grief. She was weeping under great distress of mind, but it was hard for me to extort from her the reason why she wept. She finally informed me that her master had found out that I had violated his law, and I should suffer the penalty, which was five hundred lashes, on my naked back.

I asked her how he knew that I had gone?

She said I had not long been gone before he called for me and I was not to be found. He then sent the overseer on horseback to the place where we were to meet to see if I was there. But when the overseer got to the place, the meeting was over and I had gone back home, but had gone a nearer route through the woods and the overseer happened not to meet me. He heard that I had been there and hurried back home before me and told the Deacon, who ordered him to take me on the next morning, strip off my clothes, drive down four stakes in the ground and fasten my limbs to them; then strike me five hundred lashes for going to the prayer meeting. This was what distressed my poor companion. She thought it was more than I could bear, and that it would be the death of me. I concluded then to run away—but she thought they would catch me with the blood hounds by their taking my track. But to avoid them I thought I would ride off on one of the Deacon's mules. She thought if I did, they would sell me.

"No matter, I will try it," said I, "let the consequences be what they may. The matter can be no worse than it now is." So I tackled up the Deacon's best mule with his saddle, &c., and started that night and went off eight or ten miles from home. But I found the mule to be rather troublesome, and was like to betray me by braying, especially when he would see cattle, horses, or any thing of the kind in the woods.

The second night from home I camped in a cane break down in the Red river swamp not a great way off from the road, perhaps not twenty rods, exposed to wild ferocious beasts which were numerous in that section of country. On that night about the middle of the night the mule heard the sound of horses feet on the road, and he commenced stamping and trying to break away. As the horses seemed to come nearer, the mule commenced trying to bray, and it was all that I could do to prevent him from making a loud bray there in the woods, which would have betrayed me.

I supposed that it was the overseer out with the dogs looking for me, and I found afterwards that I was not mistaken.
As soon as the people had passed by, I mounted the mule and
took him home to prevent his betraying me. When I got near
by home I stripped off the tackling and turned the mule
loose. I then slipt up to the cabin wherein my wife laid and
found her awake, much distressed about me. She informed
me that they were then out looking for me, and that the Deacon was bent on flogging me nearly to death, and then selling me off from my family. This was truly heart-rending to
my poor wife; the thought of our being torn apart in a
strange land after having been sold away from all her friends
and relations, was more than she could bear.

The Deacon had declared that I should not only suffer for
the crime of attending a prayer meeting without his permission, and for running away, but for the awful crime of stealing a jackass, which was death by the law when committed by
a negro.

But I well knew that I was regarded as property, and so was
the ass; and I thought if one piece of property took off another, there could be no law violated in the act; no more sin
committed in this than if one jackass had rode off another.

But after consultation with my wife I concluded to take her
and my little daughter with me and they would be guilty of
the same crime that I was, so far as running away was concerned; and if the Deacon sold one he might sell us all, and
perhaps to the same person.

So we started off with our child that night, and made our
way down to the Red river swamps among the buzzing insects and wild beasts of the forest. We wandered about in the
wilderness for eight or ten days before we were apprehended,
striving to make our way from slavery; but it was all in vain.
Our food was parched corn, with wild fruit such as pawpaws,
percimmons, grapes, &c. We did at one time chance to find a
sweet potato patch where we got a few potatoes; but most of
the time, while we were out, we were lost. We wanted to
cross the Red river but could find no conveyance to cross in.

I recollect one day of finding a crooked tree which bent
over the river or over one fork of the river, where it was divided by an island. I should think that the tree was at least

twenty feet from the surface of the water. I picked up my little child, and my wife followed me, saying, "if we perish let us all perish together in the stream." We succeeded in crossing over. I often look back to that dangerous event even now with astonishment, and wonder how I could have run such a risk. What would induce me to run the same risk now? What could induce me now to leave home and friends and go to the wild forest and lay out on the cold ground night after night without covering, and live on parched corn?

What would induce me to take my family and go into the Red river swamps of Louisiana among the snakes and alligators, with all the liabilities of being destroyed by them, hunted down with blood hounds, or lay myself liable to be shot down like the wild beasts of the forest? Nothing I say, nothing but the strongest love of liberty, humanity, and justice to myself and family, would induce me to run such a risk again.

When we crossed over on the tree we supposed that we had crossed over the main body of the river, but we had not proceeded far on our journey before we found that we were on an Island surrounded by water on either side. We made our bed that night in a pile of dry leaves which had fallen from off the trees. We were much rest-broken, wearied from hunger and travelling through briers, swamps and cane-brakes—consequently we soon fell asleep after lying down. About the dead hour of the night I was aroused by the awful howling of a gang of blood-thirsty wolves, which had found us out and surrounded us as their prey, there in the dark wilderness many miles from any house or settlement.

My dear little child was so dreadfully alarmed that she screamed loudly with fear—my wife trembling like a leaf on a tree, at the thought of being devoured there in the wilderness by ferocious wolves.

The wolves kept howling, and were near enough for us to see their glaring eyes, and hear their chattering teeth. I then thought that the hour of death for us was at hand; that we should not live to see the light of another day; for there was no way for our escape. My little family were looking up to me for protection, but I could afford them none. And while I was offering up my prayers to that God who never forsakes those in the hour of danger who trust in him, I thought of Deacon Whitfield; I thought of his profession, and doubted his piety. I thought of his hand-cuffs, of his whips, of his chains, of his stocks, of his thumb-screws, of his slave driver and overseer, and of his religion; I also thought of his opposition to prayer meetings, and of his five hundred lashes promised me for attending a prayer meeting. I thought of God, I thought of the devil, I thought of hell; and I thought of heaven, and wondered whether I should ever see the Deacon there. And I calculated that if heaven was made up of such Deacons, or such persons, it could not be filled with love to all mankind, and with glory and eternal happiness, as we know it is from the truth of the Bible.

The reader may perhaps think me tedious on this topic, but indeed it is one of so much interest to me, that I find myself entirely unable to describe what my own feelings were at that time. I was so much excited by the fierce howling of the savage wolves, and the frightful screams of my little family, that I thought of the future; I thought of the past; I thought the time of my departure had come at last.

My impression is, that all these thoughts and thousands of others, flashed through my mind, while I was surrounded by those wolves. But it seemed to be the will of a merciful providence, that our lives should be spared, and that we should not be destroyed by them.

I had no weapon of defence but a long bowie knife which I had slipped from the Deacon. It was a very splendid blade, about two feet in length, and about two inches in width. This used to be a part of his armor of defence while walking about the plantation among his slaves.

The plan which I took to expel the wolves was a very dangerous one, but it proved effectual. While they were advancing to me, prancing and accumulating in number, apparently of all sizes and grades, who had come to the feast, I thought just at this time, that there was no alternative left but for me to make a charge with my bowie knife. I well knew from the action of the wolves, that if I made no farther resistance, they would soon destroy us, and if I made a break at them, the matter could be no worse. I thought if I must die, I would die striving to protect my little family from destruction, die striving to escape from slavery. My wife took a club in one hand, and her child in the other, while I rushed forth with my bowie knife in hand, to fight off the savage wolves. I made one desperate charge at them, and at the same time making a loud yell at the top of my voice, that caused them to retreat and scatter, which was equivalent to a victory on our part. Our prayers were answered, and our lives spared through the night. We slept no more that night, and the next morning there were no wolves to be seen or heard, and we resolved not to stay on that island another night.

We travelled up and down the river side trying to find a place where we could cross. Finally we found a lot of drift wood clogged together, extending across the stream at a narrow place in the river, upon which we crossed over. But we had not yet surmounted our greatest difficulty. We had to meet one which was far more formidable than the first. Not many days after I had to face the Deacon.

We had been wandering about through the cane brakes, bushes, and briers, for several days, when we heard the yelping of blood hounds, a great way off, but they seemed to come nearer and nearer to us. We thought after awhile that they must be on our track; we listened attentively at the approach. We knew it was no use for us to undertake to escape from them, and as they drew nigh, we heard the voice of a man hissing on the dogs.

After awhile we saw the hounds coming in full speed on our track, and the soul drivers close after them on horse back, yelling like tigers, as they came in sight. The shrill yelling of the savage blood hounds as they drew nigh made the woods echo.

The first impulse was to run to escape the approaching danger of ferocious dogs, and blood thirsty slave hunters, who were so rapidly approaching me with loaded muskets and bowie knives, with a determination to kill or capture me and my family. I started to run with my little daughter in my arms, but stumbled and fell down and scratched the arm of little Frances with a brier, so that it bled very much; but the dear child never cried, for she seemed to know the danger to which we were exposed.

But we soon found that it was no use for us to run. The

dogs were soon at our heels, and we were compelled to stop, or be torn to pieces by them. By this time, the soul drivers came charging up on their horses, commanding us to stand still or they would shoot us down.

Of course I surrendered up for the sake of my family. The most abusive terms to be found in the English language were poured forth on us with bitter oaths. They tied my hands behind me, and drove us home before them, to suffer the penalty of a slaveholder's broken law.

As we drew nigh the plantation my heart grew faint. I was aware that we should have to suffer almost death for running off. I was filled with dreadful apprehensions at the thought of meeting a professed follower of Christ, whom I knew to be a hypocrite! No tongue, no pen can ever describe what my feelings were at that time.

CHAPTER XII.

My sad condition before Whitfield.—My terrible punishment.—
Incidents of a former attempt to escape.—Jack at a farm
house.—Six pigs and a turkey.—Our surprise and arrest.

THE reader may perhaps imagine what must have been my
feelings when I found myself surrounded on the island with
my little family, at midnight, by a gang of savage wolves. This
was one of those trying emergencies in my life when there
was apparently but one step between us and the grave. But I
had no cords wrapped about my limbs to prevent my struggling against the impending danger to which I was then exposed. I was not denied the consolation of resisting in self
defence, as was now the case. There was no Deacon standing
before me, with a loaded rifle, swearing that I should submit
to the torturing lash, or be shot down like a dumb beast.

I felt that my chance was by far better among the howling
wolves in the Red river swamp, than before Deacon Whitfield,
on the cotton plantation. I was brought before him as a criminal before a bar, without counsel, to be tried and condemned
by a tyrant's law. My arms were bound with a cord, my spirit
broken, and my little family standing by weeping. I was not
allowed to plead my own cause, and there was no one to utter
a word in my behalf.

He ordered that the field hands should be called together
to witness my punishment, that it might serve as a caution to
them never to attend a prayer meeting, or runaway as I had,
lest they should receive the same punishment.

At the sound of the overseer's horn, all the slaves came forward and witnessed my punishment. My clothing was stripped
off and I was compelled to lie down on the ground with my
face to the earth. Four stakes were driven in the ground, to
which my hands and feet were tied. Then the overseer stood
over me with the lash and laid it on according to the Deacon's order. Fifty lashes were laid on before stopping. I was
then lectured with reference to my going to prayer meeting
without his orders, and running away to escape flogging.

While I suffered under this dreadful torture, I prayed, and

wept, and implored mercy at the hand of slavery, but found none. After I was marked from my neck to my heels, the Deacon took the gory lash, and said he thought there was a spot on my back yet where he could put in a few more. He wanted to give me something to remember him by, he said.

After I was flogged almost to death in this way, a paddle was brought forward and eight or ten blows given me with it, which was by far worse than the lash. My wounds were then washed with salt brine, after which I was let up. A description of such paddles I have already given in another page. I was so badly punished that I was not able to work for several days. After being flogged as described, they took me off several miles to a shop and had a heavy iron collar riveted on my neck with prongs extending above my head, on the end of which there was a small bell. I was not able to reach the bell with my hand. This heavy load of iron I was compelled to wear for six weeks. I never was allowed to lie in the same house with my family again while I was the slave of Whitfield. I either had to sleep with my feet in the stocks, or be chained with a large log chain to a log over night, with no bed or bedding to rest my wearied limbs on, after toiling all day in the cotton field. I suffered almost death while kept in this confinement; and he had ordered the overseer never to let me loose again; saying that I thought of getting free by running off, but no negro should ever get away from him alive.

I have omitted to state that this was the second time I had run away from him; while I was gone the first time, he extorted from my wife the fact that I had been in the habit of running away, before we left Kentucky; that I had been to Canada, and that I was trying to learn the art of reading and writing. All this was against me.

It is true that I was striving to learn myself to write. I was a kind of a house servant and was frequently sent off on errands, but never without a written pass; and on Sundays I have sometimes got permission to visit our neighbor's slaves, and I have often tried to write myself a pass.

Whenever I got hold of an old letter that had been thrown away, or a piece of white paper, I would save it to write on. I have often gone off in the woods and spent the greater part of the day alone, trying to learn to write myself a pass, by writing on the backs of old letters; copying after the pass that had been written by Whitfield; by so doing I got the use of the pen and could form letters as well as I can now, but knew not what they were.

The Deacon had an old slave by the name of Jack whom he bought about the time that he bought me. Jack was born in the State of Virginia. He had some idea of freedom; had often run away, but was very ignorant; knew not where to go for refuge; but understood all about providing something to eat when unjustly deprived of it.

So for ill treatment, we concluded to take a tramp together. I was to be the pilot, while Jack was to carry the baggage and keep us in provisions. Before we started, I managed to get hold of a suit of clothes the Deacon possessed, with his gun, ammunition and bowie knife. We also procured a blanket, a joint of meat, and some bread.

We started in a northern direction, being bound for the city of Little Rock, State of Arkansas. We travelled by night and laid by in the day, being guided by the unchangeable North Star; but at length, our provisions gave out, and it was Jack's place to get more. We came in sight of a large plantation one morning, where we saw people of color, and Jack said he could get something there, among the slaves, that night, for us to eat. So we concealed ourselves, in sight of this plantation, until about bed time, when we saw the lights extinguished.

During the day we saw a female slave passing from the dwelling house to the kitchen as if she was the cook; the house being about three rods from the landlord's dwelling. After we supposed the whites were all asleep, Jack slipped up softly to the kitchen to try his luck with the cook, to see if he could get any thing from her to eat.

I would remark that the domestic slaves are often found to be traitors to their own people, for the purpose of gaining favor with their masters; and they are encouraged and trained up by them to report every plot they know of being formed about stealing any thing, or running away, or any thing of the kind; and for which they are paid. This is one of the principal causes of the slaves being divided among themselves, and without which they could not be held in bondage one year, and perhaps not half that time.

I now proceed to describe the unsuccessful attempt of poor Jack to obtain something from the female slave to satisfy hunger. The planter's house was situated on an elevated spot on the side of a hill. The fencing about the house and garden was very crookedly laid up with rails. The night was rather dark and rainy, and Jack left me with the understanding that I was to stay at a certain place until he returned. I cautioned him before he left me to be very careful—and after he started, I left the place where he was to find me when he returned, for fear something might happen which might lead to my detection, should I remain at that spot. So I left it and went off where I could see the house, and that place too.

Jack had not long been gone, before I heard a great noise; a man, crying out with a loud voice, "Catch him! Catch him!" and hissing the dogs on, and they were close after Jack. The next thing I saw, was Jack running for life, and an old white man after him, with a gun, and his dogs. The fence being on sidling ground, and wet with the rain, when Jack run against it he knocked down several pannels of it and fell, tumbling over and over to the foot of the hill; but soon recovered and ran to where he had left me; but I was gone. The dogs were still after him.

There happened to be quite a thicket of small oak shrubs and bushes in the direction he ran. I think he might have been heard running and straddling bushes a quarter of a mile! The poor fellow hurt himself considerably in straddling over bushes in that way, in making his escape.

Finally the dogs relaxed their chase and poor Jack and myself again met in the thick forest. He said when he rapped on the cook-house door, the colored woman came to the door. He asked her if she would let him have a bite of bread if she had it, that he was a poor hungry absconding slave. But she made no reply to what he said but immediately sounded the alarm by calling loudly after her master, saying, "here is a runaway negro!" Jack said that he was going to knock her down but her master was out within one moment, and he had to run for his life.

As soon as we got our eyes fixed on the North Star again, we started on our way. We travelled on a few miles and came to another large plantation, where Jack was determined to get something to eat. He left me at a certain place while he went up to the house to find something if possible.

He was gone some time before he returned, but when I saw him coming, he appeared to be very heavy loaded with a bag of something. We walked off pretty fast until we got some distance in the woods. Jack then stopped and opened his bag in which he had six small pigs. I asked him how he got them without making any noise; and he said that he found a bed of hogs, in which there were the pigs with their mother. While the pigs were sucking he crawled up to them without being discovered by the sow, and took them by their necks one after another, and choked them to death, and slipped them into his bag!

We intended to travel on all that night and lay by the next day in the forest and cook up our pigs. We fell into a large road leading on the direction which we were travelling, and had not proceeded over three miles before I found a white hat lying in the road before me. Jack being a little behind me I stopped until he came up, and showed it to him. He picked it up. We looked a few steps farther and saw a man lying by the way, either asleep or intoxicated, as we supposed.

I told Jack not to take the hat, but he would not obey me. He had only a piece of a hat himself, which he left in exchange for the other. We travelled on about five miles farther, and in passing a house discovered a large turkey sitting on the fence, which temptation was greater than Jack could resist. Notwithstanding he had six very nice fat little pigs on his back, he stepped up and took the turkey off the fence.

By this time it was getting near day-light and we left the road and went off a mile or so among the hills of the forest, where we struck camp for the day. We then picked our turkey, dressed our pigs, and cooked two of them. We got the hair off by singeing them over the fire, and after we had eaten all we wanted, one of us slept while the other watched. We had flint, punk, and powder to strike fire with. A little after dark the next night, we started on our way.

But about ten o'clock that night just as we were passing through a thick skirt of woods, five men sprang out before us with fire-arms, swearing if we moved another step, they would shoot us down; and each man having his gun drawn up

for shooting we had no chance to make any defence, and surrendered sooner than run the risk of being killed.

They had been lying in wait for us there, for several hours.
They had seen a reward out, for notices were put up in the
most public places, that fifty dollars would be paid for me,
dead or alive, if I should not return home within so many
days. And the reader will remember that neither Jack nor myself was able to read the advertisement. It was of very little
consequence with the slave catchers, whether they killed us or
took us alive, for the reward was the same to them.

After we were taken and tied, one of the men declared to
me that he would have shot me dead just as sure as he lived,
if I had moved one step after they commanded us to stop. He
had his gun levelled at my breast, already cocked, and his finger on the trigger. The way they came to find us out was from
the circumstance of Jack's taking the man's hat in connection
with the advertisement. The man whose hat was taken was
drunk; and the next morning when he came to look for his
hat it was gone and Jack's old hat lying in the place of it; and
in looking round he saw the tracks of two persons in the dust,
who had passed during the night, and one of them having but
three toes on one foot. He followed these tracks until they
came to a large mud pond in a lane on one side of which a
person might pass dry shod; but the man with three toes on
one foot had plunged through the mud. This led the man to
think there must be runaway slaves, and from out of that
neighborhood; for all persons in that settlement knew which
side of that mud hole to go. He then got others to go with
him, and they followed us until our track left the road. They
supposed that we had gone off in the woods to lay by until
night, after which we should pursue our course.

After we were captured they took us off several miles to
where one of them lived, and kept us over night. One of our
pigs was cooked for us to eat that night; and the turkey the
next morning. But we were both tied that night with our
hands behind us, and our feet were also tied. The doors were
locked, and a bedstead was set against the front door, and two
men slept in it to prevent our getting out in the night. They
said that they knew how to catch runaway negroes, and how
to keep them after they were caught.

They remarked that after they found we had stopped to lay by until night, and they saw from our tracks what direction we were travelling, they went about ten miles on that direction, and hid by the road side until we came up that night. That night after all had got fast to sleep, I thought I would try to get out, and I should have succeeded, if I could have moved the bed from the door. I managed to untie myself and crawled under the bed which was placed at the door, and strove to remove it, but in so doing I awakened the men and they got up and confined me again, and watched me until day light, each with a gun in hand.

The next morning they started with us back to Deacon Whitfield's plantation; but when they got within ten miles of where he lived they stopped at a public house to stay over night; and who should we meet there but the Deacon, who was then out looking for me.

The reader may well imagine how I felt to meet him. I had almost as soon come in contact with Satan himself. He had two long poles or sticks of wood brought in to confine us to. I was compelled to lie on my back across one of those sticks with my arms out, and have them lashed fast to the log with a cord. My feet were also tied to the other, and there I had to lie all that night with my back across this stick of wood, and my feet and hands tied. I suffered that night under the most excruciating pain. From the tight binding of the cord the circulation of the blood in my arms and feet was almost entirely stopped. If the night had been much longer I must have died in that confinement.

The next morning we were taken back to the Deacon's farm, and both flogged for going off, and set to work. But there was some allowance made for me on account of my being young. They said that they knew old Jack had persuaded me off, or I never would have gone. And the Deacon's wife begged that I might be favored some, for that time, as Jack had influenced me, so as to bring up my old habits of running away that I had entirely given up.

CHAPTER XIII.

I am sold to gamblers.—They try to purchase my family.—Our parting scene.—My good usage.—I am sold to an Indian.— His confidence in my integrity manifested.

THE reader will remember that this brings me back to the time the Deacon had ordered me to be kept in confinement until he got a chance to sell me, and that no negro should ever get away from him and live. Some days after this we were all out at the gin house ginning cotton, which was situated on the road side, and there came along a company of men, fifteen or twenty in number, who were Southern sportsmen. Their attention was attracted by the load of iron which was fastened about my neck with a bell attached. They stopped and asked the Deacon what that bell was put on my neck for? and he said it was to keep me from running away, &c.

They remarked that I looked as if I might be a smart negro, and asked if he wanted to sell me. The reply was, yes. They then got off their horses and struck a bargain with him for me. They bought me at a reduced price for speculation.

After they had purchased me, I asked the privilege of going to the house to take leave of my family before I left, which was granted by the sportsmen. But the Deacon said I should never again step my foot inside of his yard; and advised the sportsmen not to take the irons from my neck until they had sold me; that if they gave me the least chance I would run away from them, as I did from him. So I was compelled to mount a horse and go off with them as I supposed, never again to meet my family in this life.

We had not proceeded far before they informed me that they had bought me to sell again, and if they kept the irons on me it would be detrimental to the sale, and that they would therefore take off the irons and dress me up like a man, and throw away the old rubbish which I then had on; and they would sell me to some one who would treat me better than Deacon Whitfield. After they had cut off the irons and dressed me up, they crossed over Red River into Texas, where they spent some time horse racing and gambling; and although they were wicked black legs of the basest character, it is but due to them to say, that they used me far better than ever the Deacon did. They gave me plenty to eat and put nothing hard on me to do. They expressed much sympathy for me in my bereavement; and almost every day they gave me money more or less, and by my activity in waiting on them, and upright conduct, I got into the good graces of them all, but they could not get any person to buy me on account of the amount of intelligence which they supposed me to have; for many of them thought that I could read and write. When they left Texas, they intended to go to the Indian Territory west of the Mississippi, to attend a great horse race which was to take place. Not being much out of their way to go past Deacon Whitfield's again, I prevailed on them to call on him for the purpose of trying to purchase my wife and child; and I promised them that if they would buy my wife and child, I would get some person to purchase us from them. So they tried to grant my request by calling on the Deacon, and trying to make the purchase. As we approached the Deacon's plantation, my heart was filled with a thousand painful and fearful apprehensions. I had the fullest confidence in the blacklegs with whom I travelled, believing that they would do according to promise, and go to the fullest extent of their ability to restore peace and consolation to a bereaved family—to re-unite husband and wife, parent and child, who had long been severed by slavery through the agency of Deacon Whitfield. But I knew his determination in relation to myself, and I feared his wicked opposition to a restoration of myself and little family, which he had divided, and soon found that my fears were not without foundation.

When we rode up and walked into his yard, the Deacon came out and spoke to all but myself; and not finding me in tattered rags as a substitute for clothes, nor having an iron collar or bell about my neck, as was the case when he sold me, he appeared to be much displeased.

"What did you bring that negro back here for?" said he.

"We have come to try to buy his wife and child; for we can find no one who is willing to buy him alone; and we will either buy or sell so that the family may be together," said they.

While this conversation was going on, my poor bereaved

wife, who never expected to see me again in this life, spied me and came rushing to me through the crowd, throwing her arms about my neck exclaiming in the most sympathetic tones, "Oh! my dear husband! I never expected to see you again!" The poor woman was bathed with tears of sorrow and grief. But no sooner had she reached me, than the Deacon peremptorily commanded her to go to her work. This she did not obey, but prayed that her master would not separate us again, as she was there alone, far from friends and relations whom she should never meet again. And now to take away her husband, her last and only true friend, would be like taking her life!

But such appeals made no impression on the unfeeling Deacon's heart. While he was storming with abusive language, and even using the gory lash with hellish vengeance to separate husband and wife, I could see the sympathetic teardrop, stealing its way down the cheek of the profligate and black-leg, whose object it now was to bind up the broken heart of a wife, and restore to the arms of a bereaved husband, his companion.

They were disgusted at the conduct of Whitfield and cried out shame, even in his presence. They told him that they would give a thousand dollars for my wife and child, or any thing in reason. But no! he would sooner see me to the devil than indulge or gratify me after my having run away from him; and if they did not remove me from his presence very soon, he said he should make them suffer for it.

But all this, and even the gory lash had yet failed to break the grasp of poor Malinda, whose prospect of connubial, social, and future happiness was all at stake. When the dear woman saw there was no help for us, and that we should soon be separated forever, in the name of Deacon Whitfield, and American slavery to meet no more as husband and wife, parent and child—the last and loudest appeal was made on our knees. We appealed to the God of justice and to the sacred ties of humanity; but this was all in vain. The louder we prayed the harder he whipped, amid the most heart-rending shrieks from the poor slave mother and child, as little Frances stood by, sobbing at the abuse inflicted on her mother.

"Oh! how shall I give my husband the parting hand never

to meet again? This will surely break my heart," were her parting words.

I can never describe to the reader the awful reality of that separation—for it was enough to chill the blood and stir up the deepest feelings of revenge in the hearts of slaveholding black-legs, who as they stood by, were threatening, some weeping, some swearing and others declaring vengeance against such treatment being inflicted on a human being. As we left the plantation, as far as we could see and hear, the Deacon was still laying on the gory lash, trying to prevent poor Malinda from weeping over the loss of her departed husband, who was then, by the hellish laws of slavery, to her, theoretically and practically dead. One of the black-legs exclaimed that hell was full of just such Deacon's as Whitfield. This occurred in December, 1840. I have never seen Malinda, since that period. I never expect to see her again.

The sportsmen to whom I was sold, showed their sympathy for me not only by word but by deeds. They said that they had made the most liberal offer to Whitfield, to buy or sell for the sole purpose of reuniting husband and wife. But he stood out against it—they felt sorry for me. They said they had bought me to speculate on, and were not able to lose what they had paid for me. But they would make a bargain with me, if I was willing, and would lay a plan, by which I might yet get free. If I would use my influence so as to get some person to buy me while traveling about with them, they would give me a portion of the money for which they sold me, and they would also give me directions by which I might yet run away and go to Canada.

This offer I accepted, and the plot was made. They advised me to act very stupid in language and thought, but in business I must be spry; and that I must persuade men to buy me, and promise them that I would be smart.

We passed through the State of Arkansas and stopped at many places, horse-racing and gambling. My business was to drive a wagon in which they carried their gambling apparatus, clothing, &c. I had also to black boots and attend to horses. We stopped at Fayettville, where they almost lost me, betting on a horse race.

They went from thence to the Indian Territory, among the

Cherokee Indians, to attend the great races which were to take place there. During the races there was a very wealthy half Indian of that tribe, who became much attached to me, and had some notion of buying me, after hearing that I was for sale, being a slaveholder. The idea struck me rather favorable, for several reasons. First, I thought I should stand a better chance to get away from an Indian than from a white man. Second, he wanted me only for a kind of a body servant to wait on him—and in this case I knew that I should fare better than I should in the field. And my owners also told me that it would be an easy place to get away from. I took their advice for fear I might not get another chance so good as that, and prevailed on the man to buy me. He paid them nine hundred dollars, in gold and silver, for me. I saw the money counted out.

After the purchase was made, the sportsmen got me off to one side, and according to promise they gave me a part of the money, and directions how to get from there to Canada. They also advised me how to act until I got a good chance to run away. I was to embrace the earliest opportunity of getting away, before they should become acquainted with me. I was never to let it be known where I was from, nor where I was born. I was to act quite stupid and ignorant. And when I started I was to go up the boundary line, between the Indian Territory and the States of Arkansas and Missouri, and this would fetch me out on the Missouri river, near Jefferson city, the capital of Missouri. I was to travel at first by night, and to lay by in daylight, until I got out of danger.

The same afternoon that the Indian bought me, he started with me to his residence, which was fifty or sixty miles distant. And so great was his confidence in me, that he intrusted me to carry his money. The amount must have been at least five hundred dollars, which was all in gold and silver; and when we stopped over night the money and horses were all left in my charge.

It would have been a very easy matter for me to have taken one of the best horses, with the money, and run off. And the temptation was truly great to a man like myself, who was watching for the earliest opportunity to escape; and I felt confident that I should never have a better opportunity to escape full handed than then.

CHAPTER XIV.

Character of my Indian Master.—Slavery among the Indians less cruel.—Indian carousal.—Enfeebled health of my Indian Master.—His death.—My escape.—Adventure in a wigwam.—Successful progress toward liberty.

THE next morning I went home with my new master; and by the way it is only doing justice to the dead to say, that he was the most reasonable, and humane slaveholder that I have ever belonged to. He was the last man that pretended to claim property in my person; and although I have freely given the names and residences of all others who have held me as a slave, for prudential reasons I shall omit giving the name of this individual.

He was the owner of a large plantation and quite a number of slaves. He raised corn and wheat for his own consumption only. There was no cotton, tobacco, or anything of the kind produced among them for market. And I found this difference between negro slavery among the Indians, and the same thing among the white slaveholders of the South. The Indians allow their slaves enough to eat and wear. They have no overseers to whip nor drive them. If a slave offends his master, he sometimes, in a heat of passion, undertakes to chastise him; but it is as often the case as otherwise, that the slave gets the better of the fight, and even flogs his master;* for which there is no law to punish him; but when the fight is over that is the last of it. So far as religious instruction is concerned, they have it on terms of equality, the bond and the free; they have no respect of persons, they have neither slave laws nor negro pews. Neither do they separate husbands and wives, nor parents and children. All things considered, if I must be a slave, I had by far, rather be a slave to an Indian, than to a white man, from the experience I have had with both.

A majority of the Indians were uneducated, and still followed up their old heathen traditional notions. They made it a rule to have an Indian dance or frolic, about once a fort-

---

*This singular fact is corroborated in a letter read by the publisher, from an acquaintance while passing through this country in 1849.

night; and they would come together far and near to attend these dances. They would most generally commence about the middle of the afternoon; and would give notice by the blowing of horns. One would commence blowing and another would answer, and so it would go all round the neighborhood. When a number had got together, they would strike a circle about twenty rods in circumference, and kindle up fires about twenty feet apart, all around, in this circle. In the centre they would have a large fire to dance around, and at each one of the small fires there would be a squaw to keep up the fire, which looked delightful off at a distance.

But the most degrading practice of all, was the use of intoxicating drinks, which were used to a great excess by all that attended these stump dances. At almost all of these fires there was some one with rum to sell. There would be some dancing, some singing, some gambling, some fighting, and some yelling; and this was kept up often for two days and nights together.

Their dress for the dance was most generally a great bunch of bird feathers, coon tails, or something of the kind stuck in their heads, and a great many shells tied about their legs to rattle while dancing. Their manner of dancing is taking hold of each others hands and forming a ring around the large fire in the centre, and go stomping around it until they would get drunk or their heads would get to swimming, and then they would go off and drink, and another set come on. Such were some of the practises indulged in by these Indian slaveholders.

My last owner was in a declining state of health when he bought me; and not long after he bought me he went off forty or fifty miles from home to be doctored by an Indian doctor, accompanied by his wife. I was taken along also to drive the carriage and to wait upon him during his sickness. But he was then so feeble, that his life was of but short duration after the doctor commenced on him.

While he lived, I waited on him according to the best of my ability. I watched over him night and day until he died, and even prepared his body for the tomb, before I left him. He died about midnight and I understood from his friends that he was not to be buried until the second day after his death.

I pretended to be taking on at a great rate about his death, but I was more excited about running away, than I was about that, and before daylight the next morning I proved it, for I was on my way to Canada.

I never expected a better opportunity would present itself for my escape. I slipped out of the room as if I had gone off to weep for the deceased, knowing that they would not feel alarmed about me until after my master was buried and they had returned back to his residence. And even then, they would think that I was somewhere on my way home; and it would be at least four or five days before they would make any stir in looking after me. By that time, if I had no bad luck, I should be out of much danger.

After the first day, I laid by in the day and traveled by night for several days and nights, passing in this way through several tribes of Indians. I kept pretty near the boundary line. I recollect getting lost one dark rainy night. Not being able to find the road I came into an Indian settlement at the dead hour of the night. I was wet, wearied, cold and hungry; and yet I felt afraid to enter any of their houses or wigwams, not knowing whether they would be friendly or not. But I knew the Indians were generally drunkards, and that occasionally a drunken white man was found straggling among them, and that such an one would be more likely to find friends from sympathy than an upright man.

So I passed myself off that night as a drunkard among them. I walked up to the door of one of their houses, and fell up against it, making a great noise like a drunken man; but no one came to the door. I opened it and staggered in, falling about, and making a great noise. But finally an old woman got up and gave me a blanket to lie down on.

There was quite a number of them lying about on the dirt floor, but not one could talk or understand a word of the English language. I made signs so as to let them know that I wanted something to eat, but they had nothing, so I had to go without that night. I laid down and pretended to be asleep, but I slept none that night, for I was afraid that they would kill me if I went to sleep. About one hour before day, the next morning, three of the females got up and put into a tin kettle a lot of ashes with water, to boil, and then poured into it about one quart of corn. After letting it stand a few moments, they poured it into a trough, and pounded it into thin hominy. They washed it out, and boiled it down, and called me up to eat my breakfast of it.

After eating, I offered them six cents, but they refused to accept it. I then found my way to the main road, and traveled all that day on my journey, and just at night arrived at a public house kept by an Indian, who also kept a store. I walked in and asked if I could get lodging, which was granted; but I had not been there long before three men came riding up about dusk, or between sunset and dark. They were white men, and I supposed slaveholders. At any rate when they asked if they could have lodging, I trembled for fear they might be in pursuit of me. But the landlord told them that he could not lodge them, but they could get lodging about two miles off, with a white man, and they turned their horses and started.

The landlord asked me where I was traveling to, and where I was from. I told him that I had been out looking at the country; that I had thought of buying land, and that I lived in the State of Ohio, in the village of Perrysburgh. He then said that he had lived there himself, and that he had acted as an interpreter there among the Maumee tribe of Indians for several years. He then asked who I was acquainted with there? I informed him that I knew Judge Hollister, Francis Hollister, J. W. Smith, and others. At this he was so much pleased that he came up and took me by the hand, and received me joyfully, after seeing that I was acquainted with those of his old friends.

I could converse with him understandingly from personal acquaintance, for I had lived there when I first ran away from Kentucky. But I felt it to be my duty to start off the next morning before breakfast, or sunrise. I bought a dozen of eggs, and had them boiled to carry with me to eat on the way. I did not like the looks of those three men, and thought I would get on as fast as possible for fear I might be pursued by them.

I was then about to enter the territory of another slave State, Missouri. I had passed through the fiery ordeal of Sibley, Gatewood, and Garrison, and had even slipped through the fingers of Deacon Whitfield. I had doubtless gone through great peril in crossing the Indian territory, in passing through the various half civilized tribes, who seemed to look upon me with astonishment as I passed along. Their hands were almost invariably filled with bows and arrows, tomahawks, guns, butcher knives, and all the various implements of death which are used by them. And what made them look still more frightful, their faces were often painted red, and their heads muffled with birds feathers, bushes, coons tails and owls heads. But all this I had passed through, and my long enslaved limbs and spirit were then in full stretch for emancipation. I felt as if one more short struggle would set me free.

CHAPTER XV.

Adventure on the Prairie.—I borrow a horse without leave.—
Rapid traveling one whole night.—Apology for using other
men's horses.—My manner of living on the road.

Early in the morning I left the Indian territory as I have already said, for fear I might be pursued by the three white men
whom I had seen there over night; but I had not proceeded
far before my fears were magnified a hundred fold.

I always dreaded to pass through a prairie, and on coming
to one which was about six miles in width, I was careful to
look in every direction to see whether there was any person in
sight before I entered it; but I could see no one. So I started
across with a hope of crossing without coming in contact with
any one on the prairie. I walked as fast as I could, but when I
got about midway of the prairie, I came to a high spot where
the road forked, and three men came up from a low spot as if
they had been there concealed. They were all on horse back,
and I supposed them to be the same men that had tried to get
lodging where I stopped over night. Had this been in tim-
bered land, I might have stood some chance to have dodged
them, but there I was, out in the open prairie, where I could
see no possible way by which I could escape.

They came along slowly up behind me, and finally passed,
and spoke or bowed their heads on passing, but they traveled
in a slow walk and kept but a very few steps before me, until
we got nearly across the prairie. When we were coming near
a plantation a piece off from the road on the skirt of the tim-
bered land, they whipped up their horses and left the road as
if they were going across to this plantation. They soon got
out of my sight by going down into a valley which lay between us and the plantation. Not seeing them rise the hill to
go up to the farm, excited greater suspicion in my mind, so I
stepped over on the brow of the hill, where I could see what
they were doing, and to my surprise I saw them going right
back in the direction they had just came, and they were going
very fast. I was then satisfied that they were after me and that

they were only going back to get more help to assist them in taking me, for fear that I might kill some of them if they undertook it. The first impression was that I had better leave the road immediately; so I bolted from the road and ran as fast as I could for some distance in the thick forest, and concealed myself for about fifteen or twenty minutes, which were spent in prayer to God for his protecting care and guidance.

My impression was that when they should start in pursuit of me again, they would follow on in the direction which I was going when they left me; and not finding or hearing of me on the road, they would come back and hunt through the woods around, and if they could find no track they might go and get dogs to trace me out.

I thought my chance of escape would be better, if I went back to the same side of the road that they first went, for the purpose of deceiving them; as I supposed that they would not suspect my going in the same direction that they went, for the purpose of escaping from them.

So I traveled all that day square off from the road through the wild forest without any knowledge of the country whatever; for I had nothing to travel by but the sun by day, and the moon and stars by night. Just before night I came in sight of a large plantation, where I saw quite a number of horses running at large in a field, and knowing that my success in escaping depended upon my getting out of that settlement within twenty-four hours, to save myself from everlasting slavery, I thought I should be justified in riding one of those horses, that night, if I could catch one. I cut a grape vine with my knife, and made it into a bridle; and shortly after dark I went into the field and tried to catch one of the horses. I got a bunch of dry blades of fodder and walked up softly towards the horses, calling to them "cope," "cope," "cope;" but there was only one out of the number that I was able to get my hand on, and that was an old mare, which I supposed to be the mother of all the rest; and I knew that I could walk faster than she could travel. She had a bell on and was very thin in flesh; she looked gentle and walked on three legs only. The young horses pranced and galloped off. I was not able to get near them, and the old mare being of no use to me, I left them all. After fixing my eyes on the north star I pursued my journey, holding on to my bridle with a hope of finding a horse upon which I might ride that night.

I found a road leading pretty nearly in the direction which I wanted to travel, and I kept it. After traveling several miles I found another large plantation where there was a prospect of finding a horse. I stepped up to the barn-yard, wherein I found several horses. There was a little barn standing with the door open, and I found it quite an easy task to get the horses into the barn, and select out the best looking one of them. I pulled down the fence, led the noble beast out and mounted him, taking a northern direction, being able to find a road which led that way. But I had not gone over three or four miles before I came to a large stream of water which was past fording; yet I could see that it had been forded by the road track, but from high water it was then impassible. As the horse seemed willing to go in I put him through; but before he got in far, he was in water up to his sides and finally the water came over his back and he swam over. I got as wet as could be, but the horse carried me safely across at the proper place. After I got out a mile or so from the river, I came into a large prairie, which I think must have been twenty or thirty miles in width, and the road run across it about in the direction that I wanted to go. I laid whip to the horse, and I think he must have carried me not less than forty miles that night, or before sun rise the next morning. I then stopped him in a spot of high grass in an old field, and took off the bridle. I thanked God, and thanked the horse for what he had done for me, and wished him a safe journey back home.

I know the poor horse must have felt stiff, and tired from his speedy jaunt, and I felt very bad myself, riding at that rate all night without a saddle; but I felt as if I had too much at stake to favor either horse flesh or man flesh. I could indeed afford to crucify my own flesh for the sake of redeeming myself from perpetual slavery.

Some may be disposed to find fault with my taking the horse as I did; but I did nothing more than nine out of ten would do if they were placed in the same circumstances. I had no disposition to steal a horse from any man. But I ask, if a white man had been captured by the Cherokee Indians and carried away from his family for life into slavery, and could see a chance to escape and get back to his family; should the Indians pursue him with a determination to take him back or take his life, would it be a crime for the poor fugitive, whose life, liberty, and future happiness were all at stake, to mount any man's horse by the way side, and ride him without asking any questions, to effect his escape? Or who would not do the same thing to rescue a wife, child, father, or mother? Such an act committed by a white man under the same circumstances would not only be pronounced proper, but praiseworthy; and if he neglected to avail himself of such a means of escape he would be pronounced a fool. Therefore from this act I have nothing to regret, for I have done nothing more than any other reasonable person would have done under the same circumstances. But I had good luck from the morning I left the horse until I got back into the State of Ohio. About two miles from where I left the horse, I found a public house on the road, where I stopped and took breakfast. Being asked where I was traveling, I replied that I was going home to Perrysburgh, Ohio, and that I had been out to look at the land in Missouri, with a view of buying. They supposed me to be a native of Ohio, from the fact of my being so well acquainted with its location, its principal cities, inhabitants, &c.

The next night I put up at one of the best hotels in the village where I stopped, and acted with as much independence as if I was worth a million of dollars; talked about buying land, stock and village property, and contrasting it with the same kind of property in the State of Ohio. In this kind of talk they were most generally interested, and I was treated just like other travelers. I made it a point to travel about thirty miles each day on my way to Jefferson city. On several occasions I have asked the landlords where I have stopped over night, if they could tell me who kept the best house where I would stop the next night, which was most generally in a small village. But for fear I might forget, I would get them to give me the name on a piece of paper as a kind of recommend. This would serve as an introduction through which I have always been well received from one landlord to another, and I have always stopped at the best houses, eaten at the first tables, and slept in the best beds. No man ever asked me whether I was bond or free, black or white, rich or poor; but I always presented a bold front and showed the best side out, which was all the pass I had. But when I got within about one hundred miles of Jefferson city, where I expected to take a Steamboat passage to St. Louis, I stopped over night at a hotel, where I met with a young white man who was traveling on to Jefferson City on horse back, and was also leading a horse with a saddle and bridle on.

I asked him if he would let me ride the horse which he was leading, as I was going to the same city? He said that it was a hired horse, that he was paying at the rate of fifty cents per day for it, but if I would pay the same I could ride him. I accepted the offer and we rode together to the city. We were on the road together two or three days; stopped and ate and slept together at the same hotels.

CHAPTER XVI.

Stratagem to get on board the steamer.—My Irish friends.—My success in reaching Cincinnati.—Reflections on again seeing Kentucky.—I get employment in a hotel.—My fright at seeing the gambler who sold me.—I leave Ohio with Mr. Smith.—His letter.—My education.

THE greatest of my adventures came off when I arrived at Jefferson City. There I expected to meet an advertisement for my person; it was there I must cross the river or take a steamboat down; it was there I expected to be interrogated and required to prove whether I was actually a free man or a slave. If I was free, I should have to show my free papers; and if I was a slave I should be required to tell who my master was.

I stopped at a hotel, however, and ascertained that there was a steamboat expected down the river that day for St. Louis. I also found out that there were several passengers at that house who were going down on board of the first boat. I knew that the captain of a steamboat could not take a colored passenger on board of his boat from a slave state without first ascertaining whether such person was bond or free; I knew that this was more than he would dare to do by the laws of the slave states—and now to surmount this difficulty it brought into exercise all the powers of my mind. I would have got myself boxed up as freight, and have been forwarded to St. Louis, but I had no friend that I could trust to do it for me. This plan has since been adopted by some with success. But finally I thought I might possibly pass myself off as a body servant to the passengers going from the hotel down.

So I went to a store and bought myself a large trunk, and took it to the hotel. Soon, a boat came in which was bound to St. Louis, and the passengers started down to get on board. I took up my large trunk, and started along after them as if I was their servant. My heart trembled in view of the dangerous experiment which I was then about to try. It required all the moral courage that I was master of to bear me up in view of my critical condition. The white people that I was following walked on board and I after them. I acted as if

537

the trunk was full of clothes, but I had not a stitch of clothes in it. The passengers went up into the cabin and I followed them with the trunk. I suppose this made the captain think that I was their slave.

I not only took the trunk in the cabin but stood by it until after the boat had started as if it belonged to my owners, and I was taking care of it for them; but as soon as the boat got fairly under way, I knew that some account would have to be given of me; so I then took my trunk down on the deck among the deck passengers to prepare myself to meet the clerk of the boat, when he should come to collect fare from the deck passengers.

Fortunately for me there was quite a number of deck passengers on board, among whom there were many Irish. I insinuated myself among them so as to get into their good graces, believing that if I should get into a difficulty they would stand by me. I saw several of these persons going up to the saloon buying whiskey, and I thought this might be the most effectual way by which I could gain speedily their respect and sympathy. So I participated with them pretty freely for awhile, or at least until after I got my fare settled. I placed myself in a little crowd of them, and invited them all up to the bar with me, stating that it was my treat. This was responded to, and they walked up and drank and I footed the bill. This, of course, brought us into a kind of a union. We sat together and laughed and talked freely. Within ten or fifteen minutes I remarked that I was getting dry again, and invited them up and treated again. By this time I was thought to be one of the most liberal and gentlemanly men on board, by these deck passengers; they were ready to do any thing for me—they got to singing songs, and telling long yarns in which I took quite an active part; but it was all for effect.

By this time the porter came around ringing his bell for all passengers who had not paid their fare, to walk up to the captain's office and settle it. Some of my Irish friends had not yet settled, and I asked one of them if he would be good enough to take my money and get me a ticket when he was getting one for himself, and he quickly replied "yes sir, I will get you a tacket." So he relieved me of my greatest trouble. When they came round to gather the tickets before we got to St.

Louis, my ticket was taken with the rest, and no questions were asked me.

The next day the boat arrived at St. Louis; my object was to take passage on board of the first boat which was destined for Cincinnati, Ohio; and as there was a boat going out that day for Pittsburgh, I went on board to make some inquiry about the fare &c., and found the steward to be a colored man with whom I was acquainted. He lived in Cincinnati, and had rendered me some assistance in making my escape to Canada, in the summer of 1838, and he also very kindly aided me then in getting back into a land of freedom. The swift running steamer started that afternoon on her voyage, which soon wafted my body beyond the tyrannical limits of chattel slavery. When the boat struck the mouth of the river Ohio, and I had once more the pleasure of looking on that lovely stream, my heart leaped up for joy at the glorious prospect that I should again be free. Every revolution of the mighty steam-engine seemed to bring me nearer and nearer the "promised land." Only a few days had elapsed, before I was permitted by the smiles of a good providence, once more to gaze on the green hill-tops and valleys of old Kentucky, the State of my nativity. And notwithstanding I was deeply interested while standing on the deck of the steamer looking at the beauties of nature on either side of the river, as she pressed her way up the stream, my very soul was pained to look upon the slaves in the fields of Kentucky, still toiling under their task-masters without pay. It was on this soil I first breathed, the free air of Heaven, and felt the bitter pangs of slavery—it was here that I first learned to abhor it. It was here I received the first impulse of human rights—it was here that I first entered my protest against the bloody institution of slavery, by running away from it, and declared that I would no longer work for any man as I had done, without wages.

When the steamboat arrived at Portsmouth, Ohio, I took off my trunk with the intention of going to Canada. But my funds were almost exhausted, so I had to stop and go to work to get money to travel on. I hired myself at the American Hotel to a Mr. McCoy to do the work of a porter, to black boots, &c., for which he was to pay me $12 per month. I soon found the landlord to be bad pay, and not only that, but he would not allow me to charge for blacking boots, although I had to black them after everybody had gone to bed at night, and set them in the bar-room, where the gentlemen could come and get them in the morning while I was at other work. I had nothing extra for this, neither would he pay me my regular wages; so I thought this was a little too much like slavery, and devised a plan by which I got some pay for my work.

I made it a point never to blacken all the boots and shoes over night, neither would I put any of them in the bar-room, but lock them up in a room where no one could get them without calling for me. I got a piece of broken vessel, placed it in the room just before the boots, and put into it several pieces of small change, as if it had been given me for boot blacking; and almost every one that came in after their boots, would throw some small trifle into my contribution box, while I was there blacking away. In this way, I made more than my landlord paid me, and I soon got a good stock of cash again. One morning I blacked a gentleman's boots who came in during the night by a steamboat. After he had put on his boots, I was called into the bar-room to button his straps; and while I was performing this service, not thinking to see anybody that knew me, I happened to look up at the man's face and who should it be but one of the very gamblers who had recently sold me. I dropped his foot and bolted from the room as if I had been struck by an electric shock. The man happened not to recognize me, but this strange conduct on my part excited the landlord, who followed me out to see what was the matter. He found me with my hand to my breast, groaning at a great rate. He asked me what was the matter; but I was not able to inform him correctly, but said that I felt very bad indeed. He of course thought I was sick with the colic and ran in the house and got some hot stuff for me, with spice, ginger, &c. But I never got able to go into the bar-room until long after breakfast time, when I knew this man was gone; then I got well.

And yet I have no idea that the man would have hurt a hair of my head; but my first thought was that he was after me. I then made up my mind to leave Portsmouth; its location being right on the border of a slave State.

A short time after this a gentleman put up there over night

named Smith, from Perrysburgh, with whom I was acquainted in the North. He was on his way to Kentucky to buy up a drove of fine horses, and he wanted me to go and help him to drive his horses out to Perrysburgh, and said he would pay all my expenses if I would go. So I made a contract to go and agreed to meet him the next week, on a set day, in Washington, Ky., to start with his drove to the north. Accordingly at the time I took a steamboat passage down to Maysville, near where I was to meet Mr. Smith with my trunk. When I arrived at Maysville, I found that Washington was still six miles back from the river. I stopped at a hotel and took my breakfast, and who should I see there but a captain of a boat, who saw me but two years previous going down the river Ohio with handcuffs on, in a chain gang; but he happened not to know me. I left my trunk at the hotel and went out to Washington, where I found Mr. Smith, and learned that he was not going to start off with his drove until the next day.

The following letter which was addressed to the committee to investigate the truth of my narrative, will explain this part of it to the reader and corroborate my statements:

MAUMEE CITY, April 5, 1845.

CHAS. H. STEWART, ESQ.

DEAR SIR:—Your favor of 13th February, addressed to me at Perrysburgh, was not received until yesterday; having removed to this place, the letter was not forwarded as it should have been. In reply to your inquiry respecting Henry Bibb, I can only say that about the year 1838 I became acquainted with him at Perrysburgh—employed him to do some work by the job which he performed well, and from his apparent honesty and candor, I became much interested in him. About that time he went South for the purpose, as was said, of getting his wife, who was there in slavery. In the spring of 1841, I found him at Portsmouth on the Ohio river, and after much persuasion, employed him to assist my man to drive home some horses and cattle which I was about purchasing near Maysville, Ky. My confidence in him was such that when about half way home I separated the horses from the cattle, and left him with the latter, with money and instructions to hire what help he wanted to get to Perrysburgh. This he accomplished to my entire satisfaction. He worked for me during the summer, and I was unwilling to part with him, but his desire to go to school and mature plans for the liberation of his wife, were so strong that he left for Detroit, where he could enjoy the society of his colored brethren. I have heard his story and must say that I have not the least reason to suspect it being otherwise than true, and furthermore, I firmly believe, and have for a long time, that he has the foundation to make himself useful. I shall always afford him all the facilities in my power to assist him, until I hear of something in relation to him to alter my mind.

   Yours in the cause of truth.

       J. W. SMITH

When I arrived at Perrysburgh, I went to work for Mr. Smith for several months. This family I found to be one of the most kind-hearted, and unprejudiced that I ever lived with. Mr. and Mrs. Smith lived up to their profession.

I resolved to go to Detroit, that winter, and go to school, in January 1842. But when I arrived at Detroit I soon found that I was not able to give myself a very thorough education. I was among strangers, who were not disposed to show me any great favors. I had every thing to pay for, and clothing to buy, so I graduated within three weeks! And this was all the schooling that I have ever had in my life.

W. C. Monroe was my teacher; to him I went about two weeks only. My occupation varied according to circumstances, as I was not settled in mind about the condition of my bereaved family for several years, and could not settle myself down at any permanent business. I saw occasionally, fugitives from Kentucky, some of whom I knew, but none of them were my relatives; none could give me the information which I desired most.

CHAPTER XVII.

Letter from W. H. Gatewood.—My reply.—My efforts as a public lecturer.—Singular incident in Steubenville—Meeting with a friend of Whitfield in Michigan.—Outrage on a canal packet.—Fruitless efforts to find my wife.

THE first direct information that I received concerning any of my relations, after my last escape from slavery, was communicated in a letter from Wm. H. Gatewood, my former owner, which I here insert word for word, without any correction:

BEDFORD, TRIMBLE COUNTY, KY.

Mr. H. BIBB.

DEAR SIR:—After my respects to you and yours &c., I received a small book which you sent to me that I peroseed and found it was sent by H. Bibb I am a stranger in Detroit and know no man there without it is Walton H. Bibb if this be the man please to write to me and tell me all about that place and the people I will tell you the news here as well as I can your mother is still living here and she is well the people are generally well in this cuntry times are dull and produce low give my compliments to King, Jack, and all my friends in that cuntry I read that book you sent me and think it will do very well— George is sold, I do not know any thing about him I have nothing more at present, but remain yours &c

W. H GATEWOOD.

February 9th, 1844.

P. S. You will please to answer this letter.

Never was I more surprised than at the reception of this letter, it came so unexpected to me. There had just been a State Convention held in Detroit, by the free people of color, the proceedings of which were published in pamphlet form. I forwarded several of them to distinguished slaveholders in Kentucky—one among others was Mr. Gatewood, and gave him to understand who sent it. After showing this letter to several of my anti-slavery friends, and asking their opinions about the propriety of my answering it, I was advised to do it, as Mr.

Gatewood had no claim on me as a slave, for he had sold and got the money for me and my family. So I wrote him an answer, as near as I can recollect, in the following language:

DEAR SIR:—I am happy to inform you that you are not mistaken in the man whom you sold as property, and received pay for as such. But I thank God that I am not property now, but am regarded as a man like yourself, and although I live far north, I am enjoying a comfortable living by my own industry. If you should ever chance to be traveling this way, and will call on me, I will use you better than you did me while you held me as a slave. Think not that I have any malice against you, for the cruel treatment which you inflicted on me while I was in your power. As it was the custom of your country, to treat your fellow man as you did me and my little family, I can freely forgive you.

I wish to be remembered in love to my aged mother, and friends; please tell her that if we should never meet again in this life, my prayer shall be to God that we may meet in Heaven, where parting shall be no more.

You wish to be remembered to King and Jack. I am pleased, sir, to inform you that they are both here, well, and doing well. They are both living in Canada West. They are now the owners of better farms than the men are who once owned them.

You may perhaps think hard of us for running away from slavery, but as to myself, I have but one apology to make for it, which is this: I have only to regret that I did not start at an earlier period. I might have been free long before I was. But you had it in your power to have kept me there much longer than you did. I think it is very probable that I should have been a toiling slave on your plantation to-day, if you had treated me differently.

To be compelled to stand by and see you whip and slash my wife without mercy, when I could afford her no protection, not even by offering myself to suffer the lash in her place, was more than I felt it to be the duty of a slave husband to endure, while the way was open to Canada. My infant child was also frequently flogged by

Mrs. Gatewood, for crying, until its skin was bruised literally purple. This kind of treatment was what drove me from home and family, to seek a better home for them. But I am willing to forget the past. I should be pleased to hear from you again, on the reception of this, and should also be very happy to correspond with you often, if it should be agreeable to yourself. I subscribe myself a friend to the oppressed, and Liberty forever.

HENRY BIBB.

WILLIAM GATEWOOD.
Detroit, March 23d, 1844.

The first time that I ever spoke before a public audience, was to give a narration of my own sufferings and adventures, connected with slavery. I commenced in the village of Adrian, State of Michigan, May, 1844. From that up to the present period, the principle part of my time has been faithfully devoted to the cause of freedom—nerved up and encouraged by the sympathy of anti-slavery friends on the one hand, and prompted by a sense of duty to my enslaved countrymen on the other, especially, when I remembered that slavery had robbed me of my freedom—deprived me of education—banished me from my native State, and robbed me of my family.

I went from Michigan to the State of Ohio, where I traveled over some of the Southern counties of that State, in company with Samuel Brooks, and Amos Dresser, lecturing upon the subject of American Slavery. The prejudice of the people at that time was very strong against the abolitionists; so much so that they were frequently mobbed for discussing the subject.

We appointed a series of meetings along on the Ohio River, in sight of the State of Virginia; and in several places we had Virginians over to hear us upon the subject. I recollect our having appointed a meeting in the city of Steubenville, which is situated on the bank of the river Ohio. There was but one known abolitionist living in that city, named George Ore. On the day of our meeting, when we arrived in this splendid city there was not a church, school house, nor hall, that we could get for love or money, to hold our meeting in. Finally, I believe that the whigs consented to let us have the use of their club room, to hold the meeting in; but before the hour had arrived for us to commence, they re-considered the matter, and informed us that we could not have the use of their house for an abolition meeting.

We then got permission to hold forth in the public market house, and even then so great was the hostility of the rabble, that they tried to bluff us off, by threats and epithets. Our meeting was advertised to take place at nine o'clock, A. M. The pro-slavery parties hired a colored man to take a large auction bell, and go all over the city ringing it, and crying, "ho ye! ho ye! Negro auction to take place in the market house, at nine o'clock, by George Ore!" This cry was sounded all over the city, which called out many who would not otherwise have been present. They came to see if it was really the case. The object of the rabble in having the bell rung was, to prevent us from attempting to speak. But at the appointed hour, Bro. Dresser opened the meeting with prayer, and Samuel Brooks mounted the block and spoke for fifteen or twenty minutes, after which Mr. Dresser took the block and talked about one hour upon the wickedness of slaveholding. There were not yet many persons present. They were standing off I suppose to see if I was to be offered for sale. Many windows were hoisted and store doors open, and they were looking and listening to what was said. After Mr. Dresser was through, I was called to take the stand. Just at this moment there was no small stir in rushing forward; so much indeed, that I thought they were coming up to mob me. I should think that in less than fifteen minutes there were about one thousand persons standing around, listening. I saw many of them shedding tears while I related the sad story of my wrongs. At twelve o'clock we adjourned the meeting, to meet again at the same place at two P. M. Our afternoon meeting was well attended until nearly sunset, at which time, we saw some signs of a mob and adjourned. The mob followed us that night to the house of Mr. Ore, and they were yelling like tigers, until late that night, around the house, as if they wanted to tear it down.

In the fall of 1844, S. B. Treadwell, of Jackson, and myself, spent two or three months in lecturing through the State of Michigan, upon the abolition of slavery, in a section of country where abolitionists were few and far between. Our meetings were generally appointed in small log cabins, school houses, among the farmers, which were some times crowded full; and where they had no horse teams, it was often the case that there would be four or five ox teams come, loaded down with men, women and children, to attend our meetings.

But the people were generally poor, and in many places not able to give us a decent night's lodging. We most generally carried with us a few pounds of candles to light up the houses wherein we held our meetings after night; for in many places, they had neither candles nor candlesticks. After meeting was out, we have frequently gone from three to eight miles to get lodging, through the dark forest, where there was scarcely any road for a wagon to run on.

I have traveled for miles over swamps, where the roads were covered with logs, without any dirt over them, which has sometimes shook and jostled the wagon to pieces, where we could find no shop or any place to mend it. We would have to tie it up with bark, or take the lines to tie it with, and lead the horse by the bridle. At other times we were in mud up to the hubs of the wheels. I recollect one evening, we lectured in a little village where there happened to be a Southerner present, who was a personal friend of Deacon Whitfield, who became much offended at what I said about his "Bro. Whitfield," and complained about it after the meeting was out.

He told the people not to believe a word that I said, that it was all a humbug. They asked him how he knew? "Ah!" said he, "he has slandered Bro. Whitfield. I am well acquainted with him, we both belonged to one church; and Whitfield is one of the most respectable men in all that region of country." They asked if he (Whitfield) was a slaveholder?

The reply was "yes, but he treated his slaves well."

"Well," said one, "that only proves that he has told us the truth; for all we wish to know, is that there is such a man as Whitfield, as represented by Bibb, and that he is a slave holder."

On the 2d Sept., 1847, I started from Toledo on board the canal packet Erie, for Cincinnati, Ohio. But before going on board, I was waited on by one of the boat's crew, who gave me a card of the boat, upon which was printed, that no pains would be spared to render all passengers comfortable who might favor them with their patronage to Cincinnati. This card I slipped into my pocket, supposing it might be of some use to me. There were several drunken loafers on board going through as passengers, one of whom used the most vulgar language in the cabin, where there were ladies, and even vomited! But he was called a white man, and a southerner, which made it all right. I of course took my place in the cabin with the rest, and there was nothing said against it that night. When the passengers went forward to settle their fare I paid as much as any other man, which entitled me to the same privileges. The next morning at the ringing of the breakfast bell, the proprietor of the packet line, Mr. Samuel Doyle, being on board, invited the passengers to sit up to breakfast. He also invited me personally to sit up to the table. But after we were all seated, and some had began to eat, he came and ordered me up from the table, and said I must wait until the rest were done.

I left the table without making any reply, and walked out on the deck of the boat. After breakfast the passengers came up, and the cabin boy was sent after me to come to breakfast, but I refused. Shortly after, this man who had ordered me from the table, came up with the ladies. I stepped up and asked him if he was the captain of the boat. His answer was no, that he was one of the proprietors. I then informed him that I was going to leave his boat at the first stopping place, but before leaving I wanted to ask him a few questions: "Have I misbehaved to any one on board of this boat? Have I disobeyed any law of this boat?"

"No," said he.

"Have I not paid you as much as any other passenger through to Cincinnati?"

"Yes," said he.

"Then I am sure that I have been insulted and imposed upon, on board of this boat, without any just cause whatever."

"No one has misused you, for you ought to have known better than to have come to the table where there were white people."

"Sir, did you not ask me to come to the table?"

"Yes, but I did not know that you was a colored man, when I asked you; and then it was better to insult one man than all the passengers on board of the boat."

"Sir, I do not believe that there is a gentleman or lady on board of this boat who would have considered it an insult for me to have taken my breakfast, and you have imposed upon me by taking my money and promising to use me well, and then to insult me as you have."

"I don't want any of your jaw," said he.

"Sir, with all due respect to your elevated station, you have imposed upon me in a way which is unbecoming a gentleman. I have paid my money, and behaved myself as well as any other man, and I am determined that no man shall impose on me as you have, by deceiving me, without my letting the world know it. I would rather a man should rob me of my money at midnight, than to take it in that way."

I left this boat at the first stopping place, and took the next boat to Cincinnati. On the last boat I had no cause to complain of my treatment. When I arrived at Cincinnati, I published a statement of this affair in the Daily Herald.

The next day Mr. Doyle called on the editor in a great passion.—"Here," said he, "what does this mean."

"What, sir?" said the editor quietly.

"Why, the stuff here, read it and see."

"Read it yourself," answered the editor.

"Well, I want to know if you sympathize with this nigger here."

"Who, Mr. Bibb? Why yes, I think he is a gentleman, and should be used as such."

"Why this is all wrong—all of it."

"Put your finger on the place, and I will right it."

"Well, he says that we took his money, when we paid part back. And if you take his part, why I'll have nothing to do with your paper."

So ended his wrath.

In 1845, the anti-slavery friends of Michigan employed me to take the field as an anti-slavery Lecturer, in that State, during the Spring, Summer, and Fall, pledging themselves to restore to me my wife and child, if they were living, and could be reached by human agency, which may be seen by the following circular from the Signal of Liberty:

TO LIBERTY FRIENDS:—In the Signal of the 28th inst. is a report from the undersigned respecting Henry Bibb. His narrative always excites deep sympathy for himself and favorable bias for the cause, which seeks to abolish the evils he so powerfully portrays. Friends and foes attest his efficiency.

Mr. Bibb has labored much in lecturing, yet has collected but a bare pittance. He has received from Ohio lucrative offers, but we have prevailed on him to remain in this State.

We think that a strong obligation rests on the friends in this State to sustain Mr. Bibb, and restore to him his wife and child. Under the expectation that Michigan will yield to these claims: will support their laborer, and re-unite the long severed ties of husband and wife, parent and child, Mr. Bibb will lecture through the whole State.

Our object is to prepare friends for the visit of Mr. Bibb, and to suggest an effective mode of operations for the whole State.

Let friends in each vicinity appoint a collector—pay to him all contributions for the freedom of Mrs. Bibb and child: then transmit them to us. We will acknowledge them in the Signal, and be responsible for them. We will see that the proper measures for the freedom of Mrs. Bibb and child are taken, and if it be within our means we will accomplish it—nay we will accomplish it, if the objects be living and the friends sustain us. But should we fail, the contributions will be held subject to the order of the donors, less however, by a proportionate deduction of expenses from each.

The hope of this re-union will nerve the heart and body of Mr. Bibb to re-doubled effort in a cause otherwise dear to him. And as he will devote his whole time systematically to the anti-slavery cause, he must also depend on friends for the means of livelihood. We bespeak for him your hospitality, and such pecuniary contributions as you can afford, trusting that the latter may be sufficient to enable him to keep the field.

A. L. PORTER,
C. H. STEWART,
SILAS M. HOLMES

DETROIT, APRIL 22, 1845.

I have every reason to believe that they acted faithfully in the matter, but without success. They wrote letters in every quarter where they would be likely to gain any information respecting her. There were also two men sent from Michigan in the summer of 1845, down South, to find her if possible, and report—and whether they found out her condition, and refused to report, I am not able to say—but suffice it to say that they never have reported. They were respectable men and true friends of the cause, one of whom was a Methodist minister, and the other a cabinet maker, and both white men.

The small spark of hope which had still lingered about my heart had almost become extinct.

CHAPTER XVIII.

My last effort to recover my family.—Sad tidings of my wife.—
Her degradation.—I am compelled to regard our relation as
dissolved forever.

In view of the failure to hear any thing of my wife, many of
my best friends advised me to get married again, if I could
find a suitable person. They regarded my former wife as dead
to me, and all had been done that could be.

But I was not yet satisfied myself, to give up. I wanted to
know certainly what had become of her. So in the winter of
1845, I resolved to go back to Kentucky, my native State, to
see if I could hear anything from my family. And against the
advice of all my friends, I went back to Cincinnati, where I
took passage on board of a Southern steamboat to Madison,
in the State of Indiana, which was only ten miles from where
Wm. Gatewood lived, who was my former owner. No sooner
had I landed in Madison, than I learned, on inquiry, and from
good authority, that my wife was living in a state of adultery
with her master, and had been for the last three years. This
message she sent back to Kentucky, to her mother and
friends. She also spoke of the time and manner of our separation by Deacon Whitfield, my being taken off by the Southern black-legs, to where she knew not; and that she had finally
given me up. The child she said was still with her. Whitfield
had sold her to this man for the above purposes at a high
price, and she was better used than ordinary slaves. This was
a death blow to all my hopes and pleasant plans. While I was
in Madison I hired a white man to go over to Bedford, in
Kentucky, where my mother was then living, and bring her
over into a free State to see me. I hailed her approach with
unspeakable joy. She informed me too, on inquiring whether
my family had ever been heard from, that the report which I
had just heard in relation to Malinda was substantially true,
for it was the same message that she had sent to her mother
and friends. And my mother thought it was no use for me to
run any more risks, or to grieve myself any more about her.

From that time I gave her up into the hands of an all-wise

Providence. As she was then living with another man, I could no longer regard her as my wife. After all the sacrifices, sufferings, and risks which I had run, striving to rescue her from the grasp of slavery; every prospect and hope was cut off. She has ever since been regarded as theoretically and practically dead to me as a wife, for she was living in a state of adultery, according to the law of God and man.

Poor unfortunate woman, I bring no charge of guilt against her, for I know not all the circumstances connected with the case. It is consistent with slavery, however, to suppose that she became reconciled to it, from the fact of her sending word back to her friends and relatives that she was much better treated than she had ever been before, and that she had also given me up. It is also reasonable to suppose that there might have been some kind of attachment formed by living together in this way for years; and it is quite probable that they have other children according to the law of nature, which would have a tendency to unite them stronger together.

In view of all the facts and circumstances connected with this matter, I deem further comments and explanations unnecessary on my part. Finding myself thus isolated in this peculiarly unnatural state, I resolved, in 1846, to spend my days in traveling, to advance the anti-slavery cause. I spent the summer in Michigan, but in the subsequent fall I took a trip to New England, where I spent the winter. And there I found a kind reception wherever I traveled among the friends of freedom.

While traveling about in this way among strangers, I was sometimes sick, with no permanent home, or bosom friend to sympathise or take that care of me which an affectionate wife would. So I conceived the idea that it would be better for me to change my position, provided I should find a suitable person.

In the month of May, 1847, I attended the anti-slavery anniversary in the city of New York, where I had the good fortune to be introduced to the favor of a Miss Mary E. Miles, of Boston; a lady whom I had frequently heard very highly spoken of, for her activity and devotion to the anti-slavery cause, as well as her talents and learning, and benevolence in the cause of reforms, generally. I was very much impressed with the personal appearance of Miss Miles, and was deeply interested in our first interview, because I found that her principles and my own were nearly one and the same. I soon found by a few visits, as well as by letters, that she possessed moral principle, and frankness of disposition, which is often sought for but seldom found. These, in connection with other amiable qualities, soon won my entire confidence and affection. But this secret I kept to myself until I was fully satisfied that this feeling was reciprocal; that there was indeed a congeniality of principles and feeling, which time nor eternity could never change.

When I offered myself for matrimony, we mutually engaged ourselves to each other, to marry in one year, with this condition, viz: that if either party should see any reason to change their mind within that time, the contract should not be considered binding. We kept up a regular correspondence during the time, and in June, 1848, we had the happiness to be joined in holy wedlock. Not in slaveholding style, which is a mere farce, without the sanction of law or gospel; but in accordance with the laws of God and our country. My beloved wife is a bosom friend, a help-meet, a loving companion in all the social, moral, and religious relations of life. She is to me what a poor slave's wife can never be to her husband while in the condition of a slave; for she can not be true to her husband contrary to the will of her master. She can neither be pure nor virtuous, contrary to the will of her master. She dare not refuse to be reduced to a state of adultery at the will of her master; from the fact that the slaveholding law, customs and teachings are all against the poor slaves.

I presume there are no class of people in the United States who so highly appreciate the legality of marriage as those persons who have been held and treated as property. Yes, it is that fugitive who knows from sad experience, what it is to have his wife tyrannically snatched from his bosom by a slaveholding professor of religion, and finally reduced to a state of adultery, that knows how to appreciate the law that repels such high-handed villany. Such as that to which the writer has been exposed. But thanks be to God, I am now free from the hand of the cruel oppressor, no more to be plundered of my dearest rights; the wife of my bosom, and my poor unoffending offspring. Of Malinda I will only add a word in conclusion. The relation once subsisting between us, to which I clung, hoping against hope, for years, after we were torn assunder, not having been sanctioned by any loyal power, cannot be cancelled by a legal process. Voluntarily assumed without law mutually, it was by her relinquished years ago without my knowledge, as before named; during which time I was making every effort to secure her restoration. And it was not until after living alone in the world for more than eight years without a companion known in law or morals, that I changed my condition.

CHAPTER XIX.

Comments on S. Gatewood's letter about slaves stealing.—Their conduct vindicated.—Comments on W. Gatewood's letter.

BUT it seems that I am not now beyond the reach of the foul slander of slaveholders. They are not satisfied with selling and banishing me from my native State. As soon as they got news of my being in the free North, exposing their peculiar Institution, a libelous letter was written by Silas Gatewood of Kentucky, a son of one of my former owners, to a Northern Committee, for publication, which he thought would destroy my influence and character. This letter will be found in the introduction.

He has charged me with the awful crime of taking from my keeper and oppressor, some of the fruits of my own labor for the benefit of myself and family.

But while writing this letter he seems to have overlooked the disgraceful fact that he was guilty himself of what would here be regarded highway robbery, in his conduct to me as narrated on page 486 of this narrative.

A word in reply to Silas Gatewood's letter. I am willing to admit all that is true, but shall deny that which is so basely false. In the first place, he puts words in my mouth that I never used. He says that I represented that "my mother belonged to James Bibb." I deny ever having said so in private or public. He says that I stated that Bibb's daughter married a Sibley. I deny it. He also says that the first time that I left Kentucky for my liberty, I was gone about two years, before I went back to rescue my family. I deny it. I was gone from Dec. 25th, 1837, to May, or June, 1838. He says that I went back the second time for the purpose of taking off my family, and eight or ten more slaves to Canada. This I will not pretend to deny. He says I was guilty of disposing of articles from the farm for my own use, and pocketing the money, and that his father caught me stealing a sack full of wheat. I admit the fact. I acknowledge the wheat.

And who had a better right to eat of the fruits of my own hard earnings than myself? Many a long summer's day have I toiled with my wife and other slaves, cultivating his father's fields, and gathering in his harvest, under the scorching rays of the sun, without half enough to eat, or clothes to wear, and at the same time his meat-house was filled with bacon and bread stuff; his dairy with butter and cheese; his barn with grain, husbanded by the unrequited toil of the slaves. And yet if a slave presumed to take a little from the abundance which he had made by his own sweat and toil, to supply the demands of nature, to quiet the craving appetite which is sometimes almost irresistible, it is called stealing by slaveholders.

But I did not regard it as stealing then, I do not regard it as such now. I hold that a slave has a moral right to eat drink and wear all that he needs, and that it would be a sin on his part to suffer and starve in a country where there is a plenty to eat and wear within his reach. I consider that I had a just right to what I took, because it was the labor of my own hands. Should I take from a neighbor as a freeman, in a free country, I should consider myself guilty of doing wrong before God and man. But was I the slave of Wm. Gatewood to-day, or any other slaveholder, working without wages, and suffering with hunger or for clothing, I should not stop to inquire whether my master would approve of my helping myself to what I needed to eat or wear. For while the slave is regarded as property, how can he steal from his master? It is contrary to the very nature of the relation existing between master and slave, from the fact that there is no law to punish a slave for theft, but lynch law; and the way they avoid that is to hide well. For illustration, a slave from the State of Virginia, for cruel treatment left the State between daylight and dark, being borne off by one of his master's finest horses, and finally landed in Canada, where the British laws recognise no such thing as property in a human being. He was pursued by his owners, who expected to take advantage of the British law by claiming him as a fugitive from justice, and as such he was arrested and brought before the court of Queen's Bench. They swore that he was, at a certain time, the slave of Mr. A., and that he ran away at such a time and stole and brought off a horse. They enquired who the horse belonged to, and it was ascertained that the slave and horse both belonged to the same person. The court therefore decided that the horse and the man were both recognised, in the State of Virginia, alike, as articles of property, belonging to the same person—therefore, if there was theft committed on either side, the former must have stolen off the latter—the horse brought away the man, and not the man the horse. So the man was discharged and pronounced free according to the laws of Canada. There are several other letters published in this work upon the same subject, from slaveholders, which it is hardly necessary for me to notice. However, I feel thankful to the writers for the endorsement and confirmation which they have given to my story. No matter what their motives were, they have done me and the anti-slavery cause good service in writing those letters—but more especially the Gatewood's. Silas Gatewood has done more for me than all the rest. He has labored so hard in his long communication in trying to expose me, that he has proved every thing that I could have asked of him; and for which I intend to reward him by forwarding him one of my books, hoping that it may be the means of converting him from a slaveholder to an honest man, and an advocate of liberty for all mankind.

The reader will see in the introduction that Wm. Gatewood writes a more cautious letter upon the subject than his son Silas. "It is not a very easy matter to catch old birds with chaff," and I presume if Silas had the writing of his letter over again, he would not be so free in telling all he knew, and even more, for the sake of making out a strong case. The object of his writing such a letter will doubtless be understood by the reader. It was to destroy public confidence in the victims of slavery, that the system might not be exposed—it was to gag a poor fugitive who had undertaken to plead his own cause and that of his enslaved brethren. It was a feeble attempt to suppress the voice of universal freedom which is now thundering on every gale. But thank God it is too late in the day.

> Go stop the mighty thunder's roar,
> Go hush the ocean's sound,
> Or upward like the eagle soar
> To skies' remotest bound.

And when thou hast the thunder stopped,
And hushed the ocean's waves,
Then, freedom's spirit bind in chains,
And ever hold us slaves.

And when the eagle's boldest fest,
Thou canst perform with skill,
Then, think to stop proud freedom's march,
And hold the bondman still.

CHAPTER XX.

Review of my narrative.—Licentiousness a prop of slavery.—A case of mild slavery given.—Its revolting features.—Times of my purchase and sale by professed Christians.—Concluding remarks.

I NOW conclude my narrative, by reviewing briefly what I have written. This little work has been written without any personal aid or a knowledge of the English grammer, which must in part be my apology for many of its imperfections.

I find in several places, where I have spoken out the deep feelings of my soul, in trying to describe the horrid treatment which I have so often received at the hands of slaveholding professors of religion, that I might possibly make a wrong impression on the minds of some northern freemen, who are unacquainted theoretically or practically with the customs and treatment of American slaveholders to their slaves. I hope that it may not be supposed by any, that I have exaggerated in the least, for the purpose of making out the system of slavery worse than it really is, for, to exaggerate upon the cruelties of this system, would be almost impossible; and to write herein the most horrid features of it would not be in good taste for my book.

I have long thought from what has fallen under my own observation while a slave, that the strongest reason why southerners stick with such tenacity to their "peculiar institution," is because licentious white men could not carry out their wicked purposes among the defenceless colored population as they now do, without being exposed and punished by law, if slavery was abolished. Female virtue could not be trampled under foot with impunity, and marriage among the people of color kept in utter obscurity.

On the other hand, lest it should be said by slaveholders and their apologists, that I have not done them the justice to give a sketch of the best side of slavery, if there can be any best side to it; therefore in conclusion, they may have the benefit of the following case, that fell under the observation of the writer. And I challenge America to show a milder state of slavery than this. I once knew a Methodist in the state of Ky., by the name of Young, who was the owner of a large number of slaves, many of whom belonged to the same church with their master. They worshipped together in the same church.

Mr. Young never was known to flog one of his slaves or sell one. He fed and clothed them well, and never over-worked them. He allowed each family a small house to themselves with a little garden spot, whereon to raise their own vegetables; and a part of the day on Saturdays was allowed them to cultivate it.

In process of time he became deeply involved in debt by endorsing notes, and his property was all advertised to be sold by the sheriff at public auction. It consisted in slaves, many of whom were his brothers and sisters in the church.

On the day of sale there were slave traders and speculators on the ground to buy. The slaves were offered on the auction block one after another, until they were all sold before their old master's face. The first man offered on the block was an old gray-headed slave by the name of Richard. His wife followed him up to the block, and when they had bid him up to seventy or eighty dollars one of the bidders asked Mr. Young what he could do, as he looked very old and infirm? Mr. Young replied by saying, "he is not able to accomplish much manual labor, from his extreme age and hard labor in early life. Yet I would rather have him than many of those who are young and vigorous; who are able to perform twice as much labor—because I know him to be faithful and trustworthy, a Christian in good standing in my church. I can trust him anywhere with confidence. He has toiled many long years on my plantation and I have always found him faithful."

This giving him a good Christian character caused them to run him up to near two hundred dollars. His poor old companion stood by weeping and pleading that they might not be separated. But the marriage relation was soon dissolved by the sale, and they were separated never to meet again.

Another man was called up whose wife followed him with her infant in her arms, beseeching to be sold with her husband, which proved to be all in vain. After the men were all sold they then sold the women and children. They ordered the first woman to lay down her child and mount the auction block; she refused to give up her little one and clung to it as long as she could, while the cruel lash was applied to her back for disobedience. She pleaded for mercy in the name of God. But the child was torn from the arms of its mother amid the most heart-rending shrieks from the mother and child on the one hand, and bitter oaths and cruel lashes from the tyrants on the other. Finally the poor little child was torn from the mother while she was sacrificed to the highest bidder. In this way the sale was carried on from beginning to end.

There was each speculator with his hand-cuffs to bind his victims after the sale; and while they were doing their writings, the Christian portion of the slaves asked permission to kneel in prayer on the ground before they separated, which was granted. And while bathing each other with tears of sorrow on the verge of their final separation, their eloquent appeals in prayer to the Most High seemed to cause an unpleasant sensation upon the ears of their tyrants, who ordered them to rise and make ready their limbs for the caffles. And as they happened not to bound at the first sound, they were soon raised from their knees by the sound of the lash, and the rattle of the chains, in which they were soon taken off by their respective masters,—husbands from wives, and children from parents, never expecting to meet until the judgment of the great day. Then Christ shall say to the slaveholding professors of religion, "Inasmuch as ye did it unto one of the least of these little ones, my brethren, ye did it unto me."

Having thus tried to show the best side of slavery that I can conceive of, the reader can exercise his own judgment in deciding whether a man can be a Bible Christian, and yet hold his Christian brethren as property, so that they may be sold at any time in market, as sheep or oxen, to pay his debts.

During my life in slavery I have been sold by professors of religion several times. In 1836 "Bro." Albert G. Sibley, of Bedford, Kentucky, sold me for $850 to "Bro." John Sibley; and in the same year he sold me to "Bro." Wm. Gatewood of Bedford, for $850. In 1839 "Bro." Gatewood sold me to Madison Garrison, a slave trader, of Louisville, Kentucky, with my wife and child—at a depreciated price because I was a runaway. In the same year he sold me with my family to "Bro."

Whitfield, in the city of New Orleans, for $1200. In 1841 "Bro." Whitfield sold me from my family to Thomas Wilson and Co., blacklegs. In the same year they sold me to a "Bro." in the Indian Territory. I think he was a member of the Presbyterian Church. F. E. Whitfield was a deacon in regular standing in the Baptist Church. A. Sibley was a Methodist exhorter of the M. E. Church in good standing. J. Sibley was a class-leader in the same church; and Wm. Gatewood was also an acceptable member of the same church.

Is this Christianity? Is it honest or right? Is it doing as we would be done by? Is it in accordance with the principles of humanity or justice?

I believe slaveholding to be a sin against God and man under all circumstances. I have no sympathy with the person or persons who tolerate and support the system willingly and knowingly, morally, religiously or politically.

Prayerfully and earnestly relying on the power of truth, and the aid of the divine providence, I trust that this little volume will bear some humble part in lighting up the path of freedom and revolutionizing public opinion upon this great subject. And I here pledge myself, God being my helper, ever to contend for the natural equality of the human family, without regard to color, which is but fading *matter*, while *mind* makes the man.

NEW YORK CITY, *May 1, 1849.*

                                        HENRY BIBB.

INDEX.

NARRATIVE

OF

SOJOURNER TRUTH,

A

NORTHERN SLAVE,

EMANCIPATED FROM BODILY SERVITUDE BY THE STATE
OF NEW YORK, IN 1828.

WITH A PORTRAIT.

Sweet is the virgin honey, though the wild bee store it in a reed;
And bright the jewelled band that circleth an Ethiop's arm;
Pure are the grains of gold in the turbid stream of the Ganges;
And fair the living flowers that spring from the dull cold sod.
Wherefore, thou gentle student, bend thine ear to my speech,
For I also am as thou art; our hearts can commune together;
To meanest matters will I stoop, for mean is the lot of mortal;
I will rise to noblest themes, for the soul hath a heritage of glory.

BOSTON:
PUBLISHED FOR THE AUTHOR.
1850.

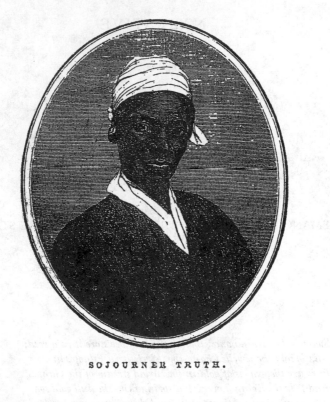

SOJOURNER TRUTH.

PREFACE.

THE following is the unpretending narrative of the life of a remarkable and meritorious woman—a life which has been checkered by strange vicissitudes, severe hardships, and singular adventures. Born a slave, and held in that brutal condition until the entire abolition of slavery in the State of New York in 1827, she has known what it is to drink to the dregs the bitterest cup of human degradation. That one thus placed on a level with cattle and swine, and for so many years subjected to the most demoralizing influences, should have retained her moral integrity to such an extent, and cherished so successfully the religious sentiment in her soul, shows a mind of no common order, while it heightens the detestation that is felt in every humane bosom, of that system of oppression which seeks to cripple the intellect, impair the understanding, and deprave the hearts of its victims—a system which has subjected to its own foul purposes, in the United States, all that is wealthy, talented, influential, and reputedly pious, in an overwhelming measure!

O the 'fantastic tricks' which the American people are 'playing before high Heaven!' O their profane use of the sacred name of Liberty! O their impious appeals to the God of the oppressed, for his divine benediction, while they are making merchandise of his image! Do they not blush? Nay, they glory in their shame! Once a year, they take special pains to exhibit themselves to the world, in all their republican deformity and Christian barbarity, insanely supposing that they thus excite the envy, admiration and applause of mankind. The nations are looking at the dreadful spectacle with disgust and amazement. However sunken and degraded they may be, they are too elevated, too virtuous, too humane to be guilty of such conduct. Their voice is heard, saying—'Americans! we hear your boasts of liberty, your shouts of independence, your declarations of hostility to every form of tyranny, your assertions that all men are created free and equal, and endowed by their Creator with an inalienable right to liberty, the merry peal of your bells, and the deafening roar of your artillery;

but, mingling with all these, and rising above them all, we also hear the clanking of chains! the shrieks and wailings of millions of your own countrymen, whom you wickedly hold in a state of slavery as much more frightful than the oppression which your fathers resisted unto blood, as the tortures of the Inquisition surpass the stings of an insect! We see your banner floating proudly in the breeze from every flag-staff and mast-head in the land; but its blood-red stripes are emblematical of your own slave-driving cruelty, as you apply the lash to the flesh of your guiltless victim, even the flesh of a wife and mother, shrieking for the restoration of the babe of her bosom, sold to the remorseless slave speculator! We catch the gleam of your illuminated hills, every where blazing with bonfires; we mark your gay processions; we note the number of your orators; we listen to the recital of your revolutionary achievements; we see you kneeling at the shrine of Freedom, as her best, her truest, her sincerest worshippers! Hypocrites! liars! adulterers! tyrants! men-stealers! atheists! Professing to believe in the natural equality of the human race—yet dooming a sixth portion of your immense population to beastly servitude, and ranking them among your goods and chattels! Professing to believe in the existence of a God—yet trading in his image, and selling those in the shambles for whose redemption the Son of God laid down his life! Professing to be Christians—yet withholding the Bible, the means of religious instruction, even the knowledge of the alphabet, from a benighted multitude, under terrible penalties! Boasting of your democracy—yet determining the rights of men by the texture of their hair and the color of their skin! Assuming to be "the land of the free and the home of the brave,"—yet keeping in chains more slaves than any other nation, not excepting slave-cursed Brazil! Prating of your morality and honesty—yet denying the rites of marriage to three millions of human beings, and plundering them of all their hard earnings! Affecting to be horror-struck in view of the foreign slave-trade—yet eagerly pursuing a domestic traffic equally cruel and unnatural, and reducing to slavery not less than seventy thousand new victims annually! Vaunting of your freedom of speech and of the press—your matchless Constitution and your glorious Union—yet denouncing as traitors, and treating as outlaws, those who have the courage and fidelity to plead for immediate, untrammelled, universal emancipation! Monsters that ye are! how can ye expect to escape the scorn of the world, and the wrath of Heaven? Emancipate your slaves, if you would redeem your tarnished character—if you would obtain forgiveness here, and salvation hereafter! Until you do so, "there will be a stain upon your national escutcheon, which all the waters of the Atlantic cannot wash out!" '

It is thus that, as a people, we are justly subjected to the reproach, the execration, the derision of mankind, and are made a proverb and a hissing among the nations. We cannot plead not guilty; every accusation that is registered against us is true; the act of violence is in our hands; the stolen property is in our possession; our fingers are stained with blood; the cup of our iniquity is full.

> Just God! and shall we calmly rest,
>   The Christian's scorn—the Heathen's mirth—
> Content to live the lingering jest
>   And by-word of a mocking earth?
> Shall our own glorious land retain
>   That curse which Europe scorns to bear?
> Shall our own brethren drag the chain,
>   Which not even Russia's menials wear?

It is useless, it is dreadful, it is impious for this nation longer to contend with the Almighty. All his attributes are against us, and on the side of the oppressed. Is it not a fearful thing to fall into the hands of the living God? Who may abide the day of his coming, and who shall stand when he appeareth as 'a swift witness against the adulterers, and against false swearers, and against those that oppress the hireling in his wages, the widow, and the fatherless, and that turn aside the stranger from his right?' Wo to this bloody land! it is all full of lies and robbery—the prey departeth not, and the sound of a whip is heard continually. 'Judgment is turned away backward, and justice standeth afar off: for truth is fallen in the street, and equity cannot enter. Yea, truth faileth; and he that departeth from evil, *maketh himself a prey*.' The Lord sees it, and is displeased that there is no judgment; and he hath put on the garments of vengeance for clothing, and is

clad with zeal as a cloak,—and, unless we repent by immediately undoing the heavy burdens and letting the oppressed go
free, according to our deeds, accordingly he will repay, fury to
his adversaries, recompense to his enemies. 'The Lord exe-
cuteth righteousness and judgment for all that are oppressed.'
'O give thanks unto the Lord; for he is good: for his mercy
endureth for ever. To him that smote Egypt in their first-
born: for his mercy endureth for ever. And overthrew
Pharaoh and his hosts in the Red sea: for his mercy endureth
for ever.' 'Sing unto the Lord, for he hath triumphed glori-
ously: the horse and his rider hath he thrown into the sea.
Thou didst blow with thy wind, the sea covered them: they
sank as lead in the mighty waters.' 'Even so, Lord God
Almighty, for so it seemeth good in thy sight.' 'Who is like
unto thee, O Lord, among the gods? who is like thee, glorious in holiness, fearful in praises, doing wonders?'

In this great contest of Right against Wrong, of Liberty
against Slavery, who are the wicked, if they be not those, who,
like vultures and vampyres, are gorging themselves with
human blood? if they be not the plunderers of the poor, the
spoilers of the defenceless, the traffickers in 'slaves and the
souls of men'? Who are the cowards, if not those who shrink
from manly argumentation, the light of truth, the concussion
of mind, and a fair field? if not those whose prowess, stimulated by whiskey potations, or the spirit of murder, grows
rampant as the darkness of night approaches; whose shouts
and yells are savage and fiend-like; who furiously exclaim,
'Down with free discussion! down with the liberty of the
press! down with the right of petition! down with constitutional law!'—who rifle mail-bags, throw types and printing-
presses into the river, burn public halls dedicated to 'Virtue,
Liberty and Independence,' and assassinate the defenders of
inalienable human rights? And who are the righteous, in this
case, if they be not those who will 'have no fellowship with
the unfruitful works of darkness, but rather reprove them;'
who maintain that the laborer is worthy of his hire, that the
marriage institution is sacred, that slavery is a system accursed
of God, that tyrants are the enemies of mankind, and that immediate emancipation should be given to all who are pining
in bondage! Who are the truly brave, if not those who de-

mand for truth and error alike, free speech, a free press, an open arena, the right of petition, AND NO QUARTERS? if not those, who, instead of skulking from the light, stand forth in the noon-tide blaze of day, and challenge their opponents to emerge from their wolf-like dens, that, by a rigid examination, it may be seen who has stolen the wedge of gold, in whose pocket are the thirty pieces of silver, and whose garments are stained with the blood of innocence?

It is hoped that the perusal of the following Narrative may increase the sympathy that is felt for the suffering colored population of this country, and inspire to renewed efforts for the liberation of all who are pining in bondage on the American soil.

NOTE.

It is due to the lady by whom the following Narrative was kindly written, to state, that she has not been able to see a single proof-sheet of it; consequently, it is very possible that divers errors in printing may have occurred, (though it is hoped none materially affecting the sense,) especially in regard to the names of individuals referred to therein. The name of Van Wagener should read Van Wagenen.

NARRATIVE
OF
SOJOURNER TRUTH.

HER BIRTH AND PARENTAGE.

THE subject of this biography, SOJOURNER TRUTH, as she now calls herself—but whose name, originally, was Isabella—was born, as near as she can now calculate, between the years 1797 and 1800. She was the daughter of James and Betsey, slaves of one Colonel Ardinburgh, Hurley, Ulster County, New York.

Colonel Ardinburgh belonged to that class of people called Low Dutch.

Of her first master, she can give no account, as she must have been a mere infant when he died; and she, with her parents and some ten or twelve other fellow human chattels, became the legal property of his son, Charles Ardinburgh. She distinctly remembers hearing her father and mother say, that their lot was a fortunate one, as Master Charles was the best of the family,—being, comparatively speaking, a kind master to his slaves.

James and Betsey having, by their faithfulness, docility, and respectful behavior, won his particular regard, received from him particular favors—among which was a lot of land, lying back on the slope of a mountain, where, by improving the pleasant evenings and Sundays, they managed to raise a little tobacco, corn, or flax; which they exchanged for extras, in the articles of food or clothing for themselves and children. She has no remembrance that Saturday afternoon was ever added to their own time, as it is by *some* masters in the Southern States.

ACCOMMODATIONS.

Among Isabella's earliest recollections was the removal of her master, Charles Ardinburgh, into his new house, which he had built for a hotel, soon after the decease of his father. A cellar, under this hotel, was assigned to his slaves, as their sleeping apartment,—all the slaves he possessed, of both sexes, sleeping (as is quite common in a state of slavery) in the same room. She carries in her mind, to this day, a vivid picture of this dismal chamber; its only lights consisting of a few panes of glass, through which she thinks the sun never shone, but with thrice reflected rays; and the space between the loose boards of the floor, and the uneven earth below, was often filled with mud and water, the uncomfortable splashings of which were as annoying as its noxious vapors must have been chilling and fatal to health. She shudders, even now, as she goes back in memory, and revisits this cellar, and sees its inmates, of both sexes and all ages, sleeping on those damp boards, like the horse, with a little straw and a blanket; and she wonders not at the rheumatisms, and fever-sores, and palsies, that distorted the limbs and racked the bodies of those fellow-slaves in after-life. Still, she does not attribute this cruelty—for cruelty it certainly is, to be so unmindful of the health and comfort of any being, leaving entirely out of sight his more important part, his everlasting interests,—so much to any innate or constitutional cruelty of the master, as to that gigantic inconsistency, that inherited habit among slaveholders, of expecting a willing and intelligent obedience from the slave, because he is a MAN—at the same time every thing belonging to the soul-harrowing system does its best to crush the last vestige of a man within him; and when it *is* crushed, and often before, he is denied the comforts of life, on the plea that he knows neither the want nor the use of them, and because he is considered to be little more or little *less* than a beast.

HER BROTHERS AND SISTERS.

Isabella's father was very tall and straight, when young, which gave him the name of 'Bomefree'—low Dutch for tree—at least, this is SOJOURNER's pronunciation of it—and by this name he usually went. The most familiar appellation of her mother was 'Mau-mau Bett.' She was the mother of some ten or twelve children; though Sojourner is far from knowing the exact number of her brothers and sisters; she being the youngest, save one, and all older than herself having been sold before her remembrance. She was privileged to behold six of them while she remained a slave.

Of the two that immediately preceded her in age, a boy of five years, and a girl of three, who were sold when she was an infant, she heard much; and she wishes that all who would fain believe that slave parents have not natural affection for their offspring could have listened as *she* did, while Bomefree and Mau-mau Bett,—their dark cellar lighted by a blazing pine-knot,—would sit for hours, recalling and recounting every endearing, as well as harrowing circumstance that taxed memory could supply, from the histories of those dear departed ones, of whom they had been robbed, and for whom their hearts still bled. Among the rest, they would relate how the little boy, on the last morning he was with them, arose with the birds, kindled a fire, calling for his Mau-mau to 'come, for all was now ready for her'—little dreaming of the dreadful separation which was so near at hand, but of which his parents had an uncertain, but all the more cruel foreboding. There was snow on the ground, at the time of which we are speaking; and a large old-fashioned sleigh was seen to drive up to the door of the late Col. Ardinburgh. This event was noticed with childish pleasure by the unsuspicious boy; but when he was taken and put into the sleigh, and saw his little sister actually shut and locked into the sleigh-box, his eyes were at once opened to their intentions; and, like a frightened deer, he sprang from the sleigh, and running into the house, concealed himself under a bed. But this availed him little. He was reconveyed to the sleigh, and separated for ever from those whom God had constituted his natural guardians and protectors, and who should have found him, in return, a stay and a staff to them in their declining years. But I make no comments on facts like these, knowing that the heart of every slave parent will make its own comments, involuntarily and correctly, as soon as each heart shall make the case its own. Those who are not parents will draw their

conclusions from the promptings of humanity and philanthropy:—these, enlightened by reason and revelation, are also
unerring.

HER RELIGIOUS INSTRUCTION.

Isabella and Peter, her youngest brother, remained, with
their parents, the legal property of Charles Ardinburgh till his
decease, which took place when Isabella was near nine years old.

After this event, she was often surprised to find her mother
in tears; and when, in her simplicity, she inquired, 'Mau-mau,
what makes you cry?' she would answer, 'Oh, my child, I am
thinking of your brothers and sisters that have been sold away
from me.' And she would proceed to detail many circumstances respecting them. But Isabella long since concluded
that it was the impending fate of her only remaining children,
which her mother but too well understood, even then, that
called up those memories from the past, and made them crucify her heart afresh.

In the evening, when her mother's work was done, she
would sit down under the sparkling vault of heaven, and calling her children to her, would talk to them of the only Being
that could effectually aid or protect them. Her teachings were
delivered in Low Dutch, her only language, and, translated
into English, ran nearly as follows:—

'My children, there is a God, who hears and sees you.' 'A
God, mau-mau! Where does he live?' asked the children. 'He
lives in the sky,' she replied; 'and when you are beaten, or cruelly treated, or fall into any trouble, you must ask help of him,
and he will always hear and help you.' She taught them to
kneel and say the Lord's prayer. She entreated them to refrain
from lying and stealing, and to strive to obey their masters.

At times, a groan would escape her, and she would break
out in the language of the Psalmist— 'Oh Lord, how long?'
'Oh Lord, how long?' And in reply to Isabella's question—
'What ails you, mau-mau?' her only answer was, 'Oh, a good
deal ails me'—'Enough ails me.' Then again, she would point
them to the stars, and say, in her peculiar language, 'Those
are the same stars, and that is the same moon, that look down

upon your brothers and sisters, and which they see as they look up to them, though they are ever so far away from us, and each other.'

Thus, in her humble way, did she endeavor to show them their Heavenly Father, as the only being who could protect them in their perilous condition; at the same time, she would strengthen and brighten the chain of family affection, which she trusted extended itself sufficiently to connect the widely scattered members of her precious flock. These instructions of the mother were treasured up and held sacred by Isabella, as our future narrative will show.

THE AUCTION.

At length, the never-to-be-forgotten day of the terrible auction arrived, when the 'slaves, horses, and other cattle' of Charles Ardinburgh, deceased, were to be put under the hammer, and again change masters. Not only Isabella and Peter, but their mother, was now destined to the auction block, and would have been struck off with the rest to the highest bidder, but for the following circumstance: A question arose among the heirs, 'Who shall be burthened with Bomefree, when we have sent away his faithful Mau-mau Bett?' He was becoming weak and infirm; his limbs were painfully rheumatic and distorted—more from exposure and hardship than from old age, though he was several years older than Mau-mau Bett; he was no longer considered of value, but must soon be a burthen and care to some one. After some contention on the point at issue, none being willing to be burthened with him, it was finally agreed, as most expedient for the heirs, that the price of Mau-mau Bett should be sacrificed, and she receive her freedom, on condition that she take care of and support her faithful James,—faithful, not only to her as a husband, but proverbially faithful as a slave to those who would not willingly sacrifice a dollar for *his* comfort, now that he had commenced his descent into the dark vale of decrepitude and suffering. This important decision was received as joyful news indeed to our ancient couple, who were the objects of it, and who were trying to prepare their hearts for a severe struggle, and one altogether new to them, as they had never before been separated; for, though ignorant, helpless, crushed in spirit, and weighed down with hardship and cruel bereavement, they were still human, and their human hearts beat within them with as true an affection as ever caused a human heart to beat. And their anticipated separation now, in the decline of life, after the last child had been torn from them, must have been truly appalling. Another privilege was granted them—that of remaining occupants of the same dark, humid cellar I have before described: otherwise, they were to support themselves as they best could. And as her mother was still able to do considerable work, and her father a little, they got on for some time very comfortably. The strangers who rented the house were humane people, and very kind to them; they were not rich, and owned no slaves. How long this state of things continued, we are unable to say, as Isabella had not then sufficiently cultivated her organ of time to calculate years, or even weeks or hours. But she thinks her mother must have lived several years after the death of Master Charles. She remembers going to visit her parents some three or four times before the death of her mother, and a good deal of time seemed to her to intervene between each visit.

At length, her mother's health began to decline—a fever-sore made its ravages on one of her limbs, and the palsy began to shake her frame; still, she and James tottered about, picking up a little here and there, which, added to the mites contributed by their kind neighbors, sufficed to sustain life, and drive famine from the door.

DEATH OF MAU-MAU BETT.

One morning, in early autumn, (from the reason above-mentioned, we cannot tell what year,) Mau-mau Bett told James she would make him a loaf of rye-bread, and get Mrs. Simmons, their kind neighbor, to bake it for them, as she would bake that forenoon. James told her he had engaged to rake after the cart for his neighbors that morning; but before he commenced, he would pole off some apples from a tree near, which they were allowed to gather; and if she could get some of them baked with the bread, it would give it a nice relish for their dinner. He beat off the apples, and soon after, saw Mau-mau Bett come out and gather them up.

At the blowing of the horn for dinner, he groped his way into his cellar, anticipating his humble, but warm and nourishing meal; when, lo! instead of being cheered by the sight and odor of fresh-baked bread and the savory apples, his cellar seemed more cheerless than usual, and at first neither sight nor sound met eye or ear. But, on groping his way through the room, his staff, which he used as a pioneer to go before, and warn him of danger, seemed to be impeded in its progress, and a low, gurgling, choaking sound proceeded from the object before him, giving him the first intimation of the truth as it was, that Mau-mau Bett, his bosom companion, the only remaining member of his large family, had fallen in a fit of the palsy, and lay helpless and senseless on the earth! Who among us, located in pleasant homes, surrounded with every comfort, and so many kind and sympathizing friends, can picture to ourselves the dark and desolate state of poor old James—penniless, weak, lame, and nearly blind, as he was at the moment he found his companion was removed from him, and he was left alone in the world, with no one to aid, comfort, or console him? for she never revived again, and lived only a few hours after being discovered senseless by her poor bereaved James.

LAST DAYS OF BOMEFREE.

Isabella and Peter were permitted to see the remains of their mother laid in their last narrow dwelling, and to make their bereaved father a little visit, ere they returned to their servitude. And most piteous were the lamentations of the poor old man, when, at last, *they* also were obliged to bid him 'Farewell!' Juan Fernandes, on his desolate island, was not so pitiable an object as this poor lame man. Blind and crippled, he was too superannuated to think for a moment of taking care of himself, and he greatly feared no persons would interest themselves in his behalf. 'Oh,' he would exclaim, 'I had thought God would take me first,—Mau-mau was so much smarter than I, and could get about and take care of herself;—and I am *so old*, and *so helpless*. What *is* to become of me? I can't do any thing more—my children are all gone, and here I am left helpless and alone.' 'And then, as I was taking leave of him,' said his daughter, in relating it, 'he raised his voice, and cried aloud like a child—*Oh, how he* DID *cry!* I HEAR it *now*—and remember it as well as if it were but yesterday—*poor old man!!!* He thought *God* had done it all—and my heart bled within me at the sight of his misery. He begged me to get permission to come and see him sometimes, which I readily and heartily promised him.' But when all had left him, the Ardinburghs, having some feeling left for their faithful and favorite slave, 'took turns about' in keeping him—permitting him to stay a few weeks at one house, and then awhile at another, and so around. If, when he made a removal, the place where he was going was not too far off, he took up his line of march, staff in hand, and asked for no assistance. If it was twelve or twenty miles, they gave him a ride. While he was living in this way, Isabella was twice permitted to visit him. Another time she walked twelve miles, and carried her infant in her arms to see him, but when she reached the place where she hoped to find him, he had just left for a place some twenty miles distant, and she never saw him more. The last time she *did* see him, she found him seated on a rock, by the road-side, alone, and far from any house. He was then migrating from the house of one Ardinburgh to that of another, several miles distant. His hair was white like wool—he was almost blind—and his gait was more a creep than a walk—but the weather was warm and pleasant, and he did not dislike the journey. When Isabella addressed him, he recognized her voice, and was exceeding glad to see her. He was assisted to mount the wagon, was carried back to the famous cellar of which we have spoken, and there they held their last earthly conversation. He again, as usual, bewailed his loneliness,—spoke in tones of anguish of his many children, saying, 'They are all taken away from me! I have now not one to give me a cup of cold water—why should I live and not die?' Isabella, whose heart yearned over her father, and who would have made any sacrifice to have been able to be with, and take care of him, tried to comfort, by telling him that 'she had heard the white folks say, that all the slaves in the State would be freed in ten years, and that then she would come and take care of him.' 'I would take just as good care of you as Mau-mau would, if she was here'—continued Isabel. 'Oh, my child,' replied he, 'I cannot *live* that long.' 'Oh *do*, daddy, do live, and I will take such *good* care of you,' was her rejoinder. She now says, 'Why, I thought then, in my ignorance, that he *could* live, if he *would*. I just as much thought so, as I ever thought *any* thing in my life—and I *insisted* on his living: but he shook his head, and insisted he could not.'

But, before Bomefree's good constitution would yield either to age, exposure, or a strong desire to die, the Ardinburghs again tired of him, and offered freedom to two old slaves—Cæsar, brother of Mau-mau Bett, and his wife Betsey—on condition that they should take care of James. (I was about to say, 'their brother-in-law'—but as slaves are neither *husbands* nor *wives* in law, the idea of their being brothers-in-law is truly ludicrous.) And although they were too old and infirm to take care of themselves, (Cæsar having been afflicted for a long time with fever-sores, and his wife with the jaundice,) they eagerly accepted the boon of freedom, which had been the life-long desire of their souls—though at a time when emancipation was to them little more than destitution, and was a freedom more to be desired by the master than the slave. Sojourner declares of the slaves in their ignorance, that 'their thoughts are no longer than her finger.'

DEATH OF BOMEFREE.

A rude cabin, in a lone wood, far from any neighbors, was granted to our freed friends, as the only assistance they were now to expect. Bomefree, from this time, found his poor needs hardly supplied, as his new providers were scarce able to administer to their *own* wants. However, the time drew near when things were to be decidedly worse rather than better; for they had not been together long, before Betty died, and shortly after, Cæsar followed her to 'that bourne from whence no traveller returns'—leaving poor James again desolate, and more helpless than ever before; as, this time, there was no kind family in the house, and the Ardinburghs no longer invited him to their homes. Yet, lone, blind and helpless as he was, James for a time lived on. One day, an aged colored woman, named Soan, called at his shanty, and James besought her, in the most moving manner, even with tears, to tarry awhile and wash and mend him up, so that he might once more be decent and comfortable; for he was suffering dreadfully with the filth and vermin that had collected upon him.

Soan was herself an emancipated slave, old and weak, with no one to care for her; and she lacked the courage to undertake a job of such seeming magnitude, fearing she might herself get sick, and perish there without assistance; and with great reluctance, and a heart swelling with pity, as she afterwards declared, she felt obliged to leave him in his wretchedness and filth. And shortly after her visit, this faithful slave, this deserted wreck of humanity, was found on his miserable pallet, frozen and stiff in death. The kind angel had come at last, and relieved him of the many miseries that his fellowman had heaped upon him. Yes, he had died, chilled and starved, with none to speak a kindly word, or do a kindly deed for him, in that last dread hour of need!

The news of his death reached the ears of John Ardinburgh, a grandson of the old Colonel; and he declared that 'Bomefree, who had ever been a kind and faithful slave, should now have a *good* funeral.' And now, gentle reader, what think you constituted a good funeral? Answer—some black paint for the coffin, and—a jug of ardent spirits! What a compensation for a life of toil, of patient submission to repeated robberies of the most aggravated kind, and, also, far more than murderous neglect!! Mankind often vainly attempt to atone for unkindness or cruelty to the living, by honoring the same after death;—but John Ardinburgh undoubtedly meant *his* pot of paint and jug of whiskey should act as an opiate on his slaves, rather than on his own seared conscience.

COMMENCEMENT OF ISABELLA'S TRIALS IN LIFE.

Having seen the sad end of her parents, so far as it relates to *this* earthly life, we will return with Isabella to that memorable auction which threatened to separate her father and mother. A slave auction is a terrible affair to its victims, and its incidents and consequences are graven on their hearts as with a pen of burning steel.

At this memorable time, Isabella was struck off, for the sum of one hundred dollars, to one John Nealy, of Ulster County, New York; and she has an impression that in this sale she was connected with a lot of sheep. She was now nine years of age, and her trials in life may be dated from this period. She says, with emphasis, '*Now the war begun.*' She could only talk Dutch—and the Nealy's could only talk English. Mr. Nealy could *understand* Dutch, but Isabel and her mistress could neither of them understand the language of the other—and this, of itself, was a formidable obstacle in the way of a *good* understanding between them, and for some time was a fruitful source of dissatisfaction to the mistress, and of punishment and suffering to Isabella. She says, 'If they sent me for a frying-pan, not knowing what they meant, perhaps I carried them the pot-hooks and trammels. Then, oh! how angry mistress would be with me!' Then she suffered '*terribly—terribly*,' with the cold. During the winter her feet were badly frozen, for want of proper covering. They gave her a plenty to eat, and also a plenty of whippings. One Sunday morning, in particular, she was told to go to the barn; on going there, she found her master with a bundle of rods, prepared in the embers, and bound together with cords. When he had tied her hands together before her, he gave her the most cruel whipping she was ever tortured with. He whipped her till the flesh was deeply lacerated, and the blood streamed from her wounds—and the scars remain to the present day, to testify to the fact. 'And now,' she says, 'when I hear 'em tell of whipping women on the bare flesh, it makes *my* flesh crawl, and my very hair rise on my head! Oh! my God!' she continues, 'what a way is this of treating human beings?' In these hours of her extremity, she did not forget the instructions of her mother, to go to God in all her trials, and every affliction; and she not only remembered, but obeyed: going to Him, 'and telling him all—and asking him if he thought it was right,' and begging him to protect and shield her from her persecutors.

She always asked with an unwavering faith that she should receive just what she plead for,—'And now,' she says, 'though it seems *curious*, I do not remember ever asking for any thing but what I got it. And I always received it as an answer to my prayers. When I got beaten, I never knew it long enough beforehand to pray; and I always thought if I only had *had* time to pray God for help, I should have escaped the beating.' She had no idea God had any knowledge of her thoughts, save what she told him; or heard her prayers, unless they were spoken audibly. And consequently, she could not pray unless she had time and opportunity to go by herself, where she could talk to God without being overheard.

TRIALS CONTINUED.

When she had been at Mr. Nealy's several months, she began to beg God most earnestly to send her father to her, and as soon as she commenced to pray, she began as confidently to look for his coming, and, ere it was long, to her great joy, he came. She had no opportunity to speak to him of the troubles that weighed so heavily on her spirit, while he remained; but when he left, she followed him to the gate, and unburdened her heart to him, inquiring if he could not do something to get her a new and better place? In this way the slaves often assist each other, by ascertaining who are kind to their slaves, comparatively; and then using their influence to get such an one to hire or buy their friends; and masters, often from policy as well as from latent humanity, allow those they are about to sell or let, to choose their own places, if the persons they happen to select for masters are considered safe *pay*. He promised to do all he could, and they parted. But, every day, as long as the snow lasted, (for there was snow on the ground at the time,) she returned to the spot where they separated, and walking in the tracks her father had made in the snow, repeated her prayer that 'God would help her father get her a new and better place.'

A long time had not elapsed, when a fisherman by the name of Scriver appeared at Mr. Nealy's, and inquired of Isabel 'if she would like to go and live with him.' She eagerly answered 'Yes,' nothing doubting but he was sent in answer to her prayer; and she soon started off with him, walking while he rode; for he had bought her at the suggestion of her father, paying one hundred and five dollars for her. He also lived in Ulster County, but some five or six miles from Mr. Nealy's.

Scriver, besides being a fisherman, kept a tavern for the accommodation of people of his own class—for his was a rude, uneducated family, exceedingly profane in their language, but, on the whole, an honest, kind and well-disposed people.

They owned a large farm, but left it wholly unimproved; attending mainly to their vocations of fishing and inn-keeping. Isabella declares she can ill describe the life she led with them. It was a wild, out-of-door kind of life. She was expected to carry fish, to hoe corn, to bring roots and herbs from the wood for beers, go to the Strand for a gallon of molasses or liquor as the case might require, and 'browse around,' as she expresses it. It was a life that suited her well for the time— being as devoid of hardship or terror as it was of improvement; a need which had not yet become a want. Instead of improving at this place, morally, she retrograded, as their example taught her to curse; and it was here that she took her first oath. After living with them about a year and a half, she was sold to one John J. Dumont, for the sum of seventy pounds. This was in 1810. Mr. Dumont lived in the same county as her former masters, in the town of New Paltz, and she remained with him till a short time previous to her emancipation by the State, in 1828.

HER STANDING WITH HER NEW MASTER AND MISTRESS.

Had Mrs. Dumont possessed that vein of kindness and consideration for the slaves, so perceptible in her husband's character, Isabella would have been as comfortable here, as one had *best* be, if one *must* be a slave. Mr. Dumont had been nursed in the very lap of slavery, and being naturally a man of kind feelings, treated his slaves with all the consideration he did his *other* animals, and *more*, perhaps. But Mrs. Dumont, who had been born and educated in a non-slaveholding family, and, like many others, used only to work-people, who, under the most stimulating of human motives, were willing to put forth their every energy, could not have patience with the creeping gait, the dull understanding, or see any cause for the listless manners and careless, slovenly habits of the poor down-trodden outcast—entirely forgetting that every high and efficient motive had been removed far from him; and that, had not his very intellect been crushed out of him, the slave would find little ground for aught but hopeless despondency. From this source arose a long series of trials in the life of our heroine, which we must pass over in silence; some, from motives of delicacy, and others, because the relation of them might inflict undeserved pain on some now living, whom Isabel remembers only with esteem and love; therefore, the reader will not be surprised if our narrative appear somewhat tame at this point, and may rest assured that it is not for want of facts, as the most thrilling incidents of this portion of her life are from various motives suppressed.

One comparatively trifling incident she wishes related, as it made a deep impression on her mind at the time—showing, as *she* thinks, how God shields the innocent, and causes them to triumph over their enemies, and also how she stood between master and mistress. In her family, Mrs. Dumont employed two white girls, one of whom, named Kate, evinced a disposition to 'lord it over' Isabel, and, in her emphatic language '*to grind her down.*' Her master often shielded her from the attacks and accusations of others, praising her for her readiness and ability to work, and these praises seemed to foster a spirit of hostility to her, in the minds of Mrs. Dumont and her white servant, the latter of whom took every opportunity to cry up her faults, lessen her in the esteem of her master, and increase against her the displeasure of her mistress, which was already more than sufficient for Isabel's comfort. Her master insisted that she could do as much work as half-a-dozen common people, and do it well, too; whilst her mistress insisted that the first was true, only because it ever came from her hand but half performed. A good deal of feeling arose from this difference of opinion, which was getting to rather an uncomfortable height, when, all at once, the potatoes that Isabel cooked for breakfast assumed a dingy, dirty look. Her mistress blamed her severely, asking her master to observe 'a fine specimen of Bell's work!'—adding, 'it is the way *all* her work is done.' Her master scolded also this time, and commanded her to be more careful in future. Kate joined with zest in the censures, and was very hard upon her. Isabella thought that she had done all she well could to have them nice; and became quite distressed at these appearances, and wondered what she should do to avoid them. In this dilemma, Gertrude Dumont, (Mr. D.'s eldest child, a good, kind-hearted girl of ten years, who pitied Isabel sincerely,) when she heard them all blame her so unsparingly, came forward, offering her sympathy and assistance; and when about to retire to bed, on the night of Isabella's humiliation, she advanced to Isabel, and told her, if she would wake her early next morning, she would get up and attend to her potatoes for her, while she (Isabella) went to milking, and they would see if they could not have them *nice*, and not have 'Poppee,' her word for father, and 'Matty,' her word for mother, and all of 'em, scolding so terribly.

Isabella gladly availed herself of this kindness, which touched her to the heart, amid so much of an opposite spirit. When Isabella had put the potatoes over to boil, Getty told her she would herself tend the fire, while Isabel milked. She had not long been seated by the fire, in performance of her promise, when Kate entered, and requested Gertrude to go out of the room and do something for her, which she refused, still keeping her place in the corner. While there, Kate came sweeping about the fire, caught up a chip, lifted some ashes with it, and dashed them into the kettle. Now the mystery was solved, the plot discovered! Kate was working a little too fast at making her mistress's words good, at showing that Mrs. Dumont and herself were on the right side of the dispute, and consequently at gaining power over Isabella. Yes, she was quite too fast, inasmuch as she had overlooked the little figure of justice, which sat in the corner, with scales nicely balanced, waiting to give all their dues.

But the time had come when she was to be overlooked no longer. It was Getty's turn to speak now. 'Oh Poppee! oh Poppee!' said she, 'Kate has been putting ashes in among the potatoes! I saw her do it! Look at those that fell on the out-side of the kettle! You can now see what made the potatoes so dingy every morning, though Bell washed them clean!' And she repeated her story to every new comer, till the fraud was made as public as the censure of Isabella had been. Her mis-tress looked blank, and remained dumb—her master mut-tered something which sounded very like an oath—and poor Kate was so chop-fallen, she looked like a convicted criminal, who would gladly have hid herself, (now that the baseness was out,) to conceal her mortified pride and deep chagrin.

It was a fine triumph for Isabella and her master, and she became more ambitious than ever to please him; and he stim-ulated her ambition by his commendation, and by boasting of her to his friends, telling them that '*that* wench' (pointing to Isabel) 'is better to me than a *man*—for she will do a good family's washing in the night, and be ready in the morning to go into the field, where she will do as much as raking and binding as my best hands.' Her ambition and desire to please were so great, that she often worked several nights in succes-sion, sleeping only short snatches, as she sat in her chair; and some nights she would not allow herself to take any sleep, save what she could get resting herself against the wall, fear-ing that if she sat down, she would sleep too long. These extra exertions to please, and the praises consequent upon them, brought upon her head the envy of her fellow-slaves, and they taunted her with being the '*white folks' nigger*.' On the other hand, she received a larger share of the confidence of her master, and many small favors that were by them unat-tainable. I asked her if her master, Dumont, ever whipped her? She answered, 'Oh yes, he sometimes whipped me soundly, though never cruelly. And the most severe whipping he ever give me was because *I* was cruel to a cat.' At this time she looked upon her master as a *God*; and believed that he knew of and could see her at all times, even as God himself. And she used sometimes to confess her delinquencies, from the conviction that he already knew them, and that she should fare better if she confessed voluntarily: and if any one talked to her of the injustice of her being a slave, she an-swered them with contempt, and immediately told her master. She then firmly believed that slavery was right and honorable. Yet she *now* sees very clearly the false position they were all in, both masters and slaves; and she looks back, with utter astonishment, at the absurdity of the claims so arrogantly set up by the masters, over beings designed by God to be as free as kings; and at the perfect stupidity of the slave, in admitting for one moment the validity of these claims.

In obedience to her mother's instructions, she had educated herself to such a sense of honesty, that, when she had become a mother, she would sometimes whip her child when it cried to her for bread, rather than give it a piece secretly, lest it should learn to take what was not its own! And the writer of this knows, from personal observation, that the slaveholders of the South feel it to be a *religious duty* to teach their slaves to be honest, and never to take what is not their own! Oh consistency, art thou not a jewel? Yet Isabella glories in the fact that she was faithful and true to her master; she says, 'It made me true to my God'—meaning, that it helped to form in her a character that loved truth, and hated a lie, and had saved her from the bitter pains and fears that are sure to follow in the wake of insincerity and hypocrisy.

As she advanced in years, an attachment sprung up between herself and a slave named Robert. But his master, an Englishman by the name of Catlin, anxious that no one's property but his own should be enhanced by the increase of his slaves, forbade Robert's visits to Isabella, and commanded him to take a wife among his fellow-servants. Notwithstanding this interdiction, Robert, following the bent of his inclinations, continued his visits to Isabel, though very stealthily, and, as he believed, without exciting the suspicion of his master; but one Saturday afternoon, hearing that Bell was ill, he took the liberty to go and see her. The first intimation *she* had of his visit was the appearance of her master, inquiring 'if she had seen Bob.' On her answering in the negative, he said to her, 'If you see him, tell him to take care of himself, for the Catlins are after him.' Almost at that instant, Bob made his appearance; and the first people he met were his old and his young masters. They were terribly enraged at finding him there, and the eldest began cursing, and calling upon his son to '*Knock down* the d——d black rascal;' at the same time, they both fell upon him like tigers, beating him with the heavy ends of their canes, bruising and mangling his head and face in the most awful manner, and causing the blood, which streamed from his wounds, to cover him like a slaughtered beast, constituting him a most shocking spectacle. Mr. Dumont interposed at this point, telling the ruffians they could no longer thus spill human blood on *his* premises—he would have 'no niggers killed there.' The Catlins then took a rope they had taken with them for the purpose, and tied Bob's hands behind him in such a manner, that Mr. Dumont insisted on loosening the cord, declaring that no brute should be tied in *that* manner, where *he* was. And as they led him away, like the greatest of criminals, the more humane Dumont followed them to their homes, as Robert's protector; and when he returned, he kindly went to Bell, as he called her, telling her he did not think they would strike him any more, as their wrath had greatly cooled before he left them. Isabella had witnessed this scene from her window, and was greatly shocked at the murderous treatment of poor Robert, whom she truly loved, and whose only crime, in the eye of his persecutors, was his affection for her. This beating, and we know not what after treatment, completely subdued the spirit of its victim, for Robert ventured no more to visit Isabella, but like an obedient and faithful chattel, took himself a wife from the house of his master. Robert did not live many years after his last visit to Isabel, but took his departure to that country, where 'they neither marry nor are given in marriage,' and where the oppressor cannot molest.

ISABELLA'S MARRIAGE.

Subsequently, Isabella was married to a fellow-slave, named Thomas, who had previously had two wives, one of whom, if not both, had been torn from him and sold far away. And it is more than probable, that he was not only allowed but encouraged to take another at each successive sale. I say it is probable, because the writer of this knows from personal observation, that such is the custom among slaveholders at the present day; and that in a twenty months' residence among them, we never knew any one to open the lip against the practice; and when we severely censured it, the slaveholder had nothing to say; and the slave pleaded that, under existing circumstances, he could do no better.

Such an abominable state of things is silently tolerated, to say the least, by slaveholders—deny it who may. And what is that religion that sanctions, even by its silence, all that is embraced in the *'Peculiar Institution?'* If there *can* be any thing more diametrically opposed to the religion of Jesus, than the working of this soul-killing system—which is as truly sanctioned by the religion of America as are her ministers and churches—we wish to be shown where it can be found.

We have said, Isabella was married to Thomas—she was, after the fashion of slavery, one of the slaves performing the ceremony for them; as no true minister of Christ *can* perform, as in the presence of God, what he knows to be a mere *farce*, a *mock* marriage, unrecognised by any civil law, and liable to be annulled any moment, when the interest or caprice of the master should dictate.

With what feelings must slaveholders expect us to listen to their horror of amalgamation in prospect, while they are well aware that we know how calmly and quietly they contemplate the present state of licentiousness their own wicked laws have created, not only as it regards the slave, but as it regards the more privileged portion of the population of the South?

Slaveholders appear to me to take the same notice of the vices of the slave, as one does of the vicious disposition of his horse. They are often an inconvenience; further than that, they care not to trouble themselves about the matter.

ISABELLA AS A MOTHER.

In process of time, Isabella found herself the mother of five children, and she rejoiced in being permitted to be the instrument of increasing the property of her oppressors! Think, dear reader, without a blush, if you can, for one moment, of a *mother* thus willingly, and with *pride*, laying her own children, the 'flesh of her flesh,' on the altar of slavery—a sacrifice to the bloody Moloch! But we must remember that beings capable of such sacrifices are not mothers; they are only 'things,' 'chattels,' 'property.'

But since that time, the subject of this narrative has made some advances from a state of chattelism towards that of a woman and a mother; and she now looks back upon her thoughts and feelings there, in her state of ignorance and degradation, as one does on the dark imagery of a fitful dream. One moment it seems but a frightful illusion; again it appears a terrible reality. I would to God it *were* but a dreamy myth, and not, as it now stands, a horrid reality to some three millions of chattelized human beings.

I have already alluded to her care not to teach her children to steal, by her example; and she says, with groanings that cannot be written, 'The Lord only knows how many times I let my children go hungry, rather than take secretly the bread I liked not to ask for.' All parents who annul their preceptive teachings by their daily practices would do well to profit by her example.

Another proof of her master's kindness of heart is found in the following fact. If her master came into the house and found her infant crying, (as she could not always attend to its wants and the commands of her mistress at the same time,) he would turn to his wife with a look of reproof, and ask her why she did not see the child taken care of; saying, most earnestly, 'I will not hear this crying; I can't bear it, and I will not hear any child cry so. Here, Bell, take care of this child, if no more work is done for a week.' And he would linger to see if his orders were obeyed, and not countermanded.

When Isabella went to the field to work, she used to put her infant in a basket, tying a rope to each handle, and suspending the basket to a branch of a tree, set another small child to swing it. It was thus secure from reptiles, and was easily administered to, and even lulled to sleep, by a child too young for other labors. I was quite struck with the ingenuity of such a baby-tender, as I have sometimes been with the swinging hammock the native mother prepares for her sick infant—apparently so much easier than aught we have in our more civilized homes; easier for the child because it gets the motion without the least jar; and easier for the nurse, because the hammock is strung so high as to supersede the necessity of stooping.

SLAVEHOLDER'S PROMISES.

After emancipation had been decreed by the State, some years before the time fixed for its consummation, Isabella's master told her if she would do well, and be faithful, he would give her 'free papers,' one year before she was legally free by statute. In the year 1826, she had a badly diseased hand, which greatly diminished her usefulness; but on the arrival of July 4, 1827, the time specified for her receiving her 'free papers,' she claimed the fulfilment of her master's promise; but he refused granting it, on account (as he alleged) of the loss he had sustained by her hand. She plead that she had worked all the time, and done many things she was not wholly able to do, although she knew she had been less useful than formerly; but her master remained inflexible. Her very faithfulness probably operated against her now, and he found it less easy than he thought to give up the profits of his faithful Bell, who had so long done him efficient service.

But Isabella inwardly determined that she would remain quietly with him only until she had spun his wool—about one hundred pounds—and then she would leave him, taking the rest of the time to herself. 'Ah!' she says, with emphasis that cannot be written, 'the slaveholders are TERRIBLE for promising to give you this or that, or such and such a privilege, if you will do thus and so; and when the time of fulfilment comes, and one claims the promise, they, forsooth, recollect nothing of the kind; and you are, like as not, taunted with being a LIAR; or, at best, the slave is accused of not having performed *his* part or condition of the contract. Oh!' said she, 'I have felt as if I could not live through the *operation* sometimes. Just think of us! *so* eager for our pleasures, and just foolish enough to keep feeding and feeding ourselves up with the idea that we should get what had been thus fairly promised; and when we think it is almost in our hands, find ourselves flatly denied! Just think! how *could* we bear it? Why, there was Charles Brodhead promised his slave Ned, that when harvesting was over, he might go and see his wife, who lived some twenty or thirty miles off. So Ned worked early and late, and as soon as the harvest was all in, he claimed the promised boon. His master said, he had merely told him he "would *see* if he could go, when the harvest was over; but now he saw that he *could not* go." But Ned, who still claimed a positive promise, on which he had fully depended, went on cleaning his shoes. His master asked him if he intended going, and on his replying "yes," took up a sled-stick that lay near him, and gave him such a blow on the head as broke his skull, killing him dead on the spot. The poor colored people all felt struck down by the blow.' Ah! and well they might. Yet it was but one of a long series of bloody, and other most effectual blows, struck against their liberty and their lives.* But to return from our digression.

The subject of this narrative was to have been free July 4, 1827, but she continued with her master till the wool was spun, and the heaviest of the 'fall's work' closed up, when she concluded to take her freedom into her own hands, and seek her fortune in some other place.

HER ESCAPE.

The question in her mind, and one not easily solved, now was, 'How can I get away?' So, as was her usual custom, she 'told God she was afraid to go in the night, and in the day every body would see her.' At length, the thought came to her that she could leave just before the day dawned, and get out of the neighborhood where she was known before the people were much astir. 'Yes,' said she, fervently, 'that's a good thought! Thank you, God, for *that* thought!' So, receiving it as coming direct from God, she acted upon it, and one fine morning, a little before day-break, she might have been seen stepping stealthily away from the rear of Master Dumont's house, her infant on one arm and her wardrobe on the other; the bulk and weight of which, probably, she never found so convenient as on the present occasion, a

*Yet no official notice was taken of this more than brutal murder.

cotton handkerchief containing both her clothes and her provisions.

As she gained the summit of a high hill, a considerable distance from her master's, the sun offended her by coming forth in all his pristine splendor. She thought it never was so light before; indeed, she thought it much too light. She stopped to look about her, and ascertain if her pursuers were yet in sight. No one appeared, and, for the first time, the question came up for settlement, 'Where, and to whom, shall I go?' In all her thoughts of getting away, she had not once asked herself whither she should direct her steps. She sat down, fed her infant, and again turning her thoughts to God, her only help, she prayed him to direct her to some safe asylum. And soon it occurred to her, that there was a man living somewhere in the direction she had been pursuing, by the name of Levi Rowe, whom she had known, and who, she thought, would be likely to befriend her. She accordingly pursued her way to his house, where she found him ready to entertain and assist her, though he was then on his death-bed. He bade her partake of the hospitalities of his house, said he knew of two good places where she might get in, and requested his wife to show her where they were to be found. As soon as she came in sight of the first house, she recollected having seen it and its inhabitants before, and instantly exclaimed, 'That's the place for me; I shall stop there.' She went there, and found the good people of the house, Mr. and Mrs. Van Wagener, absent, but was kindly received and hospitably entertained by their excellent mother, till the return of her children. When they arrived, she made her case known to them. They listened to her story, assuring her they never turned the needy away, and willingly gave her employment.

She had not been there long before her old master, Dumont, appeared, as she had anticipated; for when she took French leave of him, she resolved not to go too far from him, and not put him to as much trouble in looking her up—for the latter he was sure to do—as Tom and Jack had done when they ran away from him, a short time before. This was very considerate in her, to say the least, and a proof that 'like begets like.' He had often considered *her* feelings, though not always, and she was equally considerate.

When her master saw her, he said, 'Well, Bell, so you've run away from me.' 'No, I did not *run* away; I walked away by day-light, and all because you had promised me a year of my time.' His reply was, 'You must go back with me.' Her decisive answer was, 'No, I *wont* go back with you.' He said, 'Well, I shall take the *child.*' *This* also was as stoutly negatived.

Mr. Isaac S. Van Wagener then interposed, saying, he had never been in the practice of buying and selling slaves; he did not believe in slavery; but, rather than have Isabella taken back by force, he would buy her services for the balance of the year—for which her master charged twenty dollars, and five in addition for the child. The sum was paid, and her master Dumont departed; but not till he had heard Mr. Van Wagener tell her not to call him master—adding, 'there is but *one* master; and he who is *your* master is *my* master.' Isabella inquired what she *should* call him? He answered, 'call me Isaac Van Wagener, and my wife is Maria Van Wagener.' Isabella could not understand this, and thought it a *mighty change*, as it most truly was from a master whose word was law, to simple Isaac S. Van Wagener, who was master to *no* one. With these noble people, who, though they could not be the masters of slaves, were undoubtedly a portion of God's nobility, she resided one year, and from them she derived the name of Van Wagener; he being her last master in the eye of the law, and a slave's surname is ever the same as his master; that is, if he is allowed to have any other name than Tom, Jack, or Guffin. Slaves have sometimes been severely punished for adding their master's name to their own. But when they have no particular title to it, it is no particular offence.

ILLEGAL SALE OF HER SON.

A little previous to Isabel's leaving her old master, he had sold her child, a boy of five years, to a Dr. Gedney, who took him with him as far as New York city, on his way to England; but finding the boy too small for his service, he sent him back to his brother, Solomon Gedney. This man disposed of him to his sister's husband, a wealthy planter, by the name of Fowler, who took him to his own home in Alabama.

This illegal and fraudulent transaction had been perpetrated some months before Isabella knew of it, as she was now living at Mr. Van Wagener's. The law expressly prohibited the sale of any slave out of the State,—and all minors were to be free at twenty-one years of age; and Mr. Dumont had sold Peter with the express understanding, that he was soon to return to the State of New York, and be emancipated at the specified time.

When Isabel heard that her son had been sold South, she immediately started on foot and alone, to find the man who had thus dared, in the face of all law, human and divine, to sell her child out of the State; and if possible, to bring him to account for the deed.

Arriving at New Paltz, she went directly to her former mistress, Dumont, complaining bitterly of the removal of her son. Her mistress heard her through, and then replied— '*Ugh!* a *fine* fuss to make about a little *nigger!* Why, haven't you as many of 'em left as you can see to, and take care of? A pity 'tis, the niggers are not all in Guinea!! Making such a halloo-balloo about the neighborhood; and all for a paltry nigger!!!' Isabella heard her through, and after a moment's hesitation, answered, in tones of deep determination—'*I'll have my child again.*' 'Have *your child* again!' repeated her mistress—her tones big with contempt, and scorning the absurd idea of her getting him. 'How can you get him? And what have you to support him with, if you could? Have you any money?' 'No,' answered Bell, 'I have no money, but God has enough, or what's better! And I'll have my child again.' These words were pronounced in the most slow, solemn and determined measure and manner. And in speaking of it, she says, 'Oh my God! I know'd I'd have him agin. I was sure God would help me to get him. Why, I felt so *tall within*—I felt as if the *power of a nation* was with me!'

The impressions made by Isabella on her auditors, when moved by lofty or deep feeling, can never be transmitted to paper, (to use the words of another,) till by some Daguerrian act, we are enabled to transfer the look, the gesture, the tones of voice, in connection with the quaint, yet fit expressions used, an the spirit-stirring animation that, at such a time, pervades all she says.

After leaving her mistress, she called on Mrs. Gedney, mother of him who had sold her boy; who, after listening to her lamentatious, her grief being mingled with indignation at the sale of her son, and her declaration that she would have him again—said, 'Dear me! What a disturbance to make about your child! What is *your* child, better than *my* child? My child is gone out there, and yours is gone to live with her, to have enough of every thing, and to be treated like a gentleman!' And here she laughed at Isabel's absurd fears, as she would represent them to be. 'Yes,' said Isabel, '*your* child has gone there, but she is *married*, and my boy has gone as a *slave!* and he is too little to go so far from his mother. Oh, I must have my child.' And here the continued laugh of Mrs. G. seemed to Isabel, in this time of anguish and distress, almost demoniacal. And well it was for Mrs. Gedney, that, at that time, she could not even dream of the awful fate awaiting her own beloved daughter, at the hands of him whom she had chosen as worthy the wealth of her love and confidence, and in whose society her young heart had calculated on a happiness, purer and more elevated than was ever conferred by a kingly crown. But, alas! she was doomed to disappointment, as we shall relate by and by. At this point, Isabella earnestly begged of God that he would show to those about her that he was her helper; and she adds, in narrating, 'And he *did*; or, if he did not show them, he did me.'

IT IS OFTEN DARKEST,
JUST BEFORE DAWN.

This homely proverb was illustrated in the case of our sufferer; for, at the period at which we have arrived in our narrative, to her the darkness seemed palpable, and the waters of affliction covered her soul; yet light was about to break in upon her.

Soon after the scenes related in our last chapter, which had harrowed up her very soul to agony, she met a man, (we would like to tell you *who*, dear reader, but it would be doing him no kindness, even at the present day, to do so,) who evidently sympathized with her, and counselled her to go to the

Quakers, telling her they were already feeling very indignant at the fraudulent sale of her son, and assuring her that they would readily assist her, and direct her what to do. He pointed out to her two houses, where lived some of those people, who formerly, more than any other sect, perhaps, lived out the principles of the gospel of Christ. She wended her way to their dwellings, was listened to, unknown as she personally was to them, with patience, and soon gained their sympathies and active coöperation.

They gave her lodgings for the night; and it is very amusing to hear her tell of the 'nice, high, clean, white, *beautiful* bed' assigned her to sleep in, which contrasted so strangely with her former pallets, that she sat down and contemplated it, perfectly absorbed in wonder that *such* a bed should have been appropriated to one like herself. For some time she thought that she would lie down beneath it, on her usual bedstead, the floor. 'I did indeed,' says she, laughing heartily at her former self. However, she finally concluded to make use of the bed, for fear that not to do so might injure the feelings of her good hostess. In the morning, the Quaker saw that she was taken and set down near Kingston, with directions to go to the Court House, and enter complaint to the grand jury.

By a little inquiry, she found which was the building she sought, went into the door, and taking the first man she saw of imposing appearance for the *grand* jury, she commenced her complaint. But he very civilly informed her there was no grand jury there; she must go up stairs. When she had with some difficulty ascended the flight through the crowd that filled them, she again turned to the '*grandest*' looking man she could select, telling him she had come to enter a complaint to the grand jury. For his own amusement, he inquired what her complaint was; but, when he saw it was a serious matter, he said to her, 'This is no place to enter a complaint— go in there,' pointing in a particular direction.

She then went in, where she found the Grand Jurors indeed sitting, and again commenced to relate her injuries. After holding some conversation among themselves, one of them rose, and bidding her follow him, led the way to a side office, where he heard her story, and asked her 'if she could *swear* that the child she spoke of was her son?' 'Yes,' she answered, 'I *swear* it's my son.' 'Stop, stop!' said the lawyer, 'you must swear by this book'—giving her a book, which she thinks must have been the Bible. She took it, and putting it to her lips, began again to swear it was her child. The clerks, unable to preserve their gravity any longer, burst into an uproarious laugh; and one of them inquired of lawyer Chip of what use it could be to make *her* swear. 'It will answer the law,' replied the officer. He then made her comprehend just what he wished her to do, and she took a lawful oath, as far as the outward ceremony could make it one. All can judge how far she understood its spirit and meaning.

He now gave her a writ, directing her to take it to the constable of New Paltz, and have him serve it on Solomon Gedney. She obeyed, walking, or rather *trotting*, in her haste, some eight or nine miles.

But while the constable, through mistake, served the writ on a brother of the real culprit, Solomon Gedney slipped into a boat, and was nearly across the North River, on whose banks they were standing, before the dull Dutch constable was aware of his mistake. Solomon Gedney, meanwhile, consulted a lawyer, who advised him to go to Alabama and bring back the boy, otherwise it might cost him fourteen years' imprisonment, and a thousand dollars in cash. By this time, it is hoped he began to feel that selling slaves unlawfully was not so good a business as he had wished to find it. He secreted himself till due preparations could be made, and soon set sail for Alabama. Steamboats and railroads had not then annihilated distance to the extent they now have, and although he left in the fall of the year, spring came ere he returned, bringing the boy with him—but holding on to him as his property. It had ever been Isabella's prayer, not only that her son might be returned, but that he should be delivered from bondage, and into her own hands, lest he should be punished out of mere spite to her, who was so greatly annoying and irritating to her oppressors; and if her suit was gained, her very triumph would add vastly to their irritation.

She again sought advice of Esquire Chip, whose counsel was, that the aforesaid constable serve the before-mentioned writ upon the right person. This being done, soon brought

Solomon Gedney up to Kingston, where he gave bonds for his appearance at court, in the sum of $600.

Esquire Chip next informed his client, that her case must now lie over till the next session of the court, some months in the future. 'The law must take its course,' said he.

'What! wait another court! wait *months*?' said the persevering mother. 'Why, long before that time, he can go clear off, and take my child with him—no one knows where. I *cannot* wait; I *must* have him *now*, whilst he is to be had.' 'Well,' said the lawyer, very coolly, 'if he puts the boy out of the way, he must pay the $600—one half of which will be yours;' supposing, perhaps, that $300 would pay for a 'heap of children,' in the eye of a slave who never, in all her life, called a dollar her own. But in this instance, he was mistaken in his reckoning. She assured him, that she had not been seeking money, neither would money satisfy her; it was her son, and her son alone she wanted, and her son she must have. Neither could she wait court, not she. The lawyer used his every argument to convince her, that she ought to be very thankful for what they had done for her; that it was a great deal, and it was but reasonable that she should now wait patiently the time of the court.

Yet she never felt, for a moment, like being influenced by these suggestions. She felt confident she was to receive a full and literal answer to her prayer, the burden of which had been—'O Lord, give my son into my hands, and that speedily! Let not the spoilers have him any longer.' Notwithstanding, she very distinctly saw that those who had thus far helped her on so kindly were *wearied* of her, and she feared God was wearied also. She had a short time previous learned that Jesus was a Savior, and an intercessor; and she thought that if Jesus could but be induced to plead for her in the present trial, God would listen to *him*, though he were wearied of *her* importunities. To him, of course, she applied. As she was walking about, scarcely knowing whither she went, asking within herself, 'Who will show me any good, and lend a helping hand in this matter,' she was accosted by a perfect stranger, and one whose name she has never learned, in the following terms: 'Halloo, there; how do you get along with your boy? do they give him up to you?' She told him all, adding that now every body was tired, and she had none to help her. He said, 'Look here! I'll tell you what you'd better do. Do you see that stone house yonder?' pointing in a particular direction. 'Well, lawyer Demain lives there, and do you go to him, and lay your case before him; I think he'll help you. *Stick to him*. Don't give him peace till he does. I feel sure if you press him, he'll do it for you.' She needed no further urging, but trotted off at her peculiar gait in the direction of his house, as fast as possible,—and she was not encumbered with stockings, shoes, or any other heavy article of dress. When she had told him her story, in her impassioned manner, he looked at her a few moments, as if to ascertain if he were contemplating a new variety of the genus homo, and then told her, if she would give him five dollars, he would get her son for her, in twenty-four hours. 'Why,' she replied, '*I* have no *money*, and never had a dollar in my life!' Said he, 'If you will go to those Quakers in Poppletown, who carried you to court, they will help you to five dollars in cash, I have no doubt; and you shall have your son in twenty-four hours, from the time you bring me that sum.' She performed the journey to Poppletown, a distance of some ten miles, very expeditiously; collected considerable more than the sum specified by the barrister; then, shutting the money tightly in her hand, she trotted back, and paid the lawyer a larger fee than he had demanded. When inquired of by people what she had done with the overplus, she answered, 'Oh, I got it for lawyer Demain, and I gave it to him.' They assured her she was a *fool* to do so; that she should have kept all over five dollars, and purchased herself shoes with it. 'Oh, I do not want money or clothes now, I only want my son; and if five dollars will get him, more will *surely* get him.' And if the lawyer had returned it to her, she avers she would not have accepted it. She was perfectly willing he should have every coin she could raise, if he would but restore her lost son to her. Moreover, the five dollars he required were for the remuneration of him who should go after her son and his master, and not for his own services.

The lawyer now renewed his promise, that she should have her son in twenty-four hours. But Isabella, having no idea of this space of time, went several times in a day, to ascertain if her son had come. Once, when the servant opened the door and saw her, she said, in a tone expressive of much surprise, 'Why, this woman's come again!' She then wondered if she went too often. When the lawyer appeared, he told her the twenty-four hours would not expire till the next morning; if she would call then, she would see her son. The next morning saw Isabel at the lawyer's door, while he was yet in his bed. He now assured her it was morning till noon; and that before noon her son would be there, for he had sent the famous 'Matty Styles' after him, who would not fail to have the boy and his master on hand in due season, either dead or alive; of that he was sure. Telling her she need not come again; he would himself inform her of their arrival.

After dinner, he appeared at Mr. Rutzer's, (a place the lawyer had procured for her, while she awaited the arrival of her boy,) assuring her, her son had come; but that he stoutly denied having any mother, or any relatives in that place; and said, 'she must go over and identify him.' She went to the office, but at sight of her the boy cried aloud, and regarded her as some terrible being, who was about to take him away from a kind and loving friend. He knelt, even, and begged them, with tears, not to take him away from his dear master, who had brought him from the dreadful South, and been so kind to him.

When he was questioned relative to the bad scar on his forehead, he said, 'Fowler's horse hove him.' And of the one on his cheek, 'That was done by running against the carriage.' In answering these questions, he looked imploringly at his master, as much as to say, 'If they are falsehoods, you bade me say them; may they be satisfactory to you, at least.'

The justice, noting his appearance, bade him forget his master and attend only to him. But the boy persisted in denying his mother, and clinging to his master, saying his mother did not live in such a place as that. However, they allowed the mother to identify her son; and Esquire Demain pleaded that he claimed the boy for her, on the ground that he had been sold out of the State, contrary to the laws in such cases made and provided—spoke of the penalties annexed to said crime, and of the sum of money the delinquent was to pay, in case any one chose to prosecute him for the offence he had committed. Isabella, who was sitting in a corner, scarcely daring to breathe, thought within herself, 'If I can but get the boy, the $200 may remain for whoever else chooses to prosecute—*I* have done enough to make myself enemies already'—and she trembled at the thought of the formidable enemies she had probably arrayed against herself—helpless and despised as she was. When the pleading was at an end, Isabella understood the Judge to declare, as the sentence of the Court, that the 'boy be delivered into the hands of the mother—having no other master, no other controller, no other conductor, but his mother.' This sentence was obeyed; he was delivered into her hands, the boy meanwhile begging, most piteously, *not* to be taken from his dear master, saying she was not his mother, and that his mother did not live in such a place as that. And it was some time before lawyer Demain, the clerks, and Isabella, could collectively succeed in calming the child's fears, and in convincing him that Isabella was not some terrible monster, as he had for the last months, probably, been trained to believe; and who, in taking him away from his master, was taking him from all good, and consigning him to all evil.

When at last kind words and *bon-bons* had quieted his fears, and he could listen to their explanations, he said to Isabella—'Well, you *do* look like my mother *used* to;' and she was soon able to make him comprehend some of the obligations he was under, and the relation he stood in, both to herself and his master. She commenced as soon as practicable to examine the boy, and found, to her utter astonishment, that from the crown of his head to the sole of his foot, the callosities and indurations on his entire body were most frightful to behold. His back she described as being like her fingers, as she laid them side by side.

'Heavens! what is all *this*?' said Isabel. He answered, 'It is where Fowler whipped, kicked, and beat me.' She exclaimed, 'Oh, Lord Jesus, look! see my poor child! Oh Lord, "render unto them double" for all this! Oh my God! Pete, how *did* you bear it?'

'Oh, this is nothing, mammy—if you should see Phillis, I guess you'd *scare*! She had a little baby, and Fowler cut her till the milk as well as blood ran down *her* body. You would *scare* to see Phillis, mammy.'

When Isabella inquired, 'What did Miss Eliza* say, Pete, when you were treated so badly?' he replied, 'Oh, mammy, she said she wished I was with Bell. Sometimes I crawled under the stoop, mammy, the blood running all about me, and my back would stick to the boards; and sometimes Miss Eliza would come and grease my sores, when all were abed and asleep.'

DEATH OF MRS. ELIZA FOWLER.

As soon as possible, she procured a place for Peter, as tender of Locks, at a place called Wahkendall, near Greenkills. After he was thus disposed of, she visited her sister Sophia, who resided at Newberg, and spent the winter in several different families where she was acquainted. She remained sometime in the family of a Mr. Latin, who was a visiting relative of Solomon Gedney; and the latter, when he found Isabel with his cousin, used all his influence to persuade him she was a great mischief-maker and a very troublesome person, that she had put him to some hundreds of dollars expense, by fabricating lies about him, and especially his sister and her family, concerning her boy, when the latter was living so like a gentleman with them; and, for his part, he would not advise his friends to harbor or encourage her. However, his cousins, the Latins, could not see with the eyes of *his* feelings, and consequently his words fell powerless on them, and they retained her in their service as long as they had aught for her to do.

She then went to visit her former master, Dumont. She had scarcely arrived there, when Mr. Fred. Waring entered, and seeing Isabel, pleasantly accosted her, and asked her 'what she was driving at now-a-days.' On her answering 'nothing particular,' he requested her to go over to his place, and assist his folks, as some of them were sick, and they needed an extra hand. She very gladly assented. When Mr. W. retired, her master wanted to know why she wished to help people, that called her the 'worst of devils,' as Mr. Waring had done in the courthouse—for he was the uncle of Solomon Gedney, and

*Meaning Mrs. Eliza Fowler.

attended the trial we have described—and declared 'that she was a *fool* to; *he* wouldn't do it.' 'Oh,' she told him, 'she would not mind that, but was very glad to have people forget their anger towards her.' She went over, but too happy to feel that their resentment was passed, and commenced her work with a light heart and a strong will. She had not worked long in this frame of mind, before a young daughter of Mr. Waring rushed into the room, exclaiming, with uplifted hands— 'Heavens and earth, Isabella! Fowler's murdered Cousin Eliza!' 'Ho,' said Isabel, '*that's* nothing—he liked to have killed *my* child; nothing saved him but God.' Meaning, that she was not at all surprised at it, for a man whose heart was sufficiently hardened to treat a mere child as hers had been treated, was, in her opinion, more fiend than human, and prepared for the commission of any crime that his passions might prompt him to. The child further informed her, that a letter had arrived by mail bringing the news.

Immediately after this announcement, Solomon Gedney and his mother came in, going direct to Mrs. Waring's room, where she soon heard tones as of some one reading. She thought something said to her inwardly, 'Go up stairs and hear.' At first she hesitated, but it seemed to press her the more—'Go up and hear!' She went up, unusual as it is for slaves to leave their work and enter unbidden their mistress's room, for the sole purpose of seeing or hearing what may be seen or heard there. But on this occasion, Isabella says, she walked in at the door, shut it, placed her back against it, and listened. She saw them and heard them read—'He knocked her down with his fist, jumped on her with his knees, broke her collar-bone, and tore out her wind-pipe! He then attempted his escape, but was pursued and arrested, and put in an iron bank for safekeeping!' And the friends were requested to go down and take away the poor innocent children who had thus been made in one short day more than orphans.

If this narrative should ever meet the eye of those innocent sufferers for another's guilt, let them not be too deeply affected by the relation; but, placing their confidence in Him who sees the end from the beginning, and controls the results, rest secure in the faith, that, although they may physically suffer for the sins of others, if they remain but true to themselves, their highest and more enduring interests can never suffer from such a cause. This relation should be suppressed for their sakes, were it not even now so often denied, that slavery is fast undermining all true regard for human life. We know this one instance is not a demonstration to the contrary; but, adding this to the lists of tragedies that weekly come up to us through the Southern mails, may we not admit them as proofs irrefragable? The newspapers confirmed this account of the terrible affair.

When Isabella had heard the letter, all being too much absorbed in their own feelings to take note of her, she returned to her work, her heart swelling with conflicting emotions. She was awed at the dreadful deed; she mourned the fate of the loved Eliza, who had in such an undeserved and barbarous manner been put away from her labors and watchings as a tender mother; and, 'last though not least,' in the development of her character and spirit, her heart bled for the afflicted relatives; even those of them who 'laughed at her calamity, and mocked when her fear came.' Her thoughts dwelt long and intently on the subject, and the wonderful chain of events that had conspired to bring her that day to that house, to listen to that piece of intelligence—to that house, where she never was before or afterwards in her life, and invited there by people who had so lately been hotly incensed against her. It all seemed very remarkable to her, and she viewed it as flowing from a special providence of God. She thought she saw clearly, that their unnatural bereavement was a blow dealt in retributive justice; but she found it not in her heart to exult or rejoice over them. She felt as if God had more than answered her petition, when she ejaculated, in her anguish of mind, 'Oh, Lord, render unto them double!' She said, 'I dared not find fault with God, exactly; but the language of my heart was, "Oh, my God! that's too much—I did not mean quite so much, God!"' It was a terrible blow to the friends of the deceased; and her selfish mother (who, said Isabella, made such a 'to-do about *her* boy, not from affection, but to have her own will and way') went deranged, and walking to and fro in her delirium, called aloud for her poor murdered daughter—*'Eliza! Eliza!'*

The derangement of Mrs. G. was a matter of hearsay, as

Isabella saw her not after the trial; but she has no reason to doubt the truth of what she heard. Isabel could never learn the subsequent fate of Fowler, but heard, in the spring of '49, that his children had been seen in Kingston—one of whom was spoken of as a fine, interesting girl, albeit a halo of sadness fell like a veil about her.

ISABELLA'S RELIGIOUS EXPERIENCE.

We will now turn from the outward and temporal to the inward and spiritual life of our subject. It is ever both interesting and instructive to trace the exercises of a human mind, through the trials and mysteries of life; and especially a naturally powerful mind, left as hers was almost entirely to its own workings, and the chance influences it met on its way; and especially to note its reception of that divine 'light, that lighteth every man that cometh into the world.'

We see, as knowledge dawns upon it, truth and error strangely commingled; here, a bright spot illuminated by truth—and there, one darkened and distorted by error; and the state of such a soul may be compared to a landscape at early dawn, where the sun is seen superbly gilding some objects, and causing others to send forth their lengthened, distorted, and sometimes hideous shadows.

Her mother, as we have already said, talked to her of God. From these conversations, her incipient mind drew the conclusion, that God was 'a great man;' greatly superior to other men in power; and being located 'high in the sky,' could see all that transpired on the earth. She believed he not only saw, but noted down all her actions in a great book, even as her master kept a record of whatever he wished not to forget. But she had no idea that God knew a thought of hers till she had uttered it aloud.

As we have before mentioned, she had ever been mindful of her mother's injunctions, spreading out in detail all her troubles before God, imploring and firmly trusting him to send her deliverance from them. Whilst yet a child, she listened to a story of a wounded soldier, left alone in the trail of a flying army, helpless and starving, who hardened the very ground about him with kneeling in his supplications to God for relief, until it arrived. From this narrative, she was deeply impressed with the idea, that if *she* also were to present her petitions under the open canopy of heaven, speaking very loud, she should the more readily be heard; consequently, she sought a fitting spot for this, her rural sanctuary. The place she selected, in which to offer up her daily orisons, was a small island in a small stream, covered with large willow shrubbery, beneath which the sheep had made their pleasant winding paths; and sheltering themselves from the scorching rays of a noon-tide sun, luxuriated in the cool shadows of the graceful willows, as they listened to the tiny falls of the silver waters. It was a lonely spot, and chosen by her for its beauty, its retirement, and because she thought that there, in the noise of those waters, she could speak louder to God, without being overheard by any who might pass that way. When she had made choice of her sanctum, at a point of the island where the stream met, after having been separated, she improved it by pulling away the branches of the shrubs from the centre, and weaving them together for a wall on the outside, forming a circular arched alcove, made entirely of the graceful willow. To this place she resorted daily, and in pressing times much more frequently.

At this time, her prayers, or, more appropriately, 'talks with God,' were perfectly original and unique, and would be well worth preserving, were it possible to give the tones and manner with the words; but no adequate idea of them can be written while the tones and manner remain inexpressible.

She would sometimes repeat, 'Our Father in heaven,' in her Low Dutch, as taught her by her mother; after that, all was from the suggestions of her own rude mind. She related to God, in minute detail, all her troubles and sufferings, inquiring, as she proceeded, 'Do you think that's right, God?' and closed by begging to be delivered from the evil, whatever it might be.

She talked to God as familiarly as if he had been a creature like herself; and a thousand times more so, than if she had been in the presence of some earthly potentate. She demanded, with little expenditure of reverence or fear, a supply of all her more pressing wants, and at times her demands approached very near to commands. She felt as if God was under obligation to her, much more than she was to him. He seemed to her benighted vision in some manner bound to do her bidding.

Her heart recoils now, with very dread, when she recalls these shocking, almost blasphemous conversations with the great Jehovah. And well for herself did she deem it, that, unlike earthly potentates, his infinite character combined the tender father with the omniscient and omnipotent Creator of the universe.

She at first commenced promising God, that if he would help her out of all her difficulties, she would pay him by being very good; and this goodness she intended as a remuneration to God. She could think of no benefit that was to accrue to herself or her fellow-creatures, from her leading a life of purity and generous self-sacrifice for the good of others; as far as any but God was concerned, she saw nothing in it but heart-trying penance, sustained by the sternest exertion; and this she soon found much more easily promised than performed.

Days wore away—new trials came—God's aid was invoked, and the same promises repeated; and every successive night found her part of the contract unfulfilled. She now began to excuse herself, by telling God she could not be good in her present circumstances; but if he would give her a new place, and a good master and mistress, she could and would be good; and she expressly stipulated, that she would be good *one* day to show God how good she would be *all* of the time, when he should surround her with the right influences, and she should be delivered from the temptations that then so sorely beset her. But, alas! when night came, and she became conscious that she had yielded to all her temptations, and entirely failed of keeping her word with God, having prayed and promised one hour, and fallen into the sins of anger and profanity the next, the mortifying reflection weighed on her mind, and blunted her enjoyment. Still, she did not lay it deeply to heart, but continued to repeat her demands for aid, and her promises of pay, with full purpose of heart, at each particular time, that *that* day she would not fail to keep her plighted word.

Thus perished the inward spark, like a flame just igniting,

when one waits to see whether it will burn on or die out, till the long desired change came, and she found herself in a new place, with a good mistress, and one who never instigated an otherwise kind master to be unkind to her; in short, a place where she had literally nothing to complain of, and where, for a time, she was more happy than she could well express. 'Oh, every thing there was *so* pleasant, and kind, and good, and all so comfortable; enough of every thing; indeed, it was beautiful!' she exclaimed.

Here, at Mr. Van Wagener's,—as the reader will readily perceive she must have been,—she was so happy and satisfied, that God was entirely forgotten. Why should her thoughts turn to him, who was only known to her as a help in trouble? She had no trouble now; her every prayer had been answered in every minute particular. She had been delivered from her persecutors and temptations, her youngest child had been given her, and the others she knew she had no means of sustaining if she had them with her, and was content to leave them behind. Their father, who was much older than Isabel, and who preferred serving his time out in slavery, to the trouble and dangers of the course she pursued, remained with and could keep an eye on them—though it is comparatively little that they can do for each other while they remain in slavery; and this little the slave, like persons in every other situation of life, is not always disposed to perform. There *are* slaves, who, copying the selfishness of their superiors in power, in their conduct towards their fellows who may be thrown upon their mercy, by infirmity or illness, allow them to suffer for want of that kindness and care which it is fully in their power to render them.

The slaves in this country have ever been allowed to celebrate the principal, if not some of the lesser festivals observed by the Catholics and Church of England;—many of them not being required to do the least service for several days, and at Christmas they have almost universally an entire week to themselves, except, perhaps, the attending to a few duties, which are absolutely required for the comfort of the families they belong to. If much service is desired, they are hired to do it, and paid for it as if they were free. The more sober portion of them spend these holidays in earning a little money.

Most of them visit and attend parties and balls, and not a few of them spend it in the lowest dissipation. This respite from toil is granted them by all religionists, of whatever persuasion, and probably originated from the fact that many of the first slaveholders were members of the Church of England.

Frederick Douglass, who has devoted his great heart and noble talents entirely to the furtherance of the cause of his down-trodden race, has said—'From what I know of the effect of their holidays upon the slave, I believe them to be among the most effective means, in the hands of the slave-holder, in keeping down the spirit of insurrection. Were the slaveholders at once to abandon this practice, I have not the slightest doubt it would lead to an immediate insurrection among the slaves. These holidays serve as conductors, or safety-valves, to carry off the rebellious spirit of enslaved humanity. But for these, the slave would be forced up to the wildest desperation; and woe betide the slaveholder, the day he ventures to remove or hinder the operation of those conductors! I warn him that, in such an event, a spirit will go forth in their midst, more to be dreaded than the most appalling earthquake.'

When Isabella had been at Mr. Van Wagener's a few months, she saw in prospect one of the festivals approaching. She knows it by none but the Dutch name, Pingster, as she calls it—but I think it must have been Whitsuntide, in English. She says she 'looked back into Egypt,' and every thing looked 'so pleasant there,' as she saw retrospectively all her former companions enjoying their freedom for at least a little space, as well as their wonted convivialities, and in her heart she longed to be with them. With this picture before her mind's eye, she contrasted the quiet, peaceful life she was living with the excellent people of Wahkendall, and it seemed so dull and void of incident, that the very contrast served but to heighten her desire to return, that, at least, she might enjoy with them, once more, the coming festivities. These feelings had occupied a secret corner of her breast for some time, when, one morning, she told Mrs. Van Wagener that her old master Dumont would come that day, and that she should go home with him on his return. They expressed some surprise, and asked her where she obtained her information. She replied, that no one had told her, but she felt that he would come.

It seemed to have been one of those 'events that cast their shadows before;' for, before night, Mr. Dumont made his appearance. She informed him of her intention to accompany him home. He answered, with a smile, 'I shall not take you back again; you ran away from me.' Thinking his manner contradicted his words, she did not feel repulsed, but made herself and child ready; and when her former master had seated himself in the open dearborn, she walked towards it, intending to place herself and child in the rear, and go with him. But, ere she reached the vehicle, she says that God revealed himself to her, with all the suddenness of a flash of lightning, showing her, 'in the twinkling of an eye, that he was *all over*' —that he pervaded the universe—'and that there was no place where God was not.' She became instantly conscious of her great sin in forgetting her almighty Friend and 'ever-present help in time of trouble.' All her unfulfilled promises arose before her, like a vexed sea whose waves run mountains high; and her soul, which seemed but one mass of lies, shrunk back aghast from the 'awful look' of him whom she had formerly talked to, as if he had been a being like herself; and she would now fain have hid herself in the bowels of the earth, to have escaped his dread presence. But she plainly saw there was no place, not even in hell, where he was not; and where could she flee? Another such 'a look,' as she expressed it, and she felt that she must be extinguished forever, even as one, with the breath of his mouth, 'blows out a lamp,' so that no spark remains.

A dire dread of annihilation now seized her, and she waited to see if, by 'another look,' she was to be stricken from existence,—swallowed up, even as the fire licketh up the oil with which it comes in contact.

When at last the second look came not, and her attention was once more called to outward things, she observed her master had left, and exclaiming aloud, 'Oh, God, I did not know you were so big,' walked into the house, and made an effort to resume her work. But the workings of the inward man were too absorbing to admit of much attention to her avocations. She desired to talk to God, but her vileness utterly forbade it, and she was not able to prefer a petition. 'What!' said she, 'shall I lie again to God? I have told him nothing but lies; and shall I speak again, and tell another lie to God?' She could not; and now she began to wish for some one to speak to God for her. Then a space seemed opening between her and God, and she felt that if some one, who was worthy in the sight of heaven, would but plead *for* her in their own name, and not let God know it came from *her*, who was so unworthy, God might grant it. At length a friend appeared to stand between herself and an insulted Deity; and she felt as sensibly refreshed as when, on a hot day, an umbrella had been interposed between her scorching head and a burning sun. But who was this friend? became the next inquiry. Was it Deencia, who had so often befriended her? She looked at her, with her new power of sight—and, lo! she, too, seemed all 'bruises and putrifying sores,' like herself. No, it was some one very different from Deencia.

'Who *are* you?' she exclaimed, as the vision brightened into a form distinct, beaming with the beauty of holiness, and radiant with love. She then said, audibly addressing the mysterious visitant—'I *know* you, and I *don't* know you.' Meaning, 'You seem perfectly familiar; I feel that you not only love me, but that you always *have* loved me—yet I know you not—I cannot call you by name.' When she said, 'I know you,' the subject of the vision remained distinct and quiet. When she said, 'I don't know you,' it moved restlessly about, like agitated waters. So while she repeated, without intermission, 'I know you, I know you,' that the vision might remain—'Who are you?' was the cry of her heart, and her whole soul was in one deep prayer that this heavenly personage might be revealed to her, and remain with her. At length, after bending both soul and body with the intensity of this desire, till breath and strength seemed failing, and she could maintain her position no longer, an answer came to her, sayingly distinctly, 'It is Jesus.' 'Yes,' she responded, 'it is *Jesus*.'

Previous to these exercises of mind, she heard Jesus mentioned in reading or speaking, but had received from what she heard no impression that he was any other than an eminent man, like a Washington or a Lafayette. Now he appeared to her delighted mental vision as so mild, so good, and so every way lovely, and he loved her so much! And, how strange that he had always loved her, and she had never known it! And how great a blessing he conferred, in that he should stand between her and God! And God was no longer a terror and a dread to her.

She stopped not to argue the point, even in her own mind, whether he had reconciled her to God, or God to herself, (though she thinks the former now,) being but too happy that God was no longer to her as a consuming fire, and Jesus was 'altogether lovely.' Her heart was now full of joy and gladness, as it had been of terror, and at one time of despair. In the light of her great happiness, the world was clad in new beauty, the very air sparkled as with diamonds, and was redolent of heaven. She contemplated the unapproachable barriers that existed between herself and the great of this world, as the world calls greatness, and made surprising comparisons between them, and the union existing between herself and Jesus,—Jesus, the transcendently lovely, as well as great and powerful; for so he appeared to her, though he seemed but human; and she watched for his bodily appearance, feeling that she should know him, if she saw him; and when he came, she should go and dwell with him, as with a dear friend.

It was not given her to see that he loved any other; and she thought if others came to know and love him, as she did, she should be thrust aside and forgotten, being herself but a poor ignorant slave, with little to recommend her to his notice. And when she heard him spoken of, she said mentally— 'What! others know Jesus? I thought no one knew Jesus but me!' and she felt a sort of jealousy, lest she should be robbed of her newly found treasure.

She conceived, one day, as she listened to reading, that she heard an intimation that Jesus was married, and hastily inquired if Jesus had a wife. 'What!' said the reader, '*God* have a wife?' 'Is Jesus *God*?' inquired Isabella. 'Yes, to be sure he is,' was the answer returned. From this time, her conceptions of Jesus became more elevated and spiritual; and she sometimes spoke of him as God, in accordance with the teaching she had received.

But when she was simply told, that the Christian world was much divided on the subject of Christ's nature—some believing him to be coëqual with the Father—to be God in and of himself, 'very God, of very God;'—some, that he is the 'well-beloved,' 'only begotten Son of God;'—and others, that he is, or was, rather, but a mere man—she said, 'Of that I only know as I saw. I did not see him to be God; else, how could he stand between me and God? I saw him as a friend, standing between me and God, through whom, love flowed as from a fountain.' Now, so far from expressing her views of Christ's character and office in accordance with any system of theology extant, she says she believes Jesus is the same spirit that was in our first parents, Adam and Eve, in the beginning, when they came from the hand of their Creator. When they sinned through disobedience, this pure spirit forsook them, and fled to heaven; that there it remained, until it returned again in the person of Jesus; and that, previous to a personal union with him, man is but a brute, possessing only the spirit of an animal.

She avers that, in her darkest hours, she had no fear of any worse hell than the one she then carried in her bosom; though it had ever been pictured to her in its deepest colors, and threatened her as a reward for all her misdemeanors. Her vileness and God's holiness and all-pervading presence, which filled immensity, and threatened her with instant annihilation, composed the burden of her vision of terror. Her faith in prayer is equal to her faith in the love of Jesus. Her language is, 'Let others say what they will of the efficacy of prayer, *I* believe in it, and *I* shall pray. Thank God! Yes, *I shall always pray*,' she exclaims, putting her hands together with the greatest enthusiasm.

For sometime subsequent to the happy change we have spoken of, Isabella's prayers partook largely of their former character; and while, in deep affliction, she labored for the recovery of her son, she prayed with constancy and fervor; and the following may be taken as a specimen:—'Oh, God, you know how much I am distressed, for I have told you again and again. Now, God, help me get my son. If you were in trouble, as I am, and I could help you, as you can me, think I wouldn't do it? Yes, God, you *know* I would do it.' 'Oh, God, you know I have no money, but you can make the people do for me, and you must make the people do for me. I will never give you peace till you do, God.' 'Oh, God, make the people hear me—don't let them turn me off, without hearing and helping me.' And she has not a particle of doubt, that God heard her, and especially disposed the hearts of thoughtless clerks, eminent lawyers, and grave judges and others—between whom and herself there seemed to her almost an infinite remove—to listen to her suit with patient and respectful attention, backing it up with all needed aid. The sense of her nothingness, in the eyes of those with whom she contended for her rights, sometimes fell on her like a heavy weight, which nothing but her unwavering confidence in an arm which she believed to be stronger than all others combined could have raised from her sinking spirit. 'Oh! how little I did feel,' she repeated, with a powerful emphasis. 'Neither would you wonder, if you could have seen me, in my ignorance and destitution, trotting about the streets, meanly clad, bare-headed, and bare-footed! Oh, God only could have made such people hear me; and he did it in answer to my prayers.' And this perfect trust, based on the rock of Deity, was a soul-protecting fortress, which, raising her above the battlements of fear, and shielding her from the machinations of the enemy, impelled her onward in the struggle, till the foe was vanquished, and the victory gained.

We have now seen Isabella, her youngest daughter, and her only son, in possession of, at least, their nominal freedom. It has been said that the freedom of the most free of the colored people of this country is but nominal; but stinted and limited as it is, at best, it is an *immense* remove from chattel slavery. This fact is disputed, I know; but I have no confidence in the honesty of such questionings. If they are made in sincerity, I honor not the judgment that thus decides.

Her husband, quite advanced in age, and infirm of health, was emancipated, with the balance of the adult slaves of the State, according to law, the following summer, July 4, 1828.

For a few years after this event, he was able to earn a scanty living, and when he failed to do that, he was dependant on the 'world's cold charity,' and died in a poor-house. Isabella had herself and two children to provide for; her wages were trifling, for at that time the wages of females were at a small advance from nothing; and she doubtless had to learn the first

elements of economy—for what slaves, that were never allowed to make any stipulations or calculations for themselves,
ever possessed an adequate idea of the true value of time, or,
in fact, of any material thing in the universe? To such, 'prudent using' is meanness—and 'saving' is a word to be sneered
at. Of course, it was not in her power to make to herself a
home, around whose sacred hearth-stone she could collect
her family, as they gradually emerged from their prison-house
of bondage; a home, where she could cultivate their affection,
administer to their wants, and instil into the opening minds of
her children those principles of virtue, and that love of purity,
truth and benevolence, which must ever form the foundation
of a life of usefulness and happiness. No—all this was far beyond her power or means, in more senses than one; and it
should be taken into the account, whenever a comparison is
instituted between the progress made by her children in
virtue and goodness, and the progress of those who have
been nurtured in the genial warmth of a sunny home, where
good influences cluster, and bad ones are carefully excluded—
where 'line upon line, and precept upon precept,' are daily
brought to their quotidian tasks—and where, in short, every
appliance is brought in requisition, that self-denying parents
can bring to bear on one of the dearest objects of a parent's
life, the promotion of the welfare of their children. But God
forbid that this suggestion should be wrested from its original
intent, and made to shield any one from merited rebuke! Isabella's children are now of an age to know good from evil,
and may easily inform themselves on any point where they
may yet be in doubt; and if they now suffer themselves to be
drawn by temptation into the paths of the destroyer, or forget
what is due to the mother who has done and suffered so
much for them, and who, now that she is descending into the
vale of years, and feels her health and strength declining, will
turn her expecting eyes to them for aid and comfort, just as
instinctly as the child turns its confiding eye to its fond parent, when it seeks for succor or for sympathy—(for it is now
their turn to do the work, and hear the burdens of life, as all
must bear them in turn, as the wheel of life rolls on)—if, I say,
they forget this, their duty and their happiness, and pursue an
opposite course of sin and folly, they must lose the respect of

the wise and good, and find, when too late, that 'the way of the transgressor is hard.'

NEW TRIALS.

The reader will pardon this passing homily, while we return to our narrative.

We were saying that the day-dreams of Isabella and her husband—the plan they drew of what they would do, and the comforts they thought to have, when they should obtain their freedom, and a little home of their own—had all turned to 'thin air,' by the postponement of their freedom to so late a day. These delusive hopes were never to be realized, and a new set of trials was gradually to open before her. These were the heart-wasting trials of watching over her children, scattered, and imminently exposed to the temptations of the adversary, with few, if any, fixed principles to sustain them.

'Oh,' she says, 'how little did I know myself of the best way to instruct and counsel them! Yet I did the best I then knew, when with them. I took them to the religious meetings; I talked to, and prayed for and with them; when they did wrong, I scolded at and whipped them.'

Isabella and her son had been free about a year, when they went to reside in the city of New York; a place which she would doubtless have avoided, could she have seen what was there in store for her; for this view into the future would have taught her what she only learned by bitter experience, that the baneful influences going up from such a city were not the best helps to education, commenced as the education of *her* children had been.

Her son Peter was, at the time of which we are speaking, just at that age when no lad should be subjected to the temptations of such a place, unprotected as he was, save by the feeble arm of a mother, herself a servant there. He was growing up to be a tall, well-formed, active lad, of quick perceptions, mild and cheerful in his disposition, with much that was open, generous and winning about him, but with little power to withstand temptation, and a ready ingenuity to provide himself with ways and means to carry out his plans, and con-

ceal from his mother and her friends, all such as he knew
would not meet their approbation. As will be readily believed,
he was soon drawn into a circle of associates who did not improve either his habits or his morals.

Two years passed before Isabella knew what character Peter
was establishing for himself among his low and worthless
comrades—passing under the assumed name of Peter Williams; and she began to feel a parent's pride in the promising
appearance of her only son. But, alas! this pride and pleasure
were shortly dissipated, as distressing facts relative to him
came one by one to her astonished ear. A friend of Isabella's,
a lady, who was much pleased with the good humor, ingenuity, and open confessions of Peter, when driven into a corner,
and who, she said, 'was so smart, he ought to have an education, if any one ought'—paid ten dollars, as tuition fee, for
him to attend a navigation school. But Peter, little inclined to
spend his leisure hours in study, when he might be enjoying
himself in the dance, or otherwise, with his boon companions, went regularly and made some plausible excuses to the
teacher, who received them as genuine, along with the ten
dollars of Mrs. ——, and while his mother and her friend believed him improving at school, he was, to their latent sorrow,
improving in a very different place or places, and on entirely
opposite principles. They also procured him an excellent place
as a coachman. But, wanting money, he sold his livery, and
other things belonging to his master; who, having conceived
a kind regard for him, considered his youth, and prevented
the law from falling, with all its rigor, upon his head. Still he
continued to abuse his privileges, and to involve himself in repeated difficulties, from which his mother as often extricated
him. At each time, she talked much, and reasoned and remonstrated with him; and he would, with such perfect frankness, lay open his whole soul to her, telling her he had never
intended doing harm,—how he had been led along, little by
little, till, before he was aware, he found himself in trouble—
how he had *tried* to be good—and how, when he would have
been so, 'evil was present with him,'—indeed he knew not
how it was.

His mother, beginning to feel that the city was no place for
him, urged his going to sea, and would have shipped him on

board a man-of-war; but Peter was not disposed to consent to that proposition, while the city and its pleasures were accessible to him. Isabella now became a prey to distressing fears, dreading lest the next day or hour come fraught with the report of some dreadful crime, committed or abetted by her son. She thanks the Lord for sparing her that giant sorrow, as all his wrong doings never ranked higher, in the eye of the law, than misdemeanors. But as she could see no improvement in Peter, as a last resort, she resolved to leave him, for a time, unassisted, to bear the penalty of his conduct, and see what effect that would have on him. In the trial hour, she remained firm in her resolution. Peter again fell into the hands of the police, and sent for his mother, as usual; but she went not to his relief. In his extremity, he sent for Peter Williams, a respectable colored barber, whose name he had been wearing, and who sometimes helped young culprits out of their troubles, and sent them from city dangers, by shipping them on board of whaling vessels.

The curiosity of this man was awakened by the culprit's bearing his own name. He went to the Tombs and inquired into his case, but could not believe what Peter told him respecting his mother and family. Yet he redeemed him, and Peter promised to leave New York in a vessel that was to sail in the course of a week. He went to see his mother, and informed her of what had happened to him. She listened incredulously, as to an idle tale. He asked her to go with him and see for herself. She went, giving no credence to his story till she found herself in the presence of Mr. Williams, and heard him saying to her, 'I am very glad I have assisted your son; he stood in great need of sympathy and assistance; but I could not think he had such a mother here, although he assured me he had.'

Isabella's great trouble now was, a fear lest her son should deceive his benefactor, and be missing when the vessel sailed; but he begged her earnestly to trust him, for he said he had resolved to do better, and meant to abide by the resolve. Isabella's heart gave her no peace till the time of sailing, when Peter sent Mr. Williams and another messenger whom she knew, to tell her he had sailed. But for a month afterwards, she looked to see him emerging from some by-place in the city, and appearing before her; so afraid was she that he was still unfaithful, and doing wrong. But he did not appear, and at length she believed him really gone. He left in the summer of 1839, and his friends heard nothing further from him till his mother received the following letter, dated 'October 17, 1840':

'MY DEAR AND BELOVED MOTHER:

'I take this opportunity to write to you and inform you that I am well, and in hopes for to find you the same. I am got on board the same unlucky ship Done, of Nantucket. I am sorry for to say, that I have been punished once severely, by shoving my head in the fire for other folks. We have had bad luck, but in hopes to have better. We have about 230 on board, but in hopes, if don't have good luck, that my parents will receive me with thanks. I would like to know how my sisters are. Does my cousins live in New York yet? Have you got my letter? If not, inquire to Mr. Peirce Whiting's. I wish you would write me an answer as soon as possible. I am your only son, that is so far from your home, in the wide, briny ocean. I have seen more of the world than ever I expected, and if I ever should return home safe, I will tell you all my troubles and hardships. Mother, I hope you do not forget me, your dear and only son. I should like to know how Sophia, and Betsey, and Hannah, come on. I hope you all will forgive me for all that I have done.

'Your son,
'PETER VAN WAGENER.'

Another letter reads as follows, dated 'March 22, 1841':

'MY DEAR MOTHER:

'I take this opportunity to write to you, and inform you that I have been well and in good health. I have wrote you a letter before, but have received no answer from you, and was very anxious to see you. I hope to see you in a short time. I have had very hard luck, but are in hopes to have better in time to come. I should like if my sisters are well, and all the people round the neighborhood. I expect to be home in twenty-two months or thereabouts. I have seen Samuel Laterett. Beware! There has happened very bad news to tell you, that Peter Jackson is dead. He died within two days' sail of

Otaheite, one of the Society Islands. The Peter Jackson that used to live at Laterett's; he died on board the ship Done, of Nantucket, Captain Miller, in the latitude 15 53, and longitude 148 30 W. I have no more to say at present, but write as soon as possible.

'Your only son,
'PETER VAN WAGENER.'

Another, containing the last intelligence she has had from her son, reads as follows, and was dated 'Sept. 19, 1841':

'DEAR MOTHER:

'I take this opportunity to write to you and inform you that I am well and in good health, and in hopes to find you in the same. This is the fifth letter I have wrote you, and have received no answer, and it makes me very uneasy. So pray write as quick as you can, and tell how all the people is about the neighborhood. We are out from home twenty-three months, and in hopes to be home in fifteen months. I have not much to say; but tell me if you have been up home since I left or not. I want to know what sort of a time is at home. We had very bad luck when we first came out, but since we have had very good; so I am in hopes to do well yet; but if I don't do well, you need not expect me home these five years. So write as quick as you can, wont you? So, now I am going to put an end to my writing, at present. Notice—when this you see, remember me, and place me in your mind.

Get me to my home, that's in the far-distant west,
To the scenes of my childhood, that I like the best;
There the tall cedars grow, and the bright waters flow,
Where my parents will greet me, white man, let me go!

Let me go to the spot where the cateract plays,
Where oft I have sported in my boyish days;
And there is my poor mother, whose heart ever flows,
At the sight of her poor child, to her let me go, let me go!

'Your only son,
'PETER VAN WAGENER.'

Since the date of the last letter, Isabella has heard no tidings from her long-absent son, though ardently does her mother's heart long for such tidings, as her thoughts follow him around the world, in his perilous vocation, saying within herself—'He is good now, I have no doubt; I feel sure that he has persevered, and kept the resolve he made before he left home;—he seemed so different before he went, so determined to do better.' His letters are inserted here for preservation, in case they prove the last she ever hears from him in this world.

FINDING A BROTHER AND SISTER.

When Isabella had obtained the freedom of her son, she remained in Kingston, where she had been drawn by the judicial process, about a year, during which time she became a member of the Methodist Church there; and when she went to New York, she took a letter missive from that church to the Methodist Church in John street. Afterwards, she withdrew her connection with that church, and joined Zion's Church, in Church street, composed entirely of colored people. With the latter church she remained until she went to reside with Mr. Pierson, after which, she was gradually drawn into the 'kingdom' set up by the prophet Matthias, in the name of God the Father; for he said the spirit of God the Father dwelt in him.

While Isabella was in New York, her sister Sophia came from Newberg to reside in the former place. Isabel had been favored with occasional interviews with this sister, although at one time she lost sight of her for the space of seventeen years—almost the entire period of her being at Mr. Dumont's—and when she appeared before her again, handsomely dressed, she did not recognize her, till informed who she was. Sophia informed her that her brother Michael—a brother she had never seen—was in the city; and when she introduced him to Isabella, *he* informed her that their sister Nancy had been living in the city, and had deceased a few months before. He described her features, her dress, her manner, and said she had for some time been a member in Zion's Church, naming the class she belonged to. Isabella almost instantly recognized her as a sister in the church, with whom she had knelt at the altar, and with whom she had exchanged the speaking pressure of the hand, in recognition of their spiritual sisterhood; little thinking, at the time, that they were also children of the same earthly parents—even Bomefree and Mau-mau Bett. As inquiries and answers rapidly passed, and the conviction deepened that this was their sister, the very sister they had heard so much of, but had never seen, (for she was the self-same sister that had been locked in the great old-fashioned sleigh-box, when she was taken away, never to behold her mother's face again this side the spirit-land, and Michael, the narrator, was the brother who had shared her fate,) Isabella thought, 'D——h! here she was; we met; and was I not, at the time, struck with the peculiar feeling of her hand—the bony hardness so just like mine? and yet I could not know she was my sister; and now I see she looked *so* like my mother!' And Isabella, wept, and not alone; Sophia wept, and the strong man, Michael, mingled his tears with theirs. 'Oh Lord,' inquired Isabella, 'what is this slavery, that it can do such dreadful things? what evil can it not do?' Well may she ask; for surely the evils it can and does do, daily and hourly, can never be summed up, till we can see them as they are recorded by him who writes no errors, and reckons without mistake. This account, which now varies so widely in the estimate of different minds, will be viewed alike by all.

Think you, dear reader, when that day comes, the most 'rabid abolitionist' will say—'Behold, I saw all this while on the earth?' Will he not rather say, 'Oh, who has conceived the breadth and depth of this moral malaria, this putrescent plague-spot?' Perhaps the pioneers in the slave's cause will be as much surprised as any to find that with all *their* looking, there remained so much unseen.

GLEANINGS.

There are some hard things that crossed Isabella's life while in slavery, that she has no desire to publish, for various reasons. First, because the parties from whose hands she suffered them have rendered up their account to a higher tribunal, and their innocent friends alone are living, to have their feelings injured by the recital; secondly, because they are not all for the public ear, from their very nature; thirdly, and not least, because, she says, were she to tell all that happened to her as a slave—all that she knows is 'God's truth'—it would seem to others, especially the uninitiated, so unaccountable, so unreasonable, and what is usually called so unnatural, (though it may be questioned whether people do not always act naturally,) they would not easily believe it. 'Why, no!' she says, 'they'd call me a liar! they would, indeed! and I do not wish to say any thing to destroy my own character for veracity, though what I say is strictly true.' Some things have been omitted through forgetfulness, which not having been mentioned in their places, can only be briefly spoken of here;— such as, that her father Bomefree had had two wives before he took Mau-mau Bett; one of whom, if not both, were torn from him by the iron hand of the ruthless trafficker in human flesh;—that her husband, Thomas, after one of *his* wives had been sold away from him, ran away to New York city, where he remained a year or two, before he was discovered and taken back to the prison-house of slavery;—that her master Dumont, when he promised Isabella one year of her time, before the State should make her free, made the same promise to her husband, and in addition to freedom, they were promised a log cabin for a home of their own; all of which, with the one-thousand-and-one day-dreams resulting therefrom, went into the repository of unfulfilled promises and unrealized hopes;—that she had often heard her father repeat a thrilling story of a little slave-child, which, because it annoyed the family with its cries, was caught up by a white man, who dashed its brains out against the wall. An Indian (for Indians were plenty in that region then) passed along as the bereaved mother washed the bloody corpse of her murdered child, and learning the cause of its death, said, with characteristic vehemence, 'If I had been here, I would have put my tomahawk in his head!' meaning the murderer's.

Of the cruelty of one Hasbrouck.—He had a sick slave-woman, who was lingering with a slow consumption, whom he made to spin, regardless of her weakness and suffering; and this woman had a child, that was unable to walk or talk, at the age of five years, neither could it cry like other children, but made a constant, piteous, moaning sound. This exhibition of helplessness and imbecility, instead of exciting the master's pity, stung his cupidity, and so enraged him, that he would kick the poor thing about like a foot-ball.

Isabella's informant had seen this brute of a man, when the child was curled up under a chair, innocently amusing itself with a few sticks, drag it thence, that he might have the pleasure of tormenting it. She had seen him, with one blow of his foot, send it rolling quite across the room, and down the steps at the door. Oh, how she wished it might instantly die! 'But,' she said, 'it seemed as tough as a moccasin.' Though it *did* die at last, and made glad the heart of its friends; and its persecutor, no doubt, rejoiced with them, but from very different motives. But the day of his retribution was not far off— for he sickened, and his reason fled. It was fearful to hear his old slave soon tell how, in the day of his calamity, she treated *him*.

She was very strong, and was therefore selected to support her master, as he sat up in bed, by putting her arms around, while she stood behind him. It was then that she did her best to wreak her vengeance on him. She would clutch his feeble frame in her iron grasp, as in a vice; and, when her mistress did not see, would give him a squeeze, a shake, and lifting him up, set him down again, as *hard as possible*. If his breathing betrayed too tight a grasp, and her mistress said, 'Be careful, don't hurt him, Soan!' her ever-ready answer was, 'Oh no, Missus, no,' in her most pleasant tone—and then, as soon as Missus's eyes and ears were engaged away, another grasp— another shake—another bounce. She was afraid the disease alone would let him recover,—an event she dreaded more than to do wrong herself. Isabella asked her, if she were not afraid his spirit would haunt her. 'Oh, no,' says Soan; 'he was *so* wicked, the devil will never let him out of hell long enough for that.'

Many slaveholders boast of the love of their slaves. How would it freeze the blood of some of them to know what kind of love rankles in the bosoms of slaves for them! Witness the attempt to poison Mrs. Calhoun, and hundreds of similar cases. Most '*surprising*' to every body, because committed by slaves supposed to be so *grateful* for their chains.

These reflections bring to mind a discussion on this point, between the writer and a slaveholding friend in Kentucky, on Christmas morning, 1846. We had asserted, that until mankind were far in advance of what they now are, irresponsible power over our fellow-beings would be, as it is, abused. Our friend declared it *his* conviction, that the cruelties of slavery existed chiefly in imagination, and that no person in D—— County, where we then were, but would be above ill-treating a helpless slave. We answered, that if his belief was well-founded, the people in Kentucky were greatly in advance of the people of New England—for we would not dare say as much as that of any school-district there, letting alone counties. No, we would not answer for our own conduct even on so delicate a point.

The next evening, he very magnanimously overthrew his own position and established ours, by informing us that, on the morning previous, and as near as we could learn, at the very hour in which we were earnestly discussing the probabilities of the case, a young woman of fine appearance, and high standing in society, the pride of her husband, and the mother of an infant daughter, only a few miles from us, ay, in D—— County, too, was actually beating in the skull of a slave-woman called Tabby; and not content with that, had her tied up and whipped, after her skull was broken, and she died hanging to the bedstead, to which she had been fastened. When informed that Tabby was dead, she answered, 'I am *glad of it*, for she has worried my life out of me.' But Tabby's highest good was probably not the end proposed by Mrs. M——, for no one supposed she meant to kill her. Tabby was considered quite lacking in good sense, and no doubt belonged to that class at the South, that are silly enough to 'die of moderate correction.'

A mob collected around the house for an hour or two, in that manner expressing a momentary indignation. But was she treated as a murderess? Not at all! She was allowed to take boat (for her residence was near the beautiful Ohio) that evening, to spend a few months with her absent friends, after which she returned and remained with her husband, no one to 'molest or make her afraid.'

Had she been left to the punishment of an outraged conscience from right motives, I would have 'rejoiced with exceeding joy.' But to see the life of one woman, and she a murderess, put in the balance against the lives of three millions of innocent slaves, and to contrast her punishment with what I felt would be the punishment of one who was merely suspected of being an equal friend of all mankind, regardless of color or condition, caused my blood to stir within me, and my heart to sicken at the thought. The husband of Mrs. M—— was absent from home, at the time alluded to; and when he arrived, some weeks afterwards, bringing beautiful presents to his cherished companion, he beheld his once happy home deserted, Tabby murdered and buried in the garden, and the wife of his bosom, and the mother of his child, the doer of the dreadful deed, a *murderess!*

When Isabella went to New York city, she went in company with a Miss Gear, who introduced her to the family of Mr. James Latourette, a wealthy merchant, and a Methodist in religion; but who, the latter part of his life, felt that he had outgrown ordinances, and advocated free meetings, holding them at his own dwelling-house for several years previous to his death. She worked for them, and they generously gave her a home while she labored for others, and in their kindness made her as one of their own.

At that time, the 'moral reform' movement was awakening the attention of the benevolent in that city. Many women, among whom were Mrs. Latourette and Miss Gear, became deeply interested in making an attempt to reform their fallen sisters, even the most degraded of them; and in this enterprise of labor and danger, they enlisted Isabella and others, who for a time put forth their most zealous efforts, and performed the work of missionaries with much apparent success. Isabella accompanied those ladies to the most wretched abodes of vice and misery, and sometimes she went where they dared not follow. They even succeeded in establishing prayer-meetings in several places, where such a thing might least have been expected.

But these meetings soon became the most noisy, shouting, ranting, and boisterous of gatherings; where they became delirious with excitement, and then exhausted from over-action. Such meetings Isabel had not much sympathy with, at best. But one evening she attended one of them, where the members of it, in a fit of ecstasy, jumped upon her cloak in such a manner as to drag her to the floor—and then, thinking she had fallen in a spiritual trance, they increased their glorifications on her account,—jumping, shouting, stamping, and clapping of hands; rejoicing so much over her spirit, and so entirely overlooking her body, that she suffered much, both from fear and bruises; and ever after refused to attend any more such meetings, doubting much whether God had any thing to do with such worship.

THE MATTHIAS IMPOSTURE.

We now come to an eventful period in the life of Isabella, as identified with one of the most extraordinary religious impostures of modern times; but the limits prescribed for the present work forbid a minute narration of all the occurrences that transpired in relation to it.

After she had joined the African Church in Church street, and during her membership there, she frequently attended Mr. Latourette's meetings, at one of which, Mr. Smith invited her to go to a prayer-meeting, or to instruct the girls at the Magdalene Asylum, Bowery Hill, then under the protection of Mr. Pierson, and some other persons, chiefly respectable females. To reach the Asylum, Isabella called on Katy, Mr. Pierson's colored servant, of whom she had some knowledge. Mr. Pierson saw her there, conversed with her, asked her if she had been baptized, and was answered, characteristically, 'by the Holy Ghost.' After this, Isabella saw Katy several times, and occasionally Mr. Pierson, who engaged her to keep his house while Katy went to Virginia to see her children. This engagement was considered an answer to prayer by Mr. Pierson, who had both fasted and prayed on the subject, while Katy and Isabella appeared to see in it the hand of God.

Mr. Pierson was characterised by a strong devotional spirit, which finally became highly fanatical. He assumed the title of Prophet, asserting that God had called him in an omnibus, in these words:—'Thou art Elijah, the Tishbite. Gather unto me all the members of Israel at the foot of Mount Carmel'; which he understood as meaning the gathering of his friends at Bowery Hill. Not long afterward, he became acquainted with the notorious Matthias, whose career was as extraordinary as it was brief. Robert Matthews, or Matthias, (as he was usually called,) was of Scotch extraction, but a native of Washington county, New York, and at that time about forty-seven years of age. He was religiously brought up, among the Anti-Burghers, a sect of Presbyterians; the clergyman, the Rev. Mr. Bevridge, visiting the family after the manner of the church, and being pleased with Robert, put his hand on his head, when a boy, and pronounced a blessing, and this blessing, with his natural qualities, determined his character; for he ever after thought he should be a distinguished man. Matthias was brought up a farmer till nearly eighteen years of age, but acquired indirectly the art of a carpenter, without any regular apprenticeship, and showed considerable mechanical skill. He obtained property from his uncle, Robert Thompson, and then he went into business as a store-keeper, was considered respectable, and became a member of the Scotch Presbyterian Church. He married in 1813, and continued in business in Cambridge. In 1816, he ruined himself by a building specula-tion, and the derangement of the currency which denied bank facilities, and soon after he came to New York with his family, and worked at his trade. He afterwards removed to Albany, and became a hearer at the Dutch Reformed Church, then under Dr. Ludlow's charge. He was frequently much excited on religious subjects.

In 1829, he was well known, if not for street preaching, for loud discussions and pavement exhortations, but he did not make set sermons. In the beginning of 1830, he was only con-sidered zealous; but in the same year he prophesied the destruction of the Albanians and their capital, and while preparing to shave, with the Bible before him, he suddenly put down the soap and exclaimed, 'I have found it! I have found a text which proves that no man who shaves his beard can be a true Christian;' and shortly afterwards, without shav-ing, he went to the Mission House to deliver an address which he had promised, and in this address he proclaimed his new character, pronounced vengeance on the land, and that the law of God was the only rule of government, and that he was commanded to take possession of the world in the name of the King of kings. His harangue was cut short by the trustees putting out the lights. About this time, Matthias laid by his implements of industry, and in June, he advised his wife to fly with him from the destruction which awaited them in the city; and on her refusal, partly on account of Matthias calling himself a Jew, whom she was unwilling to retain as a husband, he left her, taking some of the children to his sister in Argyle, forty miles from Albany. At Argyle he entered the church and interrupted the minister, declaring the congregation in darkness, and warning them to repentance. He was, of course, taken out of the church, and as he was advertised in the Albany papers, he was sent back to his family. His beard had now obtained a respectable length, and thus he attracted attention, and easily obtained an audience in the streets. For this he was sometimes arrested, once by mistake for Adam Paine, who collected the crowd, and then left Matthias with it on the approach of the officers. He repeatedly urged his wife to accompany him on a mission to convert the world, declaring that food could be obtained from the roots of the forest, if not administered otherwise. At this time he assumed the name of Matthias, called himself a Jew, and set out on a mission, taking a western course, and visiting a brother at Rochester, a skilful mechanic, since dead. Leaving his brother, he proceeded on his mission over the Northern States, occasionally returning to Albany.

After visiting Washington, and passing through Pennsylvania, he came to New York. His appearance at that time was mean, but grotesque, and his sentiments were but little known.

On May the 5th, 1832, he first called on Mr. Pierson, in Fourth street, in his absence. Isabella was alone in the house, in which she had lived since the previous autumn. On opening the door, she, for the first time, beheld Matthias, and her early impression of seeing Jesus in the flesh rushed into her mind. She heard his inquiry, and invited him into the parlor; and being naturally curious, and much excited, and possessing a good deal of tact, she drew him into conversation, stated her own opinions, and heard his replies and explanations. Her faith was at first staggered by his declaring himself a Jew; but on this point she was relieved by his saying, 'Do you not re-member how Jesus prayed?' and repeated part of the Lord's prayer, in proof that the Father's kingdom was to come, and not the Son's. She then understood him to be a converted Jew, and in the conclusion she says she '*felt* as if God had sent him to set up the kingdom.' Thus Matthias at once secured the good will of Isabella, and we may suppose obtained from her some information in relation to Mr. Pierson, especially that Mrs. Pierson declared there was no true church, and ap-proved of Mr. Pierson's preaching. Matthias left the house, promising to return on Saturday evening. Mr. P. at this time had not seen Matthias.

Isabella, desirous of hearing the expected conversation be-tween Matthias and Mr. Pierson on Saturday, hurried her work, got it finished, and was permitted to be present. In-deed, the sameness of belief made her familiar with her em-ployer, while her attention to her work, and characteristic faithfulness, increased his confidence. This intimacy, the result of holding the same faith, and the principle afterwards adopted of having but one table, and all things in common, made her at once the domestic and the equal, and the depos-itory of very curious, if not valuable information. To this ob-ject, even her color assisted. Persons who have travelled in the South know the manner in which the colored people, and es-pecially slaves, are treated; they are scarcely regarded as being present. This trait in our American character has been fre-quently noticed by foreign travellers. One English lady re-marks that she discovered, in course of conversation with a Southern married gentleman, that a colored girl slept in his bedroom, in which also was his wife; and when he saw that it occasioned some surprise, he remarked, 'What would he do if he wanted a glass of water in the night?' Other travellers have remarked that the presence of colored people never seemed to interrupt conversation of any kind for one moment. Isabella, then, was present at the first interview between Matthias and Pierson. At this interview, Mr. Pierson asked Matthias if he had a family, to which he replied in the affirmative; he asked him about his beard, and he gave a scriptural reason, assert-ing also that the Jews did not shave, and that Adam had a beard. Mr. Pierson detailed to Matthias his experience, and

Matthias gave his, and they mutually discovered that they held the same sentiments, both admitting the direct influence of the Spirit, and the transmission of spirits from one body to another. Matthias admitted the call of Mr. Pierson, in the omnibus in Wall street, which, on this occasion, he gave in these words:—'Thou art Elijah the Tishbite, and thou shalt go before me in the spirit and power of Elias, to prepare my way before me.' And Mr. Pierson admitted Matthias' call, who *completed* his declaration on the 20th of June, in Argyle, which, by a curious coincidence, was the very day on which Pierson had received his call in the omnibus. Such singular coincidences have a powerful effect on excited minds. From that discovery, Pierson and Matthias rejoiced in each other, and became kindred spirits—Matthias, however, claiming to be the Father, or to possess the spirit of the Father—he was God upon earth, because the spirit of God dwelt in him; while Pierson then understood that his mission was like that of John the Baptist, which the name Elias meant. This conference ended with an invitation to supper, and Matthias and Pierson washing each other's feet. Mr. Pierson preached on the following Sunday, but after which, he declined in favor of Matthias, and some of the party believed that the 'kingdom had then come.'

As a specimen of Matthias' preaching and sentiments, the following is said to be reliable:—

'The spirit that built the Tower of Babel is now in the world—it is the spirit of the devil. The spirit of man never goes upon the clouds; all who think so are Babylonians. The only heaven is on the earth. All who are ignorant of truth are Ninevites. The Jews did not crucify Christ—it was the Gentiles. Every Jew has his guardian angel attending him in this world. God don't speak through preachers; he speaks through me, his prophet.

' "John the Baptist," (addressing Mr. Pierson,) read the tenth chapter of Revelations.' After the reading of the chapter, the prophet resumed speaking, as follows:—

'Ours is the mustard-seed kingdom which is to spread all over the earth. Our creed is truth, and no man can find truth unless he obeys John the Baptist, and comes clean into the church.

'All *real* men will be saved; all *mock* men will be damned. When a person has the Holy Ghost, then he is a man, and not till then. They who teach women are of the wicked. The communion is all nonsense; so is prayer. Eating a nip of bread and drinking a little wine won't do any good. All who admit members into their church, and suffer them to hold their lands and houses, their sentence is, "Depart, ye wicked, I know you not." All females who lecture their husbands, their sentence is the same. The sons of truth are to enjoy all the good things of this world, and must use their means to bring it about. Every thing that has the smell of woman will be destroyed. Woman is the capsheaf of the abomination of desolation—full of all deviltry. In a short time, the world will take fire and dissolve; it is combustible already. All women, not obedient, had better become so as soon as possible, and let the wicked spirit depart, and become temples of truth. Praying is all mocking. When you see any one wring the neck of a fowl, instead of cutting off its head, he has not got the Holy Ghost. (Cutting gives the least pain.)

'All who eat swine's flesh are of the devil; and just as certain as he eats it, he will tell a lie in less than half an hour. If you eat a piece of pork, it will go crooked through you, and the Holy Ghost will not stay in you, but one or the other must leave the house pretty soon. The pork will be as crooked in you as ram's horns, and as great a nuisance as the hogs in the street.

'The cholera is not the right word; it is choler, which means God's wrath. Abraham, Isaac and Jacob are now in this world; they did not go up in the clouds, as some believe—why should they go there? They don't want to go there to box the compass from one place to another. The Christians now-a-days are for setting up the *Son's* kingdom. It is not his; it is the *Father's* kingdom. It puts me in mind of the man in the country, who took his son in business, and had his sign made, "Hitchcock & Son"; but the son wanted it "Hitchcock & Father"—and that is the way with your Christians. They talk of the Son's kingdom first, and not the Father's kingdom.'

Matthias and his disciples at this time did not believe in a resurrection of the body, but that the spirits of the former saints would enter the bodies of the present generation, and thus begin heaven upon earth, of which he and Mr. Pierson were the first fruits.

Matthias made the residence of Mr. Pierson his own; but the latter, being apprehensive of popular violence in his house, if Matthias remained there proposed a monthly allowance to him, and advised him to occupy another dwelling. Matthias accordingly took a house in Clarkson street, and then sent for his family at Albany, but they declined coming to the city. However, his brother George complied with a similar offer, bringing his family with him, where they found very comfortable quarters. Isabella was employed to do the housework. In May, 1833, Matthias left his house, and placed the furniture, part of which was Isabella's, elsewhere, living himself at the hotel corner of Marketfield and West streets. Isabella found employment at Mr. Whiting's, Canal street, and did the washing for Matthias, by Mrs. Whiting's permission.

Of the subsequent removal of Matthias to the farm and residence of Mr. B. Folger, at Sing Sing, where he was joined by Mr. Pierson, and others laboring under a similar religious delusion—the sudden, melancholy and somewhat suspicious death of Mr. Pierson, and the arrest of Matthias on the charge of his murder, ending in a verdict of not guilty—the criminal connection that subsisted between Matthias, Mrs. Folger, and other members of the 'kingdom,' as 'match-spirits'—the final dispersion of this deluded company, and the voluntary exilement of Matthias in the far West, after his release—&c. &c., we do not deem it useful or necessary to give any particulars. Those who are curious to know what there transpired are referred to a work published in New York in 1835, entitled 'Fanaticism; its Sources and Influence; illustrated by the simple Narrative of Isabella, in the case of Matthias, Mr. and Mrs. B. Folger, Mr. Pierson, Mr. Mills, Catharine, Isabella, &c. &c. By G. Vale, 84 Roosevelt street.' Suffice it to say, that while Isabella was a member of the household at Sing Sing, doing much laborious service in the spirit of religious disinterestedness, and gradually getting her vision purged and her mind cured of its illusions, she happily escaped the contamination that surrounded her,—assiduously endeavoring to discharge all her duties in a becoming manner.

FASTING.

When Isabella resided with Mr. Pierson, he was in the habit of fasting every Friday; not eating or drinking any thing from Thursday evening to six o'clock on Friday evening.

Then, again, he would fast two nights and three days, neither eating nor drinking; refusing himself even a cup of cold water till the third day at night, when he took supper again, as usual.

Isabella asked him why he fasted. He answered, that fasting gave him great light in the things of God; which answer gave birth to the following train of thought in the mind of his auditor:—'Well, if fasting will give light inwardly and spiritually, *I* need it as much as any body,—and I'll fast too. If Mr. Pierson needs to fast two nights and three days, then I, who need light more than he does, ought to fast more, and I will fast three nights and three days.'

This resolution she carried out to the letter, putting not so much as a drop of water in her mouth for three whole days and nights. The fourth morning, as she arose to her feet, not having power to stand, she fell to the floor; but recovering herself sufficiently, she made her way to the pantry, and feeling herself quite voracious, and fearing that she might now offend God by her voracity, compelled herself to breakfast on dry bread and water—eating a large six-penny loaf before she felt at all stayed or satisfied. She says she did get light, but it was all in her body and none in her mind—and this lightness of body lasted a long time. Oh! she was so light, and felt so well, she could 'skim around like a gull.'

THE CAUSE OF HER LEAVING
THE CITY.

The first years spent by Isabella in the city, she accumulated more than enough to supply all her wants, and she placed all the overplus in the Savings' Bank. Afterwards, while living with Mr. Pierson, he prevailed on her to take it thence, and invest it in a common fund which he was about establishing, as a fund to be drawn from by all the faithful; the faithful, of course, were the handful that should subscribe to his peculiar creed. This fund, commenced by Mr. Pierson, afterwards became part and parcel of the kingdom of which Matthias assumed to be head; and at the breaking up of the kingdom, her little property was merged in the general ruin—or went to enrich those who profited by the loss of others, if any such there were. Mr. Pierson and others had so assured her, that the fund would supply all her wants, at all times, and in all emergencies, and to the end of life, that she became perfectly careless on the subject—asking for no interest when she drew her money from the bank, and taking no account of the sum she placed in the fund. She recovered a few articles of furniture from the wreck of the kingdom, and received a small sum of money from Mr. B. Folger, as the price of Mrs. Folger's attempt to convict her of murder. With this to start upon, she commenced anew her labors, in the hope of yet being able to accumulate a sufficiency to make a little home for herself, in her advancing age. With this stimulus before her, she toiled hard, working early and late, doing a great deal for a little money, and turning her hand to almost any thing that promised good pay. Still, she did not prosper; and somehow, could not contrive to lay by a single dollar for a 'rainy day.'

When this had been the state of her affairs some time, she suddenly paused, and taking a retrospective view of what had passed, inquired within herself, why it was that, for all her unwearied labors, she had nothing to show; why it was that others, with much less care and labor, could hoard up treasures for themselves and children? She became more and more convinced, as she reasoned, that every thing she had undertaken in the city of New York had finally proved a failure; and where her hopes had been raised the highest, there she felt the failure had been the greatest, and the disappointment most severe.

After turning it in her mind for some time, she came to the conclusion, that she had been taking part in a great drama, which was, in itself, but one great system of robbery and wrong. 'Yes,' she said, 'the rich rob the poor, and the poor rob one another.' True, she had not received labor from others, and stinted their pay, as she felt had been practised against her; but she had taken their work from them, which was their only means to get money, and was the same to them in the end. For instance—a gentleman where she lived would give her a half dollar to hire a poor man to clear the new-fallen snow from the steps and sidewalks. She would arise early, and perform the labor herself, putting the money into her own pocket. A poor man would come along, saying she ought to have let him have the job; he was poor, and needed the pay for his family. She would harden her heart against him, and answer—'I am poor, too, and I need it for mine.' But, in her retrospection, she thought of all the misery she might have been adding to, in her selfish grasping, and it troubled her conscience sorely; and this insensibility to the claims of human brotherhood, and the wants of the destitute and wretched poor, she now saw, as she never had done before, to be unfeeling, selfish and wicked. These reflections and con-victions gave rise to a sudden revulsion of feeling in the heart of Isabella, and she began to look upon money and property with great indifference, if not contempt—being at that time unable, probably, to discern any difference between a miserly grasping at and hoarding of money and means, and a true use of the good things of this life for one's own comfort, and the relief of such as she might be enabled to befriend and assist. One thing she was sure of—that the precepts, 'Do unto oth-ers as ye would that others should do unto you,' 'Love your neighbor as yourself,' and so forth, were maxims that had been but little thought of by herself, or practised by those about her.

Her next decision was, that she must leave the city; it was no place for her; yea, she felt called in spirit to leave it, and to travel east and lecture. She had never been further east than the city, neither had she any friends there of whom she had particular reason to expect any thing; yet to her it was plain that her mission lay in the east, and that she would find friends there. She determined on leaving; but these determi-nations and convictions she kept close locked in her own breast, knowing that if her children and friends were aware of it, they would make such an ado about it as would render it very unpleasant, if not distressing to all parties. Having made what preparations for leaving she deemed necessary,—which was, to put up a few articles of clothing in a pillow-case, all else being deemed an unnecessary incumbrance,—about an hour before she left, she informed Mrs. Whiting, the woman of the house where she was stopping, that her name was no longer Isabella, but SOJOURNER; and that she was going east. And to her inquiry, 'What are you going east for?' her answer was, 'The Spirit calls me there, and I must go.'

She left the city on the morning of the 1st of June, 1843, crossing over to Brooklyn, L. I.; and taking the rising sun for her only compass and guide, she 'remembered Lot's wife,' and hoping to avoid her fate, she resolved not to look back till she felt sure the wicked city from which she was fleeing was left too far behind to be visible in the distance; and when she first ventured to look back, she could just discern the blue cloud of smoke that hung over it, and she thanked the Lord that she was thus far removed from what seemed to *her* a second Sodom.

She was now fairly started on her pilgrimage; her bundle in one hand, and a little basket of provisions in the other, and two York shillings in her purse—her heart strong in the faith that her true work lay before her, and that the Lord was her director; and she doubted not he would provide for and protect her, and that it would be very censurable in her to burden herself with any thing more than a moderate supply for her then present needs. Her mission was not merely to travel east, but to 'lecture,' as she designated it; 'testifying of the hope that was in her'—exhorting the people to embrace Jesus, and refrain from sin, the nature and origin of which she explained to them in accordance with her own most curious and original views. Through her life, and all its chequered changes, she has ever clung fast to her first permanent impressions on religious subjects.

Wherever night overtook her, there she sought for lodgings—free, if she might—if not, she paid; at a tavern, if she chanced to be at one—if not, at a private dwelling; with the rich, if they would receive her—if not, with the poor.

But she soon discovered that the largest houses were nearly always full; if not quite full, company was soon expected; and that it was much easier to find an unoccupied corner in a small house than in a large one; and if a person possessed but a miserable roof over his head, you might be sure of a welcome to part of it.

But this, she had penetration enough to see, was quite as much the effect of a want of sympathy as of benevolence; and this was also very apparent in her religious conversations with people who were strangers to her. She said, 'she never could find out that the rich had any religion. If *I* had been rich and accomplished, I could; for the rich could always find religion in the rich, and *I* could find it among the poor.'

At first, she attended such meetings as she heard of, in the vicinity of her travels, and spoke to the people as she found them assembled. Afterwards, she advertised meetings of her own, and held forth to large audiences, having, as she said, 'a good time.'

When she became weary of travelling, and wished a place to stop a while and rest herself, she said some opening for her was always near at hand; and the first time she needed rest, a man accosted her as she was walking, inquiring if she was looking for work. She told him that was not the object of her travels, but that she would willingly work a few days, if any one wanted. He requested her to go to his family, who were sadly in want of assistance, which he had been thus far unable to supply. She went to the house where she was directed, and was received by his family, one of whom was ill, as a 'God-send;' and when she felt constrained to resume her journey, they were very sorry, and would fain have detained her longer; but as she urged the necessity of leaving, they offered her what seemed in her eyes a great deal of money as a remuneration for her labor, and an expression of their gratitude for her opportune assistance; but she would only receive a very little of it; enough, as she says, to enable her to pay tribute to Cæsar, if it was demanded of her; and two or three York shillings at a time were all she allowed herself to take; and then, with purse replenished, and strength renewed, she would once more set out to perform her mission.

THE CONSEQUENCES OF REFUSING A TRAVELLER A NIGHT'S LODGING.

As she drew near the centre of the Island, she commenced, one evening at nightfall, to solicit the favor of a night's lodging. She had repeated her request a great many, it seemed to her some twenty times, and as many times she received a negative answer. She walked on, the stars and the tiny horns of the new-moon shed but a dim light on her lonely way, when she was familiarly accosted by two Indians, who took her for an acquaintance. She told them they were mistaken in the person; she was a stranger there, and asked them the direction to a tavern. They informed her it was yet a long way—some two miles or so; and inquired if she were alone. Not wishing for their protection, or knowing what might be the character of their kindness, she answered, 'No, not exactly,' and passed on. At the end of a weary way, she came to the tavern,—or, rather, to a large building, which was occupied as court-house, tavern, and jail,—and on asking for a night's lodging, was informed she could stay, if she would consent to be locked in. This to her mind was an insuperable objection. To have a key turned on her was a thing not to be thought of, at least not to be endured; and she again took up her line of march, preferring to walk beneath the open sky, to being locked up by a stranger in such a place. She had not walked far, before she heard the voice of a woman under an open shed; she ventured to accost her, and inquired if she knew where she could get in for the night. The woman answered, that she did not, unless she went home with them; and turning to her 'good man,' asked him if the stranger could not share their home for the night, to which he cheerfully assented. Sojourner thought it evident he had been taking a drop too much, but as he was civil and good-natured, and she did not feel inclined to spend the night alone in the open air, she felt driven to the necessity of accepting their hospitality, whatever it might prove to be. The woman soon informed her that there was a ball in the place, at which they would like to drop in a while, before they went to their home.

Balls being no part of Sojourner's mission, she was not desirous of attending; but her hostess could be satisfied with nothing short of a taste of it, and she was forced to go with her, or relinquish their company at once, in which move there might be more exposure than in accompanying her. She went, and soon found herself surrounded by an assemblage of people, collected from the very dregs of society, too ignorant and degraded to understand, much less entertain, a high or bright idea,—in a dirty hovel, destitute of every comfort, and where the fumes of whiskey were abundant and powerful.

Sojourner's guide there was too much charmed with the combined entertainments of the place to be able to tear herself away, till she found her faculties for enjoyment failing her, from a too free use of liquor; and she betook herself to bed till she could recover them. Sojourner, seated in a corner, had time for many reflections, and refrained from lecturing them, in obedience to the recommendation, 'Cast not your pearls,' &c. When the night was far spent, the husband of the sleeping woman aroused the sleeper, and reminded her that she was not very polite to the woman she had invited to sleep at her house, and of the propriety of returning home. They once more emerged into the pure air, which to our friend Sojourner, after so long breathing the noisome air of the ballroom, was most refreshing and grateful. Just as day dawned, they reached the place they called their home. Sojourner now saw that she had lost nothing in the shape of rest by remaining so long at the ball, as their miserable cabin afforded but one bunk or pallet for sleeping; and had there been many such, she would have preferred sitting up all night to occupying one like it. They very politely offered her the bed, if she would use it; but civilly declining, she waited for morning with an eagerness of desire she never felt before on the subject, and was never more happy than when the eye of day shed its golden light once more over the earth. She was once more free, and while day-light should last, independent, and needed no invitation to pursue her journey. Let these facts teach us, that every pedestrian in the world is not a vagabond, and that it is a dangerous thing to compel any one to receive that hospitality from the vicious and abandoned which they should have received from us,—as thousands can testify, who have thus been caught in the snares of the wicked.

The fourth of July, Isabella arrived at Huntingdon; from thence she went to Cold Springs, where she found the people making preparations for a mass temperance-meeting. With her usual alacrity, she entered into their labors, getting up dishes *a la New York*, greatly to the satisfaction of those she assisted. After remaining at Cold Springs some three weeks,

she returned to Huntingdon, where she took boat for Connecticut. Landing at Bridgeport, she again resumed her
travels towards the north-east, lecturing some, and working
some, to get wherewith to pay tribute to Cæsar, as she called
it; and in this manner she presently came to the city of New
Haven, where she found many meetings, which she attended
—at some of which, she was allowed to express her views
freely, and without reservation. She also called meetings expressly to give herself an opportunity to be heard; and found
in the city many true friends of Jesus, as she judged, with
whom she held communion of spirit, having no preference for
one sect more than another, but being well satisfied with all
who gave her evidence of having known or loved the Savior.

After thus delivering her testimony in this pleasant city,
feeling she had not as yet found an abiding place, she went
from thence to Bristol, at the request of a zealous sister, who
desired her to go to the latter place, and hold a religious conversation with some friends of hers there. She went as requested, found the people kindly and religiously disposed,
and through them she became acquainted with several very
interesting persons.

A spiritually-minded brother in Bristol, becoming interested in her new views and original opinions, requested as a
favor that she would go to Hartford, to see and converse with
friends of his there. Standing ready to perform any service in
the Lord, she went to Hartford as desired, bearing in her
hand the following note from this brother:—

'SISTER, —I send you this living messenger, as I believe her
to be one that God loves. Ethiopia is stretching forth her
hands unto God. You can see by this sister, that God does by
his Spirit alone teach his own children things to come. Please
receive her, and she will tell you some new things. Let her tell
her story without interrupting her, and give close attention,
and you will see she has got the lever of truth, that God helps
her to pry where but few can. She cannot read or write, but
the law is in her heart.

'Send her to brother ——, brother ——, and where she can
do the most good.

'From your brother,
H. L. B.'

SOME OF HER VIEWS AND
REASONINGS.

As soon as Isabella saw God as an all-powerful, all-pervading spirit, she became desirous of hearing all that had been written of him, and listened to the account of the creation of the world and its first inhabitants, as contained in the first chapters of Genesis, with peculiar interest. For some time she received it all literally, though it appeared strange to her that 'God worked by the day, got tired, and stopped to rest,' &c. But after a little time, she began to reason upon it, thus— 'Why, if God works by the day, and one day's work tires him, and he is obliged to rest, either from weariness or on account of darkness, or if he waited for the "cool of the day to walk in the garden," because he was inconvenienced by the heat of the sun, why then it seems that God cannot do as much as *I* can; for *I* can bear the sun at noon, and work several days and nights in succession without being much tired. Or, if he rested nights because of the darkness, it is very queer that he should make the night so dark that he could not see himself. If *I* had been God, I would have made the night light enough for my own convenience, surely.' But the moment she placed this idea of God by the side of the impression she had once so suddenly received of his inconceivable greatness and entire spirituality, that moment she exclaimed mentally, 'No, God does not stop to rest, for he is a spirit, and cannot tire; he cannot want for light, for he hath all light in himself. And if "God is all in all," and "worketh all in all," as I have heard them read, then it is impossible he should rest at all; for if he did, every other thing would stop and rest too; the waters would not flow, and the fishes could not swim; and all motion must cease. God could have no pauses in his work, and he needed no Sabbaths of rest. Man might need them, and he should take them when he needed them, whenever he required rest. As it regarded the worship of God, he was to be worshipped at all times and in all places; and one portion of time never seemed to her more holy than another.'

These views, which were the result of the workings of her own mind, assisted solely by the light of her own experience and very limited knowledge, were, for a long time after their adoption, closely locked in her own breast, fearing lest their avowal might bring upon her the imputation of 'infidelity,'—the usual charge preferred by all religionists, against those who entertain religious views and feelings differing materially from their own. If, from their own sad experience, they are withheld from shouting the cry of 'infidel,' they fail not to see and to feel, ay, and to say, that the dissenters are not of the right spirit, and that their spiritual eyes have never been unsealed.

While travelling in Connecticut, she met a minister, with whom she held a long discussion on these points, as well as on various other topics, such as the origin of all things, especially the origin of evil, at the same time bearing her testimony strongly against a paid ministry. He belonged to that class, and, as a matter of course, as strongly advocated his own side of the question.

I had forgotten to mention, in its proper place, a very important fact, that when she was examining the scriptures, she wished to hear them without comment; but if she employed adult persons to read them to her, and she asked them to read a passage over again, they invariably commenced to explain, by giving her their version of it; and in this way, they tried her feelings exceedingly. In consequence of this, she ceased to ask adult persons to read the Bible to her, and substituted children in their stead. Children, as soon as they could read distinctly, would re-read the same sentence to her, as often as she wished, and without comment;—and in that way she was enabled to see what her own mind could make out of the record, and that, she said, was what she wanted, and not what others thought it to mean. She wished to compare the teachings of the Bible with the witness within her; and she came to the conclusion, that the spirit of truth spoke in those records, but that the recorders of those truths had intermingled with them ideas and suppositions of their own. This is one among the many proofs of her energy and independence of character.

When it became known to her children, that Sojourner had left New York, they were filled with wonder and alarm. Where could she have gone, and why had she left? were questions no one could answer satisfactorily. Now, their imaginations painted her as a wandering maniac—and again they feared she had been left to commit suicide; and many were the tears they shed at the loss of her.

But when she reached Berlin, Conn., she wrote to them by amanuensis, informing them of her whereabouts, and waiting an answer to her letter; thus quieting their fears, and gladdening their hearts once more with assurances of her continued life and her love.

THE SECOND ADVENT DOCTRINES.

In Hartford and vicinity, she met with several persons who believed in the 'Second Advent' doctrines; or, the immediate personal appearance of Jesus Christ. At first she thought she had never heard of 'Second Advent.' But when it was explained to her, she recollected having once attended Mr. Miller's meeting in New York, where she saw a great many enigmatical pictures hanging on the wall, which she could not understand, and which, being out of the reach of her understanding, failed to interest her. In this section of country, she attended two camp-meetings of the believers in these doctrines—the 'second advent' excitement being then at its greatest height. The last meeting was at Windsor Lock. The people, as a matter of course, eagerly inquired of her concerning her belief, as it regarded their most important tenet. She told them it had not been revealed to her; perhaps, if she could read, she might see it differently. Sometimes, to their eager inquiry, 'Oh, don't you believe the Lord is coming?' she answered, 'I believe the Lord is as near as he can be, and not be it.' With these evasive and non-exciting answers, she kept their minds calm as it respected her unbelief, till she could have an opportunity to hear their views fairly stated, in order to judge more understandingly of this matter, and see if, in her estimation, there was any good ground for expecting an event which was, in the minds of so many, as it were, shaking the very foundations of the universe. She was invited to join them in their religious exercises, and accepted the invitation—praying, and talking in her own peculiar style, and attracting many about her by her singing.

When she had convinced the people that she was a lover of

God and his cause, and had gained a good standing with them, so that she could get a hearing among them, she had become quite sure in her own mind that they were laboring under a delusion, and she commenced to use her influence to calm the fears of the people, and pour oil upon the troubled waters. In one part of the grounds, she found a knot of people greatly excited: she mounted a stump and called out, 'Hear! hear!' When the people had gathered around her, as they were in a state to listen to any thing new, she addressed them as 'children,' and asked them why they made such a 'To-do;—are you not commanded to "watch and pray?" You are neither watching nor praying.' And she bade them, with the tones of a kind mother, retire to their tents, and there watch and pray, without noise or tumult, for the Lord would not come to such a scene of confusion; 'the Lord came still and quiet.' She assured them, 'the Lord might come, move all through the camp, and go away again, and they never know it,' in the state they then were.

They seemed glad to seize upon any reason for being less agitated and distressed, and many of them suppressed their noisy terror, and retired to their tents to 'watch and pray;' begging others to do the same, and listen to the advice of the good sister. She felt she had done some good, and then went to listen further to the preachers. They appeared to her to be doing their utmost to agitate and excite the people, who were already too much excited; and when she had listened till her feelings would let her listen silently no longer, she arose and addressed the preachers. The following are specimens of her speech:—

'Here you are talking about being "changed in the twinkling of an eye." If the Lord should come, he'd change you to *nothing*! for there is nothing to you.

'You seem to be expecting to go to some parlor *away up* somewhere, and when the wicked have been burnt, you are coming back to walk in triumph over their ashes—this is to be your New Jerusalem!! Now, *I* can't see any thing so very *nice* in that, coming back to such a *muss* as that will be, a world covered with the ashes of the wicked! Besides, if the Lord comes and burns—as you say he will—I am not going away; *I* am going to stay here and *stand the fire*, like Shadrach,

Meshach, and Abednego! And Jesus will walk with me through the fire, and keep me from harm. Nothing belonging to God can burn, any more than God himself; such shall have no need to go away to escape the fire! No, *I* shall remain. Do you tell me that God's children *can't stand fire?*' And her manner and tone spoke louder than words, saying, 'It is *absurd* to think so!'

The ministers were taken quite aback at so unexpected an opposer, and one of them, in the kindest possible manner, commenced a discussion with her, by asking her questions, and quoting scripture to her; concluding, finally, that although she had learned nothing of the great doctrine which was so exclusively occupying their minds at the time, she had learned much that man had never taught her.

At this meeting, she received the address of different persons, residing in various places, with an invitation to visit them. She promised to go soon to Cabotville, and started, shaping her course for that place. She arrived at Springfield one evening at six o'clock, and immediately began to search for a lodging for the night. She walked from six till past nine, and was then on the road from Springfield to Cabotville, before she found any one sufficiently hospitable to give her a night's shelter under their roof. Then a man gave her twenty-five cents, and bade her go to a tavern and stay all night. She did so, returning in the morning to thank him, assuring him she had put his money to its legitimate use. She found a number of the friends she had seen at Windsor when she reached the manufacturing town of Cabotville, (which has lately taken the name of Chicopee,) and with them she spent a pleasant week or more; after which, she left them to visit the Shaker village in Enfield. She now began to think of finding a resting place, at least, for a season; for she had performed quite a long journey, considering she had walked most of the way; and she had a mind to look in upon the Shakers, and see how things were there, and whether there was any opening there for her. But on her way back to Springfield, she called at a house and asked for a piece of bread; her request was granted, and she was kindly invited to tarry all night, as it was getting late, and she would not be able to stay at every house in that vicinity, which invitation she cheerfully accepted. When the man of the house came in, he recollected having seen her at the camp-meeting, and repeated some conversations, by which she recognized him again. He soon proposed having a meeting that evening, went out and notified his friends and neighbors, who came together, and she once more held forth to them in her peculiar style. Through the agency of this meeting, she became acquainted with several people residing in Springfield, to whose houses she was cordially invited, and with whom she spent some pleasant time.

One of these friends, writing of her arrival there, speaks as follows. After saying that she and her people belonged to that class of persons who believed in the second advent doctrines; and that this class, believing also in freedom of speech and action, often found at their meetings many singular people, who did not agree with them in their principal doctrine; and that, being thus prepared to hear new and strange things, 'They listened eagerly to Sojourner, and drank in all she said;'—and also, that she 'soon became a favorite among them; that when she arose to speak in their assemblies, her commanding figure and dignified manner hushed every trifler into silence, and her singular and sometimes uncouth modes of expression never provoked a laugh, but often were the whole audience melted into tears by her touching stories.' She also adds, 'Many were the lessons of wisdom and faith I have delighted to learn from her.' . . . . 'She continued a great favorite in our meetings, both on account of her remarkable gift in prayer, and still more remarkable talent for singing, . . . and the aptness and point of her remarks, frequently illustrated by figures the most original and expressive.

'As we were walking the other day, she said she had often thought what a beautiful world this would be, when we should see every thing right side up. Now, we see every thing topsy-turvy, and all is confusion.' For a person who knows nothing of this fact in the science of optics, this seemed quite a remarkable idea.

'We also loved her for her sincere and ardent piety, her unwavering faith in God, and her contempt of what the world calls fashion, and what we call folly.

'She was in search of a quiet place, where a way-worn traveller might rest. She had heard of Fruitlands, and was inclined to go there; but the friends she found here thought it best for her to visit Northampton. She passed her time, while with us, working wherever her work was needed, and talking where work was not needed.

'She would not receive money for her work, saying she worked for the Lord; and if her wants were supplied, she received it as from the Lord.

'She remained with us till far into winter, when we introduced her at the Northampton Association.' . . . . 'She wrote to me from thence, that she had found the quiet resting place she had so long desired. And she has remained there ever since.'

ANOTHER CAMP-MEETING.

When Sojourner had been at Northampton a few months, she attended another camp-meeting, at which she performed a very important part.

A party of wild young men, with no motive but that of entertaining themselves by annoying and injuring the feelings of others, had assembled at the meeting, hooting and yelling, and in various ways interrupting the services, and causing much disturbance. Those who had the charge of the meeting, having tried their persuasive powers in vain, grew impatient and tried threatening.

The young men, considering themselves insulted, collected their friends, to the number of a hundred or more, dispersed themselves through the grounds, making the most frightful noises, and threatening to fire the tents. It was said the authorities of the meeting sat in grave consultation, decided to have the ring-leaders arrested, and sent for the constable, to the great displeasure of some of the company, who were opposed to such an appeal to force and arms. Be that as it may, Sojourner, seeing great consternation depicted in every countenance, caught the contagion, and, ere she was aware, found herself quaking with fear.

Under the impulse of this sudden emotion, she fled to the most retired corner of a tent, and secreted herself behind a trunk, saying to herself, 'I am the only colored person here, and on me, probably, their wicked mischief will fall first, and perhaps fatally.' But feeling how great was her insecurity even there, as the very tent began to shake from its foundations, she began to soliloquise as follows:—

'Shall I run away and hide from the Devil? Me, a servant of the living God? Have I not faith enough to go out and quell that mob, when I know it is written—"One shall chase a thousand, and two put ten thousand to flight"? I know there are not a thousand here; and I know I am a servant of the living God. I'll go to the rescue, and the Lord shall go with and protect me.

'Oh,' said she, 'I felt as if I had *three hearts!* and that they were so large, my body could hardly hold them!'

She now came forth from her hiding-place, and invited several to go with her and see what they could do to still the raging of the moral elements. They declined, and considered her wild to think of it.

The meeting was in the open fields—the full moon shed its saddened light over all—and the woman who was that evening to address them was trembling on the preachers' stand. The noise and confusion were now terrific. Sojourner left the tent alone and unaided, and walking some thirty rods to the top of a small rise of ground, commenced to sing, in her most fervid manner, with all the strength of her most powerful voice, the hymn on the resurrection of Christ—

'It was early in the morning—it was early in the morning,
    Just at the break of day—
  When he rose—when he rose—when he rose,
    And went to heaven on a cloud.'

All who have ever heard her sing this hymn will probably remember it as long as they remember her. The hymn, the tune, the style, are each too closely associated with to be easily separated from herself, and when sung in one of her most animated moods, in the open air, with the utmost strength of her most powerful voice, must have been truly thrilling.

As she commenced to sing, the young men made a rush towards her, and she was immediately encircled by a dense body of the rioters, many of them armed with sticks or clubs as their weapons of defence, if not of attack. As the circle narrowed around her, she ceased singing, and after a short pause, inquired, in a gentle but firm tone, 'Why do you come about me with clubs and sticks? I am not doing harm to any one.' 'We ar'n't a going to hurt you, old woman; we came to hear you sing,' cried many voices, simultaneously. 'Sing to us, old woman,' cries one. 'Talk to us, old woman,' says another. 'Pray, old woman,' says a third. 'Tell us your experience,' says a fourth. 'You stand and smoke so near me, I cannot sing or talk,' she answered.

'Stand back,' said several authoritative voices, with not the most gentle or courteous accompaniments, raising their rude weapons in the air. The crowd suddenly gave back, the circle became larger, as many voices again called for singing, talking, or praying, backed by assurances that no one should be allowed to hurt her—the speakers declaring with an oath, that they would '*knock down*' any person who should offer her the least indignity.

She looked about her, and with her usual discrimination, said inwardly—'Here must be many young men in all this assemblage, bearing within them hearts susceptible of good impressions. I will speak to them.' She did speak; they silently heard, and civilly asked her many questions. It seemed to her to be given her at the time to answer them with truth and wisdom beyond herself. Her speech had operated on the roused passions of the mob like oil on agitated waters; they were, as a whole, entirely subdued, and only clamored when she ceased to speak or sing. Those who stood in the back ground, after the circle was enlarged, cried out, 'Sing aloud, old woman, we can't hear.' Those who held the sceptre of power among them requested that she should make a pulpit of a neighboring wagon. She said, 'If I do, they'll overthrow it.' 'No, they sha'n't—he who dares hurt you, we'll knock him down instantly, d—n him,' cried the chiefs. 'No we won't, no we won't, nobody shall hurt you,' answered the many voices of the mob. They kindly assisted her to mount the wagon, from which she spoke and sung to them about an hour. Of all she said to them on the occasion, she remembers only the following:—

'Well, there are two congregations on this ground. It is written that there shall be a separation, and the sheep shall be separated from the goats. The other preachers have the sheep, *I* have the goats. And I have a few sheep among my goats, but they are *very* ragged.' This exordium produced great laughter. When she became wearied with talking, she began to cast about her to contrive some way to induce them to disperse. While she paused, they loudly clamored for 'more,' 'more,'—'sing,' 'sing more.' She motioned them to be quiet, and called out to them: 'Children, I have talked and sung to you, as you asked me; and now I have a request to make of you; will you grant it?' 'Yes, yes, yes,' resounded from every quarter. 'Well, it is this,' she answered; 'if I will sing one more hymn for you, will you then go away, and leave us this night in peace?' 'Yes, yes,' came faintly, feebly from a few. 'I repeat it,' says Sojourner, 'and I want an answer from you all, as of one accord. If I will sing you one more, will you go away, and leave us this night in peace?' 'Yes, yes, yes,' shouted many voices, with hearty emphasis. 'I repeat my request once more,' said she, 'and I want you *all* to answer.' And she reiterated the words again. This time a long, loud 'Yes—yes—yes,' came up, as from the multitudinous mouth of the entire mob. 'AMEN! it is SEALED,' repeated Sojourner, in the deepest and most solemn tones of her powerful and sonorous voice. Its effect ran through the multitude, like an electric shock; and the most of them considered themselves bound by their promise, as they might have failed to do under less imposing circumstances. Some of them began instantly to leave; others said, 'Are we not to have one more hymn?' 'Yes,' answered their entertainer, and she commenced to sing:

'I bless the Lord I've got my seal—to-day and to-day—
To slay Goliath in the field—to-day and to-day;
The good old way is a righteous way,
I mean to take the kingdom in the good old way.'

While singing, she heard some enforcing obedience to their promise, while a few seemed refusing to abide by it. But before she had quite concluded, she saw them turn from her, and in the course of a few minutes, they were running as fast as they well could in a solid body; and she says she can compare them to nothing but a swarm of bees, so dense was their phalanx, so straight their course, so hurried their march. As they passed with a rush very near the stand of the other preachers, the hearts of the people were smitten with fear, thinking that their entertainer had failed to enchain them longer with her spell, and that they were coming upon them with redoubled and remorseless fury. But they found they were mistaken, and that their fears were groundless; for, before they could well recover from their surprise, every rioter was gone, and not one was left on the grounds, or seen there again during the meeting. Sojourner was informed that as her audience reached the main road, some distance from the tents, a few of the rebellious spirits refused to go on, and proposed returning; but their leaders said, 'No—we have promised to leave—all promised, and we must go, all go, and you shall none of you return again.'

She did not fall in love at first sight with the Northampton Association, for she arrived there at a time when appearances did not correspond with the ideas of associationists, as they had been spread out in their writings; for their phalanx was a factory, and they were wanting in means to carry out their ideas of beauty and elegance, as they would have done in different circumstances. But she thought she would make an effort to tarry with them one night, though that seemed to her no desirable affair. But as soon as she saw that accomplished, literary and refined persons were living in that plain and simple manner, and submitting to the labors and privations incident to such an infant institution, she said, 'Well, if these can live here, *I* can.' Afterwards, she gradually became pleased with, and attached to, the place and the people, as well she might; for it must have been no small thing to have found a home in a 'Community composed of some of the choicest spirits of the age,' where all was characterised by an equality of feeling, a liberty of thought and speech, and a largeness of soul, she could not have before met with, to the same extent, in any of her wanderings.

Our first knowledge of her was derived from a friend who had resided for a time in the 'Community,' and who, after describing her, and singing one of her hymns, wished that we might see her. But we little thought, at that time, that we should ever pen these 'simple annals' of this child of nature.

When we first saw her, she was working with a hearty good will; saying she would not be induced to take regular wages, believing, as once before, that now Providence had provided her with a never-failing fount, from which her every want might be perpetually supplied through her mortal life. In this, she had calculated too fast. For the Associationists found, that, taking every thing into consideration, they would find it most expedient to act individually; and again, the subject of this sketch found her dreams unreal, and herself flung back upon her own resources for the supply of her needs. This she might have found more inconvenient at her time of life—for labor, exposure and hardship had made sad inroads upon her iron constitution, by inducing chronic disease and premature old age—had she not remained under the shadow of one,* who never wearies in doing good, giving to the needy, and supplying the wants of the destitute. She has now set her heart upon having a little home of her own, even at this late hour of life, where she may feel a greater freedom than she can in the house of another, and where she can repose a little, after her day of action has passed by. And for such a 'home' she is now dependant on the charities of the benevolent, and to them we appeal with confidence.

Through all the scenes of her eventful life may be traced the energy of a naturally powerful mind—the fearlessness and child-like simplicity of one untrammelled by education or conventional customs—purity of character—an unflinching adherence to principle—and a native enthusiasm, which, under different circumstances, might easily have produced another Joan of Arc.

With all her fervor, and enthusiasm, and speculation, her religion is not tinctured in the least with gloom. No doubt, no hesitation, no despondency, spreads a cloud over her soul; but all is bright, clear, positive, and at times ecstatic. Her trust is in God, and from him she looks for good, and not evil. She feels that 'perfect love casteth out fear.'

*GEORGE W. BENSON.

Having more than once found herself awaking from a mortifying delusion,—as in the case of the Sing-Sing kingdom,—and resolving not to be thus deluded again, she has set suspicion to guard the door of her heart, and allows it perhaps to be aroused by too slight causes, on certain subjects—her vivid imagination assisting to magnify the phantoms of her fears into gigantic proportions, much beyond their real size; instead of resolutely adhering to the rule we all like best, when it is to be applied to ourselves—that of placing every thing we see to the account of the best possible motive, until time and circumstance prove that we were wrong. Where no good motive can be assigned, it may become our duty to suspend our judgment till evidence can be had.

In the application of this rule, it is an undoubted duty to exercise a commendable prudence, by refusing to repose any important trust to the keeping of persons who may be strangers to us, and whose trustworthiness we have never seen tried. But no possible good, but incalculable evil may and does arise from the too common practice of placing all conduct, the source of which we do not fully understand, to the worst of intentions. How often is the gentle, timid soul discouraged, and driven perhaps to despondency, by finding its 'good evil spoken of;' and a well-meant but mistaken action loaded with an evil design!

If the world would but sedulously set about reforming itself on this one point, who can calculate the change it would produce—the evil it would annihilate, and the happiness it would confer! None but an all-seeing eye could at once embrace so vast a result. A result, how desirable! and one that can be brought about only by the most simple process—that of every individual seeing to it that he commit not this sin himself. For why should we allow in ourselves, the very fault we most dislike, when committed against us? Shall we not at least aim at consistency?

Had she possessed less generous self-sacrifice, more knowledge of the world and of business matters in general, and had she failed to take it for granted that others were like herself, and would, when her turn came to need, do as she had done, and find it 'more blessed to give than to receive,' she might have laid by something for the future. For few, perhaps, have ever possessed the power and inclination, in the same degree, at one and the same time, to labor as she has done, both day and night, for so long a period of time. And had these energies been well-directed, and the proceeds well husbanded, since she has been her own mistress, they would have given her an independence during her natural life. But her constitutional biases, and her early training, or rather want of training, prevented this result; and it is too late now to remedy the great mistake. Shall she then be left to want? Who will not answer, 'No!'

LAST INTERVIEW WITH HER MASTER.

In the spring of 1849, Sojourner made a visit to her eldest daughter, Diana, who has ever suffered from ill health, and remained with Mr. Dumont, Isabella's humane master. She found him still living, though advanced in age, and reduced in property, (as he had been for a number of years,) but greatly enlightened on the subject of slavery. He said he could then see, that 'slavery was the wickedest thing in the world, the greatest curse the earth had ever felt'—that it was then very clear to his mind that it was so, though, while he was a slaveholder himself, he did not see it so, and thought it was as right as holding any other property. Sojourner remarked to him, that it might be the same with those who are now slaveholders. 'O, no,' replied he, with warmth, 'it cannot be. For, now, the sin of slavery is so clearly written out, and so much talked against,—(why, the whole world cries out against it!)—that if any one says he don't know, and has not heard, he must, I think, be a liar. In my slaveholding days, there were few that spoke against it, and these few made little impression on any one. Had it been as it is now, think you I could have held slaves? No! I should not have dared to do it, but should have emancipated every one of them. Now, it is very different; all may hear if they will.'

Yes, reader, if any one feels that the tocsin of alarm, or the anti-slavery trump, must sound a louder note before they can hear it, one would think they must be very hard of hearing,—yea, that they belong to that class, of whom it may be truly said, 'they have stopped their ears that they may not hear.'

She received a letter from her daughter Diana, dated Hyde Park, December 19, 1849, which informed her that Mr. Dumont had 'gone West' with some of his sons—that he had taken along with him, probably through mistake, the few articles of furniture she had left with him. 'Never mind,' says Sojourner, 'what we give to the poor, we lend to the Lord.' She thanked the Lord with fervor, that she had lived to hear her master say such blessed things! She recalled the lectures he used to give his slaves, on speaking the truth and being honest, and laughing, she says he taught us not to lie and steal, when *he* was stealing all the time himself, and did not know it! Oh! how sweet to my mind was this confession! And what a confession for a master to make to a slave! A slaveholding master turned to a brother! Poor old man, may the Lord bless him, and all slaveholders partake of his spirit!

END OF THE NARRATIVE.

APPENDIX.

[Extract from 'Slavery as It Is.']
SLAVERY A SYSTEM OF INHERENT CRUELTY.
BY THEODORE D. WELD.

THIRTY hundred thousand persons in this country, men, women and children, are in SLAVERY. Is slavery, as a condition for human beings, good, bad, or indifferent? We submit the question without argument. You have common sense, and conscience, and a human heart;—pronounce upon it. You have a wife, or a husband, a child, a father, a mother, a brother or a sister—make the case your own, make it theirs, and bring in your verdict. The case of Human Rights against Slavery has been adjudicated in the court of conscience times innumerable. The same verdict has always been rendered—'Guilty;' the same sentence has always been pronounced, 'Let it be accursed!' and human nature, with her million echoes, has rung it round the world in every language under heaven, 'Let it be accursed! Let it be accursed!' His heart is false to human nature, who will not say 'Amen.' There is not a man on earth who does not believe that slavery is a curse. Human beings may be inconsistent, but human *nature* is true to herself. She has uttered her testimony against slavery with a shriek ever since the monster was begotten; and till it perishes amidst the execrations of the universe, she will traverse the world on its track, dealing her bolts upon its head, and dashing against it her condemning brand. We repeat it, every man knows that slavery is a curse. Whoever denies this, his lips libel his heart. Try him; clank the chains in his ears, and tell him they are for *him*; give him an hour to prepare his wife and children for a life of slavery; bid him make haste and get ready their necks for the yoke, and their wrists for the coffle chains, then look at his pale lips and trembling knees, and you have *nature's* testimony against slavery.

At least thirty hundred thousand persons in these States are in this condition. They were made slaves and are held such by force, and by being put in fear, and this for no crime! Reader, what have you to say of such treatment? Is it right, just, benevolent? Suppose I should seize you, rob you of your liberty, drive you into the field, and make you work without pay as long as you live, would that be justice and kindness, or monstrous injustice and cruelty? Now, every body knows that the slaveholders do these things to the slaves every day, and yet it is stoutly affirmed that they treat them well and kindly, and that their tender regard for their slaves restrains their masters from inflicting cruelties upon them. We shall go into no metaphysics to show the absurdity of this pretence. The man who *robs* you every day, is, forsooth, quite too tender-hearted ever to cuff or kick you! True, he can snatch your money, but he does it gently, lest he should hurt you. He can empty your pockets without qualms, but if your *stomach* is empty, it cuts him to the quick. He can make you work a life-time without pay, but loves you too well to let you go hungry. He fleeces you of your *rights* with a relish, but is shocked if you work bareheaded in summer, or in winter without warm stockings. He can make you go without your *liberty*, but never without a shirt. He can crush, in you, all hope of bettering your condition, by vowing that you shall die his slave, but though he can coolly torture your feelings, he is too compassionate to lacerate your back—he can break your heart, but he is very tender of your skin. He can strip you of all protection and thus expose you to all outrages, but if you are exposed to the *weather*, half clad and half sheltered, how yearn his tender bowels! What! slaveholders talk of treating men well, and yet not only rob them of all they get, and as fast as they get it, but rob them of *themselves*, also; their very hands and feet, all their muscles, and limbs, and senses, their bodies and minds, their time and liberty and earnings, their free speech and rights of conscience, their right to acquire knowledge, and property, and reputation;—and yet they, who plunder them of all these, would fain make us believe that their soft hearts ooze out so lovingly toward their slaves, that they always keep them well housed and well clad, never push them too hard in the field, never make their dear backs smart, nor let their dear stomachs get empty.

But there is no end to these absurdities. Are slaveholders dunces, or do they take all the rest of the world to be, that they think to bandage our eyes with such thin gauzes? Protesting their kind regard for those whom they hourly plunder of all they have and all they get! What! when they have seized their victims, and annihilated all their *rights*, still claim to be the special guardians of their *happiness*? Plunderers of their liberty, yet the careful suppliers of their wants? Robbers of their earnings, yet watchful sentinels round their interests, and kind providers for their comfort? Filching all their time, yet granting generous donations for rest and sleep? Stealing the use of their muscles, yet thoughtful of their ease? Putting them under *drivers*, yet careful that they are not hard-pushed? Too humane, forsooth, to stint the stomachs of their slaves, yet force their *minds* to starve, and brandish over them pains and penalties, if they dare to reach forth for the smallest crumb of knowledge, even a letter of the alphabet!

It is no marvel that slaveholders are always talking of their *kind treatment* of their slaves. The only marvel is, that men of sense can be gulled by such professions. Despots always insist that they are merciful. The greatest tyrants that ever dripped with blood have assumed the titles of 'most gracious,' 'most clement,' 'most merciful,' &c., and have ordered their crouching vassals to accost them thus. When did not vice lay claim to those virtues which are the opposites of its habitual crimes? The guilty, according to their own showing, are always innocent, and cowards brave, and drunkards sober, and harlots chaste, and pickpockets honest to a fault. Every body understands this. When a man's tongue grows thick, and he begins to hiccough and walk cross-legged, we expect him, as a matter of course, to protest that he is not drunk; so when a man is always singing the praises of his own honesty, we instinctively watch his movements and look out for our pocket-books. Whoever is simple enough to be hoaxed by such professions, should never be trusted in the streets without somebody to take care of him. Human nature works out in slaveholders just as it does in other men, and in American slaveholders just as in English, French, Turkish, Algerine, Roman and Grecian. The Spartans boasted of their kindness to their slaves, while they whipped them to death by thousands at the altars of their gods. The Romans lauded their own mild treatment of their bondsmen, while they branded their names on their flesh with hot irons, and when old, threw them into their fish ponds, or like Cato 'the Just,' starved them to death. It is the boast of the Turks, that they treat their slaves as though they were their children, yet their common name for them is 'dogs,' and for the merest trifles, their feet are bastinadoed to a jelly, or their heads clipped off with a scimetar. The Portuguese pride themselves on their gentle bearing towards their slaves, yet the streets of Rio Janeiro are filled with naked men and women yoked in pairs to carts and wagons, and whipped by drivers like beasts of burden.

Slaveholders, the world over, have sung the praises of their tender mercies towards their slaves. Even the wretches that plied the African slave trade tried to rebut Clarkson's proofs of their cruelties, by speeches, affidavits, and published pamphlets, setting forth the accommodations of the 'middle passage,' and their kind attentions to the comfort of those whom they had stolen from their homes, and kept stowed away under hatches, during a voyage of four thousand miles. So, according to the testimony of the autocrat of the Russias, he exercises great clemency towards the Poles, though he exiles them by thousands to the snows of Siberia, and tramples them down by millions at home. Who discredits the atrocities perpetrated by Ovando in Hispaniola, Pizarro in Peru, and Cortez in Mexico,—because they filled the ears of the Spanish Court with protestations of their benignant rule? While they were yoking the enslaved natives like beasts to the draught, working them to death by thousands in their mines, hunting them with bloodhounds, torturing them on racks, and broiling them on beds of coals, their representations to the mother country teemed with eulogies of their parental sway! The bloody atrocities of Philip II., in the expulsion of his Moorish subjects, are matters of imperishable history. Who disbelieves or doubts them? And yet his courtiers magnified his virtues and chanted his clemency and his mercy, while the wail of a million victims, smitten down by a tempest of fire and slaughter let loose at his bidding, rose above the *Te Deums* that thundered from all Spain's cathedrals. When Louis XIV. revoked the edict of Nantes, and proclaimed two millions of his subjects free plunder for persecution,—when from the English channel to the Pyrennees the mangled bodies of the Protestants were dragged on reeking hurdles by a shouting populace,—he claimed to be 'the father of his people,' and wrote himself 'His most *Christian* Majesty.'

That the slaves in the United States are treated with barbarous inhumanity; that they are over-worked, under-fed, wretchedly clad and lodged, and have insufficient sleep; that they are often made to wear round their necks iron collars armed with prongs, to drag heavy chains and weights at their feet while working in the field, and to wear yokes, and bells, and iron horns; that they are often kept confined in the stocks day and night for weeks together, made to wear gags in their mouths for hours or days, have some of their front teeth torn out or broken off, that they may be easily detected when they run away; that they are frequently flogged with terrible severity, have red pepper rubbed into their lacerated flesh, and hot brine, spirits of turpentine, &c., poured over the gashes to increase the torture; that they are often stripped naked, their backs and limbs cut with knives, bruised and mangled by scores and hundreds of blows with the paddle, and terribly torn by the claws of cats, drawn over them by their tormentors; that they are often hunted with bloodhounds and shot down like beasts, or torn in pieces by dogs; that they are often suspended by the arms and whipped and beaten till they faint, and when revived by restoratives, beaten again till they faint, and sometimes till they die; that their ears are often cut off, their eyes knocked out, their bones broken, their flesh branded with red hot irons; that they are maimed, mutilated and burned to death over slow fires; are undeniable facts.

The enormities inflicted by slaveholders upon their slaves will never be discredited, except by those who overlook the simple fact, that he who holds human beings as his *bona fide* property, regards them as property, and not as *persons*; this is his permanent state of mind toward them. He does not contemplate slaves as human beings, consequently does not treat them as such; and with entire indifference sees them suffer privations and writhe under blows, which, if inflicted upon whites, would fill him with horror and indignation. He regards that as good treatment of slaves, which would seem to him insufferable abuse, if practised upon others; and would denounce that as a monstrous outrage and horrible cruelty, if perpetrated upon white men and women, which he sees every day meted out to black slaves, without perhaps ever thinking it cruel. Accustomed all his life to regard them rather as domestic animals, to hear them stormed at, and to see them cuffed and caned; and being himself in constant habit of treating them thus, such practices have become to him a mere matter of course, and make no impression on his mind. True, it is incredible that men should treat as *chattels* those whom they truly regard as *human beings*; but that they should treat as chattels and working animals those whom they *regard* as such, is no marvel. The common treatment of dogs, when they are in the way, is to kick them out of it; we see them every day kicked off of sidewalks, and on Sabbaths out of churches—yet, as they are but dogs, these do not strike us as outrages; yet if we were to see men, women and children—our neighbors and friends—kicked out of stores by merchants, or out of churches by the deacons and sexton, we should call the perpetrators inhuman wretches.

We have said that slaveholders regard their slaves not as human beings, but as mere working animals, or merchandise. The whole vocabulary of slaveholders, their laws, their usages, and their entire treatment of their slaves, fully establish this. The same terms are applied to slaves that are given to cattle. They are called 'stock.' So, when the children of slaves are spoken of prospectively, they are called their 'increase;' the same term that is applied to flocks and herds. So the female slaves that are mothers are called 'breeders,' till past child-bearing; and often the same terms are applied to the different sexes that are applied to the males and females among cattle. Those who compel the labor of slaves and cattle have the same appellation, 'drivers;' the names which they call them are the same, and similar to those given to their horses and oxen. The laws of slave States make them property, equally with goats and swine; they are levied upon for debt in the same way; they are included in the same advertisements of public sales with cattle, swine and asses; when moved from one part of the country to another, they are herded in droves like cattle, and like them urged on by drivers; their labor is compelled in the same way. They are bought and sold, and separated like cattle; when exposed for sale, their good qualities are described as jockeys show off the good points of their horses; their strength, activity, skill, power of endurance, &c., are lauded, and those who bid upon them examine their persons, just as purchasers inspect horses and oxen; they open their mouths to see if their teeth are sound; strip their backs to see if they are badly scarred, and handle their limbs and muscles to see if they are firmly knit. Like horses, they are warranted to be 'sound,' or to be returned to the owner if 'unsound.' A father gives his son a horse and *slave*; by his will he distributes among them his racehorses, hounds, game-cocks and *slaves*. We leave the reader to carry out the parallel which we have only begun. Its details would cover many pages.

That slaveholders do not practically regard slaves as *human beings* is abundantly shown by their own voluntary testimony. In a recent work entitled, 'The South Vindicated from the Treason and Fanaticism of Northern Abolitionists,' which was written, we are informed, by Colonel Dayton, late member of Congress from South Carolina, the writer, speaking of the awe with which the slaves regard the whites, says—

'The Northerner looks upon a band of negroes as upon so many *men*, but the planter or Southerner *views them in a very different light!*'

Extract from a speech of Mr. SUMMERS, of Virginia, in the Legislature of that State, January 26, 1832. See the Richmond Whig: –

'When, in the sublime lessons of Christianity, he (the slaveholder) is taught to "do unto others as he would have others do unto him," HE NEVER DREAMS THAT THE DEGRADED NEGRO IS WITHIN THE PALE OF THAT HOLY CANON.'

PRESIDENT JEFFERSON, in his letter to GOVERNOR COLES, of Illinois, dated August 25, 1814, asserts that slaveholders regard their slaves as brutes, in the following remarkable language:—

'Nursed and educated in the daily habit of seeing the degraded condition, both bodily and mental, of these unfortunate beings, [the slaves,] FEW MINDS HAVE YET DOUBTED BUT THAT THEY WERE AS LEGITIMATE SUBJECTS OF PROPERTY AS THEIR HORSES OR CATTLE.'

Having shown that slaveholders regard their slaves as mere working animals and cattle, we now proceed to show that their actual treatment of them is *worse* than it would be if they were brutes. We repeat it, SLAVEHOLDERS TREAT THEIR SLAVES WORSE THAN THEY DO THEIR BRUTES. Whoever heard of cows or sheep being deliberately tied up and beaten and lacerated till they died? or horses coolly tortured by the hour, till covered with mangled flesh? or of swine having their legs tied and being suspended from a tree and lacerated with thongs for hours? or of hounds stretched and made fast at full length, flayed with whips, red pepper rubbed into their bleeding gashes, and hot brine dashed on to aggravate the torture? Yet, just such forms and degrees of torture are *daily* perpetrated upon the slaves. Now, no man that knows human nature will marvel at this. Though great cruelties have always been inflicted by men upon brutes, yet incomparably the most horrid ever perpetrated have been those of men upon *their own species*. Any leaf of history turned over at random has proof enough of this. Every reflecting mind perceives that when men hold *human beings* as *property*, they must, from the nature of the case, treat them worse than they treat their horses and oxen. It is impossible for *cattle* to excite in men such tempests of fury as men excite in each other. Men are often provoked if their horses or hounds refuse to do, or their pigs refuse to go where they wish to drive them, but the feeling is rarely intense and never permanent. It is vexation and impatience, rather than settled rage, malignity, or revenge. If horses and dogs were intelligent beings, and still held as property, their opposition to the wishes of their owners would exasperate them immeasurably more than it would be possible for them to do, with the minds of brutes. None but little children and idiots get angry at sticks and stones that lie in their way or hurt them; but put into sticks and stones intelligence, and will, and power of feeling and motion, while they remain as now, articles of property, and what a towering rage would men be in, if bushes whipped them in the face when they walked among them, or stones rolled over their toes when they climbed hills! and what exemplary vengeance would be inflicted upon door-stops and hearth-stones, if they were to move out of their places, instead of lying still where they were put for their owners to tread upon. The greatest provocation to human nature is *opposition to its will*. If a man's will be resisted by one far *below* him, the provocation is vastly greater, than when it is resisted by an acknowledged superior. In the former case, it inflames strong passions, which in the latter lie dormant. The rage of proud Haman knew no bounds against the poor Jew who would not do as he wished, and so he built a gallows for him. If the person opposing the will of another be so far below him as to be on a level with chattels, and be actually held and used as an article of property, pride, scorn, lust of power, rage and revenge explode together upon the hapless victim. The idea of *property* having a will, and that too in opposition to the will of its *owner*, and counteracting it, is a stimulant of terrible power to the most relentless human passions; and from the nature of slavery, and the constitution of the human mind, this fierce stimulant must, with various degrees of strength, act upon slaveholders almost without ceasing. The slave, however abject and crushed, is an intelligent being: he has a *will*, and that will cannot be annihilated, *it will show itself;* if for a moment it is smothered, like pent up fires, when vent is found, it flames the fiercer. Make intelligence *property*, and its manager will have his match; he is met at every turn by an *opposing will*, not in the form of downright rebellion and defiance, but yet, visibly, an *ever-opposing will*. He sees it in the dissatisfied look, and reluctant air, and unwilling movement; the constrained strokes of labor, the drawling tones, the slow hearing, the feigned stupidity, the sham pains and sickness, the short memory; and he *feels* it every hour, in innumerable forms, frustrating his designs by a ceaseless, though perhaps invisible countermining. This unceasing opposition to the will of its 'owner,' on the part of his rational 'property,' is to the slaveholder as the hot iron to the nerve. He raves under it, and storms, and gnashes, and smites; but the more he smites, the hotter it gets, and the more it burns him. Further, this opposition of the slave's will to his owner's, not only excites him to severity, that he may gratify his rage, but makes it necessary for him to use violence in breaking down this resistance— thus subjecting the slave to additional tortures. There is another inducement to cruel inflictions upon the slave, and a necessity for it, which does not exist in the case of brutes. Offenders must be made an example to others, to strike them with terror. If a slave runs away and is caught, his master flogs him with terrible severity, not merely to gratify his resentment, and to keep him from running away again, but as a warning to others. So in every case of disobedience, neglect, stubbornness, unfaithfulness, indolence, insolence, theft, feigned sickness, when his directions are forgotten, or slighted, or supposed to be, or his wishes crossed, or his property injured, or left exposed, or his work ill-executed, the master is tempted to inflict cruelties, not merely to wreak his own vengeance upon him, and to make the slave more circumspect in future, but to sustain his authority over the other slaves, to restrain them from like practices, and to preserve his own property.

A multitude of facts, illustrating the position that slaveholders treat their slaves *worse* than they do their cattle, will occur to all who are familiar with slavery. When cattle break through their owners' inclosures and escape, if found, they are driven back and fastened in again; and even slaveholders would execrate as a wretch, the man who should tie them up, and bruise and lacerate them for straying away; but when *slaves* that have escaped are caught, they are flogged with the most terrible severity. When herds of cattle are driven to market, they are suffered to go in the easiest way, each by himself; but when slaves are driven to market, they are fastened together with handcuffs, galled by iron collars and chains, and thus forced to travel on foot hundreds of miles, sleeping at night in their chains. Sheep, and sometimes horned cattle, are marked with their owners' initials—but this is generally done with paint, and of course produces no pain. Slaves, too, are often marked with their owners' initials, but the letters are stamped into their flesh with a hot iron. Cattle are suffered to graze their pastures without stint; but the slaves are restrained in their food to a fixed allowance. The slaveholders' horses are notoriously far better fed, more moderately worked, have fewer hours of labor, and longer intervals of rest, than their slaves; and their valuable horses are far more comfortably housed and lodged, and their stables more effectually defended from the weather, than the slaves' huts.

These objectors can really believe the fact, that in the city of New York, less than a hundred years since, thirteen persons were publicly burned to death, over a slow fire: and that the legislature of the same State took under its paternal care the African slave-trade, and declared that 'all encouragement should be given to the *direct* importation of slaves; that all *smuggling* of slaves should be condemned, as *an eminent discouragement to the fair trader.*'

They do not call in question the fact that the African slave-trade was carried on from the ports of the free States till within thirty years; that even members of the Society of Friends were actively engaged in it, shortly before the revolutionary war;* that as late as 1807, no less than fifty-nine of the vessels engaged in that trade were sent out from the little State of Rhode Island, which had then only about seventy thousand inhabitants; that among those most largely engaged in those foul crimes, are the men whom the people of Rhode Island delight to honor: that the man who dipped most deeply in that trade of blood, (James De Wolf,) and amassed a most princely fortune by it, was not long since their Senator in Congress; and another, who was captain of one of his vessels, was recently Lieutenant Governor of the State.

They can believe, too, all the horrors of the middle passage, the chains, suffocation, maimings, stranglings, starvation, and cold-blooded murders, atrocities perpetrated on board these slave-ships by their own citizens, perhaps by their own townsmen and neigh-

*See Life and Travels of John Woolman, page 92.

bors—possibly by their own *fathers*: but, O! they 'can't believe that the slaveholders can be so hard-hearted towards their slaves as to treat them with great cruelty.' They can believe that His Holiness the Pope, with his cardinals, bishops and priests, have tortured, broken on the wheel, and burned to death thousands of Protestants—that eighty thousand of the Anabaptists were slaughtered in Germany—that hundreds of thousands of the blameless Waldenses, Huguenots and Lollards, were torn in pieces by the most titled dignitaries of church and state, and that *almost every professedly Christian sect has, at some period of its history, persecuted unto blood* those who dissented from their creed. They can believe, also, that in Boston, New York, Utica, Philadelphia, Cincinnati, Alton, and scores of other cities and villages of the free States, 'gentlemen of property and standing,' led on by civil officers, by members of State legislatures, and of Congress, by judges and attorneys-general, by editors of newspapers, and by professed ministers of the gospel, have organized mobs, broken up lawful meetings of peaceable citizens, committed assault and battery upon their persons, knocked them down with stones, led them about with ropes, dragged them from their beds at midnight, gagged and forced them into vehicles, and driven them into unfrequented places, and there tormented and disfigured them—that they have rifled their houses, made bonfires of their furniture in the streets, burned to the ground, or torn in pieces the halls or churches in which they were assembled—attacked them with deadly weapons, stabbed some, shot others, and killed one. They can believe all this—and further, that a majority of the citizens in the places where these outrages have been committed, connived at them; and by refusing to indict the perpetrators, or, if they were indicted, by combining to secure their acquittal, and rejoicing in it, have publicly adopted these felonies as their own. All these things they can believe without hesitation, and that they have been been done by their own acquaintances, neighbors, relatives; perhaps those with whom they interchange courtesies, those for whom they *vote*, or to whose *salaries they contribute*—but yet, O! they can never believe that slaveholders inflict cruelties upon their slaves!

They can give full credence to the kidnapping, imprisonment, and deliberate murder of WILLIAM MORGAN, and that by men of high standing in society; they can believe that this deed was aided and abetted, and the murderers screened from justice, by a large number of influential persons, who were virtually accomplices, either before or after the fact; and that this combination was so effectual, as successfully to defy and triumph over the combined powers of the government;—yet that those who constantly rob men of their time, liberty and wages, and all their *rights*, should rob them of bits of flesh, and occasionally of a tooth, make their backs bleed, and put fetters on their legs, is too monstrous to be credited! Further, these same persons, who 'can't believe' that slaveholders are so iron-hearted as to ill-treat their slaves, believe that the very *elite* of these slaveholders, those most highly esteemed and honored among them, are continually daring each other to mortal conflict, and in the presence of mutual friends, taking deadly aim at each other's hearts, with settled purpose to *kill*, if possible. That among the most distinguished Governors of slave States, among their most celebrated judges, senators, and representatives in Congress, there is hardly *one* who has not either killed, or tried to kill, or aided and abetted his friends in trying to kill, one or more individuals. That pistols, dirks, bowie-knives, or other instruments of death, are generally carried throughout the slave States—and that deadly affrays with them, in the streets of their cities and villages, are matters of daily occurrence; that the sons of slaveholders in southern colleges bully, threaten, and fire upon their teachers, and their teachers upon them; that, during the last summer, in the most celebrated seat of science and literature in the South, the University of Virginia, the professors were attacked by more than seventy armed students, and, in the words of a Virginia paper, were obliged 'to conceal themselves from their fury;' also, that almost all the riots and violence that occur in northern colleges are produced by the turbulence and lawless passions of southern students. That such are the furious passions of slaveholders, no considerations of personal respect, none for the proprieties of life, none for the honor of our national legislature, none for the character of our country abroad, can restrain the slaveholding members of Congress from the most disgraceful personal encounters on the floor of our nation's legislature—smiting their fists in each other's faces, throttling, and even *kicking* and trying to *gouge* each other; that, during the session of the Congress just closed, no less than six slaveholders, taking fire at words spoken in debate, have either rushed at each other's throats, or kicked, or struck, or attempted to knock each other down; and that in all these instances, they would doubtless have killed each other, if their friends had not separated them. Further, they know full well, these were not insignificant, vulgar blackguards, elected because they were the head bullies and bottle-holders in a boxing ring, or because their constituents went drunk to the ballot-box; but they were some of the most conspicuous members of the House—one of them a former Speaker.

Our newspapers are full of these and similar daily occurrences among slaveholders, copied verbatim from their own accounts of them in their own papers, and all this we fully credit; no man is simpleton enough to cry out, 'O, I can't believe that slaveholders do such things,'—and yet, when we turn to the treatment which these men mete out to their *slaves*, and show that they are in the habitual practice of striking, kicking, knocking down, and shooting *them*, as well as each other—the look of blank incredulity that comes over northern dough-faces is a study for a painter: and then the sentimental outcry, with eyes and hands uplifted, 'Oh, indeed, I can't believe the slaveholders are so cruel to their slaves.' Most amiable and touching charity!

Arbitrary power is to the mind what alcohol is to the body; it intoxicates. Man loves power. It is perhaps the strongest human passion; and the more absolute the power, the stronger the desire for it; and the more it is desired, the more its exercise is enjoyed: this enjoyment is to human nature a fearful temptation,—generally an overmatch for it. Hence it is true, with hardly an exception, that arbitrary power is abused in proportion as it is *desired*. The fact that a person intensely desires power over others, *without restraint*, shows the absolute necessity of restraint. What woman would marry a man who made it a condition that he should have the power to divorce her whenever he pleased? Oh! he might never wish to exercise it, but the *power* he would have! No woman, not stark mad, would trust her happiness in such hands.

Would a father apprentice his son to a master, who insisted that his power over the lad should be *absolute*? The master might, perhaps, never *wish* to commit a battery upon the boy, but if he should, he insists upon having full swing! He who would leave his son in the clutches of such a wretch, would be bled and blistered for a lunatic as soon as his friends could get their hands upon him.

The possession of power, even when greatly restrained, is such a fiery stimulant, that its lodgment in human hands is always perilous. Give men the handling of immense sums of money, and all the eyes of Argus and the hands of Briareus can hardly prevent embezzlement.

That American slaveholders possess a power over their slaves which is virtually absolute, none will deny.* That they *desire* this absolute power, is shown from the fact of their holding and exercising it, and making laws to confirm and enlarge it. That the desire to pos-

---

*The following extracts from the laws of slave States are proofs sufficient:—

'The slave is ENTIRELY subject to the WILL of his master. Louisiana Civil Code, Art. 273.

'Slaves shall be deemed, sold, taken, reputed, and adjudged in law to be *chattels personal*, in the hands of their owners and possessors, and their executors, administrators and assigns, TO ALL INTENTS, CONSTRUCTIONS, AND PURPOSES, WHATSOEVER.'—Laws of South Carolina, 2 Brev. Dig. 229; Prince's Digest, 446, &c.

sess this power, every tittle of it, is *intense*, is proved by the fact, that slaveholders cling to it with such obstinate tenacity, as well as by all their doings and sayings, their threats, cursings and gnashings against all who denounce the exercise of such power as usurpation and outrage, and counsel its immediate abrogation.

From the nature of the case, from the laws of mind, such power, so intensely desired, griped with such a death-clutch, and with such fierce spurnings of all curtailment or restraint, *cannot but be abused*. Privations and inflictions must be its natural, habitual products, with ever and anon, terror, torture and despair, let loose to do their worst upon their helpless victims.

Slaveholders organize themselves into a tribunal to adjudicate upon their own conduct, and give us, in their decisions, their estimate of their own character; informing us with characteristic modesty, that they have a high opinion of themselves; that in their own judgment, they are very mild, kind, and merciful gentlemen! In these conceptions of their own merits, and of the eminent propriety of their bearing towards their slaves,—slaveholders remind us of the Spaniard, who always took off his hat whenever he spoke of himself, and of the Governor of Schiraz, who, from a sense of justice to his own character, added to his other titles those of 'Flower of Courtesy,' 'Nutmeg of Consolation,' and 'Rose of Delight.'

When men speak of the treatment of others as being either good or bad, their declarations are not generally to be taken as testimony to matters of *fact*, so much as expressions of *their own feelings* towards those persons or classes who are the subjects of such treatment. If those persons are their fellow citizens; if they are in the same class of society with themselves; of the same language, creed, and color; similar in their habits, pursuits, and sympathies; they will keenly feel any wrong done to them, and denounce it as base, outrageous treatment; but let the same wrongs be done to persons of a condition in all respects the reverse, persons whom they habitually despise, and regard only in the light of mere conveniences, to be used for their pleasure, and the idea that such treatment is barbarous will be laughed at as ridiculous. When we hear slaveholders say that their slaves are *well treated*, we have only to remember that they are not speaking of *persons*, but of *property*; not of men and women, but of *chattels* and *things*; not of friends and associates, but of *vassals* and *victims*; not of those whom they respect and honor, but of those whom they *scorn* and trample on; not of those with whom they sympathize, and co-operate, and interchange courtesies, but of those whom they regard with contempt and aversion, and disdainfully set with the dogs of their flock. Reader, keep this fact in your mind, and you will have a clue to the slaveholder's definition of '*good treatment*.'

CERTIFICATES OF CHARACTER.

HURLEY, ULSTER Co., Oct. 13th, 1834.
This is to certify, that I am well acquainted with Isabella, this colored woman; I have been acquainted with her from her infancy; she has been in my employ for one year, and she was a faithful servant, honest, and industrious; and have always known her to be in good report by all who employed her.

ISAAC S. VAN WAGENEN.

———

NEW PALTZ, ULSTER Co., Oct. 13th, 1834.
This is to certify, that Isabella, this colored woman, lived with me since the year 1810, and that she has always been a good and faithful servant; and the eighteen years that she was with me, I always found her to be perfectly honest. I have always heard her well spoken of by every one that has employed her.

JOHN J. DUMONT.

———

NORTHAMPTON, March, 1850.
We, the undersigned, having known Isabella (or Sojourner Truth) for several years, most cheerfully bear testimony to her uniform good character, her untiring industry, kind deportment, unwearied benevolence, and the many social and excellent traits which make her worthy to bear her adopted name.

GEO. W. BENSON,
S. L. HILL,
A. W. THAYER.

———

BOSTON, March, 1850.
My acquaintance with the subject of the accompanying Narrative, Sojourner Truth, for several years past, has led me

to form a very high appreciation of her understanding, moral integrity, disinterested kindness, and religious sincerity and enlightenment. Any assistance or co-operation that she may receive in the sale of her Narrative, or in any other manner, I am sure will be meritoriously bestowed.

WM. LLOYD GARRISON.

RUNNING A THOUSAND MILES FOR FREEDOM;

OR, THE ESCAPE

OF

WILLIAM AND ELLEN CRAFT

FROM SLAVERY.

"Slaves cannot breathe in England: if their lungs
Receive our air, that moment they are free;
They touch our country, and their shackles fall."
COWPER.

LONDON:
WILLIAM TWEEDIE, 337, STRAND.
1860.

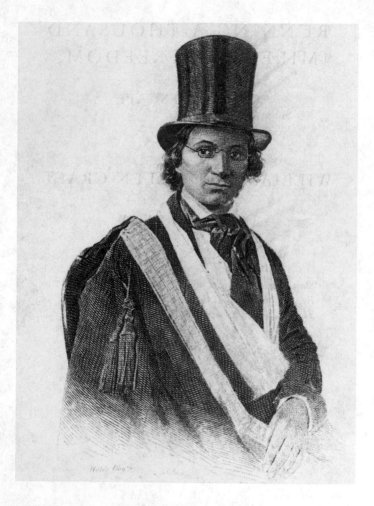

Ellen Craft, the fugitive slave.

PREFACE.

HAVING heard while in Slavery that "God made of one blood all nations of men," and also that the American Declaration of Independence says, that "We hold these truths to be self-evident, that all men are created equal; that they are endowed by their Creator with certain inalienable rights; that among these, are life, liberty, and the pursuit of happiness;" we could not understand by what right we were held as "chattels." Therefore, we felt perfectly justified in undertaking the dangerous and exciting task of "running a thousand miles" in order to obtain those rights which are so vividly set forth in the Declaration.

I beg those who would know the particulars of our journey, to peruse these pages.

This book is not intended as a full history of the life of my wife, nor of myself; but merely as an account of our escape; together with other matter which I hope may be the means of creating in some minds a deeper abhorrence of the sinful and abominable practice of enslaving and brutifying our fellow-creatures.

Without stopping to write a long apology for offering this little volume to the public, I shall commence at once to pursue my simple story.

W. CRAFT.

12, CAMBRIDGE ROAD,
    HAMMERSMITH,
        LONDON.

RUNNING A THOUSAND MILES FOR FREEDOM.

PART I.

> "God gave us only over beast, fish, fowl,
> Dominion absolute; that right we hold
> By his donation. But man over man
> He made not lord; such title to himself
> Reserving, human left from human free."
>
> MILTON.

My wife and myself were born in different towns in the State of Georgia, which is one of the principal slave States. It is true, our condition as slaves was not by any means the worst; but the mere idea that we were held as chattels, and deprived of all legal rights—the thought that we had to give up our hard earnings to a tyrant, to enable him to live in idleness and luxury—the thought that we could not call the bones and sinews that God gave us our own: but above all, the fact that another man had the power to tear from our cradle the new-born babe and sell it in the shambles like a brute, and then scourge us if we dared to lift a finger to save it from such a fate, haunted us for years.

But in December, 1848, a plan suggested itself that proved quite successful, and in eight days after it was first thought of we were free from the horrible trammels of slavery, rejoicing and praising God in the glorious sunshine of liberty.

My wife's first master was her father, and her mother his slave, and the latter is still the slave of his widow.

Notwithstanding my wife being of African extraction on her mother's side, she is almost white—in fact, she is so nearly so that the tyrannical old lady to whom she first belonged became so annoyed, at finding her frequently mistaken for a child of the family, that she gave her when eleven years of age to a daughter, as a wedding present. This separated my wife from her mother, and also from several other dear friends. But the incessant cruelty of her old mistress made the change

681

of owners or treatment so desirable, that she did not grumble much at this cruel separation.

It may be remembered that slavery in America is not at all confined to persons of any particular complexion; there are a very large number of slaves as white as any one; but as the evidence of a slave is not admitted in court against a free white person, it is almost impossible for a white child, after having been kidnapped and sold into or reduced to slavery, in a part of the country where it is not known (as often is the case), ever to recover its freedom.

I have myself conversed with several slaves who told me that their parents were white and free; but that they were stolen away from them and sold when quite young. As they could not tell their address, and also as the parents did not know what had become of their lost and dear little ones, of course all traces of each other were gone.

The following facts are sufficient to prove, that he who has the power, and is inhuman enough to trample upon the sacred rights of the weak, cares nothing for race or colour:—

In March, 1818, three ships arrived at New Orleans, bringing several hundred German emigrants from the province of Alsace, on the lower Rhine. Among them were Daniel Muller and his two daughters, Dorothea and Salomé, whose mother had died on the passage. Soon after his arrival, Muller, taking with him his two daughters, both young children, went up the river to Attakapas parish, to work on the plantation of John F. Miller. A few weeks later, his relatives, who had remained at New Orleans, learned that he had died of the fever of the country. They immediately sent for the two girls; but they had disappeared, and the relatives, notwithstanding repeated and persevering inquiries and researches, could find no traces of them. They were at length given up for dead. Dorothea was never again heard of; nor was any thing known of Salomé from 1818 till 1843.

In the summer of that year, Madame Karl, a German woman who had come over in the same ship with the Mullers, was passing through a street in New Orleans, and accidentally saw Salomé in a wine-shop, belonging to Louis Belmonte, by whom she was held as a slave. Madame Karl recognised her at once, and carried her to the house of another German woman, Mrs. Schubert, who was Salomé's cousin and god-mother, and who no sooner set eyes on her than, without having any intimation that the discovery had been previously made, she unhesitatingly exclaimed, "My God! here is the long-lost Salomé Muller."

The *Law Reporter*, in its account of this case, says:—

"As many of the German emigrants of 1818 as could be gathered together were brought to the house of Mrs. Schubert, and every one of the number who had any recollection of the little girl upon the passage, or any acquaintance with her father and mother, immediately identified the woman before them as the long-lost Salomé Muller. By all these witnesses, who appeared at the trial, the identity was fully established. The family resemblance in every feature was declared to be so remarkable, that some of the witnesses did not hesitate to say that they should know her among ten thousand; that they were as certain the plaintiff was Salomé Muller, the daughter of Daniel and Dorothea Muller, as of their own existence."

Among the witnesses who appeared in Court was the midwife who had assisted at the birth of Salomé. She testified to the existence of certain peculiar marks upon the body of the child, which were found, exactly as described, by the surgeons who were appointed by the Court to make an examination for the purpose.

There was no trace of African descent in any feature of Salomé Muller. She had long, straight, black hair, hazel eyes, thin lips, and a Roman nose. The complexion of her face and neck was as dark as that of the darkest brunette. It appears, however, that, during the twenty-five years of her servitude, she had been exposed to the sun's rays in the hot climate of Louisiana, with head and neck unsheltered, as is customary with the female slaves, while labouring in the cotton or the sugar field. Those parts of her person which had been shielded from the sun were comparatively white.

Belmonte, the pretended owner of the girl, had obtained possession of her by an act of sale from John F. Miller, the planter in whose service Salomé's father died. This Miller was a man of consideration and substance, owning large sugar estates, and bearing a high reputation for honour and honesty, and for indulgent treatment of his slaves. It was testified on the trial that he had said to Belmonte, a few weeks after the sale of Salomé, "that she was white, and had as much right to her freedom as any one, and was only to be retained in slavery by care and kind treatment." The broker who negotiated the sale from Miller to Belmonte, in 1838, testified in Court that he then thought, and still thought, that the girl was white!

The case was elaborately argued on both sides, but was at length decided in favour of the girl, by the Supreme Court declaring that "she was free and white, and therefore unlawfully held in bondage."

The Rev. George Bourne, of Virginia, in his *Picture of Slavery*, published in 1834, relates the case of a white boy who, at the age of seven, was stolen from his home in Ohio, tanned and stained in such a way that he could not be distinguished from a person of colour, and then sold as a slave in Virginia. At the age of twenty, he made his escape, by running away, and happily succeeded in rejoining his parents.

I have known worthless white people to sell their own free children into slavery; and, as there are good-for-nothing white as well as coloured persons everywhere, no one, perhaps, will wonder at such inhuman transactions: particularly in the Southern States of America, where I believe there is a greater want of humanity and high principle amongst the whites, than among any other civilized people in the world.

I know that those who are not familiar with the working of "the peculiar institution," can scarcely imagine any one so totally devoid of all natural affection as to sell his own offspring into returnless bondage. But Shakspeare, that great observer of human nature, says:—

> "With caution judge of probabilities.
> Things deemed unlikely, e'en impossible,
> Experience often shows us to be true."

My wife's new mistress was decidedly more humane than the majority of her class. My wife has always given her credit for not exposing her to many of the worst features of slavery. For instance, it is a common practice in the slave States for ladies, when angry with their maids, to send them to the calybuce sugar-house, or to some other place established for the purpose of punishing slaves, and have them severely flogged; and I am sorry it is a fact, that the villains to whom those defenceless creatures are sent, not only flog them as they are ordered, but frequently compel them to submit to the greatest indignity. Oh! if there is any one thing under the wide canopy of heaven, horrible enough to stir a man's soul, and to make his very blood boil, it is the thought of his dear wife, his unprotected sister, or his young and virtuous daughters, struggling to save themselves from falling a prey to such demons!

It always appears strange to me that any one who was not born a slaveholder, and steeped to the very core in the demoralizing atmosphere of the Southern States, can in any way palliate slavery. It is still more surprising to see virtuous ladies looking with patience upon, and remaining indifferent to, the existence of a system that exposes nearly two millions of their own sex in the manner I have mentioned, and that too in a professedly free and Christian country. There is, however, great consolation in knowing that God is just, and will not let the oppressor of the weak, and the spoiler of the virtuous, escape unpunished here and hereafter.

I believe a similar retribution to that which destroyed Sodom is hanging over the slaveholders. My sincere prayer is that they may not provoke God, by persisting in a reckless course of wickedness, to pour out his consuming wrath upon them.

I must now return to our history.

My old master had the reputation of being a very humane and Christian man, but he thought nothing of selling my poor old father, and dear aged mother, at separate times, to different persons, to be dragged off never to behold each other again, till summoned to appear before the great tribunal of heaven. But, oh! what a happy meeting it will be on that great day for those faithful souls. I say a happy meeting, because I never saw persons more devoted to the service of God than they. But how will the case stand with those reckless traffickers in human flesh and blood, who plunged the poisonous dagger of separation into those loving hearts which God had for so many years closely joined together—nay, sealed as it were with his own hands for the eternal courts of heaven? It is not for me to say what will become of those heartless tyrants. I must leave them in the hands of an all-wise and just God, who will, in his own good time, and in his own way, avenge the wrongs of his oppressed people.

My old master also sold a dear brother and a sister, in the same manner as he did my father and mother. The reason he assigned for disposing of my parents, as well as of several other aged slaves, was, that "they were getting old, and would soon become valueless in the market, and therefore he intended to sell off all the old stock, and buy in a young lot." A most disgraceful conclusion for a man to come to, who made such great professions of religion!

This shameful conduct gave me a thorough hatred, not for true Christianity, but for slaveholding piety.

My old master, then, wishing to make the most of the rest of his slaves, apprenticed a brother and myself out to learn trades: he to a blacksmith, and myself to a cabinet-maker. If a slave has a good trade, he will let or sell for more than a person without one, and many slaveholders have their slaves taught trades on this account. But before our time expired, my old master wanted money; so he sold my brother, and then mortgaged my sister, a dear girl about fourteen years of age, and myself, then about sixteen, to one of the banks, to get money to speculate in cotton. This we knew nothing of at the moment; but time rolled on, the money became due, my master was unable to meet his payments; so the bank had us placed upon the auction stand and sold to the highest bidder.

My poor sister was sold first: she was knocked down to a planter who resided at some distance in the country. Then I was called upon the stand. While the auctioneer was crying the bids, I saw the man that had purchased my sister getting her into a cart, to take her to his home. I at once asked a slave friend who was standing near the platform, to run and ask the gentleman if he would please to wait till I was sold, in order that I might have an opportunity of bidding her good-bye. He sent me word back that he had some distance to go, and could not wait.

I then turned to the auctioneer, fell upon my knees, and humbly prayed him to let me just step down and bid my last sister farewell. But, instead of granting me this request, he grasped me by the neck, and in a commanding tone of voice, and with a violent oath, exclaimed, "Get up! You can do the wench no good; therefore there is no use in your seeing her."

On rising, I saw the cart in which she sat moving slowly off; and, as she clasped her hands with a grasp that indicated despair, and looked pitifully round towards me, I also saw the large silent tears trickling down her cheeks. She made a farewell bow, and buried her face in her lap. This seemed more than I could bear. It appeared to swell my aching heart to its utmost. But before I could fairly recover, the poor girl was gone;—gone, and I have never had the good fortune to see her from that day to this! Perhaps I should have never heard of her again, had it not been for the untiring efforts of my good old mother, who became free a few years ago by purchase, and, after a great deal of difficulty, found my sister residing with a family in Mississippi. My mother at once wrote to me, informing me of the fact, and requesting me to do something to get her free; and I am happy to say that, partly by lecturing occasionally, and through the sale of an engraving of my wife in the disguise in which she escaped, together with the extreme kindness and generosity of Miss Burdett Coutts, Mr. George Richardson of Plymouth, and a few other friends, I have nearly accomplished this. It would be to me a great and ever-glorious achievement to restore my sister to our dear mother, from whom she was forcibly driven in early life.

I was knocked down to the cashier of the bank to which we were mortgaged, and ordered to return to the cabinet shop where I previously worked.

But the thought of the harsh auctioneer not allowing me to bid my dear sister farewell, sent red-hot indignation darting like lightning through every vein. It quenched my tears, and appeared to set my brain on fire, and made me crave for power to avenge our wrongs! But, alas! we were only slaves, and had no legal rights; consequently we were compelled to smother our wounded feelings, and crouch beneath the iron heel of despotism.

I must now give the account of our escape; but, before doing so, it may be well to quote a few passages from the fundamental laws of slavery; in order to give some idea of the legal as well as the social tyranny from which we fled.

According to the law of Louisiana, "A slave is one who is in the power of a master to whom he belongs. The master may sell him, dispose of his person, his industry, and his labour; he can do nothing, possess nothing, nor acquire anything but what must belong to his master."—*Civil Code, art.* 35.

In South Carolina it is expressed in the following language:—"Slaves shall be deemed, sold, taken, reputed and judged in law to be *chattels personal* in the hands of their owners and possessors, and their executors, administrators, and assigns, *to all intents, constructions, and purposes whatsoever.*"—2 *Brevard's Digest,* 229.

The Constitution of Georgia has the following (Art. 4, sec. 12):—"Any person who shall maliciously dismember or deprive a slave of life, shall suffer such punishment as would be inflicted in case the like offence had been committed on a free white person, and on the like proof, except in case of insurrection of such slave, and unless SUCH DEATH SHOULD HAPPEN BY ACCIDENT IN GIVING SUCH SLAVE MODERATE CORRECTION."—*Prince's Digest,* 559.

I have known slaves to be beaten to death, but as they died under "moderate correction," it was quite lawful; and of course the murderers were not interfered with.

"If any slave, who shall be out of the house or plantation where such slave shall live, or shall be usually employed, or without some white person in company with such slave, shall *refuse to submit* to undergo the examination of *any white* person, (let him be ever so drunk or crazy), it shall be lawful for such white person to pursue, apprehend, and moderately correct such slave; and if such slave shall assault and strike such white person, such slave may be *lawfully killed.*"—2 *Brevard's Digest,* 231.

"Provided always," says the law, "that such striking be not done by the command and in the defence of the person or property of the owner, or other person having the government of such slave; in which case the slave shall be wholly excused."

According to this law, if a slave, by the direction of his overseer, strike a white person who is beating said overseer's pig, "the slave shall be wholly excused." But, should the bondman, of his own accord, fight to defend his wife, or should his terrified daughter instinctively raise her hand and strike the wretch who attempts to violate her chastity, he or she shall, saith the model republican law, suffer death.

From having been myself a slave for nearly twenty-three years, I am quite prepared to say, that the practical working of slavery is worse than the odious laws by which it is governed.

At an early age we were taken by the persons who held us as property to Maçon, the largest town in the interior of the State of Georgia, at which place we became acquainted with each other for several years before our marriage; in fact, our marriage was postponed for some time simply because one of the unjust and worse than Pagan laws under which we lived compelled all children of slave mothers to follow their condition. That is to say, the father of the slave may be the President of the Republic; but if the mother should be a slave at the infant's birth, the poor child is ever legally doomed to the same cruel fate.

It is a common practice for gentlemen (if I may call them such), moving in the highest circles of society, to be the fathers of children by their slaves, whom they can and do sell with the greatest impunity; and the more pious, beautiful, and virtuous the girls are, the greater the price they bring, and that too for the most infamous purposes.

Any man with money (let him be ever such a rough brute), can buy a beautiful and virtuous girl, and force her to live with him in a criminal connexion; and as the law says a slave shall have no higher appeal than the mere will of the master, she cannot escape, unless it be by flight or death.

In endeavouring to reconcile a girl to her fate, the master sometimes says that he would marry her if it was not unlawful.* However, he will always consider her to be his wife, and will treat her as such; and she, on the other hand, may regard him as her lawful husband; and if they have any children, they will be free and well educated.

---

*It is unlawful in the slave States for any one of purely European descent to intermarry with a person of African extraction; though a white man may live with as many coloured women as he pleases without materially damaging his reputation in Southern society.

I am in duty bound to add, that while a great majority of such men care nothing for the happiness of the women with whom they live, nor for the children of whom they are the fathers, there are those to be found, even in that heterogeneous mass of licentious monsters, who are true to their pledges. But as the woman and her children are legally the property of the man, who stands in the anomalous relation to them of husband and father, as well as master, they are liable to be seized and sold for his debts, should he become involved.

There are several cases on record where such persons have been sold and separated for life. I know of some myself, but I have only space to glance at one.

I knew a very humane and wealthy gentleman, that bought a woman, with whom he lived as his wife. They brought up a family of children, among whom were three nearly white, well educated, and beautiful girls.

On the father being suddenly killed it was found that he had not left a will; but, as the family had always heard him say that he had no surviving relatives, they felt that their liberty and property were quite secured to them, and, knowing the insults to which they were exposed, now their protector was no more, they were making preparations to leave for a free State.

But, poor creatures, they were soon sadly undeceived. A villain residing at a distance, hearing of the circumstance, came forward and swore that he was a relative of the deceased; and as this man bore, or assumed, Mr. Slator's name, the case was brought before one of those horrible tribunals, presided over by a second Judge Jeffreys, and calling itself a court of justice, but before whom no coloured person, nor an abolitionist, was ever known to get his full rights.

A verdict was given in favour of the plaintiff, whom the better portion of the community thought had wilfully conspired to cheat the family.

The heartless wretch not only took the ordinary property, but actually had the aged and friendless widow, and all her fatherless children, except Frank, a fine young man about twenty-two years of age, and Mary, a very nice girl, a little younger than her brother, brought to the auction stand and sold to the highest bidder. Mrs. Slator had cash enough, that

her husband and master left, to purchase the liberty of herself
and children; but on her attempting to do so, the pusillani-
mous scoundrel, who had robbed them of their freedom,
claimed the money as his property; and, poor creature, she
had to give it up. According to law, as will be seen hereafter,
a slave cannot own anything. The old lady never recovered
from her sad affliction.

At the sale she was brought up first, and after being vul-
garly criticised, in the presence of all her distressed family, was
sold to a cotton planter, who said he wanted the "proud old
critter to go to his plantation, to look after the little woolly
heads, while their mammies were working in the field."

When the sale was over, then came the separation, and

> "O, deep was the anguish of that slave mother's heart,
>   When called from her darlings for ever to part;
>   The poor mourning mother of reason bereft,
>   Soon ended her sorrows, and sank cold in death."

Antoinette, the flower of the family, a girl who was much
beloved by all who knew her, for her Christ-like piety, dignity
of manner, as well as her great talents and extreme beauty,
was bought by an uneducated and drunken slave-dealer.

I cannot give a more correct description of the scene, when
she was called from her brother to the stand, than will be
found in the following lines—

> "Why stands she near the auction stand?
>   That girl so young and fair;
>   What brings her to this dismal place?
>   Why stands she weeping there?
>
>   Why does she raise that bitter cry?
>   Why hangs her head with shame,
>   As now the auctioneer's rough voice
>   So rudely calls her name!
>
>   But see! she grasps a manly hand,
>   And in a voice so low,
>   As scarcely to be heard, she says,
>   'My brother, must I go?'

A moment's pause: then, midst a wail
    Of agonizing woe,
His answer falls upon the ear,—
    'Yes, sister, you must go!

No longer can my arm defend,
    No longer can I save
My sister from the horrid fate
    That waits her as a SLAVE!'

Blush, Christian, blush! for e'en the dark
    Untutored heathen see
Thy inconsistency, and lo!
    They scorn thy God, and thee!"

The low trader said to a kind lady who wished to purchase Antoinette out of his hands, "I reckon I'll not sell the smart critter for ten thousand dollars; I always wanted her for my own use." The lady, wishing to remonstrate with him, commenced by saying, "You should remember, Sir, that there is a just God." Hoskens not understanding Mrs. Huston, interrupted her by saying, "I does, and guess its monstrous kind an' him to send such likely niggers for our convenience." Mrs. Huston finding that a long course of reckless wickedness, drunkenness, and vice, had destroyed in Hoskens every noble impulse, left him.

Antoinette, poor girl, also seeing that there was no help for her, became frantic. I can never forget her cries of despair, when Hoskens gave the order for her to be taken to his house, and locked in an upper room. On Hoskens entering the apartment, in a state of intoxication, a fearful struggle ensued. The brave Antoinette broke loose from him, pitched herself head foremost through the window, and fell upon the pavement below.

Her bruised but unpolluted body was soon picked up—restoratives brought—doctor called in; but, alas! it was too late: her pure and noble spirit had fled away to be at rest in those realms of endless bliss, "where the wicked cease from troubling, and the weary are at rest."

Antoinette like many other noble women who are deprived of liberty, still

"Holds something sacred, something undefiled;
Some pledge and keepsake of their higher nature.
And, like the diamond in the dark, retains
Some quenchless gleam of the celestial light."

On Hoskens fully realizing the fact that his victim was no more, he exclaimed "By thunder I am a used-up man!" The sudden disappointment, and the loss of two thousand dollars, was more than he could endure: so he drank more than ever, and in a short time died, raving mad with *delirium tremens.*

The villain Slator said to Mrs. Huston, the kind lady who endeavoured to purchase Antoinette from Hoskins, "Nobody needn't talk to me 'bout buying them ar likely niggers, for I'm not going to sell em." "But Mary is rather delicate," said Mrs. Huston, "and, being unaccustomed to hard work, cannot do you much service on a plantation." "I don't want her for the field," replied Slator, "but for another purpose." Mrs. Huston understood what this meant, and instantly exclaimed, "Oh, but she is your cousin!" "The devil she is!" said Slator; and added, "Do you mean to insult me Madam, by saying that I am related to niggers?" "No," replied Mrs. Huston, "I do not wish to offend you, Sir. But wasn't Mr. Slator, Mary's father, your uncle?" "Yes, I calculate he was," said Slator; "but I want you and everybody to understand that I'm no kin to his niggers." "Oh, very well," said Mrs. Huston; adding, "Now what will you take for the poor girl?" "Nothin'," he replied; "for, as I said before, I'm not goin' to sell, so you needn't trouble yourself no more. If the critter behaves herself, I'll do as well by her as any man."

Slator spoke up boldly, but his manner and sheepish look clearly indicated that

"His heart within him was at strife
With such accursed gains;
For he knew whose passions gave her life,
Whose blood ran in her veins."

"The monster led her from the door,
He led her by the hand,
To be his slave and paramour
In a strange and distant land!"

Poor Frank and his sister were handcuffed together, and confined in prison. Their dear little twin brother and sister were sold, and taken where they knew not. But it often happens that misfortune causes those whom we counted dearest to shrink away; while it makes friends of those whom we least expected to take any interest in our affairs. Among the latter class Frank found two comparatively new but faithful friends to watch the gloomy paths of the unhappy little twins.

In a day or two after the sale, Slator had two fast horses put to a large light van, and placed in it a good many small but valuable things belonging to the distressed family. He also took with him Frank and Mary, as well as all the money for the spoil; and after treating all his low friends and bystanders, and drinking deeply himself, he started in high glee for his home in South Carolina. But they had not proceeded many miles, before Frank and his sister discovered that Slator was too drunk to drive. But he, like most tipsy men, thought he was all right; and as he had with him some of the ruined family's best brandy and wine, such as he had not been accustomed to, and being a thirsty soul, he drank till the reins fell from his fingers, and in attempting to catch them he tumbled out of the vehicle, and was unable to get up. Frank and Mary there and then contrived a plan by which to escape. As they were still handcuffed by one wrist each, they alighted, took from the drunken assassin's pocket the key, undid the iron bracelets, and placed them upon Slator, who was better fitted to wear such ornaments. As the demon lay unconscious of what was taking place, Frank and Mary took from him the large sum of money that was realized at the sale, as well as that which Slator had so very meanly obtained from their poor mother. They then dragged him into the woods, tied him to a tree, and left the inebriated robber to shift for himself, while they made good their escape to Savannah. The fugitives being white, of course no one suspected that they were slaves.

Slator was not able to call any one to his rescue till late the next day; and as there were no railroads in that part of the country at that time, it was not until late the following day that Slator was able to get a party to join him for the chase.

A person informed Slator that he had met a man and woman, in a trap, answering to the description of those whom he had lost, driving furiously towards Savannah. So Slator and several slavehunters on horseback started off in full tilt, with their bloodhounds, in pursuit of Frank and Mary.

On arriving at Savannah, the hunters found that the fugitives had sold the horses and trap, and embarked as free white persons, for New York. Slator's disappointment and rascality so preyed upon his base mind, that he, like Judas, went and hanged himself.

As soon as Frank and Mary were safe, they endeavoured to redeem their good mother. But, alas! she was gone; she had passed on to the realm of spirit life.

In due time Frank learned from his friends in Georgia where his little brother and sister dwelt. So he wrote at once to purchase them, but the persons with whom they lived would not sell them. After failing in several attempts to buy them, Frank cultivated large whiskers and moustachios, cut off his hair, put on a wig and glasses, and went down as a white man, and stopped in the neighborhood where his sister was; and after seeing her and also his little brother, arrangements were made for them to meet at a particular place on a Sunday, which they did, and got safely off.

I saw Frank myself, when he came for the little twins. Though I was then quite a lad, I well remember being highly delighted by hearing him tell how nicely he and Mary had served Slator.

Frank had so completely disguised or changed his appearance that his little sister did not know him, and would not speak till he showed their mother's likeness; the sight of which melted her to tears,—for she knew the face. Frank might have said to her

> "'O, Emma! O, my sister, speak to me!
> Dost thou not know me, that I am thy brother!
> Come to me, little Emma, thou shalt dwell
> With me henceforth, and know no care or want.'
> Emma was silent for a space, as if
> 'Twere hard to summon up a human voice."

Frank and Mary's mother was my wife's own dear aunt.

After this great diversion from our narrative, which I hope, dear reader, you will excuse, I shall return at once to it.

My wife was torn from her mother's embrace in childhood, and taken to a distant part of the country. She had seen so many other children separated from their parents in this cruel manner, that the mere thought of her ever becoming the mother of a child, to linger out a miserable existence under the wretched system of American slavery, appeared to fill her very soul with horror; and as she had taken what I felt to be an important view of her condition, I did not, at first, press the marriage, but agreed to assist her in trying to devise some plan by which we might escape from our unhappy condition, and then be married.

We thought of plan after plan, but they all seemed crowded with insurmountable difficulties. We knew it was unlawful for any public conveyance to take us as passengers, without our master's consent. We were also perfectly aware of the startling fact, that had we left without this consent the professional slave-hunters would have soon had their ferocious blood-hounds baying on our track, and in a short time we should have been dragged back to slavery, not to fill the more favourable situations which we had just left, but to be separated for life, and put to the very meanest and most laborious drudgery; or else have been tortured to death as examples, in order to strike terror into the hearts of others, and thereby prevent them from even attempting to escape from their cruel taskmasters. It is a fact worthy of remark, that nothing seems to give the slaveholders so much pleasure as the catching and torturing of fugitives. They had much rather take the keen and poisonous lash, and with it cut their poor trembling victims to atoms, than allow one of them to escape to a free country, and expose the infamous system from which he fled.

The greatest excitement prevails at a slave-hunt. The slave-holders and their hired ruffians appear to take more pleasure in this inhuman pursuit than English sportsmen do in chasing a fox or a stag. Therefore, knowing what we should have been compelled to suffer, if caught and taken back, we were more than anxious to hit upon a plan that would lead us safely to a land of liberty.

But, after puzzling our brains for years, we were reluctantly driven to the sad conclusion, that it was almost impossible to escape from slavery in Georgia, and travel 1,000 miles across the slave States. We therefore resolved to get the consent of our owners, be married, settle down in slavery, and endeavour to make ourselves as comfortable as possible under that system; but at the same time ever to keep our dim eyes steadily fixed upon the glimmering hope of liberty, and earnestly pray God mercifully to assist us to escape from our unjust thraldom.

We were married, and prayed and toiled on till December, 1848, at which time (as I have stated) a plan suggested itself that proved quite successful, and in eight days after it was first thought of we were free from the horrible trammels of slavery, and glorifying God who had brought us safely out of a land of bondage.

Knowing that slaveholders have the privilege of taking their slaves to any part of the country they think proper, it occurred to me that, as my wife was nearly white, I might get her to disguise herself as an invalid gentleman, and assume to be my master, while I could attend as his slave, and that in this manner we might effect our escape. After I thought of the plan, I suggested it to my wife, but at first she shrank from the idea. She thought it was almost impossible for her to assume that disguise, and travel a distance of 1,000 miles across the slave States. However, on the other hand, she also thought of her condition. She saw that the laws under which we lived did not recognize her to be a woman, but a mere chattel, to be bought and sold, or otherwise dealt with as her owner might see fit. Therefore the more she contemplated her helpless condition, the more anxious she was to escape from it. So she said, "I think it is almost too much for us to undertake; however, I feel that God is on our side, and with his assistance, notwithstanding all the difficulties, we shall be able to succeed. Therefore, if you will purchase the disguise, I will try to carry out the plan."

But after I concluded to purchase the disguise, I was afraid to go to any one to ask him to sell me the articles. It is unlawful in Georgia for a white man to trade with slaves without the master's consent. But, notwithstanding this, many persons will sell a slave any article that he can get the money to buy. Not that they sympathize with the slave, but merely because his testimony is not admitted in court against a free white person.

Therefore, with little difficulty I went to different parts of the town, at odd times, and purchased things piece by piece, (except the trowsers which she found necessary to make,) and took them home to the house where my wife resided. She being a ladies' maid, and a favourite slave in the family, was allowed a little room to herself; and amongst other pieces of furniture which I had made in my overtime, was a chest of drawers; so when I took the articles home, she locked them up carefully in these drawers. No one about the premises knew that she had anything of the kind. So when we fancied we had everything ready the time was fixed for the flight. But we knew it would not do to start off without first getting our master's consent to be away for a few days. Had we left without this, they would soon have had us back into slavery, and probably we should never have got another fair opportunity of even attempting to escape.

Some of the best slaveholders will sometimes give their favourite slaves a few days' holiday at Christmas time; so, after no little amount of perseverance on my wife's part, she obtained a pass from her mistress, allowing her to be away for a few days. The cabinet-maker with whom I worked gave me a similar paper, but said that he needed my services very much, and wished me to return as soon as the time granted was up. I thanked him kindly; but somehow I have not been able to make it convenient to return yet; and, as the free air of good old England agrees so well with my wife and our dear little ones, as well as with myself, it is not at all likely we shall return at present to the "peculiar institution" of chains and stripes.

On reaching my wife's cottage she handed me her pass, and I showed mine, but at that time neither of us were able to read them. It is not only unlawful for slaves to be taught to read, but in some of the States there are heavy penalties attached, such as fines and imprisonment, which will be vigorously enforced upon any one who is humane enough to violate the so-called law.

The following case will serve to show how persons are treated in the most enlightened slaveholding community.

"INDICTMENT.

COMMONWEALTH OF VIRGINIA, }   *In the Circuit*
    NORFOLK COUNTY, *ss.*   }   *Court.*

The Grand Jurors empannelled and sworn to inquire of offences committed in the body of the said County on their oath present, that Margaret Douglass, being an evil disposed person, not having the fear of God before her eyes, but moved and instigated by the devil, wickedly, maliciously, and feloniously, on the fourth day of July, in the year of our Lord one thousand eight hundred and fifty-four, at Norfolk, in said County, did teach a certain black girl named Kate to read in the Bible, to the great displeasure of Almighty God, to the pernicious example of others in like case offending, contrary to the form of the statute in such case made and provided, and against the peace and dignity of the Commonwealth of Virginia.

"VICTOR VAGABONE, *Prosecuting Attorney.*"

"On this indictment Mrs. Douglass was arraigned as a necessary matter of form, tried, found guilty of course; and Judge Scalawag, before whom she was tried, having consulted with Dr. Adams, ordered the sheriff to place Mrs. Douglass in the prisoner's box, when he addressed her as follows: 'Margaret Douglass, stand up. You are guilty of one of the vilest crimes that ever disgraced society; and the jury have found you so. You have taught a slave girl to read in the Bible. No enlightened society can exist where such offences go unpunished. The Court, in your case, do not feel for you one solitary ray of sympathy, and they will inflict on you the utmost penalty of the law. In any other civilized country you would have paid the forfeit of your crime with your life, and the Court have only to regret that such is not the law in this country. The sentence for your offence is, that you be imprisoned one month in the county jail, and that you pay the costs of this prosecution. Sheriff, remove the prisoner to jail.' On the publication of these proceedings, the Doctors of Divinity preached each a sermon on the necessity of obeying the laws; the *New York Observer* noticed with much pious gladness a revival of religion on Dr. Smith's plantation in Georgia, among his slaves; while the *Journal of Commerce* commended this political preaching of the Doctors of Divinity because it favoured slavery. Let us do nothing to offend our Southern brethren."

However, at first, we were highly delighted at the idea of having gained permission to be absent for a few days; but when the thought flashed across my wife's mind, that it was customary for travellers to register their names in the visitors' book at hotels, as well as in the clearance or Custom-house book at Charleston, South Carolina—it made our spirits droop within us.

So, while sitting in our little room upon the verge of despair, all at once my wife raised her head, and with a smile upon her face, which was a moment before bathed in tears, said, "I think I have it!" I asked what it was. She said, "I think I can make a poultice and bind up my right hand in a sling, and with propriety ask the officers to register my name for me." I thought that would do.

It then occurred to her that the smoothness of her face might betray her; so she decided to make another poultice, and put it in a white handkerchief to be worn under the chin, up the cheeks, and to tie over the head. This nearly hid the expression of the countenance, as well as the beardless chin.

The poultice is left off in the engraving, because the likeness could not have been taken well with it on.

My wife, knowing that she would be thrown a good deal into the company of gentlemen, fancied that she could get on better if she had something to go over the eyes; so I went to a shop and bought a pair of green spectacles. This was in the evening.

We sat up all night discussing the plan, and making preparations. Just before the time arrived, in the morning, for us to leave, I cut off my wife's hair square at the back of the head, and got her to dress in the disguise and stand out on the floor. I found that she made a most respectable looking gentleman.

My wife had no ambition whatever to assume this disguise, and would not have done so had it been possible to have obtained our liberty by more simple means; but we knew it was not customary in the South for ladies to travel with male servants; and therefore, notwithstanding my wife's fair complexion, it would have been a very difficult task for her to have come off as a free white lady, with me as her slave; in fact, her not being able to write would have made this quite impossible. We knew that no public conveyance would take us, or any other slave, as a passenger, without our master's consent. This consent could never be obtained to pass into a free State. My wife's being muffled in the poultices, &c., furnished a plausible excuse for avoiding general conversation, of which most Yankee travellers are passionately fond.

There are a large number of free negroes residing in the southern States; but in Georgia (and I believe in all the slave States,) every coloured person's complexion is *primâ facie* evidence of his being a slave; and the lowest villain in the country, should he be a white man, has the legal power to arrest, and question, in the most inquisitorial and insulting manner, any coloured person, male or female, that he may find at large, particularly at night and on Sundays, without a written pass, signed by the master or some one in authority; or stamped free papers, certifying that the person is the rightful owner of himself.

If the coloured person refuses to answer questions put to him, he may be beaten, and his defending himself against this attack makes him an outlaw, and if he be killed on the spot, the murderer will be exempted from all blame; but after the coloured person has answered the questions put to him, in a most humble and pointed manner, he may then be taken to prison; and should it turn out, after further examination, that he was caught where he had no permission or legal right to be, and that he has not given what they term a satisfactory account of himself, the master will have to pay a fine. On his refusing to do this, the poor slave may be legally and severely flogged by public officers. Should the prisoner prove to be a free man, he is most likely to be both whipped and fined.

The great majority of slaveholders hate this class of persons with a hatred that can only be equalled by the condemned spirits of the infernal regions. They have no mercy upon, nor sympathy for, any negro whom they cannot enslave. They say that God made the black man to be a slave for the white, and act as though they really believed that all free persons of colour are in open rebellion to a direct command from heaven, and that they (the whites) are God's chosen agents to pour out upon them unlimited vengeance. For instance, a Bill has been introduced in the Tennessee Legislature to prevent free negroes from travelling on the railroads in that State. It has passed the first reading. The bill provides that the President who shall permit a free negro to travel on any road within the jurisdiction of the State under his supervision shall pay a fine of 500 dollars; any conductor permitting a violation of the Act shall pay 250 dollars; provided such free negro is not under the control of a free white citizen of Tennessee, who will vouch for the character of said free negro in a penal bond of one thousand dollars. The State of Arkansas has passed a law to banish all free negroes from its bounds, and it came into effect on the 1st day of January, 1860. Every free negro found there after that date will be liable to be sold into slavery, the crime of freedom being unpardonable. The Missouri Senate has before it a bill providing that all free negroes above the age of eighteen years who shall be found in the State after September, 1860, shall be sold into slavery; and that all such negroes as shall enter the State after September, 1861, and remain there twenty-four hours, shall also be sold into slavery for ever. Mississippi, Kentucky, and Georgia, and in fact, I believe, all the slave States, are legislating in the same manner. Thus the slaveholders make it almost impossible for free persons of colour to get out of the slave States, in order that they may sell them into slavery if they don't go. If no white persons travelled upon railroads except those who could get some one to vouch for their character in a penal bond of one thousand dollars, the railroad companies would soon go to the "wall." Such mean legislation is too low for comment; therefore I leave the villanous acts to speak for themselves.

But the Dred Scott decision is the crowning act of infamous Yankee legislation. The Supreme Court, the highest tribunal of the Republic, composed of nine Judge Jeffries's, chosen both from the free and slave States, has decided that no coloured person, or persons of African extraction, can ever become a citizen of the United States, or have any rights which white men are bound to respect. That is to say, in the opinion of this Court, robbery, rape, and murder are not crimes when committed by a white upon a coloured person.

Judges who will sneak from their high and honourable position down into the lowest depths of human depravity, and scrape up a decision like this, are wholly unworthy the confidence of any people. I believe such men would, if they had the power, and were it to their temporal interest, sell their country's independence, and barter away every man's birthright for a mess of pottage. Well may Thomas Campbell say—

> United States, your banner wears,
> Two emblems,—one of fame;
> Alas, the other that it bears
> Reminds us of your shame!
> The white man's liberty in types
> Stands blazoned by your stars;
> But what's the meaning of your stripes?
> They mean your Negro-scars.

When the time had arrived for us to start, we blew out the lights, knelt down, and prayed to our Heavenly Father mercifully to assist us, as he did his people of old, to escape from cruel bondage; and we shall ever feel that God heard and answered our prayer. Had we not been sustained by a kind, and I sometimes think special, providence, we could never have overcome the mountainous difficulties which I am now about to describe.

After this we rose and stood for a few moments in breathless silence,—we were afraid that some one might have been about the cottage listening and watching our movements. So I took my wife by the hand, stepped softly to the door, raised the latch, drew it open, and peeped out. Though there were trees all around the house, yet the foliage scarcely moved; in fact, everything appeared to be as still as death. I then whispered to my wife, "Come my dear, let us make a desperate leap for liberty!" But poor thing, she shrank back, in a state of trepidation. I turned and asked what was the matter; she made no reply, but burst into violent sobs, and threw her head upon my breast. This appeared to touch my very heart, it caused me to enter into her feelings more fully than ever.

We both saw the many mountainous difficulties that rose one after the other before our view, and knew far too well what our sad fate would have been, were we caught and forced back into our slavish den. Therefore on my wife's fully realizing the solemn fact that we had to take our lives, as it were, in our hands, and contest every inch of the thousand miles of slave territory over which we had to pass, it made her heart almost sink within her, and, had I known them at that time, I would have repeated the following encouraging lines, which may not be out of place here—

"The hill, though high, I covet to ascend,
The *difficulty will not me offend*;
For I perceive the way to life lies here:
Come, pluck up heart, let's neither faint nor fear;
Better, though difficult, the right way to go,—
Than wrong, though easy, where the end is woe."

However, the sobbing was soon over, and after a few moments of silent prayer she recovered her self-possession, and said, "Come, William, it is getting late, so now let us venture upon our perilous journey."

We then opened the door, and stepped as softly out as "moonlight upon the water." I locked the door with my own key, which I now have before me, and tiptoed across the yard into the street. I say tiptoed, because we were like persons near a tottering avalanche, afraid to move, or even breathe freely, for fear the sleeping tyrants should be aroused, and come down upon us with double vengeance, for daring to attempt to escape in the manner which we contemplated.

We shook hands, said farewell, and started in different directions for the railway station. I took the nearest possible way to the train, for fear I should be recognized by some one, and got into the negro car in which I knew I should have to ride; but my *master* (as I will now call my wife) took a longer way round, and only arrived there with the bulk of the passengers. He obtained a ticket for himself and one for his slave to Savannah, the first port, which was about two hundred miles off. My master then had the luggage stowed away, and stepped into one of the best carriages.

But just before the train moved off I peeped through the

window, and, to my great astonishment, I saw the cabinet-maker with whom I had worked so long, on the platform. He stepped up to the ticket-seller, and asked some question, and then commenced looking rapidly through the passengers, and into the carriages. Fully believing that we were caught, I shrank into a corner, turned my face from the door, and expected in a moment to be dragged out. The cabinet-maker looked into my master's carriage, but did not know him in his new attire, and, as God would have it, before he reached mine the bell rang, and the train moved off.

I have heard since that the cabinet-maker had a presentiment that we were about to "make tracks for parts unknown;" but, not seeing me, his suspicions vanished, until he received the startling intelligence that we had arrived safely in a free State.

As soon as the train had left the platform, my master looked round in the carriage, and was terror-stricken to find a Mr. Cray—an old friend of my wife's master, who dined with the family the day before, and knew my wife from childhood—sitting on the same seat.

The doors of the American railway carriages are at the ends. The passengers walk up the aisle, and take seats on either side; and as my master was engaged in looking out of the window, he did not see who came in.

My master's first impression, after seeing Mr. Cray, was, that he was there for the purpose of securing him. However, my master thought it was not wise to give any information respecting himself, and for fear that Mr. Cray might draw him into conversation and recognise his voice, my master resolved to feign deafness as the only means of self-defence.

After a little while, Mr. Cray said to my master, "It is a very fine morning, sir." The latter took no notice, but kept looking out of the window. Mr. Cray soon repeated this remark, in a little louder tone, but my master remained as before. This indifference attracted the attention of the passengers near, one of whom laughed out. This, I suppose, annoyed the old gentleman; so he said, "I will make him hear;" and in a loud tone of voice repeated, "It is a very fine morning, sir."

My master turned his head, and with a polite bow said, "Yes," and commenced looking out of the window again.

One of the gentlemen remarked that it was a very great deprivation to be deaf. "Yes," replied Mr. Cray, "and I shall not trouble that fellow any more." This enabled my master to breathe a little easier, and to feel that Mr. Cray was not his pursuer after all.

The gentlemen then turned the conversation upon the three great topics of discussion in first-class circles in Georgia, namely, Niggers, Cotton, and the Abolitionists.

My master had often heard of abolitionists, but in such a connection as to cause him to think that they were a fearful kind of wild animal. But he was highly delighted to learn, from the gentlemen's conversation, that the abolitionists were persons who were opposed to oppression; and therefore, in his opinion, not the lowest, but the very highest, of God's creatures.

Without the slightest objection on my master's part, the gentlemen left the carriage at Gordon, for Milledgeville (the capital of the State).

We arrived at Savannah early in the evening, and got into an omnibus, which stopped at the hotel for the passengers to take tea. I stepped into the house and brought my master something on a tray to the omnibus, which took us in due time to the steamer, which was bound for Charleston, South Carolina.

Soon after going on board, my master turned in; and as the captain and some of the passengers seemed to think this strange, and also questioned me respecting him, my master thought I had better get out the flannels and opodeldoc which we had prepared for the rheumatism, warm them quickly by the stove in the gentleman's saloon, and bring them to his berth. We did this as an excuse for my master's retiring to bed so early.

While at the stove one of the passengers said to me, "Buck, what have you got there?" "Opodeldoc, sir," I replied. "I should think it's opo*devil*," said a lanky swell, who was leaning back in a chair with his heels upon the back of another, and chewing tobacco as if for a wager; "it stinks enough to kill or cure twenty men. Away with it, or I reckon I will throw it overboard!"

It was by this time warm enough, so I took it to my master's berth, remained there a little while, and then went on deck and asked the steward where I was to sleep. He said there was no place provided for coloured passengers, whether slave or free. So I paced the deck till a late hour, then mounted some cotton bags, in a warm place near the funnel, sat there till morning, and then went and assisted my master to get ready for breakfast.

He was seated at the right hand of the captain, who, together with all the passengers, inquired very kindly after his health. As my master had one hand in a sling, it was my duty to carve his food. But when I went out the captain said, "You have a very attentive boy, sir; but you had better watch him like a hawk when you get on to the North. He seems all very well here, but he may act quite differently there. I know several gentlemen who have lost their valuable niggers among them d——d cut-throat abolitionists."

Before my master could speak, a rough slave-dealer, who was sitting opposite, with both elbows on the table, and with a large piece of broiled fowl in his fingers, shook his head with emphasis, and in a deep Yankee tone, forced through his crowded mouth the words, "Sound doctrine, captain, very sound." He then dropped the chicken into the plate, leant back, placed his thumbs in the armholes of his fancy waistcoat, and continued, "I would not take a nigger to the North under no consideration. I have had a deal to do with niggers in my time, but I never saw one who ever had his heel upon free soil that was worth a d——n." "Now stranger," addressing my master, "if you have made up your mind to sell that ere nigger, I am your man; just mention your price, and if it isn't out of the way, I will pay for him on this board with hard silver dollars." This hard-featured, bristly-bearded, wire-headed, red-eyed monster, staring at my master as the serpent did at Eve, said, "What do you say, stranger?" He replied, "I don't wish to sell, sir; I cannot get on well without him."

"You will have to get on without him if you take him to the North," continued this man; "for I can tell ye, stranger, as a friend, I am an older cove than you, I have seen lots of this ere world, and I reckon I have had more dealings with niggers than any man living or dead. I was once employed by General Wade Hampton, for ten years, in doing nothing but breaking

'em in; and everybody knows that the General would not
have a man that didn't understand his business. So I tell ye,
stranger, again, you had better sell, and let me take him down
to Orleans. He will do you no good if you take him across
Mason's and Dixon's line; he is a keen nigger, and I can see
from the cut of his eye that he is certain to run away." My
master said, "I think not, sir; I have great confidence in his fidelity." "Fi*devil*," indignantly said the dealer, as his fist came
down upon the edge of the saucer and upset a cup of hot coffee in a gentleman's lap. (As the scalded man jumped up the
trader quietly said, "Don't disturb yourself, neighbour; accidents will happen in the best of families.") "It always makes
me mad to hear a man talking about fidelity in niggers. There
isn't a d——d one on 'em who wouldn't cut sticks, if he had
half a chance."

By this time we were near Charleston; my master thanked
the captain for his advice, and they all withdrew and went on
deck, where the trader fancied he became quite eloquent. He
drew a crowd around him, and with emphasis said, "Cap'en,
if I was the President of this mighty United States of America, the greatest and freest country under the whole univarse,
I would never let no man, I don't care who he is, take a nigger into the North and bring him back here, filled to the
brim, as he is sure to be, with d——d abolition vices, to taint
all quiet niggers with the hellish spirit of running away. These
air, cap'en, my flat-footed, every day, right up and down sentiments, and as this is a free country, cap'en, I don't care who
hears 'em; for I am a Southern man, every inch on me to the
backbone." "Good!" said an insignificant-looking individual
of the slave-dealer stamp. "Three cheers for John C. Calhoun
and the whole fair sunny South!" added the trader. So off
went their hats, and out burst a terrific roar of irregular but
continued cheering. My master took no more notice of the
dealer. He merely said to the captain that the air on deck was
too keen for him, and he would therefore return to the cabin.

While the trader was in the zenith of his eloquence, he
might as well have said, as one of his kit did, at a great Fili-
bustering meeting, that "When the great American Eagle gets
one of his mighty claws upon Canada and the other into
South America, and his glorious and starry wings of liberty

extending from the Atlantic to the Pacific, oh! then, where will England be, ye gentlemen? I tell ye, she will only serve as a pocket-handkerchief for Jonathan to wipe his nose with."

On my master entering the cabin he found at the breakfast-table a young southern military officer, with whom he had travelled some distance the previous day.

After passing the usual compliments the conversation turned upon the old subject,—niggers.

The officer, who was also travelling with a manservant, said to my master, "You will excuse me, Sir, for saying I think you are very likely to spoil your boy by saying 'thank you' to him. I assure you, sir, nothing spoils a slave so soon as saying, 'thank you' and 'if you please' to him. The only way to make a nigger toe the mark, and to keep him in his place, is to storm at him like thunder, and keep him trembling like a leaf. Don't you see, when I speak to my Ned, he darts like lightning; and if he didn't I'd skin him."

Just then the poor dejected slave came in, and the officer swore at him fearfully, merely to teach my master what he called the proper way to treat me.

After he had gone out to get his master's luggage ready, the officer said, "That is the way to speak to them. If every nigger was drilled in this manner, they would be as humble as dogs, and never dare to run away.

The gentleman urged my master not to go to the North for the restoration of his health, but to visit the Warm Springs in Arkansas.

My master said, he thought the air of Philadelphia would suit his complaint best; and, not only so, he thought he could get better advice there.

The boat had now reached the wharf. The officer wished my master a safe and pleasant journey, and left the saloon.

There were a large number of persons on the quay waiting the arrival of the steamer: but we were afraid to venture out for fear that some one might recognize me; or that they had heard that we were gone, and had telegraphed to have us stopped. However, after remaining in the cabin till all the other passengers were gone, we had our luggage placed on a fly, and I took my master by the arm, and with a little difficulty he hobbled on shore, got in and drove off to the best

hotel, which John C. Calhoun, and all the other great southern fire-eating statesmen, made their head-quarters while in
Charleston.

On arriving at the house the landlord ran out and opened
the door: but judging, from the poultices and green glasses,
that my master was an invalid, he took him very tenderly by
one arm and ordered his man to take the other.

My master then eased himself out, and with their assistance
found no trouble in getting up the steps into the hotel. The
proprietor made me stand on one side, while he paid my master the attention and homage he thought a gentleman of his
high position merited.

My master asked for a bed-room. The servant was ordered
to show a good one, into which we helped him. The servant
returned. My master then handed me the bandages, I took
them downstairs in great haste, and told the landlord my master wanted two hot poultices as quickly as possible. He rang
the bell, the servant came in, to whom he said, "Run to the
kitchen and tell the cook to make two hot poultices right off,
for there is a gentleman upstairs very badly off indeed!"

In a few minutes the smoking poultices were brought in. I
placed them in white handkerchiefs, and hurried upstairs,
went into my master's apartment, shut the door, and laid
them on the mantel-piece. As he was alone for a little while,
he thought he could rest a great deal better with the poultices
off. However, it was necessary to have them to complete the
remainder of the journey. I then ordered dinner, and took my
master's boots out to polish them. While doing so I entered
into conversation with one of the slaves. I may state here, that
on the sea-coast of South Carolina and Georgia the slaves
speak worse English than in any other part of the country.
This is owing to the frequent importation, or smuggling in,
of Africans, who mingle with the natives. Consequently the
language cannot properly be called English or African, but a
corruption of the two.

The shrewd son of African parents to whom I referred said
to me, "Say, brudder, way you come from, and which side
you goin day wid dat ar little don up buckra" (white man)?

I replied, "To Philadelphia."

"What!" he exclaimed, with astonishment, "to Philuma-delphy?"

"Yes," I said.

"By squash! I wish I was going wid you! I hears um say dat dare's no slaves way over in dem parts; is um so?"

I quietly said, "I have heard the same thing."

"Well," continued he, as he threw down the boot and brush, and, placing his hands in his pockets, strutted across the floor with an air of independence—"Gorra Mighty, dem is de parts for Pompey; and I hope when you get dare you will stay, and nebber follow dat buckra back to dis hot quarter no more, let him be eber so good."

I thanked him; and just as I took the boots up and started off, he caught my hand between his two, and gave it a hearty shake, and, with tears streaming down his cheeks, said:—

"God bless you, broder, and may de Lord be wid you. When you gets de freedom, and sitin under your own wine and fig-tree, don't forget to pray for poor Pompey."

I was afraid to say much to him, but I shall never forget his earnest request, nor fail to do what little I can to release the millions of unhappy bondmen, of whom he was one.

At the proper time my master had the poultices placed on, came down, and seated himself at a table in a very brilliant dining-room, to have his dinner. I had to have something at the same time, in order to be ready for the boat; so they gave me my dinner in an old broken plate, with a rusty knife and fork, and said, "Here, boy, you go in the kitchen." I took it and went out, but did not stay more than a few minutes, because I was in a great hurry to get back to see how the invalid was getting on. On arriving I found two or three servants waiting on him; but as he did not feel able to make a very hearty dinner, he soon finished, paid the bill, and gave the servants each a trifle, which caused one of them to say to me, "Your massa is a big bug"—meaning a gentleman of distinction—"he is the greatest gentleman dat has been dis way for dis six months." I said, "Yes, he is some pumpkins," meaning the same as "big bug."

When we left Maçon, it was our intention to take a steamer at Charleston through to Philadelphia; but on arriving there we found that the vessels did not run during the winter, and I have no doubt it was well for us they did not; for on the very last voyage the steamer made that we intended to go by, a fugitive was discovered secreted on board, and sent back to slavery. However, as we had also heard of the Overland Mail Route, we were all right. So I ordered a fly to the door, had the luggage placed on; we got in, and drove down to the Custom-house Office, which was near the wharf where we had to obtain tickets, to take a steamer for Wilmington, North Carolina. When we reached the building, I helped my master into the office, which was crowded with passengers. He asked for a ticket for himself and one for his slave to Philadelphia. This caused the principal officer—a very mean-looking, cheese-coloured fellow, who was sitting there—to look up at us very suspiciously, and in a fierce tone of voice he said to me, "Boy, do you belong to that gentleman?" I quickly replied, "Yes, sir" (which was quite correct). The tickets were handed out, and as my master was paying for them the chief man said to him, "I wish you to register your name here, sir, and also the name of your nigger, and pay a dollar duty on him."

My master paid the dollar, and pointing to the hand that was in the poultice, requested the officer to register his name for him. This seemed to offend the "high-bred" South Carolinian. He jumped up, shaking his head; and, cramming his hands almost through the bottom of his trousers pockets, with a slave-bullying air, said, "I shan't do it."

This attracted the attention of all the passengers. Just then the young military officer with whom my master travelled and conversed on the steamer from Savannah stepped in, somewhat the worse for brandy; he shook hands with my master, and pretended to know all about him. He said, "I know his kin (friends) like a book;" and as the officer was known in Charleston, and was going to stop there with friends, the recognition was very much in my master's favour.

The captain of the steamer, a good-looking jovial fellow, seeing that the gentleman appeared to know my master, and perhaps not wishing to lose us as passengers, said in an off-hand sailor-like manner, "I will register the gentleman's name, and take the responsibility upon myself." He asked my master's name. He said, "William Johnson." The names were put down, I think, "Mr. Johnson and slave." The captain said, "It's all right now, Mr. Johnson." He thanked him kindly, and the young officer begged my master to go with him, and have something to drink and a cigar; but as he had not acquired these accomplishments, he excused himself, and we went on board and came off to Wilmington, North Carolina. When the gentleman finds out his mistake, he will, I have no doubt, be careful in future not to pretend to have an intimate acquaintance with an entire stranger. During the voyage the captain said, "It was rather sharp shooting this morning, Mr. Johnson. It was not out of any disrespect to you, sir; but they make it a rule to be very strict at Charleston. I have known families to be detained there with their slaves till reliable information could be received respecting them. If they were not very careful, any d——d abolitionist might take off a lot of valuable niggers."

My master said, "I suppose so," and thanked him again for helping him over the difficulty.

We reached Wilmington the next morning, and took the train for Richmond, Virginia. I have stated that the American railway carriages (or cars, as they are called), are constructed differently to those in England. At one end of some of them, in the South, there is a little apartment with a couch on both sides for the convenience of families and invalids; and as they thought my master was very poorly, he was allowed to enter one of these apartments at Petersburg, Virginia, where an old gentleman and two handsome young ladies, his daughters, also got in, and took seats in the same carriage. But before the train started, the gentleman stepped into my car, and questioned me respecting my master. He wished to know what was the matter with him, where he was from, and where he was going. I told him where he came from, and said that he was suffering from a complication of complaints, and was going to Philadelphia, where he thought he could get more suitable advice than in Georgia.

The gentleman said my master could obtain the very best advice in Philadelphia. Which turned out to be quite correct, though he did not receive it from physicians, but from kind abolitionists who understood his case much better. The gentleman also said, "I reckon your master's father hasn't any more such faithful and smart boys as you." "O, yes, sir, he has," I replied, "lots on 'em." Which was literally true. This seemed all he wished to know. He thanked me, gave me a ten-cent piece, and requested me to be attentive to my good master. I promised that I would do so, and have ever since endeavoured to keep my pledge. During the gentleman's absence, the ladies and my master had a little cosy chat. But on his return, he said, "You seem to be very much afflicted, sir." "Yes, sir," replied the gentleman in the poultices. "What seems to be the matter with you, sir; may I be allowed to ask?" "Inflammatory rheumatism, sir." "Oh! that is very bad, sir," said the kind gentleman: "I can sympathise with you; for I know from bitter experience what the rheumatism is." If he did, he knew a good deal more than Mr. Johnson.

The gentleman thought my master would feel better if he would lie down and rest himself; and as he was anxious to avoid conversation, he at once acted upon this suggestion. The ladies politely rose, took their extra shawls, and made a nice pillow for the invalid's head. My master wore a fashionable cloth cloak, which they took and covered him comfortably on the couch. After he had been lying a little while the ladies, I suppose, thought he was asleep; so one of them gave a long sigh, and said, in a quiet fascinating tone, "Papa, he seems to be a very nice young gentleman." But before papa could speak, the other lady quickly said, "Oh! dear me, I never felt so much for a gentleman in my life!" To use an American expression, "they fell in love with the wrong chap."

After my master had been lying a little while he got up, the gentleman assisted him in getting on his cloak, the ladies took their shawls, and soon all were seated. They then insisted upon Mr. Johnson taking some of their refreshments, which of course he did, out of courtesy to the ladies. All went on enjoying themselves until they reached Richmond, where the ladies and their father left the train. But, before doing so, the good old Virginian gentleman, who appeared to be much pleased with my master, presented him with a recipe, which he said was a perfect cure for the inflammatory rheumatism. But the invalid not being able to read it, and fearing he should hold it upside down in pretending to do so, thanked the donor kindly, and placed it in his waistcoat pocket. My master's new friend also gave him his card, and requested him the next time he travelled that way to do him the kindness to call; adding, "I shall be pleased to see you, and so will my daughters." Mr. Johnson expressed his gratitude for the proffered hospitality, and said he should feel glad to call on his return. I have not the slightest doubt that he will fulfil the promise whenever that return takes place. After changing trains we went on a little beyond Fredericksburg, and took a steamer to Washington.

At Richmond, a stout elderly lady, whose whole demeanour indicated that she belonged (as Mrs. Stowe's Aunt Chloe expresses it) to one of the "firstest families," stepped into the carriage, and took a seat near my master. Seeing me passing quickly along the platform, she sprang up as if taken by a fit, and exclaimed, "Bless my soul! there goes my nigger, Ned!"

My master said, "No; that is my boy."

The lady paid no attention to this; she poked her head out of the window, and bawled to me, "You Ned, come to me, sir, you runaway rascal!"

On my looking round she drew her head in, and said to my master, "I beg your pardon, sir, I was sure it was my nigger; I never in my life saw two black pigs more alike than your boy and my Ned."

After the disappointed lady had resumed her seat, and the train had moved off, she closed her eyes, slightly raising her hands, and in a sanctified tone said to my master, "Oh! I hope, sir, your boy will not turn out to be so worthless as my Ned has. Oh! I was as kind to him as if he had been my own son. Oh! sir, it grieves me very much to think that after all I did for him he should go off without having any cause whatever."

"When did he leave you?" asked Mr. Johnson.

"About eighteen months ago, and I have never seen hair or hide of him since."

"Did he have a wife?" enquired a very respectable-looking young gentleman, who was sitting near my master and opposite to the lady.

"No, sir; not when he left, though he did have one a little before that. She was very unlike him; she was as good and as faithful a nigger as any one need wish to have. But, poor thing! she became so ill, that she was unable to do much work; so I thought it would be best to sell her, to go to New Orleans, where the climate is nice and warm."

"I suppose she was very glad to go South for the restoration of her health?" said the gentleman.

"No; she was not," replied the lady, "for niggers never know what is best for them. She took on a great deal about leaving Ned and the little nigger; but, as she was so weakly, I let her go."

"Was she good-looking?" asked the young passenger, who was evidently not of the same opinion as the talkative lady, and therefore wished her to tell all she knew.

"Yes; she was very handsome, and much whiter than I am; and therefore will have no trouble in getting another husband. I am sure I wish her well. I asked the speculator who bought her to sell her to a good master. Poor thing! she has my prayers, and I know she prays for me. She was a good Christian, and always used to pray for my soul. It was through her earliest prayers," continued the lady, "that I was first led to seek forgiveness of my sins, before I was converted at the great camp-meeting."

This caused the lady to snuffle and to draw from her pocket a richly embroidered handkerchief, and apply it to the corner of her eyes. But my master could not see that it was at all soiled.

The silence which prevailed for a few moments was broken by the gentleman's saying, "As your 'July' was such a very good girl, and had served you so faithfully before she lost her health, don't you think it would have been better to have emancipated her?"

"No, indeed I do not!" scornfully exclaimed the lady, as she impatiently crammed the fine handkerchief into a little work-bag. "I have no patience with people who set niggers at liberty. It is the very worst thing you can do for them. My dear husband just before he died willed all his niggers free. But I and all our friends knew very well that he was too good a man to have ever thought of doing such an unkind and foolish thing, had he been in his right mind, and, therefore we had the will altered as it should have been in the first place."

"Did you mean, madam," asked my master, "that willing the slaves free was unjust to yourself, or unkind to them?"

"I mean that it was decidedly unkind to the servants themselves. It always seems to me such a cruel thing to turn niggers loose to shift for themselves, when there are so many good masters to take care of them. As for myself," continued the considerate lady, "I thank the Lord my dear husband left me and my son well provided for. Therefore I care nothing for the niggers, on my own account, for they are a great deal more trouble than they are worth, I sometimes wish that there was not one of them in the world; for the ungrateful wretches are always running away. I have lost no less than ten since my poor husband died. It's ruinous, sir!"

"But as you are well provided for, I suppose you do not feel the loss very much," said the passenger.

"I don't feel it at all," haughtily continued the good soul; "but that is no reason why property should be squandered. If my son and myself had the money for those valuable niggers, just see what a great deal of good we could do for the poor, and in sending missionaries abroad to the poor heathen, who have never heard the name of our blessed Redeemer. My dear son who is a good Christian minister has advised me not to worry and send my soul to hell for the sake of niggers; but to sell every blessed one of them for what they will fetch, and go and live in peace with him in New York. This I have concluded to do. I have just been to Richmond and made arrangements with my agent to make clean work of the forty that are left."

"Your son being a good Christian minister," said the gentleman, "it's strange he did not advise you to let the poor negroes have their liberty and go North."

"It's not at all strange, sir; it's not at all strange. My son knows what's best for the niggers; he has always told me that they were much better off than the free niggers in the North. In fact, I don't believe there are any white labouring people in the world who are as well off as the slaves."

"You are quite mistaken, madam," said the young man. "For instance, my own widowed mother, before she died, emancipated all her slaves, and sent them to Ohio, where they are getting along well. I saw several of them last summer myself."

"Well," replied the lady, "freedom may do for your ma's niggers, but it will never do for mine; and, plague them, they shall never have it; that is the word, with the bark on it."

"If freedom will not do for your slaves," replied the passenger, "I have no doubt your Ned and the other nine negroes will find out their mistake, and return to their old home."

"Blast them!" exclaimed the old lady, with great emphasis, "if I ever get them, I will cook their infernal hash, and tan their accursed black hides well for them! God forgive me," added the old soul, "the niggers will make me lose all my religion!"

By this time the lady had reached her destination. The gentleman got out at the next station beyond. As soon as she was gone, the young Southerner said to my master, "What a d——d shame it is for that old whining hypocritical humbug to cheat the poor negroes out of their liberty! If she has religion, may the devil prevent me from ever being converted!"

For the purpose of somewhat disguising myself, I bought and wore a very good second-hand white beaver, an article which I had never indulged in before. So just before we arrived at Washington, an uncouth planter, who had been watching me very closely, said to my master, "I reckon, stranger, you are '*spiling*' that ere nigger of yourn, by letting him wear such a devilish fine hat. Just look at the quality on it; the President couldn't wear a better. I should just like to go and kick it overboard." His friend touched him, and said, "Don't speak so to a gentleman." "Why not?" exclaimed the fellow. He grated his short teeth, which appeared to be nearly worn away by the incessant chewing of tobacco, and said, "It always makes me itch all over, from head to toe, to get hold of every d——d nigger I see dressed like a white man. Washington is run away with *spiled* and free niggers. If I had my way I would sell every d——d rascal of 'em way down South, where the devil would be whipped out on 'em."

This man's fierce manner made my master feel rather nervous, and therefore he thought the less he said the better; so he walked off without making any reply. In a few minutes we were landed at Washington, where we took a conveyance and hurried off to the train for Baltimore.

We left our cottage on Wednesday morning, the 21st of December, 1848, and arrived at Baltimore, Saturday evening, the 24th (Christmas Eve). Baltimore was the last slave port of any note at which we stopped.

On arriving there we felt more anxious than ever, because we knew not what that last dark night would bring forth. It is true we were near the goal, but our poor hearts were still as if tossed at sea; and, as there was another great and dangerous bar to pass, we were afraid our liberties would be wrecked, and, like the ill-fated *Royal Charter*, go down for ever just off the place we longed to reach.

They are particularly watchful at Baltimore to prevent slaves from escaping into Pennsylvania, which is a free State. After I had seen my master into one of the best carriages, and was just about to step into mine, an officer, a full-blooded Yankee of the lower order, saw me. He came quickly up, and, tapping me on the shoulder, said in his unmistakable native twang, together with no little display of his authority, "Where are you going, boy?" "To Philadelphia, sir," I humbly replied. "Well, what are you going there for?" "I am travelling with my master, who is in the next carriage, sir." "Well, I calculate you had better get him out; and be mighty quick about it, because the train will soon be starting. It is against my rules to let any man take a slave past here, unless he can satisfy them in the office that he has a right to take him along."

The officer then passed on and left me standing upon the platform, with my anxious heart apparently palpitating in the throat. At first I scarcely knew which way to turn. But it soon occurred to me that the good God, who had been with us thus far, would not forsake us at the eleventh hour. So with renewed hope I stepped into my master's carriage, to inform him of the difficulty. I found him sitting at the farther end, quite alone. As soon as he looked up and saw me, he smiled. I also tried to wear a cheerful countenance, in order to break the shock of the sad news. I knew what made him smile. He was aware that if we were fortunate we should reach our destination at five o'clock the next morning, and this made it the more painful to communicate what the officer had said; but, as there was no time to lose, I went up to him and asked him how he felt. He said "Much better," and that he thanked God we were getting on so nicely. I then said we were not getting on quite so well as we had anticipated. He anxiously and quickly asked what was the matter. I told him. He started as if struck by lightning, and exclaimed, "Good Heavens! William, is it possible that we are, after all, doomed to hopeless bondage?" I could say nothing, my heart was too full to speak, for at first I did not know what to do. However we knew it would never do to turn back to the "City of Destruction," like Bunyan's *Mistrust* and *Timorous*, because they saw lions in the narrow way after ascending the hill Difficulty; but press on, like noble *Christian* and *Hopeful*, to the great city in which dwelt a few "shining ones." So, after a few moments, I did all I could to encourage my companion, and we stepped out and made for the office: but how or where my master obtained sufficient courage to face the tyrants who had power to blast all we held dear, heaven only knows! Queen Elizabeth could not have been more terror-stricken, on being forced to land at the traitors' gate leading to the Tower, than we were on entering that office. We felt that our very existence was at stake, and that we must either sink or swim. But, as God was our present and mighty helper in this as well as in all former trials, we were able to keep our heads up and press forwards.

On entering the room we found the principal man, to whom my master said, "Do you wish to see me, sir?" "Yes," said this eagle-eyed officer; and he added, "It is against our rules, sir, to allow any person to take a slave out of Baltimore into Philadelphia, unless he can satisfy us that he has a right to take him along." "Why is that?" asked my master, with more firmness than could be expected. "Because, sir," continued he, in a voice and manner that almost chilled our blood, "if we should suffer any gentleman to take a slave past here into Philadelphia; and should the gentleman with whom the slave might be travelling turn out not to be his rightful owner; and should the proper master come and prove that his slave escaped on our road, we shall have him to pay for; and, therefore, we cannot let any slave pass here without receiving security to show, and to satisfy us, that it is all right."

This conversation attracted the attention of the large number of bustling passengers. After the officer had finished, a few of them said, "Chit, chit, chit;" not because they thought we were slaves endeavouring to escape, but merely because they thought my master was a slaveholder and invalid gentleman, and therefore it was wrong to detain him. The officer, observing that the passengers sympathised with my master, asked him if he was not acquainted with some gentleman in Baltimore that he could get to endorse for him, to show that I was his property, and that he had a right to take me off. He said, "No;" and added, "I bought tickets in Charleston to pass us through to Philadelphia, and therefore you have no right to detain us here." "Well, sir," said the man, indignantly, "right or no right, we shan't let you go." These sharp words fell upon our anxious hearts like the crack of doom, and made us feel that hope only smiles to deceive.

For a few moments perfect silence prevailed. My master looked at me, and I at him, but neither of us dared to speak a word, for fear of making some blunder that would tend to our detection. We knew that the officers had power to throw us into prison, and if they had done so we must have been detected and driven back, like the vilest felons, to a life of slavery, which we dreaded far more than sudden death.

We felt as though we had come into deep waters and were about being overwhelmed, and that the slightest mistake would clip asunder the last brittle thread of hope by which we were suspended, and let us down for ever into the dark and horrible pit of misery and degradation from which we were straining every nerve to escape. While our hearts were crying lustily unto Him who is ever ready and able to save, the conductor of the train that we had just left stepped in. The officer asked if we came by the train with him from Washington; he said we did, and left the room. Just then the bell rang for the train to leave; and had it been the sudden shock of an earthquake it could not have given us a greater thrill. The sound of the bell caused every eye to flash with apparent interest, and to be more steadily fixed upon us than before. But, as God would have it, the officer all at once thrust his fingers through his hair, and in a state of great agitation said, "I really don't know what to do; I calculate it is all right." He then told the clerk to run and tell the conductor to "let this gentleman and slave pass;" adding, "As he is not well, it is a pity to stop him here. We will let him go." My master thanked him, and stepped out and hobbled across the platform as quickly as possible. I tumbled him unceremoniously into one of the best carriages, and leaped into mine just as the train was gliding off towards our happy destination.

We thought of this plan about four days before we left Maçon; and as we had our daily employment to attend to, we only saw each other at night. So we sat up the four long nights talking over the plan and making preparations.

We had also been four days on the journey; and as we travelled night and day, we got but very limited opportunities for sleeping. I believe nothing in the world could have kept us awake so long but the intense excitement, produced by the fear of being retaken on the one hand, and the bright anticipation of liberty on the other.

We left Baltimore about eight o'clock in the evening; and not being aware of a stopping-place of any consequence between there and Philadelphia, and also knowing that if we were fortunate we should be in the latter place early the next morning, I thought I might indulge in a few minutes' sleep in the car; but I, like Bunyan's Christian in the arbour, went to sleep at the wrong time, and took too long a nap. So, when the train reached Havre de Grace, all the first-class passengers had to get out of the carriages and into a ferry-boat, to be ferried across the Susquehanna river, and take the train on the opposite side.

The road was constructed so as to be raised or lowered to suit the tide. So they rolled the luggage-vans on to the boat, and off on the other side; and as I was in one of the apartments adjoining a baggage-car, they considered it unnecessary to awaken me, and tumbled me over with the luggage. But when my master was asked to leave his seat, he found it very dark, and cold, and raining. He missed me for the first time on the journey. On all previous occasions, as soon as the train stopped, I was at hand to assist him. This caused many slave-holders to praise me very much: they said they had never before seen a slave so attentive to his master: and therefore my absence filled him with terror and confusion; the children of Israel could not have felt more troubled on arriving at the

Red Sea. So he asked the conductor if he had seen anything of his slave. The man being somewhat of an abolitionist, and believing that my master was really a slaveholder, thought he would tease him a little respecting me. So he said, "No, sir; I haven't seen anything of him for some time: I have no doubt he has run away, and is in Philadelphia, free, long before now." My master knew that there was nothing in this; so he asked the conductor if he would please to see if he could find me. The man indignantly replied, "I am no slave-hunter; and as far as I am concerned everybody must look after their own niggers." He went off and left the confused invalid to fancy whatever he felt inclined. My master at first thought I must have been kidnapped into slavery by some one, or left, or perhaps killed on the train. He also thought of stopping to see if he could hear anything of me, but he soon remembered that he had no money. That night all the money we had was consigned to my own pocket, because we thought, in case there were any pickpockets about, a slave's pocket would be the last one they would look for. However, hoping to meet me some day in a land of liberty, and as he had the tickets, he thought it best upon the whole to enter the boat and come off to Philadelphia, and endeavour to make his way alone in this cold and hollow world as best he could. The time was now up, so he went on board and came across with feelings that can be better imagined than described.

After the train had got fairly on the way to Philadelphia, the guard came into my car and gave me a violent shake, and bawled out at the same time, "Boy, wake up!" I started, almost frightened out of my wits. He said, "Your master is scared half to death about you." That frightened me still more—I thought they had found him out; so I anxiously inquired what was the matter. The guard said, "He thinks you have run away from him." This made me feel quite at ease. I said, "No, sir; I am satisfied my good master doesn't think that." So off I started to see him. He had been fearfully nervous, but on seeing me he at once felt much better. He merely wished to know what had become of me.

On returning to my seat, I found the conductor and two or three other persons amusing themselves very much respecting my running away. So the guard said, "Boy, what did your master want?* I replied, "He merely wished to know what had become of me." "No," said the man, "that was not it; he thought you had taken French leave, for parts unknown. I never saw a fellow so badly scared about losing his slave in my life. Now," continued the guard, "let me give you a little friendly advice. When you get to Philadelphia, run away and leave that cripple, and have your liberty." "No, sir," I indifferently replied, "I can't promise to do that." "Why not?" said the conductor, evidently much surprised; "don't you want your liberty?" "Yes, sir," I replied; "but I shall never run away from such a good master as I have at present."

One of the men said to the guard, "Let him alone; I guess he will open his eyes when he gets to Philadelphia, and see things in another light." After giving me a good deal of information, which I afterwards found to be very useful, they left me alone.

I also met with a coloured gentleman on this train, who recommended me to a boarding-house that was kept by an abolitionist, where he thought I would be quite safe, if I wished to run away from my master. I thanked him kindly, but of course did not let him know who we were. Late at night, or rather early in the morning, I heard a fearful whistling of the steam-engine; so I opened the window and looked out, and saw a large number of flickering lights in the distance, and heard a passenger in the next carriage—who also had his head out of the window—say to his companion, "Wake up, old horse, we are at Philadelphia!"

The sight of those lights and that announcement made me feel almost as happy as Bunyan's Christian must have felt when he first caught sight of the cross. I, like him, felt that the straps that bound the heavy burden to my back began to pop, and the load to roll off. I also looked, and looked again, for it appeared very wonderful to me how the mere sight of our first city of refuge should have all at once made my hitherto sad and heavy heart become so light and happy. As the

*I may state here that every man slave is called boy till he is very old, then the more respectable slaveholders call him uncle. The women are all girls till they are aged, then they are called aunts. This is the reason why Mrs. Stowe calls her characters Uncle Tom, Aunt Chloe, Uncle Tiff, &c.

train speeded on, I rejoiced and thanked God with all my heart and soul for his great kindness and tender mercy, in watching over us, and bringing us safely through.

As soon as the train had reached the platform, before it had fairly stopped, I hurried out of my carriage to my master, whom I got at once into a cab, placed the luggage on, jumped in myself, and we drove off to the boarding-house which was so kindly recommended to me. On leaving the station, my master—or rather my wife, as I may now say—who had from the commencement of the journey borne up in a manner that much surprised us both, grasped me by the hand, and said, "Thank God, William, we are safe!" then burst into tears, leant upon me, and wept like a child. The reaction was fearful. So when we reached the house, she was in reality so weak and faint that she could scarcely stand alone. However, I got her into the apartments that were pointed out, and there we knelt down, on this Sabbath, and Christmas-day,—a day that will ever be memorable to us,—and poured out our heartfelt gratitude to God, for his goodness in enabling us to overcome so many perilous difficulties, in escaping out of the jaws of the wicked.

PART II.

After my wife had a little recovered herself, she threw off the disguise and assumed her own apparel. We then stepped into the sitting-room, and asked to see the landlord. The man came in, but he seemed thunderstruck on finding a fugitive slave and his wife, instead of a "young cotton planter and his nigger." As his eyes travelled round the room, he said to me. "Where is your master?" I pointed him out. The man gravely replied, "I am not joking, I really wish to see your master." I pointed him out again, but at first he could not believe his eyes; he said "he knew that was not the gentleman that came with me."

But, after some conversation, we satisfied him that we were fugitive slaves, and had just escaped in the manner I have described. We asked him if he thought it would be safe for us to stop in Philadelphia. He said he thought not, but he would call in some persons who knew more about the laws than himself. He then went out, and kindly brought in several of the leading abolitionists of the city, who gave us a most hearty and friendly welcome amongst them. As it was in December, and also as we had just left a very warm climate, they advised us not to go to Canada as we had intended, but to settle at Boston in the United States. It is true that the constitution of the Republic has always guaranteed the slaveholders the right to come into any of the so-called free States, and take their fugitives back to southern Egypt. But through the untiring, uncompromising, and manly efforts of Mr. Garrison, Wendell Phillips, Theodore Parker, and a host of other noble abolitionists of Boston and the neighbourhood, public opinion in Massachusetts had become so much opposed to slavery and to kidnapping, that it was almost impossible for any one to take a fugitive slave out of that State.

So we took the advice of our good Philadelphia friends, and settled at Boston. I shall have something to say about our sojourn there presently.

Among other friends we met with at Philadelphia, was Robert Purves, Esq., a well educated and wealthy coloured gentleman, who introduced us to Mr. Barkley Ivens, a member of the Society of Friends, and a noble and generous-hearted farmer, who lived at some distance in the country.

This good Samaritan at once invited us to go and stop quietly with his family, till my wife could somewhat recover from the fearful reaction of the past journey. We most gratefully accepted the invitation, and at the time appointed we took a steamer to a place up the Delaware river, where our new and dear friend met us with his snug little cart, and took us to his happy home. This was the first act of great and disinterested kindness we had ever received from a white person.

The gentleman was not of the fairest complexion, and therefore, as my wife was not in the room when I received the information respecting him and his anti-slavery character, she thought of course he was a quadroon like herself. But on arriving at the house, and finding out her mistake, she became more nervous and timid than ever.

As the cart came into the yard, the dear good old lady, and her three charming and affectionate daughters, all came to the door to meet us. We got out, and the gentleman said, "Go in, and make yourselves at home; I will see after the baggage." But my wife was afraid to approach them. She stopped in the yard, and said to me, "William, I thought we were coming among coloured people?" I replied, "It is all right; these are the same." "No," she said, "it is not all right, and I am not going to stop here; I have no confidence whatever in white people, they are only trying to get us back to slavery." She turned round and said, "I am going right off." The old lady then came out, with her sweet, soft, and winning smile, shook her heartily by the hand, and kindly said, "How art thou, my dear? We are all very glad to see thee and thy husband. Come in, to the fire; I dare say thou art cold and hungry after thy journey."

We went in, and the young ladies asked if she would like to go upstairs and "fix" herself before tea. My wife said, "No, I thank you; I shall only stop a little while." "But where art thou going this cold night?" said Mr. Ivens, who had just stepped in. "I don't know," was the reply. "Well, then," he continued, "I think thou hadst better take off thy things and sit near the fire; tea will soon be ready." "Yes, come Ellen," said Mrs. Ivens, "let me assist thee;" (as she commenced undoing my wife's bonnet-strings;) "don't be frightened, Ellen, I shall not hurt a single hair of thy head. We have heard with much pleasure of the marvellous escape of thee and thy husband, and deeply sympathise with thee in all that thou hast undergone. I don't wonder at thee, poor thing, being timid; but thou needs not fear us; we would as soon send one of our own daughters into slavery as thee; so thou mayest make thyself quite at ease!" These soft and soothing words fell like balm upon my wife's unstrung nerves, and melted her to tears; her fears and prejudices vanished, and from that day she has firmly believed that there are good and bad persons of every shade of complexion.

After seeing Sally Ann and Jacob, two coloured domestics, my wife felt quite at home. After partaking of what Mrs. Stowe's Mose and Pete called a "busting supper," the ladies wished to know whether we could read. On learning we could not, they said if we liked they would teach us. To this kind offer, of course, there was no objection. But we looked rather knowingly at each other, as much as to say that they would have rather a hard task to cram anything into our thick and matured sculls.

However, all hands set to and quickly cleared away the tea-things, and the ladies and their good brother brought out the spelling and copy books and slates, &c., and commenced with their new and green pupils. We had, by stratagem, learned the alphabet while in slavery, but not the writing characters; and, as we had been such a time learning so little, we at first felt that it was a waste of time for any one at our ages to undertake to learn to read and write. But, as the ladies were so anxious that we should learn, and so willing to teach us, we concluded to give our whole minds to the work, and see what could be done. By so doing, at the end of the three weeks we remained with the good family we could spell and write our names quite legibly. They all begged us to stop longer; but, as we were not safe in the State of Pennsylvania, and also as we wished to commence doing something for a livelihood, we did not remain.

When the time arrived for us to leave for Boston, it was like parting with our relatives. We have since met with many very kind and hospitable friends, both in America and England; but we have never been under a roof where we were made to feel more at home, or where the inmates took a deeper interest in our well-being, than Mr. Barkley Ivens and his dear family. May God ever bless them, and preserve each one from every reverse of fortune!

We finally, as I have stated, settled at Boston, where we remained nearly two years, I employed as cabinet-maker and furniture broker, and my wife at her needle; and, as our little earnings in slavery were not all spent on the journey, we were getting on very well, and would have made money, if we had not been compelled by the General Government, at the bidding of the slaveholders, to break up business, and fly from under the Stars and Stripes to save our liberties and our lives.

In 1850, Congress passed the Fugitive Slave Bill, an enactment too infamous to have been thought of or tolerated by any people in the world, except the unprincipled and tyrannical Yankees. The following are a few of the leading features of the above law; which requires, under heavy penalties, that the inhabitants of the *free* States should not only refuse food and shelter to a starving, hunted human being, but also should assist, if called upon by the authorities, to seize the unhappy fugitive and send him back to slavery.

In no case is a person's evidence admitted in Court, in defence of his liberty, when arrested under this law.

If the judge decides that the prisoner is a slave, he gets ten dollars; but if he sets him at liberty, he only receives five.

After the prisoner has been sentenced to slavery, he is handed over to the United States Marshal, who has the power, at the expense of the General Government, to summon a sufficient force to take the poor creature back to slavery, and to the lash, from which he fled.

Our old masters sent agents to Boston after us. They took out warrants, and placed them in the hands of the United States Marshal to execute. But the following letter from our highly esteemed and faithful friend, the Rev. Samuel May, of Boston, to our equally dear and much lamented friend, Dr. Estlin of Bristol, will show why we were not taken into custody.

> "*21, Cornhill, Boston,*
> "*November 6th, 1850.*

"My dear Mr Estlin,
      "I trust that in God's good providence this letter will be handed to you in safety by our good friends, William and Ellen Craft. They have lived amongst us about two years, and have proved themselves worthy, in all respects, of our confidence and regard. The laws of this republican and Christian land (tell it not in Moscow, nor in Constantinople) regard them only as slaves—chattels—personal property. But they nobly vindicated their title and right to freedom, two years since, by winning their way to it; at least, so they thought. But now, the slave power, with the aid of Daniel Webster and a band of lesser traitors, has enacted a law, which puts their dearly-bought liberties in the most imminent peril; holds out a strong temptation to every mercenary and unprincipled ruffian to become their kidnapper; and has stimulated the slaveholders generally to such desperate acts for the recovery

of their fugitive property, as have never before been enacted in the history of this government.

"Within a fortnight, two fellows from Maçon, Georgia, have been in Boston for the purpose of arresting our friends William and Ellen. A writ was served against them from the United States District Court; but it was not served by the United States Marshal; why not, is not certainly known: perhaps through fear, for a general feeling of indignation, and a cool determination not to allow this young couple to be taken from Boston into slavery, was aroused, and pervaded the city. It is understood that one of the judges told the Marshal that he would not be authorised in breaking the door of Craft's house. Craft kept himself close within the house, armed himself, and awaited with remarkable composure the event. Ellen, in the meantime, had been taken to a retired place out of the city. The Vigilance Committee (appointed at a late meeting in Fanueil Hall) enlarged their numbers, held an almost permanent session, and appointed various subcommittees to act in different ways. One of these committees called repeatedly on Messrs. Hughes and Knight, the slave-catchers, and requested and advised them to leave the city. At first they peremptorily refused to do so, ''til they got hold of the niggers.' On complaint of different persons, these two fellows were several times arrested, carried before one of our county courts, and held to bail on charges of 'conspiracy to kidnap,' and of 'defamation,' in calling William and Ellen '*slaves*.' At length, they became so alarmed, that they left the city by an indirect route, evading the vigilance of many persons who were on the look-out for them. Hughes, at one time, was near losing his life at the hands of an infuriated coloured man. While these men remained in the city, a prominent whig gentleman sent word to William Craft, that if he would submit peaceably to an arrest, he and his wife should be bought from their owners, cost what it might. Craft replied, in effect, that he was in a measure the representative of all the other fugitives in Boston, some 200 or 300 in number; that, if he gave up, they would all be at the mercy of the slave-catchers, and must fly from the city at any sacrifice; and that, if his freedom could be bought for two cents, he would not consent to compromise the matter in such a way. This event has stirred up the slave spirit of the country, south and north; the United States government is determined to try its hand in enforcing the Fugitive Slave law; and William and Ellen Craft would be prominent objects of the slaveholders' vengeance. Under these circumstances, it is the almost unanimous opinion of their best friends, that they should quit America as speedily as possible, and seek an asylum in England! Oh! shame, shame upon us, that Americans, whose fathers fought against Great Britain, in order to be FREE, should have to acknowledge this disgraceful fact! God gave us a fair and goodly heritage in this land, but man has cursed it with his devices and crimes against human souls and human rights. Is America the 'land of the free, and the home of the brave?' God knows it is not; and we know it too. A brave young man and a virtuous young woman must fly the American shores, and seek, under the shadow of the British throne, the enjoyment of 'life, liberty, and the pursuit of happiness.'

"But I must pursue my plain, sad story. All day long, I have been busy planning a safe way for William and Ellen to leave Boston. We dare not allow them to go on board a vessel, even in the port of Boston; for the writ is yet in the Marshal's hands, and he *may* be waiting an opportunity to serve it; so I am expecting to accompany them to-morrow to Portland, Maine, which is beyond the reach of the Marshal's authority; and there I hope to see them on board a British steamer.

"This letter is written to introduce them to you. I know your infirm health; but I am sure, if you were stretched on your bed in your last illness, and could lift your hand at all, you would extend it to welcome these poor hunted fellow-creatures. Henceforth, England is their nation and their home. It is with real regret for our personal loss in their departure, as well as burning shame for the land that is not worthy of them, that we send them away, or rather allow them to go. But, with all the resolute courage they have shown in a most trying hour, they themselves see it is the part of a foolhardy rashness to attempt to stay here longer.

"I must close; and with many renewed thanks for all your kind words and deeds towards us,

"I am, very respectfully yours,

"SAMUEL MAY, JUN."

Our old masters, having heard how their agents were treated at Boston, wrote to Mr. Filmore, who was then President of the States, to know what he could do to have us sent back to slavery. Mr. Filmore said that we should be returned. He gave instructions for military force to be sent to Boston to assist the officers in making the arrest. Therefore we, as well as our friends (among whom was George Thompson, Esq., late M.P. for the Tower Hamlets—the slave's long-tried, self-sacrificing friend, and eloquent advocate) thought it best, at any sacrifice, to leave the mock-free Republic, and come to a country where we and our dear little ones can be truly free.— "No one daring to molest or make us afraid." But, as the officers were watching every vessel that left the port to prevent us from escaping, we had to take the expensive and tedious overland route to Halifax.

We shall always cherish the deepest feelings of gratitude to the Vigilance Committee of Boston (upon which were many of the leading abolitionists), and also to our numerous friends, for the very kind and noble manner in which they assisted us to preserve our liberties and to escape from Boston, as it were like Lot from Sodom, to a place of refuge, and finally to this truly free and glorious country; where no tyrant, let his power be ever so absolute over his poor trembling victims at home, dare come and lay violent hands upon us or upon our dear little boys (who had the good fortune to be born upon British soil), and reduce us to the legal level of the beast that perisheth. Oh! may God bless the thousands of unflinching, disinterested abolitionists of America, who are labouring through evil as well as through good report, to cleanse their country's escutcheon from the foul and destructive blot of slavery, and to restore to every bondman his God-given rights; and may God ever smile upon England and upon England's good, much-beloved, and deservedly-honoured Queen, for the generous protection that is given to unfortunate refugees of every rank, and of every colour and clime.

On the passing of the Fugitive Slave Bill, the following learned doctors, as well as a host of lesser traitors, came out strongly in its defence.

The Rev. Dr. Gardiner Spring, an eminent Presbyterian

Clergyman of New York, well known in this country by his religious publications, declared from the pulpit that, "if by one prayer he could liberate every slave in the world he would not dare to offer it."

The Rev. Dr. Joel Parker, of Philadelphia, in the course of a discussion on the nature of Slavery, says, "What, then, are the evils inseparable from slavery? There is not one that is not equally inseparable from depraved human nature in other lawful relations."

The Rev. Moses Stuart, D.D., (late Professor in the Theological College of Andover), in his vindication of this Bill, reminds his readers that "many Southern slaveholders are true *Christians.*" That "sending back a fugitive to them is not like restoring one to an idolatrous people." That "though we may *pity* the fugitive, yet the Mosaic Law does not authorize the rejection of the claims of the slaveholders to their stolen or strayed *property.*"

The Rev. Dr. Spencer, of Brooklyn, New York, has come forward in support of the "Fugitive Slave Bill," by publishing a sermon entitled the "Religious Duty of Obedience to the Laws," which has elicited the highest encomiums from Dr. Samuel H. Cox, the Presbyterian minister of Brooklyn (notorious both in this country and America for his sympathy with the slaveholder).

The Rev. W. M. Rogers, an orthodox minister of Boston, delivered a sermon in which he says, "When the slave asks me to stand between him and his master, what does he ask? He asks me to murder a nation's life; and I will not do it, because I have a conscience,—because there is a God." He proceeds to affirm that if resistance to the carrying out of the "Fugitive Slave Law" should lead the magistracy to call the citizens to arms, their duty was to obey and "if ordered to take human life, in the name of God to take it;" and he concludes by admonishing the fugitives to "hearken to the Word of God, and to count their own masters worthy of all honour."

The Rev. William Crowell, of Waterfield, State of Maine, printed a Thanksgiving Sermon of the same kind, in which he calls upon his hearers not to allow "excessive sympathies for a few hundred fugitives to blind them so as that they may risk increased suffering to the millions already in chains."

The Rev. Dr. Taylor, an Episcopal Clergyman of New Haven, Connecticut, made a speech at a Union Meeting, in which he deprecates the agitation on the law, and urges obedience to it; asking,—"Is that article in the Constitution contrary to the law of Nature, of nations, or to the will of God? Is it so? Is there a shadow of reason for saying it? I have not been able to discover it. Have I not shown you it is lawful to deliver up, in compliance with the laws, fugitive slaves, for the high, the great, the momentous interests of those [Southern] States?"

The Right Rev. Bishop Hopkins, of Vermont, in a Lecture at Lockport, says, "It was warranted by the Old Testament;" and inquires, "What effect had the Gospel in doing away with slavery? None whatever." Therefore he argues, as it is expressly permitted by the Bible, it does not in itself involve any sin; but that every Christian is authorised by the Divine Law to own slaves, provided they were not treated with unnecessary cruelty.

The Rev. Orville Dewey, D.D., of the Unitarian connexion, maintained in his lectures that the safety of the Union is not to be hazarded for the sake of the African race. He declares that, for his part, he would send his own brother or child into slavery, if needed to preserve the Union between the free and the slaveholding States; and, counselling the slave to similar magnanimity, thus exhorts him:—"*Your right to be free is not absolute, unqualified, irrespective of all consequences.* If my espousal of your claim is likely to involve your race and mine together in disasters infinitely greater than your personal servitude, then you ought not to be free. In such a case personal rights ought to be sacrificed to the general good. You yourself ought to see this, and be willing to suffer for a while—one for many."

If the Doctor is prepared, he is quite at liberty to sacrifice his "personal rights to the general good." But, as I have suffered a long time in slavery, it is hardly fair for the Doctor to advise me to go back. According to his showing, he ought rather to take my place. That would be practically carrying out his logic, as respects "suffering awhile—one for many."

In fact, so eager were they to prostrate themselves before the great idol of slavery, and, like Baalam, to curse instead of blessing the people whom God had brought out of bondage, that they in bringing up obsolete passages from the Old Testament to justify their downward course, overlooked, or would not see, the following verses, which show very clearly, according to the Doctor's own textbook, that the slaves have a right to run away, and that it is unscriptural for any one to send them back.

In the 23rd chapter of Deuteronomy, 15th and 16th verses, it is thus written:—"Thou shalt not deliver unto his master the servant which is escaped from his master unto thee. He shall dwell with thee, even among you, in that place which he shall choose in one of thy gates, where it liketh him best: thou shalt not oppress him."

"Hide the outcast. Bewray not him that wandereth. Let mine outcasts dwell with thee. Be thou a covert to them from the face of the spoiler."—(Isa. xvi. 3, 4.)

The great majority of the American ministers are not content with uttering sentences similar to the above, or remaining wholly indifferent to the cries of the poor bondman; but they do all they can to blast the reputation, and to muzzle the mouths, of the few good men who dare to beseech the God of mercy "to loose the bonds of wickedness, to undo the heavy burdens, and let the oppressed go free." These reverend gentlemen pour a terrible cannonade upon "Jonah," for refusing to carry God's message against Nineveh, and tell us about the whale in which he was entombed; while they utterly overlook the existence of the whales which trouble their republican waters, and know not that they themselves are the "Jonahs" who threaten to sink their ship of state, by steering in an unrighteous direction. We are told that the whale vomited up the runaway prophet. This would not have seemed so strange, had it been one of the above lukewarm Doctors of Divinity whom he had swallowed; for even a whale might find such a morsel difficult of digestion.

> "I venerate the man whose heart is warm,
>   Whose hands are pure; whose doctrines and whose life
>   Coincident, exhibit lucid proof
>   That he is honest in the sacred cause."

> "But grace abused brings forth the foulest deeds,
>   As richest soil the most luxuriant weeds."

I must now leave the reverend gentlemen in the hands of Him who knows best how to deal with a recreant ministry.

I do not wish it to be understood that all the ministers of the States are of the Baalam stamp. There are those who are as uncompromising with slaveholders as Moses was with Pharaoh, and, like Daniel, will never bow down before the great false God that has been set up.

On arriving at Portland, we found that the steamer we intended to take had run into a schooner the previous night, and was lying up for repairs; so we had to wait there, in fearful suspense, for two or three days. During this time, we had the honour of being the guest of the late and much lamented Daniel Oliver, Esq., one of the best and most hospitable men in the State. By simply fulfilling the Scripture injunction, to take in the stranger, &c., he ran the risk of incurring a penalty of 2,000 dollars, and twelve months' imprisonment.

But neither the Fugitive Slave Law, nor any other Satanic enactment, can ever drive the spirit of liberty and humanity out of such noble and generous-hearted men.

May God ever bless his dear widow, and eventually unite them in His courts above!

We finally got off to St. John's, New Brunswick, where we had to wait two days for the steamer that conveyed us to Windsor, Nova Scotia.

On going into a hotel at St. John's, we met the butler in the hall, to whom I said, "We wish to stop here to-night." He turned round, scratching his head, evidently much put about. But thinking that my wife was white, he replied, "We have plenty of room for the lady, but I don't know about yourself; we never take in coloured folks." "Oh, don't trouble about me," I said; "if you have room for the lady, that will do; so please have the luggage taken to a bed-room." Which was immediately done, and my wife went upstairs into the apartment.

After taking a little walk in the town, I returned, and asked to see the "lady." On being conducted to the little sitting-room, where she then was, I entered without knocking, much to the surprise of the whole house." The "lady" then rang the bell, and ordered dinner for two. "Dinner for two, mum!" exclaimed the waiter, as he backed out of the door. "Yes, for two," said my wife. In a little while the stout, red-nosed butler, whom we first met, knocked at the door. I called out, "Come in." On entering, he rolled his whisky eyes at me, and then at my wife, and said, in a very solemn tone, "Did you order dinner for two, mum?" "Yes, for two," my wife again replied. This confused the chubby butler more than ever; and, as the landlord was not in the house, he seemed at a loss what to do.

When dinner was ready, the maid came in and said, "Please mum, the Missis wishes to know whether you will have dinner up now, or wait till your friend arrives?" "I will have it up at once, if you please." "Thank you, mum," continued the maid, and out she glided.

After a good deal of giggling in the passage, some one said, "You are in for it, butler, after all; so you had better make the best of a bad job." But before dinner was sent up, the landlord returned, and having heard from the steward of the steamer by which we came that we were bound for England, the proprietor's native country, he treated us in the most respectful manner.

At the above house, the boots (whose name I forget) was a fugitive slave, a very intelligent and active man, about forty-five years of age. Soon after his marriage, while in slavery, his bride was sold away from him, and he could never learn where the poor creature dwelt. So after remaining single for many years, both before and after his escape, and never expecting to see again, nor even to hear from, his long-lost partner, he finally married a woman at St. John's. But, poor fellow, as he was passing down the street one day, he met a woman; at the first glance they nearly recognized each other; they both turned round and stared, and unconsciously advanced, till she screamed and flew into his arms. Her first words were, "Dear, are you married?" On his answering in the affirmative, she shrank from his embrace, hung her head, and wept. A person who witnessed this meeting told me it was most affecting.

This couple knew nothing of each other's escape or whereabouts. The woman had escaped a few years before to the free States, by secreting herself in the hold of a vessel; but as they tried to get her back to bondage, she fled to New Brunswick for that protection which her native country was too mean to afford.

The man at once took his old wife to see his new one, who was also a fugitive slave, and as they all knew the workings of the infamous system of slavery, they could (as no one else can,) sympathise with each other's misfortune.

According to the rules of slavery, the man and his first wife were already divorced, but not morally; and therefore it was arranged between the three that he should live only with the lastly married wife, and allow the other one so much a week, as long she requested his assistance.

After staying at St. John's two days, the steamer arrived, which took us to Windsor, where we found a coach bound for Halifax. Prejudice against colour forced me on the top in the rain. On arriving within about seven miles of the town, the coach broke down and was upset. I fell upon the big crotchety driver, whose head stuck in the mud; and as he "always objected to niggers riding inside with white folks," I was not particularly sorry to see him deeper in the mire than myself. All of us were scratched and bruised more or less. After the passengers had crawled out as best they could, we all set off, and paddled through the deep mud and cold and rain, to Halifax.

On leaving Boston, it was our intention to reach Halifax at least two or three days before the steamer from Boston touched there, *en route* for Liverpool; but, having been detained so long at Portland and St. John's, we had the misfortune to arrive at Halifax at dark, just two hours after the steamer had gone; consequently we had to wait there a fortnight, for the *Cambria*.

The coach was patched up, and reached Halifax with the luggage, soon after the passengers arrived. The only respectable hotel that was then in the town had suspended business, and was closed; so we went to the inn, opposite the market, where the coach stopped: a most miserable, dirty hole it was.

Knowing that we were still under the influence of the low Yankee prejudice, I sent my wife in with the other passengers, to engage a bed for herself and husband. I stopped outside in the rain till the coach came up. If I had gone in and asked for a bed they would have been quite full. But as they thought my wife was white, she had no difficulty in securing apartments, into which the luggage was afterwards carried. The landlady, observing that I took an interest in the baggage, became somewhat uneasy, and went into my wife's room, and said to her, "Do you know the dark man downstairs?" "Yes, he is my husband." "Oh! I mean the black man—the *nigger*?" "I quite understand you; he is my husband." "My God!" exclaimed the woman as she flounced out and banged to the door. On going upstairs, I heard what had taken place: but, as we were there, and did not mean to leave that night, we did not disturb ourselves. On our ordering tea, the landlady sent word back to say that we must take it in the kitchen, or in our bed-room, as she had no other room for "niggers." We replied that we were not particular, and that they could send it up to our room,—which they did.

After the pro-slavery persons who were staying there heard that we were in, the whole house became agitated, and all sorts of oaths and fearful threats were heaped upon the "d——d niggers, for coming among white folks" Some of them said they would not stop there a minute if there was another house to go to.

The mistress came up the next morning to know how long we wished to stop. We said a fortnight. "Oh! dear me, it is impossible for us to accommodate you, and I think you had better go: you must understand, I have no prejudice myself; I think a good deal of the coloured people, and have always been their friend; but if you stop here we shall lose all our customers, which we can't do nohow." We said we were glad to hear that she had "no prejudice," and was such a staunch friend to the coloured people. We also informed her that we would be sorry for her "customers" to leave on our account; and as it was not our intention to interfere with anyone, it was foolish for them to be frightened away. However, if she would get us a comfortable place, we would be glad to leave. The landlady said she would go out and try. After spending the whole morning in canvassing the town, she came to our room and said, "I have been from one end of the place to the other, but everybody is full." Having a little foretaste of the vulgar prejudice of the town, we did not wonder at this result.

However, the landlady gave me the address of some respectable coloured families, whom she thought, "under the circumstances," might be induced to take us. And, as we were not at all comfortable—being compelled to sit, eat and sleep, in the same small room—we were quite willing to change our quarters.

I called upon the Rev. Mr. Cannady, a truly good-hearted Christian man, who received us at a word; and both he and his kind lady treated us handsomely, and for a nominal charge.

My wife and myself were both unwell when we left Boston, and, having taken fresh cold on the journey to Halifax, we were laid up there under the doctor's care, nearly the whole fortnight. I had much worry about getting tickets, for they baffled us shamefully at the Cunard office. They at first said that they did not book till the steamer came; which was not the fact. When I called again, they said they knew the steamer would come full from Boston, and therefore we had "better try to get to Liverpool by other means." Other mean Yankee excuses were made; and it was not till an influential gentleman, to whom Mr. Francis Jackson, of Boston, kindly gave us a letter, went and rebuked them, that we were able to secure our tickets. So when we went on board my wife was very poorly, and was also so ill on the voyage that I did not believe she could live to see Liverpool.

However, I am thankful to say she arrived; and, after laying up at Liverpool very ill for two or three weeks, gradually recovered.

It was not until we stepped upon the shore at Liverpool that we were free from every slavish fear.

We raised our thankful hearts to Heaven, and could have knelt down, like the Neapolitan exiles, and kissed the soil; for we felt that from slavery

"Heaven sure had kept this spot of earth uncurs'd,
    To show how all things were created first."

In a few days after we landed, the Rev. Francis Bishop and his lady came and invited us to be their guests; to whose unlimited kindness and watchful care my wife owes, in a great degree, her restoration to health.

We enclosed our letter from the Rev. Mr. May to Mr. Est-lin, who at once wrote to invite us to his house at Bristol. On arriving there, both Mr. and Miss Estlin received us as cordially as did our first good Quaker friends in Pennsylvania. It grieves me much to have to mention that he is no more. Everyone who knew him can truthfully say—

"Peace to the memory of a man of worth,
A man of letters, and of manners too!
Of manners sweet as Virtue always wears
When gay Good-nature dresses her in smiles."

It was principally through the extreme kindness of Mr. Estlin, the Right Hon. Lady Noel Byron, Miss Harriet Martineau, Mrs. Reid, Miss Sturch, and a few other good friends, that my wife and myself were able to spend a short time at a school in this country, to acquire a little of that education which we were so shamefully deprived of while in the house of bondage. The school is under the supervision of the Misses Lushington, daughters of the Right Hon. Stephen Lushington, D.C.L. During our stay at the school we received the greatest attention from every one, and I am particularly indebted to Thomas Wilson, Esq., of Bradmore House, Chiswick, (who was then the master,) for the deep interest he took in trying to get me on in my studies. We shall ever fondly and gratefully cherish the memory of our endeared and departed friend, Mr. Estlin. We, as well as the Anti-Slavery cause, lost a good friend in him. However, if departed spirits in Heaven are conscious of the wickedness of this world, and are allowed to speak, he will never fail to plead in the presence of the angelic host, and before the great and just Judge, for down-trodden and outraged humanity.

"Therefore I cannot think thee wholly gone;
The better part of thee is with us still;
Thy soul its hampering clay aside hath thrown,
And only freer wrestles with the ill.

"Thou livest in the life of all good things;
What words thou spak'st for Freedom shall not die;
Thou sleepest not, for now thy Love hath wings
To soar where hence thy hope could hardly fly.

"And often, from that other world, on this
　　Some gleams from great souls gone before may shine,
To shed on struggling hearts a clearer bliss,
　　And clothe the Right with lustre more divine.

"Farewell! good man, good angel now! this hand
　　Soon, like thine own, shall lose its cunning, too;
Soon shall this soul, like thine, bewildered stand,
　　Then leap to thread the free unfathomed blue."

JAMES RUSSELL LOWELL.

————

In the preceding pages I have not dwelt upon the great barbarities which are practised upon the slaves; because I wish to present the system in its mildest form, and to show that the "tender mercies of the wicked are cruel." But I do now, however, most solemnly declare, that a very large majority of the American slaves are over-worked, under-fed, and frequently unmercifully flogged.

I have often seen slaves tortured in every conceivable manner. I have seen them hunted down and torn by bloodhounds. I have seen them shamefully beaten, and branded with hot irons. I have seen them hunted, and even burned alive at the stake, frequently for offences that would be applauded if committed by white persons for similar purposes.

In short, it is well known in England, if not all over the world, that the Americans, as a people, are notoriously mean and cruel towards all coloured persons, whether they are bond or free.

"Oh, tyrant, thou who sleepest
　　On a volcano, from whose pent-up wrath,
　　Already some red flashes bursting up,
Beware!"

INCIDENTS

IN THE

LIFE OF A SLAVE GIRL.

WRITTEN BY HERSELF.

"Northerners know nothing at all about Slavery. They think it is perpetual bondage only. They have no conception of the depth of degradation involved in that word, SLAVERY; if they had, they would never cease their efforts until so horrible a system was overthrown."
A WOMAN OF NORTH CAROLINA.

"Rise up, ye women that are at ease! Hear my voice, ye careless daughters! Give ear unto my speech."
ISAIAH xxxii. 9.

EDITED BY L. MARIA CHILD.

BOSTON:
PUBLISHED FOR THE AUTHOR.
1861.

PREFACE BY THE AUTHOR.

Reader, be assured this narrative is no fiction. I am aware that some of my adventures may seem incredible; but they are, nevertheless, strictly true. I have not exaggerated the wrongs inflicted by Slavery; on the contrary, my descriptions fall far short of the facts. I have concealed the names of places, and given persons fictitious names. I had no motive for secrecy on my own account, but I deemed it kind and considerate towards others to pursue this course.

I wish I were more competent to the task I have undertaken. But I trust my readers will excuse deficiencies in consideration of circumstances. I was born and reared in Slavery; and I remained in a Slave State twenty-seven years. Since I have been at the North, it has been necessary for me to work diligently for my own support and the education of my children. This has not left me much leisure to make up for the loss of early opportunities to improve myself; and it has compelled me to write these pages at irregular intervals, whenever I could snatch an hour from household duties.

When I first arrived in Philadelphia, Bishop Paine advised me to publish a sketch of my life, but I told him I was altogether incompetent to such an undertaking. Though I have improved my mind somewhat since that time, I still remain of the same opinion; but I trust my motives will excuse what might otherwise seem presumptuous. I have not written my experiences in order to attract attention to myself; on the contrary, it would have been more pleasant to me to have been silent about my own history. Neither do I care to excite sympathy for my own sufferings. But I do earnestly desire to arouse the women of the North to a realizing sense of the condition of two millions of women at the South, still in bondage, suffering what I suffered, and most of them far worse. I want to add my testimony to that of abler pens to convince the people of the Free States what Slavery really is.

Only by experience can any one realize how deep, and dark, and foul is that pit of abominations. May the blessing of God rest on this imperfect effort in behalf of my persecuted people!

LINDA BRENT.

INTRODUCTION BY THE EDITOR.

THE author of the following autobiography is personally known to me, and her conversation and manners inspire me with confidence. During the last seventeen years, she has lived the greater part of the time with a distinguished family in New York, and has so deported herself as to be highly esteemed by them. This fact is sufficient, without further credentials of her character. I believe those who know her will not be disposed to doubt her veracity, though some incidents in her story are more romantic than fiction.

At her request, I have revised her manuscript; but such changes as I have made have been mainly for purposes of condensation and orderly arrangement. I have not added any thing to the incidents, or changed the import of her very pertinent remarks. With trifling exceptions, both the ideas and the language are her own. I pruned excrescences a little, but otherwise I had no reason for changing her lively and dramatic way of telling her own story. The names of both persons and places are known to me; but for good reasons I suppress them.

It will naturally excite surprise that a woman reared in Slavery should be able to write so well. But circumstances will explain this. In the first place, nature endowed her with quick perceptions. Secondly, the mistress, with whom she lived till she was twelve years old, was a kind, considerate friend, who taught her to read and spell. Thirdly, she was placed in favorable circumstances after she came to the North; having frequent intercourse with intelligent persons, who felt a friendly interest in her welfare, and were disposed to give her opportunities for self-improvement.

I am well aware that many will accuse me of indecorum for presenting these pages to the public; for the experiences of this intelligent and much-injured woman belong to a class which some call delicate subjects, and others indelicate. This peculiar phase of Slavery has generally been kept veiled; but the public ought to be made acquainted with its monstrous features, and I willingly take the responsibility of presenting them with the veil withdrawn. I do this for the sake of my sisters in bondage, who are suffering wrongs so foul, that our ears are too delicate to listen to them. I do it with the hope of arousing conscientious and reflecting women at the North to a sense of their duty in the exertion of moral influence on the question of Slavery, on all possible occasions. I do it with the hope that every man who reads this narrative will swear solemnly before God that, so far as he has power to prevent it, no fugitive from Slavery shall ever be sent back to suffer in that loathsome den of corruption and cruelty.

L. MARIA CHILD.

Contents.

INCIDENTS
IN THE
LIFE OF A SLAVE GIRL,
SEVEN YEARS CONCEALED.

I.

CHILDHOOD.

I WAS born a slave; but I never knew it till six years of happy childhood had passed away. My father was a carpenter, and considered so intelligent and skilful in his trade, that, when buildings out of the common line were to be erected, he was sent for from long distances, to be head workman. On condition of paying his mistress two hundred dollars a year, and supporting himself, he was allowed to work at his trade, and manage his own affairs. His strongest wish was to purchase his children; but, though he several times offered his hard earnings for that purpose, he never succeeded. In complexion my parents were a light shade of brownish yellow, and were termed mulattoes. They lived together in a comfortable home; and, though we were all slaves, I was so fondly shielded that I never dreamed I was a piece of merchandise, trusted to them for safe keeping, and liable to be demanded of them at any moment. I had one brother, William, who was two years younger than myself—a bright, affectionate child. I had also a great treasure in my maternal grandmother, who was a remarkable woman in many respects. She was the daughter of a planter in South Carolina, who, at his death, left her mother and his three children free, with money to go to St. Augustine, where they had relatives. It was during the Revolutionary War; and they were captured on their passage, carried back, and sold to different purchasers. Such was the story my grandmother used to tell me; but I do not remember all the particulars. She was a little girl when she was captured and sold to the keeper of a large hotel. I have often heard her tell how hard she fared during childhood. But as she grew older she evinced so much intelligence, and was so faithful, that her master and mistress could not help seeing it was for their interest to take care of such a valuable piece of property. She became an indispensable personage in the household, officiating in all capacities, from cook and wet nurse to seamstress. She was much praised for her cooking; and her nice crackers became so famous in the neighborhood that many people were desirous of obtaining them. In consequence of numerous requests of this kind, she asked permission of her mistress to bake crackers at night, after all the household work was done; and she obtained leave to do it, provided she would clothe herself and her children from the profits. Upon these terms, after working hard all day for her mistress, she began her midnight bakings, assisted by her two oldest children. The business proved profitable; and each year she laid by a little, which was saved for a fund to purchase her children. Her master died, and the property was divided among his heirs. The widow had her dower in the hotel, which she continued to keep open. My grandmother remained in her service as a slave; but her children were divided among her master's children. As she had five, Benjamin, the youngest one, was sold, in order that each heir might have an equal portion of dollars and cents. There was so little difference in our ages that he seemed more like my brother than my uncle. He was a bright, handsome lad, nearly white; for he inherited the complexion my grandmother had derived from Anglo-Saxon ancestors. Though only ten years old, seven hundred and twenty dollars were paid for him. His sale was a terrible blow to my grandmother; but she was naturally hopeful, and she went to work with renewed energy, trusting in time to be able to purchase some of her children. She had laid up three hundred dollars, which her mistress one day begged as a loan, promising to pay her soon. The reader probably knows that no promise or writing given to a slave is legally binding; for, according to Southern laws, a slave, *being* property, can *hold* no property. When my grandmother lent her hard earnings to her mistress, she trusted solely to her honor. The honor of a slaveholder to a slave!

To this good grandmother I was indebted for many comforts. My brother Willie and I often received portions of the crackers, cakes, and preserves, she made to sell; and after we ceased to be children we were indebted to her for many more important services.

Such were the unusually fortunate circumstances of my early childhood. When I was six years old, my mother died; and then, for the first time, I learned, by the talk around me, that I was a slave. My mother's mistress was the daughter of my grandmother's mistress. She was the foster sister of my mother; they were both nourished at my grandmother's breast. In fact, my mother had been weaned at three months old, that the babe of the mistress might obtain sufficient food. They played together as children; and, when they became women, my mother was a most faithful servant to her whiter foster sister. On her death-bed her mistress promised that her children should never suffer for any thing; and during her lifetime she kept her word. They all spoke kindly of my dead mother, who had been a slave merely in name, but in nature was noble and womanly. I grieved for her, and my young mind was troubled with the thought who would now take care of me and my little brother. I was told that my home was now to be with her mistress; and I found it a happy one. No toilsome or disagreeable duties were imposed upon me. My mistress was so kind to me that I was always glad to do her bidding, and proud to labor for her as much as my young years would permit. I would sit by her side for hours, sewing diligently, with a heart as free from care as that of any free-born white child. When she thought I was tired, she would send me out to run and jump; and away I bounded, to gather berries or flowers to decorate her room. Those were happy days—too happy to last. The slave child had no thought for the morrow; but there came that blight, which too surely waits on every human being born to be a chattel.

When I was nearly twelve years old, my kind mistress sickened and died. As I saw the cheek grow paler, and the eye more glassy, how earnestly I prayed in my heart that she might live! I loved her; for she had been almost like a mother to me. My prayers were not answered. She died, and they buried her in the little churchyard, where, day after day, my tears fell upon her grave.

I was sent to spend a week with my grandmother. I was now old enough to begin to think of the future; and again and again I asked myself what they would do with me. I felt sure I should never find another mistress so kind as the one who was gone. She had promised my dying mother that her children should never suffer for any thing; and when I remembered that, and recalled her many proofs of attachment to me, I could not help having some hopes that she had left me free. My friends were almost certain it would be so. They thought she would be sure to do it, on account of my mother's love and faithful service. But, alas! we all know that the memory of a faithful slave does not avail much to save her children from the auction block.

After a brief period of suspense, the will of my mistress was read, and we learned that she had bequeathed me to her sister's daughter, a child of five years old. So vanished our hopes. My mistress had taught me the precepts of God's Word: "Thou shalt love thy neighbor as thyself." "Whatsoever ye would that men should do unto you, do ye even so unto them." But I was her slave, and I suppose she did not recognize me as her neighbor. I would give much to blot out from my memory that one great wrong. As a child, I loved my mistress; and, looking back on the happy days I spent with her, I try to think with less bitterness of this act of injustice. While I was with her, she taught me to read and spell; and for this privilege, which so rarely falls to the lot of a slave, I bless her memory.

She possessed but few slaves; and at her death those were all distributed among her relatives. Five of them were my grandmother's children, and had shared the same milk that nourished her mother's children. Notwithstanding my grandmother's long and faithful service to her owners, not one of her children escaped the auction block. These God-breathing machines are no more, in the sight of their masters, than the cotton they plant, or the horses they tend.

II.

THE NEW MASTER AND MISTRESS.

Dr. Flint, a physician in the neighborhood, had married the sister of my mistress, and I was now the property of their little daughter. It was not without murmuring that I prepared for my new home; and what added to my unhappiness, was the fact that my brother William was purchased by the same family. My father, by his nature, as well as by the habit of transacting business as a skilful mechanic, had more of the feelings of a freeman than is common among slaves. My brother was a spirited boy; and being brought up under such influences, he early detested the name of master and mistress. One day, when his father and his mistress both happened to call him at the same time, he hesitated between the two; being perplexed to know which had the strongest claim upon his obedience. He finally concluded to go to his mistress. When my father reproved him for it, he said, "You both called me, and I didn't know which I ought to go to first."

"You are *my* child," replied our father, "and when I call you, you should come immediately, if you have to pass through fire and water."

Poor Willie! He was now to learn his first lesson of obedience to a master. Grandmother tried to cheer us with hopeful words, and they found an echo in the credulous hearts of youth.

When we entered our new home we encountered cold looks, cold words, and cold treatment. We were glad when the night came. On my narrow bed I moaned and wept, I felt so desolate and alone.

I had been there nearly a year, when a dear little friend of mine was buried. I heard her mother sob, as the clods fell on the coffin of her only child, and I turned away from the grave, feeling thankful that I still had something left to love. I met my grandmother, who said, "Come with me, Linda;" and from her tone I knew that something sad had happened. She led me apart from the people, and then said, "My child, your father is dead." Dead! How could I believe it? He had died so suddenly I had not even heard that he was sick. I went home with my grandmother. My heart rebelled against God, who had taken from me mother, father, mistress, and friend. The good grandmother tried to comfort me. "Who knows the ways of God?" said she. "Perhaps they have been kindly taken from the evil days to come." Years afterwards I often thought of this. She promised to be a mother to her grandchildren, so far as she might be permitted to do so; and strengthened by her love, I returned to my master's. I thought I should be allowed to go to my father's house the next morning; but I was ordered to go for flowers, that my mistress's house might be decorated for an evening party. I spent the day gathering flowers and weaving them into festoons, while the dead body of my father was lying within a mile of me. What cared my owners for that? he was merely a piece of property. Moreover, they thought he had spoiled his children, by teaching them to feel that they were human beings. This was blasphemous doctrine for a slave to teach; presumptuous in him, and dangerous to the masters.

The next day I followed his remains to a humble grave beside that of my dear mother. There were those who knew my father's worth, and respected his memory.

My home now seemed more dreary than ever. The laugh of the little slave-children sounded harsh and cruel. It was selfish to feel so about the joy of others. My brother moved about with a very grave face. I tried to comfort him, by saying, "Take courage, Willie; brighter days will come by and by."

"You don't know any thing about it, Linda," he replied. "We shall have to stay here all our days; we shall never be free."

I argued that we were growing older and stronger, and that perhaps we might, before long, be allowed to hire our own time, and then we could earn money to buy our freedom. William declared this was much easier to say than to do; moreover, he did not intend to *buy* his freedom. We held daily controversies upon this subject.

Little attention was paid to the slaves' meals in Dr. Flint's house. If they could catch a bit of food while it was going, well and good. I gave myself no trouble on that score, for on my various errands I passed my grandmother's house, where there was always something to spare for me. I was frequently threatened with punishment if I stopped there; and my grandmother, to avoid detaining me, often stood at the gate with something for my breakfast or dinner. I was indebted to *her* for all my comforts, spiritual or temporal. It was *her* labor that supplied my scanty wardrobe. I have a vivid recollection of the linsey-woolsey dress given me every winter by Mrs. Flint. How I hated it! It was one of the badges of slavery.

While my grandmother was thus helping to support me from her hard earnings, the three hundred dollars she had lent her mistress were never repaid. When her mistress died, her son-in-law, Dr. Flint, was appointed executor. When grandmother applied to him for payment, he said the estate was insolvent, and the law prohibited payment. It did not, however, prohibit him from retaining the silver candelabra, which had been purchased with that money. I presume they will be handed down in the family, from generation to generation.

My grandmother's mistress had always promised her that, at her death, she should be free; and it was said that in her will she made good the promise. But when the estate was settled, Dr. Flint told the faithful old servant that, under existing circumstances, it was necessary she should be sold.

On the appointed day, the customary advertisement was posted up, proclaiming that there would be a "public sale of negroes, horses, &c." Dr. Flint called to tell my grandmother that he was unwilling to wound her feelings by putting her up at auction, and that he would prefer to dispose of her at private sale. My grandmother saw through his hypocrisy; she understood very well that he was ashamed of the job. She was a very spirited woman, and if he was base enough to sell her, when her mistress intended she should be free, she was determined the public should know it. She had for a long time supplied many families with crackers and preserves; consequently, "Aunt Marthy," as she was called, was generally known, and every body who knew her respected her intelligence and good character. Her long and faithful service in the family was also well known, and the intention of her mistress to leave her free. When the day of sale came, she took her place among the chattels, and at the first call she sprang upon the auction-block. Many voices called out, "Shame! Shame! Who is going to sell *you*, aunt Marthy? Don't stand there! That is no place for *you*." Without saying a word, she quietly awaited her fate. No one bid for her. At last, a feeble voice said, "Fifty dollars." It came from a maiden lady, seventy years old, the sister of my grandmother's deceased mistress. She had lived forty years under the same roof with my grandmother; she knew how faithfully she had served her owners, and how cruelly she had been defrauded of her rights; and she resolved to protect her. The auctioneer waited for a higher bid; but her wishes were respected; no one bid above her. She could neither read nor write; and when the bill of sale was made out, she signed it with a cross. But what consequence was that, when she had a big heart overflowing with human kindness? She gave the old servant her freedom.

At that time, my grandmother was just fifty years old. Laborious years had passed since then; and now my brother and I were slaves to the man who had defrauded her of her money, and tried to defraud her of her freedom. One of my mother's sisters, called Aunt Nancy, was also a slave in his family. She was a kind, good aunt to me; and supplied the place of both housekeeper and waiting maid to her mistress. She was, in fact, at the beginning and end of every thing.

Mrs. Flint, like many southern women, was totally deficient in energy. She had not strength to superintend her household affairs; but her nerves were so strong, that she could sit in her easy chair and see a woman whipped, till the blood trickled from every stroke of the lash. She was a member of the church; but partaking of the Lord's supper did not seem to put her in a Christian frame of mind. If dinner was not served at the exact time on that particular Sunday, she would station herself in the kitchen, and wait till it was dished, and then spit in all the kettles and pans that had been used for cooking. She did this to prevent the cook and her children from eking out their meagre fare with the remains of the gravy and other scrapings. The slaves could get nothing to eat except what she chose to give them. Provisions were weighed out by the pound and ounce, three times a day. I can assure you she gave them no chance to eat wheat bread from her flour barrel. She knew how many biscuits a quart of flour would make, and exactly what size they ought to be.

Dr. Flint was an epicure. The cook never sent a dinner to his table without fear and trembling; for if there happened to be a dish not to his liking, he would either order her to be whipped, or compel her to eat every mouthful of it in his presence. The poor, hungry creature might not have objected to eating it; but she did object to having her master cram it down her throat till she choked.

They had a pet dog, that was a nuisance in the house. The cook was ordered to make some Indian mush for him. He refused to eat, and when his head was held over it, the froth flowed from his mouth into the basin. He died a few minutes after. When Dr. Flint came in, he said the mush had not been well cooked, and that was the reason the animal would not eat it. He sent for the cook, and compelled her to eat it. He thought that the woman's stomach was stronger than the dog's; but her sufferings afterwards proved that he was mistaken. This poor woman endured many cruelties from her master and mistress; sometimes she was locked up, away from her nursing baby, for a whole day and night.

When I had been in the family a few weeks, one of the plantation slaves was brought to town, by order of his master. It was near night when he arrived, and Dr. Flint ordered him to be taken to the work house, and tied up to the joist, so that his feet would just escape the ground. In that situation he was to wait till the doctor had taken his tea. I shall never forget that night. Never before, in my life, had I heard hundreds of blows fall, in succession, on a human being. His piteous groans, and his "O, pray don't, massa," rang in my ear for months afterwards. There were many conjectures as to the cause of this terrible punishment. Some said master accused him of stealing corn; others said the slave had quarrelled with his wife, in presence of the overseer, and had accused his master of being the father of her child. They were both black, and the child was very fair.

I went into the work house next morning, and saw the cowhide still wet with blood, and the boards all covered with gore. The poor man lived, and continued to quarrel with his wife. A few months afterwards Dr. Flint handed them both over to a slave-trader. The guilty man put their value into his pocket, and had the satisfaction of knowing that they were out of sight and hearing. When the mother was delivered into the trader's hands, she said, "You *promised* to treat me well." To which he replied, "You have let your tongue run too far; damn you!" She had forgotten that it was a crime for a slave to tell who was the father of her child.

From others than the master persecution also comes in such cases. I once saw a young slave girl dying soon after the birth of a child nearly white. In her agony she cried out, "O Lord, come and take me!" Her mistress stood by, and mocked at her like an incarnate fiend. "You suffer, do you?" she exclaimed. "I am glad of it. You deserve it all, and more too."

The girl's mother said, "The baby is dead, thank God; and I hope my poor child will soon be in heaven, too."

"Heaven!" retorted the mistress. "There is no such place for the like of her and her bastard."

The poor mother turned away, sobbing. Her dying daughter called her, feebly, and as she bent over her, I heard her say, "Don't grieve so, mother; God knows all about it; and HE will have mercy upon me."

Her sufferings, afterwards, became so intense, that her mistress felt unable to stay; but when she left the room, the scornful smile was still on her lips. Seven children called her mother. The poor black woman had but the one child, whose eyes she saw closing in death, while she thanked God for taking her away from the greater bitterness of life.

III.

THE SLAVES' NEW YEAR'S DAY.

DR. FLINT owned a fine residence in town, several farms, and about fifty slaves, besides hiring a number by the year.

Hiring-day at the south takes place on the 1st of January. On the 2d, the slaves are expected to go to their new masters. On a farm, they work until the corn and cotton are laid. They then have two holidays. Some masters give them a good dinner under the trees. This over, they work until Christmas eve. If no heavy charges are meantime brought against them, they are given four or five holidays, whichever the master or overseer may think proper. Then comes New Year's eve; and they gather together their little alls, or more properly speaking, their little nothings, and wait anxiously for the dawning of day. At the appointed hour the grounds are thronged with men, women, and children, waiting, like criminals, to hear their doom pronounced. The slave is sure to know who is the most humane, or cruel master, within forty miles of him.

It is easy to find out, on that day, who clothes and feeds his slaves well; for he is surrounded by a crowd, begging, "Please, massa, hire me this year. I will work *very* hard, massa."

If a slave is unwilling to go with his new master, he is whipped, or locked up in jail, until he consents to go, and promises not to run away during the year. Should he chance to change his mind, thinking it justifiable to violate an extorted promise, woe unto him if he is caught! The whip is used till the blood flows at his feet; and his stiffened limbs are put in chains, to be dragged in the field for days and days!

If he lives until the next year, perhaps the same man will hire him again, without even giving him an opportunity of going to the hiring-ground. After those for hire are disposed of, those for sale are called up.

O, you happy free women, contrast *your* New Year's day with that of the poor bond-woman! With you it is a pleasant season, and the light of the day is blessed. Friendly wishes meet you every where, and gifts are showered upon you. Even hearts that have been estranged from you soften at this season, and lips that have been silent echo back, "I wish you a happy New Year." Children bring their little offerings, and raise their rosy lips for a caress. They are your own, and no hand but that of death can take them from you.

But to the slave mother New Year's day comes laden with peculiar sorrows. She sits on her cold cabin floor, watching the children who may all be torn from her the next morning; and often does she wish that she and they might die before the day dawns. She may be an ignorant creature, degraded by the system that has brutalized her from childhood; but she has a mother's instincts, and is capable of feeling a mother's agonies.

On one of these sale days, I saw a mother lead seven children to the auction-block. She knew that *some* of them would be taken from her; but they took *all*. The children were sold to a slave-trader, and their mother was bought by a man in her own town. Before night her children were all far away. She begged the trader to tell her where he intended to take them; this he refused to do. How *could* he, when he knew he would sell them, one by one, wherever he could command the highest price? I met that mother in the street, and her wild, haggard face lives to-day in my mind. She wrung her hands in anguish, and exclaimed, "Gone! All gone! Why *don't* God kill me?" I had no words wherewith to comfort her. Instances of this kind are of daily, yea, of hourly occurrence.

Slaveholders have a method, peculiar to their institution, of getting rid of *old* slaves, whose lives have been worn out in their service. I knew an old woman, who for seventy years faithfully served her master. She had become almost helpless, from hard labor and disease. Her owners moved to Alabama, and the old black woman was left to be sold to any body who would give twenty dollars for her.

IV.

THE SLAVE WHO DARED TO FEEL LIKE A MAN.

Two years had passed since I entered Dr. Flint's family, and those years had brought much of the knowledge that comes from experience, though they had afforded little opportunity for any other kinds of knowledge.

My grandmother had, as much as possible, been a mother to her orphan grandchildren. By perseverance and unwearied industry, she was now mistress of a snug little home, surrounded with the necessaries of life. She would have been happy could her children have shared them with her. There remained but three children and two grandchildren, all slaves. Most earnestly did she strive to make us feel that it was the will of God: that He had seen fit to place us under such circumstances; and though it seemed hard, we ought to pray for contentment.

It was a beautiful faith, coming from a mother who could not call her children her own. But I, and Benjamin, her youngest boy, condemned it. We reasoned that it was much more the will of God that we should be situated as she was. We longed for a home like hers. There we always found sweet balsam for our troubles. She was so loving, so sympathizing!

She always met us with a smile, and listened with patience to all our sorrows. She spoke so hopefully, that unconsciously the clouds gave place to sunshine. There was a grand big oven there, too, that baked bread and nice things for the town, and we knew there was always a choice bit in store for us.

But, alas! even the charms of the old oven failed to reconcile us to our hard lot. Benjamin was now a tall, handsome lad, strongly and gracefully made, and with a spirit too bold and daring for a slave. My brother William, now twelve years old, had the same aversion to the word master that he had when he was an urchin of seven years. I was his confidant. He came to me with all his troubles. I remember one instance in particular. It was on a lovely spring morning, and when I marked the sunlight dancing here and there, its beauty seemed to mock my sadness. For my master, whose restless, craving, vicious nature roved about day and night, seeking whom to devour, had just left me, with stinging, scorching words; words that scathed ear and brain like fire. O, how I despised him! I thought how glad I should be, if some day when he walked the earth, it would open and swallow him up, and disencumber the world of a plague.

When he told me that I was made for his use, made to obey his command in *every* thing; that I was nothing but a slave, whose will must and should surrender to his, never before had my puny arm felt half so strong.

So deeply was I absorbed in painful reflections afterwards, that I neither saw nor heard the entrance of any one, till the voice of William sounded close beside me. "Linda," said he, "what makes you look so sad? I love you. O, Linda, isn't this a bad world? Every body seems so cross and unhappy. I wish I had died when poor father did."

I told him that every body was *not* cross, or unhappy; that those who had pleasant homes, and kind friends, and who were not afraid to love them, were happy. But we, who were slave-children, without father or mother, could not expect to be happy. We must be good; perhaps that would bring us contentment.

"Yes," he said, "I try to be good; but what's the use? They are all the time troubling me." Then he proceeded to relate his afternoon's difficulty with young master Nicholas. It seemed that the brother of master Nicholas had pleased himself with making up stories about William. Master Nicholas said he should be flogged, and he would do it. Whereupon he went to work; but William fought bravely, and the young master, finding he was getting the better of him, undertook to tie his hands behind him. He failed in that likewise. By dint of kicking and fisting, William came out of the skirmish none the worse for a few scratches.

He continued to discourse on his young master's *meanness*; how he whipped the *little* boys, but was a perfect coward when a tussle ensued between him and white boys of his own size. On such occasions he always took to his legs. William had other charges to make against him. One was his rubbing up pennies with quicksilver, and passing them off for quarters of a dollar on an old man who kept a fruit stall. William was often sent to buy fruit, and he earnestly inquired of me what he ought to do under such circumstances. I told him it was certainly wrong to deceive the old man, and that it was his duty to tell him of the impositions practised by his young master. I assured him the old man would not be slow to comprehend the whole, and there the matter would end. William thought it might with the old man, but not with *him*. He said he did not mind the smart of the whip, but he did not like the *idea* of being whipped.

While I advised him to be good and forgiving I was not unconscious of the beam in my own eye. It was the very knowledge of my own shortcomings that urged me to retain, if possible, some sparks of my brother's God-given nature. I had not lived fourteen years in slavery for nothing. I had felt, seen, and heard enough, to read the characters, and question the motives, of those around me. The war of my life had begun; and though one of God's most powerless creatures, I resolved never to be conquered. Alas, for me!

If there was one pure, sunny spot for me, I believed it to be in Benjamin's heart, and in another's, whom I loved with all the ardor of a girl's first love. My owner knew of it, and sought in every way to render me miserable. He did not resort to corporal punishment, but to all the petty, tyrannical ways that human ingenuity could devise.

I remember the first time I was punished. It was in the

month of February. My grandmother had taken my old shoes, and replaced them with a new pair. I needed them; for several inches of snow had fallen, and it still continued to fall. When I walked through Mrs. Flint's room, their creaking grated harshly on her refined nerves. She called me to her, and asked what I had about me that made such a horrid noise. I told her it was my new shoes. "Take them off," said she; "and if you put them on again, I'll throw them into the fire."

I took them off, and my stockings also. She then sent me a long distance, on an errand. As I went through the snow, my bare feet tingled. That night I was very hoarse; and I went to bed thinking the next day would find me sick, perhaps dead. What was my grief on waking to find myself quite well!

I had imagined if I died, or was laid up for some time, that my mistress would feel a twinge of remorse that she had so hated "the little imp," as she styled me. It was my ignorance of that mistress that gave rise to such extravagant imaginings.

Dr. Flint occasionally had high prices offered for me; but he always said, "She don't belong to me. She is my daughter's property, and I have no right to sell her." Good, honest man! My young mistress was still a child, and I could look for no protection from her. I loved her, and she returned my affection. I once heard her father allude to her attachment to me; and his wife promptly replied that it proceeded from fear. This put unpleasant doubts into my mind. Did the child feign what she did not feel? or was her mother jealous of the mite of love she bestowed on me? I concluded it must be the latter. I said to myself, "Surely, little children are true."

One afternoon I sat at my sewing, feeling unusual depression of spirits. My mistress had been accusing me of an offence, of which I assured her I was perfectly innocent; but I saw, by the contemptuous curl of her lip, that she believed I was telling a lie.

I wondered for what wise purpose God was leading me through such thorny paths, and whether still darker days were in store for me. As I sat musing thus, the door opened softly, and William came in. "Well, brother," said I, "what is the matter this time?"

"O Linda, Ben and his master have had a dreadful time!" said he.

My first thought was that Benjamin was killed. "Don't be frightened, Linda," said William; "I will tell you all about it."

It appeared that Benjamin's master had sent for him, and he did not immediately obey the summons. When he did, his master was angry, and began to whip him. He resisted. Master and slave fought, and finally the master was thrown. Benjamin had cause to tremble; for he had thrown to the ground his master—one of the richest men in town. I anxiously awaited the result.

That night I stole to my grandmother's house, and Benjamin also stole thither from his master's. My grandmother had gone to spend a day or two with an old friend living in the country.

"I have come," said Benjamin, "to tell you good by. I am going away."

I inquired where.

"To the north," he replied.

I looked at him to see whether he was in earnest. I saw it all in his firm, set mouth. I implored him not to go, but he paid no heed to my words. He said he was no longer a boy, and every day made his yoke more galling. He had raised his hand against his master, and was to be publicly whipped for the offence. I reminded him of the poverty and hardships he must encounter among strangers. I told him he might be caught and brought back; and that was terrible to think of.

He grew vexed, and asked if poverty and hardships with freedom, were not preferable to our treatment in slavery. "Linda," he continued, "we are dogs here; foot-balls, cattle, every thing that's mean. No, I will not stay. Let them bring me back. We don't die but once."

He was right; but it was hard to give him up. "Go," said I, "and break your mother's heart."

I repented of my words ere they were out.

"Linda," said he, speaking as I had not heard him speak that evening, "how *could* you say that? Poor mother! be kind to her, Linda; and you, too, cousin Fanny."

Cousin Fanny was a friend who had lived some years with us.

Farewells were exchanged, and the bright, kind boy, endeared to us by so many acts of love, vanished from our sight.

It is not necessary to state how he made his escape. Suffice it to say, he was on his way to New York when a violent storm overtook the vessel. The captain said he must put into the nearest port. This alarmed Benjamin, who was aware that he would be advertised in every port near his own town. His embarrassment was noticed by the captain. To port they went. There the advertisement met the captain's eye. Benjamin so exactly answered its description, that the captain laid hold on him, and bound him in chains. The storm passed, and they proceeded to New York. Before reaching that port Benjamin managed to get off his chains and throw them overboard. He escaped from the vessel, but was pursued, captured, and carried back to his master.

When my grandmother returned home and found her youngest child had fled, great was her sorrow; but, with characteristic piety, she said, "God's will be done." Each morning, she inquired if any news had been heard from her boy. Yes, news *was* heard. The master was rejoicing over a letter, announcing the capture of his human chattel.

That day seems but as yesterday, so well do I remember it I saw him led through the streets in chains, to jail. His face was ghastly pale, yet full of determination. He had begged one of the sailors to go to his mother's house and ask her not to meet him. He said the sight of her distress would take from him all self-control. She yearned to see him, and she went; but she screened herself in the crowd, that it might be as her child had said.

We were not allowed to visit him; but we had known the jailer for years, and he was a kind-hearted man. At midnight he opened the jail door for my grandmother and myself to enter, in disguise. When we entered the cell not a sound broke the stillness. "Benjamin, Benjamin!" whispered my grandmother. No answer. "Benjamin!" she again faltered. There was a jingle of chains. The moon had just risen, and cast an uncertain light through the bars of the window. We knelt down and took Benjamin's cold hands in ours. We did not speak. Sobs were heard, and Benjamin's lips were unsealed; for his mother was weeping on his neck. How vividly does memory bring back that sad night! Mother and son talked together. He asked her pardon for the suffering he had caused her. She said she had nothing to forgive; she could not blame his desire for freedom. He told her that when he was captured, he broke away, and was about casting himself into the river, when thoughts of *her* came over him, and he desisted. She asked if he did not also think of God. I fancied I saw his face grow fierce in the moonlight. He answered, "No, I did not think of him. When a man is hunted like a wild beast he forgets there is a God, a heaven. He forgets every thing in his struggle to get beyond the reach of the bloodhounds."

"Don't talk so, Benjamin," said she. "Put your trust in God. Be humble, my child, and your master will forgive you."

"Forgive me for *what*, mother? For not letting him treat me like a dog? No! I will never humble myself to him. I have worked for him for nothing all my life, and I am repaid with stripes and imprisonment. Here I will stay till I die, or till he sells me."

The poor mother shuddered at his words. I think he felt it; for when he next spoke, his voice was calmer. "Don't fret about me, mother. I ain't worth it," said he. "I wish I had some of your goodness. You bear every thing patiently, just as though you thought it was all right. I wish I could."

She told him she had not always been so; once, she was like him; but when sore troubles came upon her, and she had no arm to lean upon, she learned to call on God, and he lightened her burdens. She besought him to do likewise.

We overstaid our time, and were obliged to hurry from the jail.

Benjamin had been imprisoned three weeks, when my grandmother went to intercede for him with his master. He was immovable. He said Benjamin should serve as an example to the rest of his slaves; he should be kept in jail till he was subdued, or be sold if he got but one dollar for him. However, he afterwards relented in some degree. The chains were taken off, and we were allowed to visit him.

As his food was of the coarsest kind, we carried him as often as possible a warm supper, accompanied with some little luxury for the jailer.

Three months elapsed, and there was no prospect of release or of a purchaser. One day he was heard to sing and laugh.

This piece of indecorum was told to his master, and the over-seer was ordered to re-chain him. He was now confined in an apartment with other prisoners, who were covered with filthy rags. Benjamin was chained near them, and was soon covered with vermin. He worked at his chains till he succeeded in getting out of them. He passed them through the bars of the window, with a request that they should be taken to his master, and he should be informed that he was covered with vermin.

This audacity was punished with heavier chains, and prohibition of our visits.

My grandmother continued to send him fresh changes of clothes. The old ones were burned up. The last night we saw him in jail his mother still begged him to send for his master, and beg his pardon. Neither persuasion nor argument could turn him from his purpose. He calmly answered, "I am waiting his time."

Those chains were mournful to hear.

Another three months passed, and Benjamin left his prison walls. We that loved him waited to bid him a long and last farewell. A slave trader had bought him. You remember, I told you what price he brought when ten years of age. Now he was more than twenty years old, and sold for three hundred dollars. The master had been blind to his own interest. Long confinement had made his face too pale, his form too thin; moreover, the trader had heard something of his character, and it did not strike him as suitable for a slave. He said he would give any price if the handsome lad was a girl. We thanked God that he was not.

Could you have seen that mother clinging to her child, when they fastened the irons upon his wrists; could you have heard her heart-rending groans, and seen her bloodshot eyes wander wildly from face to face, vainly pleading for mercy; could you have witnessed that scene as I saw it, you would exclaim, *Slavery is damnable!*

Benjamin, her youngest, her pet, was forever gone! She could not realize it. She had had an interview with the trader for the purpose of ascertaining if Benjamin could be purchased. She was told it was impossible, as he had given bonds not to sell him till he was out of the state. He promised that he would not sell him till he reached New Orleans.

With a strong arm and unvaried trust, my grandmother began her work of love. Benjamin must be free. If she succeeded, she knew they would still be separated; but the sacrifice was not too great. Day and night she labored. The trader's price would treble that he gave; but she was not discouraged.

She employed a lawyer to write to a gentleman, whom she knew, in New Orleans. She begged him to interest himself for Benjamin, and he willingly favored her request. When he saw Benjamin, and stated his business, he thanked him; but said he preferred to wait a while before making the trader an offer. He knew he had tried to obtain a high price for him, and had invariably failed. This encouraged him to make another effort for freedom. So one morning, long before day, Benjamin was missing. He was riding over the blue billows, bound for Baltimore.

For once his white face did him a kindly service. They had no suspicion that it belonged to a slave; otherwise, the law would have been followed out to the letter, and the *thing* rendered back to slavery. The brightest skies are often overshadowed by the darkest clouds. Benjamin was taken sick, and compelled to remain in Baltimore three weeks. His strength was slow in returning; and his desire to continue his journey seemed to retard his recovery. How could he get strength without air and exercise? He resolved to venture on a short walk. A by-street was selected, where he thought himself secure of not being met by any one that knew him; but a voice called out, "Halloo, Ben, my boy! what are you doing *here?*"

His first impulse was to run; but his legs trembled so that he could not stir. He turned to confront his antagonist, and behold, there stood his old master's next door neighbor! He thought it was all over with him now; but it proved otherwise. That man was a miracle. He possessed a goodly number of slaves, and yet was not quite deaf to that mystic clock, whose ticking is rarely heard in the slaveholder's breast.

"Ben, you are sick," said he. "Why, you look like a ghost. I guess I gave you something of a start. Never mind, Ben, I am not going to touch you. You had a pretty tough time of it, and you may go on your way rejoicing for all me. But I would advise you to get out of this place plaguy quick, for there are several gentlemen here from our town." He described the nearest and safest route to New York, and added, "I shall be glad to tell your mother I have seen you. Good by, Ben."

Benjamin turned away, filled with gratitude, and surprised that the town he hated contained such a gem—a gem worthy of a purer setting.

This gentleman was a Northerner by birth, and had married a southern lady. On his return, he told my grandmother that he had seen her son, and of the service he had rendered him.

Benjamin reached New York safely, and concluded to stop there until he had gained strength enough to proceed further. It happened that my grandmother's only remaining son had sailed for the same city on business for his mistress. Through God's providence, the brothers met. You may be sure it was a happy meeting. "O Phil," exclaimed Benjamin, "I am here at last." Then he told him how near he came to dying, almost in sight of free land, and how he prayed that he might live to get one breath of free air. He said life was worth something now, and it would be hard to die. In the old jail he had not valued it; once, he was tempted to destroy it; but something, he did not know what, had prevented him; perhaps it was fear. He had heard those who profess to be religious declare there was no heaven for self-murderers; and as his life had been pretty hot here, he did not desire a continuation of the same in another world. "If I die now," he exclaimed, "thank God, I shall die a freeman!"

He begged my uncle Phillip not to return south; but stay and work with him, till they earned enough to buy those at home. His brother told him it would kill their mother if he deserted her in her trouble. She had pledged her house, and with difficulty had raised money to buy him. Would he be bought?

"No, never!" he replied. "Do you suppose, Phil, when I have got so far out of their clutches, I will give them one red cent? No! And do you suppose I would turn mother out of her home in her old age? That I would let her pay all those hard-earned dollars for me, and never to see me? For you know she will stay south as long as her other children are slaves. What a good mother! Tell her to buy *you*, Phil. You have been a comfort to her, and I have been a trouble. And Linda, poor Linda; what'll become of her? Phil, you don't know what a life they lead her. She has told me something about it, and I wish old Flint was dead, or a better man. When I was in jail, he asked her if she didn't want *him* to ask my master to forgive me, and take me home again. She told him, No; that I didn't want to go back. He got mad, and said we were all alike. I never despised my own master half as much as I do that man. There is many a worse slaveholder than my master; but for all that I would not be his slave."

While Benjamin was sick, he had parted with nearly all his clothes to pay necessary expenses. But he did not part with a little pin I fastened in his bosom when we parted. It was the most valuable thing I owned, and I thought none more worthy to wear it. He had it still.

His brother furnished him with clothes, and gave him what money he had.

They parted with moistened eyes; and as Benjamin turned away, he said, "Phil, I part with all my kindred." And so it proved. We never heard from him again.

Uncle Phillip came home; and the first words he uttered when he entered the house were, "Mother, Ben is free! I have seen him in New York." She stood looking at him with a bewildered air. "Mother, don't you believe it?" he said, laying his hand softly upon her shoulder. She raised her hands, and exclaimed, "God be praised! Let us thank him." She dropped on her knees, and poured forth her heart in prayer. Then Phillip must sit down and repeat to her every word Benjamin had said. He told her all; only he forbore to mention how sick and pale her darling looked. Why should he distress her when she could do him no good?

The brave old woman still toiled on, hoping to rescue some of her other children. After a while she succeeded in buying Phillip. She paid eight hundred dollars, and came home with the precious document that secured his freedom. The happy mother and son sat together by the old hearthstone that night, telling how proud they were of each other, and how they would prove to the world that they could take care of

themselves, as they had long taken care of others. We all concluded by saying, "He that is *willing* to be a slave, let him be
a slave."

V.

THE TRIALS OF GIRLHOOD.

DURING the first years of my service in Dr. Flint's family, I
was accustomed to share some indulgences with the children
of my mistress. Though this seemed to me no more than
right, I was grateful for it, and tried to merit the kindness by
the faithful discharge of my duties. But I now entered on my
fifteenth year—a sad epoch in the life of a slave girl. My master began to whisper foul words in my ear. Young as I was, I
could not remain ignorant of their import. I tried to treat
them with indifference or contempt. The master's age, my extreme youth, and the fear that his conduct would be reported
to my grandmother, made him bear this treatment for many
months. He was a crafty man, and resorted to many means to
accomplish his purposes. Sometimes he had stormy, terrific
ways, that made his victims tremble; sometimes he assumed a
gentleness that he thought must surely subdue. Of the two, I
preferred his stormy moods, although they left me trembling.
He tried his utmost to corrupt the pure principles my grandmother had instilled. He peopled my young mind with unclean images, such as only a vile monster could think of. I
turned from him with disgust and hatred. But he was my
master. I was compelled to live under the same roof with
him—where I saw a man forty years my senior daily violating
the most sacred commandments of nature. He told me I was
his property; that I must be subject to his will in all things.
My soul revolted against the mean tyranny. But where could
I turn for protection? No matter whether the slave girl be as
black as ebony or as fair as her mistress. In either case, there
is no shadow of law to protect her from insult, from violence,
or even from death; all these are inflicted by fiends who bear
the shape of men. The mistress, who ought to protect the
helpless victim, has no other feelings towards her but those of
jealousy and rage. The degradation, the wrongs, the vices, that

grow out of slavery, are more than I can describe. They are greater than you would willingly believe. Surely, if you credited one half the truths that are told you concerning the helpless millions suffering in this cruel bondage, you at the north would not help to tighten the yoke. You surely would refuse to do for the master, on your own soil, the mean and cruel work which trained bloodhounds and the lowest class of whites do for him at the south.

Every where the years bring to all enough of sin and sorrow; but in slavery the very dawn of life is darkened by these shadows. Even the little child, who is accustomed to wait on her mistress and her children, will learn, before she is twelve years old, why it is that her mistress hates such and such a one among the slaves. Perhaps the child's own mother is among those hated ones. She listens to violent outbreaks of jealous passion, and cannot help understanding what is the cause. She will become prematurely knowing in evil things. Soon she will learn to tremble when she hears her master's footfall. She will be compelled to realize that she is no longer a child. If God has bestowed beauty upon her, it will prove her greatest curse. That which commands admiration in the white woman only hastens the degradation of the female slave. I know that some are too much brutalized by slavery to feel the humiliation of their position; but many slaves feel it most acutely, and shrink from the memory of it. I cannot tell how much I suffered in the presence of these wrongs, nor how I am still pained by the retrospect. My master met me at every turn, reminding me that I belonged to him, and swearing by heaven and earth that he would compel me to submit to him. If I went out for a breath of fresh air, after a day of unwearied toil, his footsteps dogged me. If I knelt by my mother's grave, his dark shadow fell on me even there. The light heart which nature had given me became heavy with sad forebodings. The other slaves in my master's house noticed the change. Many of them pitied me; but none dared to ask the cause. They had no need to inquire. They knew too well the guilty practices under that roof; and they were aware that to speak of them was an offence that never went unpunished.

I longed for some one to confide in. I would have given the world to have laid my head on my grandmother's faithful bosom, and told her all my troubles. But Dr. Flint swore he would kill me, if I was not as silent as the grave. Then, although my grandmother was all in all to me, I feared her as well as loved her. I had been accustomed to look up to her with a respect bordering upon awe. I was very young, and felt shamefaced about telling her such impure things, especially as I knew her to be very strict on such subjects. Moreover, she was a woman of a high spirit. She was usually very quiet in her demeanor; but if her indignation was once roused, it was not very easily quelled. I had been told that she once chased a white gentleman with a loaded pistol, because he insulted one of her daughters. I dreaded the consequences of a violent outbreak; and both pride and fear kept me silent. But though I did not confide in my grandmother, and even evaded her vigilant watchfulness and inquiry, her presence in the neighborhood was some protection to me. Though she had been a slave, Dr. Flint was afraid of her. He dreaded her scorching rebukes. Moreover, she was known and patronized by many people; and he did not wish to have his villany made public. It was lucky for me that I did not live on a distant plantation, but in a town not so large that the inhabitants were ignorant of each other's affairs. Bad as are the laws and customs in a slaveholding community, the doctor, as a professional man, deemed it prudent to keep up some outward show of decency.

O, what days and nights of fear and sorrow that man caused me! Reader, it is not to awaken sympathy for myself that I am telling you truthfully what I suffered in slavery. I do it to kindle a flame of compassion in your hearts for my sisters who are still in bondage, suffering as I once suffered.

I once saw two beautiful children playing together. One was a fair white child; the other was her slave, and also her sister. When I saw them embracing each other, and heard their joyous laughter, I turned sadly away from the lovely sight. I foresaw the inevitable blight that would fall on the little slave's heart. I knew how soon her laughter would be changed to sighs. The fair child grew up to be a still fairer woman. From childhood to womanhood her pathway was blooming with flowers, and overarched by a sunny sky. Scarcely one day of her life had been clouded when the sun rose on her happy bridal morning.

How had those years dealt with her slave sister, the little playmate of her childhood? She, also, was very beautiful; but the flowers and sunshine of love were not for her. She drank the cup of sin, and shame, and misery, whereof her persecuted race are compelled to drink.

In view of these things, why are ye silent, ye free men and women of the north? Why do your tongues falter in maintenance of the right? Would that I had more ability! But my heart is so full, and my pen is so weak! There are noble men and women who plead for us, striving to help those who cannot help themselves. God bless them! God give them strength and courage to go on! God bless those, every where, who are laboring to advance the cause of humanity!

VI.
THE JEALOUS MISTRESS.

I WOULD ten thousand times rather that my children should be the half-starved paupers of Ireland than to be the most pampered among the slaves of America. I would rather drudge out my life on a cotton plantation, till the grave opened to give me rest, than to live with an unprincipled master and a jealous mistress. The felon's home in a penitentiary is preferable. He may repent, and turn from the error of his ways, and so find peace; but it is not so with a favorite slave. She is not allowed to have any pride of character. It is deemed a crime in her to wish to be virtuous.

Mrs. Flint possessed the key to her husband's character before I was born. She might have used this knowledge to counsel and to screen the young and the innocent among her slaves; but for them she had no sympathy. They were the objects of her constant suspicion and malevolence. She watched her husband with unceasing vigilance; but he was well practised in means to evade it. What he could not find opportunity to say in words he manifested in signs. He invented more than were ever thought of in a deaf and dumb asylum. I let them pass, as if I did not understand what he meant; and many were the curses and threats bestowed on me for my stupidity. One day he caught me teaching myself to write. He frowned, as if he was not well pleased; but I suppose he came to the conclusion that such an accomplishment might help to advance his favorite scheme. Before long, notes were often slipped into my hand. I would return them, saying, "I can't read them, sir." "Can't you?" he replied; "then I must read them to you." He always finished the reading by asking, "Do you understand?" Sometimes he would complain of the heat of the tea room, and order his supper to be placed on a small table in the piazza. He would seat himself there with a well-satisfied smile, and tell me to stand by and brush away the flies. He would eat very slowly, pausing between the mouthfuls. These intervals were employed in describing the happiness I was so foolishly throwing away, and in threatening me with the penalty that finally awaited my stubborn disobedience. He boasted much of the forbearance he had exercised towards me, and reminded me that there was a limit to his patience. When I succeeded in avoiding opportunities for him to talk to me at home, I was ordered to come to his office, to do some errand. When there, I was obliged to stand and listen to such language as he saw fit to address to me. Sometimes I so openly expressed my contempt for him that he would become violently enraged, and I wondered why he did not strike me. Circumstanced as he was, he probably thought it was better policy to be forbearing. But the state of things grew worse and worse daily. In desperation I told him that I must and would apply to my grandmother for protection. He threatened me with death, and worse than death, if I made any complaint to her. Strange to say, I did not despair. I was naturally of a buoyant disposition, and always I had a hope of somehow getting out of his clutches. Like many a poor, simple slave before me, I trusted that some threads of joy would yet be woven into my dark destiny.

I had entered my sixteenth year, and every day it became more apparent that my presence was intolerable to Mrs. Flint. Angry words frequently passed between her and her husband. He had never punished me himself, and he would not allow any body else to punish me. In that respect, she was never satisfied; but, in her angry moods, no terms were too vile for her to bestow upon me. Yet I, whom she detested so bitterly, had

far more pity for her than he had, whose duty it was to make
her life happy. I never wronged her, or wished to wrong her;
and one word of kindness from her would have brought me
to her feet.

After repeated quarrels between the doctor and his wife, he
announced his intention to take his youngest daughter, then
four years old, to sleep in his apartment. It was necessary that
a servant should sleep in the same room, to be on hand if the
child stirred. I was selected for that office, and informed for
what purpose that arrangement had been made. By managing
to keep within sight of people, as much as possible, during
the day time, I had hitherto succeeded in eluding my master,
though a razor was often held to my throat to force me to
change this line of policy. At night I slept by the side of my
great aunt, where I felt safe. He was too prudent to come
into her room. She was an old woman, and had been in the
family many years. Moreover, as a married man, and a professional man, he deemed it necessary to save appearances in
some degree. But he resolved to remove the obstacle in the
way of his scheme; and he thought he had planned it so that
he should evade suspicion. He was well aware how much I
prized my refuge by the side of my old aunt, and he determined to dispossess me of it. The first night the doctor had
the little child in his room alone. The next morning, I was ordered to take my station as nurse the following night. A kind
Providence interposed in my favor. During the day Mrs. Flint
heard of this new arrangement, and a storm followed. I rejoiced to hear it rage.

After a while my mistress sent for me to come to her room.
Her first question was, "Did you know you were to sleep in
the doctor's room?"

"Yes, ma'am."

"Who told you?"

"My master."

"Will you answer truly all the questions I ask?"

"Yes, ma'am."

"Tell me, then, as you hope to be forgiven, are you innocent of what I have accused you?"

"I am."

She handed me a Bible, and said, "Lay your hand on your

heart, kiss this holy book, and swear before God that you tell me the truth."

I took the oath she required, and I did it with a clear conscience.

"You have taken God's holy word to testify your innocence," said she. "If you have deceived me, beware! Now take this stool, sit down, look me directly in the face, and tell me all that has passed between your master and you."

I did as she ordered. As I went on with my account her color changed frequently, she wept, and sometimes groaned. She spoke in tones so sad, that I was touched by her grief. The tears came to my eyes; but I was soon convinced that her emotions arose from anger and wounded pride. She felt that her marriage vows were desecrated, her dignity insulted; but she had no compassion for the poor victim of her husband's perfidy. She pitied herself as a martyr; but she was incapable of feeling for the condition of shame and misery in which her unfortunate, helpless slave was placed.

Yet perhaps she had some touch of feeling for me; for when the conference was ended, she spoke kindly, and promised to protect me. I should have been much comforted by this assurance if I could have had confidence in it; but my experiences in slavery had filled me with distrust. She was not a very refined woman, and had not much control over her passions. I was an object of her jealousy, and, consequently, of her hatred; and I knew I could not expect kindness or confidence from her under the circumstances in which I was placed. I could not blame her. Slaveholders' wives feel as other women would under similar circumstances. The fire of her temper kindled from small sparks, and now the flame became so intense that the doctor was obliged to give up his intended arrangement.

I knew I had ignited the torch, and I expected to suffer for it afterwards; but I felt too thankful to my mistress for the timely aid she rendered me to care much about that. She now took me to sleep in a room adjoining her own. There I was an object of her especial care, though not of her especial comfort, for she spent many a sleepless night to watch over me. Sometimes I woke up, and found her bending over me. At other times she whispered in my ear, as though it was her husband who was speaking to me, and listened to hear what I would answer. If she startled me, on such occasions, she would glide stealthily away; and the next morning she would tell me I had been talking in my sleep, and ask who I was talking to. At last, I began to be fearful for my life. It had been often threatened; and you can imagine, better than I can describe, what an unpleasant sensation it must produce to wake up in the dead of night and find a jealous woman bending over you. Terrible as this experience was, I had fears that it would give place to one more terrible.

My mistress grew weary of her vigils; they did not prove satisfactory. She changed her tactics. She now tried the trick of accusing my master of crime, in my presence, and gave my name as the author of the accusation. To my utter astonishment, he replied, "I don't believe it; but if she did acknowledge it, you tortured her into exposing me." Tortured into exposing him! Truly, Satan had no difficulty in distinguishing the color of his soul! I understood his object in making this false representation. It was to show me that I gained nothing by seeking the protection of my mistress; that the power was still all in his own hands. I pitied Mrs. Flint. She was a second wife, many years the junior of her husband; and the hoary-headed miscreant was enough to try the patience of a wiser and better woman. She was completely foiled, and knew not how to proceed. She would gladly have had me flogged for my supposed false oath; but, as I have already stated, the doctor never allowed any one to whip me. The old sinner was politic. The application of the lash might have led to remarks that would have exposed him in the eyes of his children and grandchildren. How often did I rejoice that I lived in a town where all the inhabitants knew each other! If I had been on a remote plantation, or lost among the multitude of a crowded city, I should not be a living woman at this day.

The secrets of slavery are concealed like those of the Inquisition. My master was, to my knowledge, the father of eleven slaves. But did the mothers dare to tell who was the father of their children? Did the other slaves dare to allude to it, except in whispers among themselves? No, indeed! They knew too well the terrible consequences.

My grandmother could not avoid seeing things which excited her suspicions. She was uneasy about me, and tried various ways to buy me; but the never-changing answer was always repeated: "Linda does not belong to *me*. She is my daughter's property, and I have no legal right to sell her." The conscientious man! He was too scrupulous to *sell* me; but he had no scruples whatever about committing a much greater wrong against the helpless young girl placed under his guardianship, as his daughter's property. Sometimes my persecutor would ask me whether I would like to be sold. I told him I would rather be sold to any body than to lead such a life as I did. On such occasions he would assume the air of a very injured individual, and reproach me for my ingratitude. "Did I not take you into the house, and make you the companion of my own children?" he would say. "Have I ever treated you like a negro? I have never allowed you to be punished, not even to please your mistress. And this is the recompense I get, you ungrateful girl!" I answered that he had reasons of his own for screening me from punishment, and that the course he pursued made my mistress hate me and persecute me. If I wept, he would say, "Poor child! Don't cry! don't cry! I will make peace for you with your mistress. Only let me arrange matters in my own way. Poor, foolish girl! you don't know what is for your own good. I would cherish you. I would make a lady of you. Now go, and think of all I have promised you."

I did think of it.

Reader, I draw no imaginary pictures of southern homes. I am telling you the plain truth. Yet when victims make their escape from this wild beast of Slavery, northerners consent to act the part of bloodhounds, and hunt the poor fugitive back into his den, "full of dead men's bones, and all uncleanness." Nay, more, they are not only willing, but proud, to give their daughters in marriage to slaveholders. The poor girls have romantic notions of a sunny clime, and of the flowering vines that all the year round shade a happy home. To what disappointments are they destined! The young wife soon learns that the husband in whose hands she has placed her happiness pays no regard to his marriage vows. Children of every shade of complexion play with her own fair babies, and too well she knows that they are born unto him of his own household.

Jealousy and hatred enter the flowery home, and it is ravaged of its loveliness.

Southern women often marry a man knowing that he is the father of many little slaves. They do not trouble themselves about it. They regard such children as property, as marketable as the pigs on the plantation; and it is seldom that they do not make them aware of this by passing them into the slavetrader's hands as soon as possible, and thus getting them out of their sight. I am glad to say there are some honorable exceptions.

I have myself known two southern wives who exhorted their husbands to free those slaves towards whom they stood in a "parental relation;" and their request was granted. These husbands blushed before the superior nobleness of their wives' natures. Though they had only counselled them to do that which it was their duty to do, it commanded their respect, and rendered their conduct more exemplary. Concealment was at an end, and confidence took the place of distrust.

Though this bad institution deadens the moral sense, even in white women, to a fearful extent, it is not altogether extinct. I have heard southern ladies say of Mr. Such a one, "He not only thinks it no disgrace to be the father of those little niggers, but he is not ashamed to call himself their master. I declare, such things ought not to be tolerated in any decent society!"

VII.

THE LOVER.

WHY does the slave ever love? Why allow the tendrils of the heart to twine around objects which may at any moment be wrenched away by the hand of violence? When separations come by the hand of death, the pious soul can bow in resignation, and say, "Not my will, but thine be done, O Lord!" But when the ruthless hand of man strikes the blow, regardless of the misery he causes, it is hard to be submissive. I did not reason thus when I was a young girl. Youth will be youth. I loved, and I indulged the hope that the dark clouds around me would turn out a bright lining. I forgot that in the land of my birth the shadows are too dense for light to penetrate. A land

"Where laughter is not mirth; nor thought the mind;
Nor words a language; nor e'en men mankind.
Where cries reply to curses, shrieks to blows,
And each is tortured in his separate hell."

There was in the neighborhood a young colored carpenter; a free born man. We had been well acquainted in childhood, and frequently met together afterwards. We became mutually attached, and he proposed to marry me. I loved him with all the ardor of a young girl's first love. But when I reflected that I was a slave, and that the laws gave no sanction to the marriage of such, my heart sank within me. My lover wanted to buy me; but I knew that Dr. Flint was too wilful and arbitrary a man to consent to that arrangement. From him, I was sure of experiencing all sorts of opposition, and I had nothing to hope from my mistress. She would have been delighted to have got rid of me, but not in that way. It would have relieved her mind of a burden if she could have seen me sold to some distant state, but if I was married near home I should be just as much in her husband's power as I had previously been,— for the husband of a slave has no power to protect her. Moreover, my mistress, like many others, seemed to think that slaves had no right to any family ties of their own; that they were created merely to wait upon the family of the mistress. I once heard her abuse a young slave girl, who told her that a colored man wanted to make her his wife. "I will have you peeled and pickled, my lady," said she, "if I ever hear you mention that subject again. Do you suppose that I will have you tending *my* children with the children of that nigger?" The girl to whom she said this had a mulatto child, of course not acknowledged by its father. The poor black man who loved her would have been proud to acknowledge his helpless offspring.

Many and anxious were the thoughts I revolved in my mind. I was at a loss what to do. Above all things, I was desirous to spare my lover the insults that had cut so deeply into my own soul. I talked with my grandmother about it, and partly told her my fears. I did not dare to tell her the worst. She had long suspected all was not right, and if I confirmed her suspicions I knew a storm would rise that would prove the overthrow of all my hopes.

This love-dream had been my support through many trials; and I could not bear to run the risk of having it suddenly dissipated. There was a lady in the neighborhood, a particular friend of Dr. Flint's, who often visited the house. I had a great respect for her, and she had always manifested a friendly interest in me. Grandmother thought she would have great influence with the doctor. I went to this lady, and told her my story. I told her I was aware that my lover's being a free-born man would prove a great objection; but he wanted to buy me; and if Dr. Flint would consent to that arrangement, I felt sure he would be willing to pay any reasonable price. She knew that Mrs. Flint disliked me; therefore, I ventured to suggest that perhaps my mistress would approve of my being sold, as that would rid her of me. The lady listened with kindly sympathy, and promised to do her utmost to promote my wishes. She had an interview with the doctor, and I believe she pleaded my cause earnestly; but it was all to no purpose.

How I dreaded my master now! Every minute I expected to be summoned to his presence; but the day passed, and I heard nothing from him. The next morning, a message was brought to me: "Master wants you in his study." I found the door ajar, and I stood a moment gazing at the hateful man who claimed a right to rule me, body and soul. I entered, and tried to appear calm. I did not want him to know how my heart was bleeding. He looked fixedly at me, with an expression which seemed to say, "I have half a mind to kill you on the spot." At last he broke the silence, and that was a relief to both of us.

"So you want to be married, do you?" said he, "and to a free nigger."

"Yes, sir."

"Well, I'll soon convince you whether I am your master, or the nigger fellow you honor so highly. If you *must* have a husband, you may take up with one of my slaves."

What a situation I should be in, as the wife of one of *his* slaves, even if my heart had been interested!

I replied, "Don't you suppose, sir, that a slave can have some preference about marrying? Do you suppose that all men are alike to her?"

"Do you love this nigger?" said he, abruptly.

"Yes, sir."

"How dare you tell me so!" he exclaimed, in great wrath. After a slight pause, he added, "I supposed you thought more of yourself; that you felt above the insults of such puppies."

I replied, "If he is a puppy I am a puppy, for we are both of the negro race. It is right and honorable for us to love each other. The man you call a puppy never insulted me, sir; and he would not love me if he did not believe me to be a virtuous woman."

He sprang upon me like a tiger, and gave me a stunning blow. It was the first time he had ever struck me; and fear did not enable me to control my anger. When I had recovered a little from the effects, I exclaimed, "You have struck me for answering you honestly. How I despise you!"

There was silence for some minutes. Perhaps he was deciding what should be my punishment; or, perhaps, he wanted to give me time to reflect on what I had said, and to whom I had said it. Finally, he asked, "Do you know what you have said?"

"Yes, sir; but your treatment drove me to it."

"Do you know that I have a right to do as I like with you,—that I can kill you, if I please?"

"You have tried to kill me, and I wish you had; but you have no right to do as you like with me."

"Silence!" he exclaimed, in a thundering voice. "By heavens, girl, you forget yourself too far! Are you mad? If you are, I will soon bring you to your senses. Do you think any other master would bear what I have borne from you this morning? Many masters would have killed you on the spot. How would you like to be sent to jail for your insolence?"

"I know I have been disrespectful, sir," I replied; "but you drove me to it; I couldn't help it. As for the jail, there would be more peace for me there than there is here."

"You deserve to go there," said he, "and to be under such treatment, that you would forget the meaning of the word *peace*. It would do you good. It would take some of your high notions out of you. But I am not ready to send you there yet, notwithstanding your ingratitude for all my kindness and forbearance. You have been the plague of my life. I have wanted to make you happy, and I have been repaid with the basest ingratitude; but though you have proved yourself incapable of appreciating my kindness, I will be lenient towards you, Linda. I will give you one more chance to redeem your character. If you behave yourself and do as I require, I will forgive you and treat you as I always have done; but if you disobey me, I will punish you as I would the meanest slave on my plantation. Never let me hear that fellow's name mentioned again. If I ever know of your speaking to him, I will cowhide you both; and if I catch him lurking about my premises, I will shoot him as soon as I would a dog. Do you hear what I say? I'll teach you a lesson about marriage and free niggers! Now go, and let this be the last time I have occasion to speak to you on this subject."

Reader, did you ever hate? I hope not. I never did but once; and I trust I never shall again. Somebody has called it "the atmosphere of hell;" and I believe it is so.

For a fortnight the doctor did not speak to me. He thought to mortify me; to make me feel that I had disgraced myself by receiving the honorable addresses of a respectable colored man, in preference to the base proposals of a white man. But though his lips disdained to address me, his eyes were very loquacious. No animal ever watched its prey more narrowly than he watched me. He knew that I could write, though he had failed to make me read his letters; and he was now troubled lest I should exchange letters with another man. After a while he became weary of silence; and I was sorry for it. One morning, as he passed through the hall, to leave the house, he contrived to thrust a note into my hand. I thought I had better read it, and spare myself the vexation of having him read it to me. It expressed regret for the blow he had given me, and reminded me that I myself was wholly to blame for it. He hoped I had become convinced of the injury I was doing myself by incurring his displeasure. He wrote that he had made up his mind to go to Louisiana; that he should take several slaves with him, and intended I should be one of the number. My mistress would remain where she was;

therefore I should have nothing to fear from that quarter. If I merited kindness from him, he assured me that it would be lavishly bestowed. He begged me to think over the matter, and answer the following day.

The next morning I was called to carry a pair of scissors to his room. I laid them on the table, with the letter beside them. He thought it was my answer, and did not call me back. I went as usual to attend my young mistress to and from school. He met me in the street, and ordered me to stop at his office on my way back. When I entered, he showed me his letter, and asked me why I had not answered it. I replied, "I am your daughter's property, and it is in your power to send me, or take me, wherever you please." He said he was very glad to find me so willing to go, and that we should start early in the autumn. He had a large practice in the town, and I rather thought he had made up the story merely to frighten me. However that might be, I was determined that I would never go to Louisiana with him.

Summer passed away, and early in the autumn Dr. Flint's eldest son was sent to Louisiana to examine the country, with a view to emigrating. That news did not disturb me. I knew very well that I should not be sent with *him*. That I had not been taken to the plantation before this time, was owing to the fact that his son was there. He was jealous of his son; and jealousy of the overseer had kept him from punishing me by sending me into the fields to work. Is it strange that I was not proud of these protectors? As for the overseer, he was a man for whom I had less respect than I had for a bloodhound.

Young Mr. Flint did not bring back a favorable report of Louisiana, and I heard no more of that scheme. Soon after this, my lover met me at the corner of the street, and I stopped to speak to him. Looking up, I saw my master watching us from his window. I hurried home, trembling with fear. I was sent for, immediately, to go to his room. He met me with a blow. "When is mistress to be married?" said he, in a sneering tone. A shower of oaths and imprecations followed. How thankful I was that my lover was a free man! that my tyrant had no power to flog him for speaking to me in the street!

Again and again I revolved in my mind how all this would

end. There was no hope that the doctor would consent to sell me on any terms. He had an iron will, and was determined to keep me, and to conquer me. My lover was an intelligent and religious man. Even if he could have obtained permission to marry me while I was a slave, the marriage would give him no power to protect me from my master. It would have made him miserable to witness the insults I should have been subjected to. And then, if we had children, I knew they must "follow the condition of the mother." What a terrible blight that would be on the heart of a free, intelligent father! For *his* sake, I felt that I ought not to link his fate with my own unhappy destiny. He was going to Savannah to see about a little property left him by an uncle; and hard as it was to bring my feelings to it, I earnestly entreated him not to come back. I advised him to go to the Free States, where his tongue would not be tied, and where his intelligence would be of more avail to him. He left me, still hoping the day would come when I could be bought. With me the lamp of hope had gone out. The dream of my girlhood was over. I felt lonely and desolate.

Still I was not stripped of all. I still had my good grandmother, and my affectionate brother. When he put his arms round my neck, and looked into my eyes, as if to read there the troubles I dared not tell, I felt that I still had something to love. But even that pleasant emotion was chilled by the reflection that he might be torn from me at any moment, by some sudden freak of my master. If he had known how we loved each other, I think he would have exulted in separating us. We often planned together how we could get to the north. But, as William remarked, such things are easier said than done. My movements were very closely watched, and we had no means of getting any money to defray our expenses. As for grandmother, she was strongly opposed to her children's undertaking any such project. She had not forgotten poor Benjamin's sufferings, and she was afraid that if another child tried to escape, he would have a similar or a worse fate. To me, nothing seemed more dreadful than my present life. I said to myself, "William *must* be free. He shall go to the north, and I will follow him." Many a slave sister has formed the same plans.

VIII.

WHAT SLAVES ARE TAUGHT TO THINK OF THE NORTH.

SLAVEHOLDERS pride themselves upon being honorable men; but if you were to hear the enormous lies they tell their slaves, you would have small respect for their veracity. I have spoken plain English. Pardon me. I cannot use a milder term. When they visit the north, and return home, they tell their slaves of the runaways they have seen, and describe them to be in the most deplorable condition. A slaveholder once told me that he had seen a runaway friend of mine in New York, and that she besought him to take her back to her master, for she was literally dying of starvation; that many days she had only one cold potato to eat, and at other times could get nothing at all. He said he refused to take her, because he knew her master would not thank him for bringing such a miserable wretch to his house. He ended by saying to me, "This is the punishment she brought on herself for running away from a kind master."

This whole story was false. I afterwards staid with that friend in New York, and found her in comfortable circumstances. She had never thought of such a thing as wishing to go back to slavery. Many of the slaves believe such stories, and think it is not worth while to exchange slavery for such a hard kind of freedom. It is difficult to persuade such that freedom could make them useful men, and enable them to protect their wives and children. If those heathen in our Christian land had as much teaching as some Hindoos, they would think otherwise. They would know that liberty is more valuable than life. They would begin to understand their own capabilities, and exert themselves to become men and women.

But while the Free States sustain a law which hurls fugitives back into slavery, how can the slaves resolve to become men? There are some who strive to protect wives and daughters from the insults of their masters; but those who have such sentiments have had advantages above the general mass of slaves. They have been partially civilized and Christianized by favorable circumstances. Some are bold enough to *utter* such sentiments to their masters. O, that there were more of them!

Some poor creatures have been so brutalized by the lash that they will sneak out of the way to give their masters free access to their wives and daughters. Do you think this proves the black man to belong to an inferior order of beings? What would *you* be, if you had been born and brought up a slave, with generations of slaves for ancestors? I admit that the black man *is* inferior. But what is it that makes him so? It is the ignorance in which white men compel him to live; it is the torturing whip that lashes manhood out of him; it is the fierce bloodhounds of the South, and the scarcely less cruel human bloodhounds of the north, who enforce the Fugitive Slave Law. *They* do the work.

Southern gentlemen indulge in the most contemptuous expressions about the Yankees, while they, on their part, consent to do the vilest work for them, such as the ferocious bloodhounds and the despised negro-hunters are employed to do at home. When southerners go to the north, they are proud to do them honor; but the northern man is not welcome south of Mason and Dixon's line, unless he suppresses every thought and feeling at variance with their "peculiar institution." Nor is it enough to be silent. The masters are not pleased, unless they obtain a greater degree of subservience than that; and they are generally accommodated. Do they respect the northerner for this? I trow not. Even the slaves despise "a northern man with southern principles;" and that is the class they generally see. When northerners go to the south to reside, they prove very apt scholars. They soon imbibe the sentiments and disposition of their neighbors, and generally go beyond their teachers. Of the two, they are proverbially the hardest masters.

They seem to satisfy their consciences with the doctrine that God created the Africans to be slaves. What a libel upon the heavenly Father, who "made of one blood all nations of men!" And then who *are* Africans? Who can measure the amount of Anglo-Saxon blood coursing in the veins of American slaves?

I have spoken of the pains slaveholders take to give their slaves a bad opinion of the north; but, notwithstanding this, intelligent slaves are aware that they have many friends in the Free States. Even the most ignorant have some confused notions about it. They knew that I could read; and I was often asked if I had seen any thing in the newspapers about white folks over in the big north, who were trying to get their freedom for them. Some believe that the abolitionists have already made them free, and that it is established by law, but that their masters prevent the law from going into effect. One woman begged me to get a newspaper and read it over. She said her husband told her that the black people had sent word to the queen of 'Merica that they were all slaves; that she didn't believe it, and went to Washington city to see the president about it. They quarrelled; she drew her sword upon him, and swore that he should help her to make them all free.

That poor, ignorant woman thought that America was governed by a Queen, to whom the President was subordinate. I wish the President was subordinate to Queen Justice.

IX.

SKETCHES OF NEIGHBORING SLAVEHOLDERS.

THERE was a planter in the country, not far from us, whom I will call Mr. Litch. He was an ill-bred, uneducated man, but very wealthy. He had six hundred slaves, many of whom he did not know by sight. His extensive plantation was managed by well-paid overseers. There was a jail and a whipping post on his grounds; and whatever cruelties were perpetrated there, they passed without comment. He was so effectually screened by his great wealth that he was called to no account for his crimes, not even for murder.

Various were the punishments resorted to. A favorite one was to tie a rope round a man's body, and suspend him from the ground. A fire was kindled over him, from which was suspended a piece of fat pork. As this cooked, the scalding drops of fat continually fell on the bare flesh. On his own plantation, he required very strict obedience to the eighth commandment. But depredations on the neighbors were allowable, provided the culprit managed to evade detection or suspicion. If a neighbor brought a charge of theft against any of his slaves, he was browbeaten by the master, who assured him that his slaves had enough of every thing at home, and had no inducement to steal. No sooner was the neighbor's back turned, than the accused was sought out, and whipped for his lack of discretion. If a slave stole from him even a pound of meat or a peck of corn, if detection followed, he was put in chains and imprisoned, and so kept till his form was attenuated by hunger and suffering.

A freshet once bore his wine cellar and meat house miles away from the plantation. Some slaves followed, and secured bits of meat and bottles of wine. Two were detected; a ham and some liquor being found in their huts. They were summoned by their master. No words were used, but a club felled them to the ground. A rough box was their coffin, and their interment was a dog's burial. Nothing was said.

Murder was so common on his plantation that he feared to be alone after nightfall. He might have believed in ghosts.

His brother, if not equal in wealth, was at least equal in cruelty. His bloodhounds were well trained. Their pen was spacious, and a terror to the slaves. They were let loose on a runaway, and, if they tracked him, they literally tore the flesh from his bones. When this slaveholder died, his shrieks and groans were so frightful that they appalled his own friends. His last words were, "I am going to hell; bury my money with me."

After death his eyes remained open. To press the lids down, silver dollars were laid on them. These were buried with him. From this circumstance, a rumor went abroad that his coffin was filled with money. Three times his grave was opened, and his coffin taken out. The last time, his body was found on the ground, and a flock of buzzards were pecking at it. He was again interred, and a sentinel set over his grave. The perpetrators were never discovered.

Cruelty is contagious in uncivilized communities. Mr. Conant, a neighbor of Mr. Litch, returned from town one evening in a partial state of intoxication. His body servant gave him some offence. He was divested of his clothes, except his shirt, whipped, and tied to a large tree in front of the house. It was a stormy night in winter. The wind blew bitterly cold, and the boughs of the old tree crackled under falling sleet. A member of the family, fearing he would freeze to death, begged that he might be taken down; but the master would not relent. He remained there three hours; and, when he was cut down, he was more dead than alive. Another slave, who stole a pig from this master, to appease his hunger, was terribly flogged. In desperation, he tried to run away. But at the end of two miles, he was so faint with loss of blood, he thought he was dying. He had a wife, and he longed to see her once more. Too sick to walk, he crept back that long distance on his hands and knees. When he reached his master's, it was night. He had not strength to rise and open the gate. He moaned, and tried to call for help. I had a friend living in the same family. At last his cry reached her. She went out and found the prostrate man at the gate. She ran back to the house for assistance, and two men returned with her. They carried him in, and laid him on the floor. The back of his shirt was one clot of blood. By means of lard, my friend loosened it from the raw flesh. She bandaged him, gave him cool drink, and left him to rest. The master said he deserved a hundred more lashes. When his own labor was stolen from him, he had stolen food to appease his hunger. This was his crime.

Another neighbor was a Mrs. Wade. At no hour of the day was there cessation of the lash on her premises. Her labors began with the dawn, and did not cease till long after nightfall. The barn was her particular place of torture. There she lashed the slaves with the might of a man. An old slave of hers once said to me, "It is hell in missis's house. 'Pears I can never get out. Day and night I prays to die."

The mistress died before the old woman, and, when dying, entreated her husband not to permit any one of her slaves to look on her after death. A slave who had nursed her children, and had still a child in her care, watched her chance, and stole with it in her arms to the room where lay her dead mistress. She gazed a while on her, then raised her hand and dealt two blows on her face, saying, as she did so, "The devil is got you *now!*" She forgot that the child was looking on. She had just begun to talk; and she said to her father, "I did see ma, and

mammy did strike ma, so," striking her own face with her little hand. The master was startled. He could not imagine how
the nurse could obtain access to the room where the corpse
lay; for he kept the door locked. He questioned her. She confessed that what the child had said was true, and told how she
had procured the key. She was sold to Georgia.

In my childhood I knew a valuable slave, named Charity,
and loved her, as all children did. Her young mistress married, and took her to Louisiana. Her little boy, James, was
sold to a good sort of master. He became involved in debt,
and James was sold again to a wealthy slaveholder, noted for
his cruelty. With this man he grew up to manhood, receiving
the treatment of a dog. After a severe whipping, to save himself from further infliction of the lash, with which he was
threatened, he took to the woods. He was in a most miserable
condition—cut by the cowskin, half naked, half starved, and
without the means of procuring a crust of bread.

Some weeks after his escape, he was captured, tied, and carried back to his master's plantation. This man considered
punishment in his jail, on bread and water, after receiving
hundreds of lashes, too mild for the poor slave's offence.
Therefore he decided, after the overseer should have whipped
him to his satisfaction, to have him placed between the screws
of the cotton gin, to stay as long as he had been in the woods.
This wretched creature was cut with the whip from his head
to his feet, then washed with strong brine, to prevent the
flesh from mortifying, and make it heal sooner than it otherwise would. He was then put into the cotton gin, which was
screwed down, only allowing him room to turn on his side
when he could not lie on his back. Every morning a slave was
sent with a piece of bread and bowl of water, which were
placed within reach of the poor fellow. The slave was charged,
under penalty of severe punishment, not to speak to him.

Four days passed, and the slave continued to carry the
bread and water. On the second morning, he found the bread
gone, but the water untouched. When he had been in the
press four days and five nights, the slave informed his master
that the water had not been used for four mornings, and that
a horrible stench came from the gin house. The overseer was
sent to examine into it. When the press was unscrewed, the

dead body was found partly eaten by rats and vermin. Perhaps the rats that devoured his bread had gnawed him before life was extinct. Poor Charity! Grandmother and I often asked each other how her affectionate heart would bear the news, if she should ever hear of the murder of her son. We had known her husband, and knew that James was like him in manliness and intelligence. These were the qualities that made it so hard for him to be a plantation slave. They put him into a rough box, and buried him with less feeling than would have been manifested for an old house dog. Nobody asked any questions. He was a slave; and the feeling was that the master had a right to do what he pleased with his own property. And what did *he* care for the value of a slave? He had hundreds of them. When they had finished their daily toil, they must hurry to eat their little morsels, and be ready to extinguish their pine knots before nine o'clock, when the overseer went his patrol rounds. He entered every cabin, to see that men and their wives had gone to bed together, lest the men, from over-fatigue, should fall asleep in the chimney corner, and remain there till the morning horn called them to their daily task. Women are considered of no value, unless they continually increase their owner's stock. They are put on a par with animals. This same master shot a woman through the head, who had run away and been brought back to him. No one called him to account for it. If a slave resisted being whipped, the bloodhounds were unpacked, and set upon him, to tear his flesh from his bones. The master who did these things was highly educated, and styled a perfect gentleman. He also boasted the name and standing of a Christian, though Satan never had a truer follower.

I could tell of more slaveholders as cruel as those I have described. They are not exceptions to the general rule. I do not say there are no humane slaveholders. Such characters do exist, notwithstanding the hardening influences around them. But they are "like angels' visits—few and far between."

I knew a young lady who was one of these rare specimens. She was an orphan, and inherited as slaves a woman and her six children. Their father was a free man. They had a comfortable home of their own, parents and children living together. The mother and eldest daughter served their mistress during the day, and at night returned to their dwelling, which was on the premises. The young lady was very pious, and there was some reality in her religion. She taught her slaves to lead pure lives, and wished them to enjoy the fruit of their own industry. *Her* religion was not a garb put on for Sunday, and laid aside till Sunday returned again. The eldest daughter of the slave mother was promised in marriage to a free man; and the day before the wedding this good mistress emancipated her, in order that her marriage might have the sanction of *law*.

Report said that this young lady cherished an unrequited affection for a man who had resolved to marry for wealth. In the course of time a rich uncle of hers died. He left six thousand dollars to his two sons by a colored woman, and the remainder of his property to this orphan niece. The metal soon attracted the magnet. The lady and her weighty purse became his. She offered to manumit her slaves—telling them that her marriage might make unexpected changes in their destiny, and she wished to insure their happiness. They refused to take their freedom, saying that she had always been their best friend, and they could not be so happy any where as with her. I was not surprised. I had often seen them in their comfortable home, and thought that the whole town did not contain a happier family. They had never felt slavery; and, when it was too late, they were convinced of its reality.

When the new master claimed this family as his property, the father became furious, and went to his mistress for protection. "I can do nothing for you now, Harry," said she. "I no longer have the power I had a week ago. I have succeeded in obtaining the freedom of your wife; but I cannot obtain it for your children." The unhappy father swore that nobody should take his children from him. He concealed them in the woods for some days; but they were discovered and taken. The father was put in jail, and the two oldest boys sold to Georgia. One little girl, too young to be of service to her master, was left with the wretched mother. The other three were carried to their master's plantation. The eldest soon became a mother; and, when the slaveholder's wife looked at the babe, she wept bitterly. She knew that her own husband had violated the purity she had so carefully inculcated. She had a second child by her master, and then he sold her and his offspring to his brother. She bore two children to the brother, and was sold again. The next sister went crazy. The life she was compelled to lead drove her mad. The third one became the mother of five daughters. Before the birth of the fourth the pious mistress died. To the last, she rendered every kindness to the slaves that her unfortunate circumstances permitted. She passed away peacefully, glad to close her eyes on a life which had been made so wretched by the man she loved.

This man squandered the fortune he had received, and sought to retrieve his affairs by a second marriage; but, having retired after a night of drunken debauch, he was found dead in the morning. He was called a good master; for he fed and clothed his slaves better than most masters, and the lash was not heard on his plantation so frequently as on many others. Had it not been for slavery, he would have been a better man, and his wife a happier woman.

No pen can give an adequate description of the all-pervading corruption produced by slavery. The slave girl is reared in an atmosphere of licentiousness and fear. The lash and the foul talk of her master and his sons are her teachers. When she is fourteen or fifteen, her owner, or his sons, or the overseer, or perhaps all of them, begin to bribe her with presents. If these fail to accomplish their purpose, she is whipped or starved into submission to their will. She may have had religious principles inculcated by some pious mother or grandmother, or some good mistress; she may have a lover, whose good opinion and peace of mind are dear to her heart; or the profligate men who have power over her may be exceedingly odious to her. But resistance is hopeless.

> "The poor worm
> Shall prove her contest vain. Life's little day
> Shall pass, and she is gone!"

The slaveholder's sons are, of course, vitiated, even while boys, by the unclean influences every where around them. Nor do the master's daughters always escape. Severe retributions sometimes come upon him for the wrongs he does to the daughters of the slaves. The white daughters early hear their parents quarrelling about some female slave. Their curiosity is excited, and they soon learn the cause. They are attended by the young slave girls whom their father has corrupted; and they hear such talk as should never meet youthful ears, or any other ears. They know that the women slaves are subject to their father's authority in all things; and in some cases they exercise the same authority over the men slaves. I have myself seen the master of such a household whose head was bowed down in shame; for it was known in the neighborhood that his daughter had selected one of the meanest slaves on his plantation to be the father of his first grandchild. She did not make her advances to her equals, nor even to her father's more intelligent servants. She selected the most brutalized, over whom her authority could be exercised with less fear of exposure. Her father, half frantic with rage, sought to revenge himself on the offending black man; but his daughter, foreseeing the storm that would arise, had given him free papers, and sent him out of the state.

In such cases the infant is smothered, or sent where it is never seen by any who know its history. But if the white parent is the *father*, instead of the mother, the offspring are unblushingly reared for the market. If they are girls, I have indicated plainly enough what will be their inevitable destiny.

You may believe what I say; for I write only that whereof I know. I was twenty-one years in that cage of obscene birds. I can testify, from my own experience and observation, that slavery is a curse to the whites as well as to the blacks. It makes the white fathers cruel and sensual; the sons violent and licentious; it contaminates the daughters, and makes the wives wretched. And as for the colored race, it needs an abler pen than mine to describe the extremity of their sufferings, the depth of their degradation.

Yet few slaveholders seem to be aware of the widespread moral ruin occasioned by this wicked system. Their talk is of blighted cotton crops—not of the blight on their children's souls.

If you want to be fully convinced of the abominations of slavery, go on a southern plantation, and call yourself a negro trader. Then there will be no concealment; and you will see and hear things that will seem to you impossible among human beings with immortal souls.

X.

A PERILOUS PASSAGE IN THE SLAVE GIRL'S LIFE.

AFTER my lover went away, Dr. Flint contrived a new plan. He seemed to have an idea that my fear of my mistress was his greatest obstacle. In the blandest tones, he told me that he was going to build a small house for me, in a secluded place, four miles away from the town. I shuddered; but I was constrained to listen, while he talked of his intention to give me a home of my own, and to make a lady of me. Hitherto, I had escaped my dreaded fate, by being in the midst of people. My grandmother had already had high words with my master about me. She had told him pretty plainly what she thought of his character, and there was considerable gossip in the neighborhood about our affairs, to which the open-mouthed jealousy of Mrs. Flint contributed not a little. When my master said he was going to build a house for me, and that he could do it with little trouble and expense, I was in hopes something would happen to frustrate his scheme; but I soon heard that the house was actually begun. I vowed before my Maker that I would never enter it. I had rather toil on the plantation from dawn till dark; I had rather live and die in jail, than drag on, from day to day, through such a living death. I was determined that the master, whom I so hated and loathed, who had blighted the prospects of my youth, and made my life a desert, should not, after my long struggle with him, succeed at last in trampling his victim under his feet. I would do any thing, every thing, for the sake of defeating him. What *could* I do? I thought and thought, till I became desperate, and made a plunge into the abyss.

And now, reader, I come to a period in my unhappy life, which I would gladly forget if I could. The remembrance fills me with sorrow and shame. It pains me to tell you of it; but I have promised to tell you the truth, and I will do it honestly, let it cost me what it may. I will not try to screen myself behind the plea of compulsion from a master; for it was not so. Neither can I plead ignorance or thoughtlessness. For years, my master had done his utmost to pollute my mind with foul images, and to destroy the pure principles inculcated by my grandmother, and the good mistress of my childhood. The influences of slavery had had the same effect on me that they had on other young girls; they had made me prematurely knowing, concerning the evil ways of the world. I knew what I did, and I did it with deliberate calculation.

But, O, ye happy women, whose purity has been sheltered from childhood, who have been free to choose the objects of your affection, whose homes are protected by law, do not judge the poor desolate slave girl too severely! If slavery had been abolished, I, also, could have married the man of my choice; I could have had a home shielded by the laws; and I should have been spared the painful task of confessing what I am now about to relate; but all my prospects had been blighted by slavery. I wanted to keep myself pure; and, under the most adverse circumstances, I tried hard to preserve my self-respect; but I was struggling alone in the powerful grasp of the demon Slavery; and the monster proved too strong for me. I felt as if I was forsaken by God and man; as if all my efforts must be frustrated; and I became reckless in my despair.

I have told you that Dr. Flint's persecutions and his wife's jealousy had given rise to some gossip in the neighborhood. Among others, it chanced that a white unmarried gentleman had obtained some knowledge of the circumstances in which I was placed. He knew my grandmother, and often spoke to me in the street. He became interested for me, and asked questions about my master, which I answered in part. He expressed a great deal of sympathy, and a wish to aid me. He constantly sought opportunities to see me, and wrote to me frequently. I was a poor slave girl, only fifteen years old.

So much attention from a superior person was, of course, flattering; for human nature is the same in all. I also felt grateful for his sympathy, and encouraged by his kind words. It seemed to me a great thing to have such a friend. By degrees, a more tender feeling crept into my heart. He was an educated and eloquent gentleman; too eloquent, alas, for the poor slave girl who trusted in him. Of course I saw whither all this was tending. I knew the impassable gulf between us; but to be an object of interest to a man who is not married, and who is not her master, is agreeable to the pride and feelings of a slave, if her miserable situation has left her any pride or sentiment. It seems less degrading to give one's self, than to submit to compulsion. There is something akin to freedom in having a lover who has no control over you, except that which he gains by kindness and attachment. A master may treat you as rudely as he pleases, and you dare not speak; moreover, the wrong does not seem so great with an unmarried man, as with one who has a wife to be made unhappy. There may be sophistry in all this; but the condition of a slave confuses all principles of morality, and, in fact, renders the practice of them impossible.

When I found that my master had actually begun to build the lonely cottage, other feelings mixed with those I have described. Revenge, and calculations of interest, were added to flattered vanity and sincere gratitude for kindness. I knew nothing would enrage Dr. Flint so much as to know that I favored another; and it was something to triumph over my tyrant even in that small way. I thought he would revenge himself by selling me, and I was sure my friend, Mr. Sands, would buy me. He was a man of more generosity and feeling than my master, and I thought my freedom could be easily obtained from him. The crisis of my fate now came so near that I was desperate. I shuddered to think of being the mother of children that should be owned by my old tyrant. I knew that as soon as a new fancy took him, his victims were sold far off to get rid of them; especially if they had children. I had seen several women sold, with his babies at the breast. He never allowed his offspring by slaves to remain long in sight of himself and his wife. Of a man who was not my master I could ask to have my children well supported; and in this case, I felt confident I should obtain the boon. I also felt quite sure that they would be made free. With all these thoughts revolving in my mind, and seeing no other way of escaping the doom I so much dreaded, I made a headlong plunge. Pity me, and pardon me, O virtuous reader! You never knew what it is to be a slave; to be entirely unprotected by law or custom; to have the laws reduce you to the condition of a chattel, entirely subject to the will of another. You never exhausted your ingenuity in avoiding the snares, and eluding the power of a hatred tyrant; you never shuddered at the sound of his footsteps, and trembled within hearing of his voice. I know I did wrong. No one can feel it more sensibly than I do. The painful and humiliating memory will haunt me to my dying day. Still, in looking back, calmly, on the events of my life, I feel that the slave woman ought not to be judged by the same standard as others.

The months passed on. I had many unhappy hours. I secretly mourned over the sorrow I was bringing on my grandmother, who had so tried to shield me from harm. I knew that I was the greatest comfort of her old age, and that it was a source of pride to her that I had not degraded myself, like most of the slaves. I wanted to confess to her that I was no longer worthy of her love; but I could not utter the dreaded words.

As for Dr. Flint, I had a feeling of satisfaction and triumph in the thought of telling *him*. From time to time he told me of his intended arrangements, and I was silent. At last, he came and told me the cottage was completed, and ordered me to go to it. I told him I would never enter it. He said, "I have heard enough of such talk as that. You shall go, if you are carried by force; and you shall remain there."

I replied, "I will never go there. In a few months I shall be a mother."

He stood and looked at me in dumb amazement, and left the house without a word. I thought I should be happy in my triumph over him. But now that the truth was out, and my relatives would hear of it, I felt wretched. Humble as were their circumstances, they had pride in my good character. Now, how could I look them in the face? My self-respect was gone! I had resolved that I would be virtuous, though I was a slave. I had said, "Let the storm beat! I will brave it till I die." And now, how humiliated I felt!

I went to my grandmother. My lips moved to make confession, but the words stuck in my throat. I sat down in the shade of a tree at her door and began to sew. I think she saw something unusual was the matter with me. The mother of slaves is very watchful. She knows there is no security for her children. After they have entered their teens she lives in daily expectation of trouble. This leads to many questions. If the girl is of a sensitive nature, timidity keeps her from answering truthfully, and this well-meant course has a tendency to drive her from maternal counsels. Presently, in came my mistress, like a mad woman, and accused me concerning her husband. My grandmother, whose suspicions had been previously awakened, believed what she said. She exclaimed, "O Linda! has it come to this? I had rather see you dead than to see you as you now are. You are a disgrace to your dead mother." She tore from my fingers my mother's wedding ring and her silver thimble. "Go away!" she exclaimed, "and never come to my house, again." Her reproaches fell so hot and heavy, that they left me no chance to answer. Bitter tears, such as the eyes never shed but once, were my only answer. I rose from my seat, but fell back again, sobbing. She did not speak to me; but the tears were running down her furrowed cheeks, and they scorched me like fire. She had always been so kind to me! *So* kind! How I longed to throw myself at her feet, and tell her all the truth! But she had ordered me to go, and never to come there again. After a few minutes, I mustered strength, and started to obey her. With what feelings did I now close that little gate, which I used to open with such an eager hand in my childhood! It closed upon me with a sound I never heard before.

Where could I go? I was afraid to return to my master's. I walked on recklessly, not caring where I went, or what would become of me. When I had gone four or five miles, fatigue compelled me to stop. I sat down on the stump of an old tree. The stars were shining through the boughs above me. How they mocked me, with their bright, calm light! The hours passed by, and as I sat there alone a chilliness and deadly sickness came over me. I sank on the ground. My mind was full of horrid thoughts. I prayed to die; but the prayer was not answered. At last, with great effort I roused myself, and walked some distance further, to the house of a woman who had been a friend of my mother. When I told her why I was there, she spoke soothingly to me; but I could not be comforted. I thought I could bear my shame if I could only be reconciled to my grandmother. I longed to open my heart to her. I thought if she could know the real state of the case, and all I had been bearing for years, she would perhaps judge me less harshly. My friend advised me to send for her. I did so; but days of agonizing suspense passed before she came. Had she utterly forsaken me? No. She came at last. I knelt before her, and told her the things that had poisoned my life; how long I had been persecuted; that I saw no way of escape; and in an hour of extremity I had become desperate. She listened in silence. I told her I would bear any thing and do any thing, if in time I had hopes of obtaining her forgiveness. I begged of her to pity me, for my dead mother's sake. And she did pity me. She did not say, "I forgive you;" but she looked at me lovingly, with her eyes full of tears. She laid her old hand gently on my head, and murmured, "Poor child! Poor child!"

XI.
THE NEW TIE TO LIFE.

I RETURNED to my good grandmother's house. She had an interview with Mr. Sands. When she asked him why he could not have left her one ewe lamb,— whether there were not plenty of slaves who did not care about character,—he made no answer; but he spoke kind and encouraging words. He promised to care for my child, and to buy me, be the conditions what they might.

I had not seen Dr. Flint for five days. I had never seen him since I made the avowal to him. He talked of the disgrace I had brought on myself; how I had sinned against my master, and mortified my old grandmother. He intimated that if I had accepted his proposals, he, as a physician, could have saved me from exposure. He even condescended to pity me. Could he have offered wormwood more bitter? He, whose persecutions had been the cause of my sin!

"Linda," said he, "though you have been criminal towards me, I feel for you, and I can pardon you if you obey my wishes. Tell me whether the fellow you wanted to marry is the father of your child. If you deceive me, you shall feel the fires of hell."

I did not feel as proud as I had done. My strongest weapon with him was gone. I was lowered in my own estimation, and had resolved to bear his abuse in silence. But when he spoke contemptuously of the lover who had always treated me honorably; when I remembered that but for *him* I might have been a virtuous, free, and happy wife, I lost my patience. "I have sinned against God and myself," I replied; "but not against you."

He clinched his teeth, and muttered, "Curse you!" He came towards me, with ill-suppressed rage, and exclaimed, "You obstinate girl! I could grind your bones to powder! You have thrown yourself away on some worthless rascal. You are weak-minded, and have been easily persuaded by those who don't care a straw for you. The future will settle accounts between us. You are blinded now; but hereafter you will be convinced that your master was your best friend. My lenity towards you is a proof of it. I might have punished you in many ways. I might have had you whipped till you fell dead under the lash. But I wanted you to live; I would have bettered your condition. Others cannot do it. You are my slave. Your mistress, disgusted by your conduct, forbids you to return to the house; therefore I leave you here for the present; but I shall see you often. I will call tomorrow."

He came with frowning brows, that showed a dissatisfied state of mind. After asking about my health, he inquired whether my board was paid, and who visited me. He then went on to say that he had neglected his duty; that as a physician there were certain things that he ought to have explained to me. Then followed talk such as would have made the most shameless blush. He ordered me to stand up before him. I obeyed. "I command you," said he, "to tell me whether the father of your child is white or black." I hesitated. "Answer me this instant!" he exclaimed. I did answer. He sprang upon me like a wolf, and grabbed my arm as if he would have broken it. "Do you love him?" said he, in a hissing tone.

"I am thankful that I do not despise him," I replied.

He raised his hand to strike me; but it fell again. I don't know what arrested the blow. He sat down, with lips tightly compressed. At last he spoke. "I came here," said he, "to make you a friendly proposition; but your ingratitude chafes me beyond endurance. You turn aside all my good intentions towards you. I don't know what it is that keeps me from killing you." Again he rose, as if he had a mind to strike me.

But he resumed. "On one condition I will forgive your insolence and crime. You must henceforth have no communication of any kind with the father of your child. You must not ask any thing from him, or receive any thing from him. I will take care of you and your child. You had better promise this at once, and not wait till you are deserted by him. This is the last act of mercy I shall show towards you."

I said something about being unwilling to have my child supported by a man who had cursed it and me also. He rejoined, that a woman who had sunk to my level had no right to expect any thing else. He asked, for the last time, would I accept his kindness? I answered that I would not.

"Very well," said he; "then take the consequences of your wayward course. Never look to me for help. You are my slave, and shall always be my slave. I will never sell you, that you may depend upon."

Hope died away in my heart as he closed the door after him. I had calculated that in his rage he would sell me to a slave-trader; and I knew the father of my child was on the watch to buy me.

About this time my uncle Phillip was expected to return from a voyage. The day before his departure I had officiated as bridesmaid to a young friend. My heart was then ill at ease, but my smiling countenance did not betray it. Only a year had passed; but what fearful changes it had wrought! My heart had grown gray in misery. Lives that flash in sunshine, and lives that are born in tears, receive their hue from circumstances. None of us know what a year may bring forth.

I felt no joy when they told me my uncle had come. He wanted to see me, though he knew what had happened. I shrank from him at first; but at last consented that he should come to my room. He received me as he always had done. O, how my heart smote me when I felt his tears on my burning cheeks! The words of my grandmother came to my mind,— "Perhaps your mother and father are taken from the evil days to come." My disappointed heart could now praise God that it was so. But why, thought I, did my relatives ever cherish hopes for me? What was there to save me from the usual fate of slave girls? Many more beautiful and more intelligent than I had experienced a similar fate, or a far worse one. How could they hope that I should escape?

My uncle's stay was short, and I was not sorry for it. I was too ill in mind and body to enjoy my friends as I had done. For some weeks I was unable to leave my bed. I could not have any doctor but my master, and I would not have him sent for. At last, alarmed by my increasing illness, they sent for him. I was very weak and nervous; and as soon as he entered the room, I began to scream. They told him my state was very critical. He had no wish to hasten me out of the world, and he withdrew.

When my babe was born, they said it was premature. It weighed only four pounds; but God let it live. I heard the doctor say I could not survive till morning. I had often prayed for death; but now I did not want to die, unless my child could die too. Many weeks passed before I was able to leave my bed. I was a mere wreck of my former self. For a year there was scarcely a day when I was free from chills and fever. My babe also was sickly. His little limbs were often racked with pain. Dr. Flint continued his visits, to look after my health; and he did not fail to remind me that my child was an addition to his stock of slaves.

I felt too feeble to dispute with him, and listened to his re-marks in silence. His visits were less frequent; but his busy spirit could not remain quiet. He employed my brother in his office, and he was made the medium of frequent notes and messages to me. William was a bright lad, and of much use to the doctor. He had learned to put up medicines, to leech, cup, and bleed. He had taught himself to read and spell. I was proud of my brother; and the old doctor suspected as much. One day, when I had not seen him for several weeks, I heard his steps approaching the door. I dreaded the encounter, and hid myself. He inquired for me, of course; but I was nowhere to be found. He went to his office, and despatched William with a note. The color mounted to my brother's face when he gave it to me; and he said, "Don't you hate me, Linda, for bringing you these things?" I told him I could not blame him; he was a slave, and obliged to obey his master's will. The note ordered me to come to his office. I went. He demanded

to know where I was when he called. I told him I was at
home. He flew into a passion, and said he knew better. Then
he launched out upon his usual themes,—my crimes against
him, and my ingratitude for his forbearance. The laws were
laid down to me anew, and I was dismissed. I felt humiliated
that my brother should stand by, and listen to such language
as would be addressed only to a slave. Poor boy! He was powerless to defend me; but I saw the tears, which he vainly
strove to keep back. This manifestation of feeling irritated the
doctor. William could do nothing to please him. One morning he did not arrive at the office so early as usual; and that
circumstance afforded his master an opportunity to vent his
spleen. He was put in jail. The next day my brother sent a
trader to the doctor, with a request to be sold. His master was
greatly incensed at what he called his insolence. He said he
had put him there to reflect upon his bad conduct, and he
certainly was not giving any evidence of repentance. For two
days he harassed himself to find somebody to do his office
work; but every thing went wrong without William. He was
released, and ordered to take his old stand, with many threats,
if he was not careful about his future behavior.

As the months passed on, my boy improved in health.
When he was a year old, they called him beautiful. The little
vine was taking deep root in my existence, though its clinging
fondness excited a mixture of love and pain. When I was most
sorely oppressed I found a solace in his smiles. I loved to
watch his infant slumbers; but always there was a dark cloud
over my enjoyment. I could never forget that he was a slave.
Sometimes I wished that he might die in infancy. God tried
me. My darling became very ill. The bright eyes grew dull,
and the little feet and hands were so icy cold that I thought
death had already touched them. I had prayed for his death,
but never so earnestly as I now prayed for his life; and my
prayer was heard. Alas, what mockery it is for a slave mother
to try to pray back her dying child to life! Death is better than
slavery. It was a sad thought that I had no name to give my
child. His father caressed him and treated him kindly, whenever he had a chance to see him. He was not unwilling that
he should bear his name; but he had no legal claim to it; and
if I had bestowed it upon him, my master would have re-

garded it as a new crime, a new piece of insolence, and would, perhaps, revenge it on the boy. O, the serpent of Slavery has many and poisonous fangs!

XII.

FEAR OF INSURRECTION.

NOT far from this time Nat Turner's insurrection broke out; and the news threw our town into great commotion. Strange that they should be alarmed, when their slaves were so "contented and happy"! But so it was.

It was always the custom to have a muster every year. On that occasion every white man shouldered his musket. The citizens and the so-called country gentlemen wore military uniforms. The poor whites took their places in the ranks in every-day dress, some without shoes, some without hats. This grand occasion had already passed; and when the slaves were told there was to be another muster, they were surprised and rejoiced. Poor creatures! They thought it was going to be a holiday. I was informed of the true state of affairs, and imparted it to the few I could trust. Most gladly would I have proclaimed it to every slave; but I dared not. All could not be relied on. Mighty is the power of the torturing lash.

By sunrise, people were pouring in from every quarter within twenty miles of the town. I knew the houses were to be searched; and I expected it would be done by country bullies and the poor whites. I knew nothing annoyed them so much as to see colored people living in comfort and respectability; so I made arrangements for them with especial care. I arranged every thing in my grandmother's house as neatly as possible. I put white quilts on the beds, and decorated some of the rooms with flowers. When all was arranged, I sat down at the window to watch. Far as my eye could reach, it rested on a motley crowd of soldiers. Drums and fifes were discoursing martial music. The men were divided into companies of sixteen, each headed by a captain. Orders were given, and the wild scouts rushed in every direction, wherever a colored face was to be found.

It was a grand opportunity for the low whites, who had no negroes of their own to scourge. They exulted in such a chance to exercise a little brief authority, and show their subserviency to the slaveholders; not reflecting that the power which trampled on the colored people also kept themselves in poverty, ignorance, and moral degradation. Those who never witnessed such scenes can hardly believe what I know was inflicted at this time on innocent men, women, and children, against whom there was not the slightest ground for suspicion. Colored people and slaves who lived in remote parts of the town suffered in an especial manner. In some cases the searchers scattered powder and shot among their clothes, and then sent other parties to find them, and bring them forward as proof that they were plotting insurrection. Every where men, women, and children were whipped till the blood stood in puddles at their feet. Some received five hundred lashes; others were tied hands and feet, and tortured with a bucking paddle, which blisters the skin terribly. The dwellings of the colored people, unless they happened to be protected by some influential white person, who was nigh at hand, were robbed of clothing and every thing else the marauders thought worth carrying away. All day long these unfeeling wretches went round, like a troop of demons, terrifying and tormenting the helpless. At night, they formed themselves into patrol bands, and went wherever they chose among the colored people, acting out their brutal will. Many women hid themselves in woods and swamps, to keep out of their way. If any of the husbands or fathers told of these outrages, they were tied up to the public whipping post, and cruelly scourged for telling lies about white men. The consternation was universal. No two people that had the slightest tinge of color in their faces dared to be seen talking together.

I entertained no positive fears about our household, because we were in the midst of white families who would protect us. We were ready to receive the soldiers whenever they came. It was not long before we heard the tramp of feet and the sound of voices. The door was rudely pushed open; and in they tumbled, like a pack of hungry wolves. They snatched at every thing within their reach. Every box, trunk, closet, and corner underwent a thorough examination. A box in one of the drawers containing some silver change was eagerly pounced upon. When I stepped forward to take it from them, one of the soldiers turned and said angrily, "What d'ye foller us fur? D'ye s'pose white folks is come to steal?"

I replied, "You have come to search; but you have searched that box, and I will take it, if you please."

At that moment I saw a white gentleman who was friendly to us; and I called to him, and asked him to have the goodness to come in and stay till the search was over. He readily complied. His entrance into the house brought in the captain of the company, whose business it was to guard the outside of the house, and see that none of the inmates left it. This officer was Mr. Litch, the wealthy slaveholder whom I mentioned, in the account of neighboring planters, as being notorious for his cruelty. He felt above soiling his hands with the search. He merely gave orders; and, if a bit of writing was discovered, it was carried to him by his ignorant followers, who were unable to read.

My grandmother had a large trunk of bedding and table cloths. When that was opened, there was a great shout of surprise; and one exclaimed, "Where'd the damned niggers git all dis sheet an' table clarf?"

My grandmother, emboldened by the presence of our white protector, said, "You may be sure we didn't pilfer 'em from *your* houses."

"Look here, mammy," said a grim-looking fellow without any coat, "you seem to feel mighty gran' 'cause you got all them 'ere fixens. White folks oughter have 'em all."

His remarks were interrupted by a chorus of voices shouting, "We's got 'em! We's got 'em! Dis 'ere yaller gal's got letters!"

There was a general rush for the supposed letter, which, upon examination, proved to be some verses written to me by a friend. In packing away my things, I had overlooked them. When their captain informed them of their contents, they seemed much disappointed. He inquired of me who wrote them. I told him it was one of my friends. "Can you read them?" he asked. When I told him I could, he swore, and raved, and tore the paper into bits. "Bring me all your letters!" said he, in a commanding tone. I told him I had none.

"Don't be afraid," he continued, in an insinuating way. "Bring them all to me. Nobody shall do you any harm." Seeing I did not move to obey him, his pleasant tone changed to oaths and threats. "Who writes to you? half free niggers?" inquired he. I replied, "O, no; most of my letters are from white people. Some request me to burn them after they are read, and some I destroy without reading."

An exclamation of surprise from some of the company put a stop to our conversation. Some silver spoons which ornamented an old-fashioned buffet had just been discovered. My grandmother was in the habit of preserving fruit for many ladies in the town, and of preparing suppers for parties; consequently she had many jars of preserves. The closet that contained these was next invaded, and the contents tasted. One of them, who was helping himself freely, tapped his neighbor on the shoulder, and said, "Wal done! Don't wonder de niggers want to kill all de white folks, when dey live on 'sarves" [meaning preserves]. I stretched out my hand to take the jar, saying, "You were not sent here to search for sweetmeats."

"And what *were* we sent for?" said the captain, bristling up to me. I evaded the question.

The search of the house was completed, and nothing found to condemn us. They next proceeded to the garden, and knocked about every bush and vine, with no better success. The captain called his men together, and, after a short consultation, the order to march was given. As they passed out of the gate, the captain turned back, and pronounced a malediction on the house. He said it ought to be burned to the ground, and each of its inmates receive thirty-nine lashes. We came out of this affair very fortunately; not losing any thing except some wearing apparel.

Towards evening the turbulence increased. The soldiers, stimulated by drink, committed still greater cruelties. Shrieks and shouts continually rent the air. Not daring to go to the door, I peeped under the window curtain. I saw a mob dragging along a number of colored people, each white man, with his musket upraised, threatening instant death if they did not stop their shrieks. Among the prisoners was a respectable old colored minister. They had found a few parcels of shot in his house, which his wife had for years used to balance her scales.

For this they were going to shoot him on Court House Green. What a spectacle was that for a civilized country! A rabble, staggering under intoxication, assuming to be the administrators of justice!

The better class of the community exerted their influence to save the innocent, persecuted people; and in several instances they succeeded, by keeping them shut up in jail till the excitement abated. At last the white citizens found that their own property was not safe from the lawless rabble they had summoned to protect them. They rallied the drunken swarm, drove them back into the country, and set a guard over the town.

The next day, the town patrols were commissioned to search colored people that lived out of the city; and the most shocking outrages were committed with perfect impunity. Every day for a fortnight, if I looked out, I saw horsemen with some poor panting negro tied to their saddles, and compelled by the lash to keep up with their speed, till they arrived at the jail yard. Those who had been whipped too unmercifully to walk were washed with brine, tossed into a cart, and carried to jail. One black man, who had not fortitude to endure scourging, promised to give information about the conspiracy. But it turned out that he knew nothing at all. He had not even heard the name of Nat Turner. The poor fellow had, however, made up a story, which augmented his own sufferings and those of the colored people.

The day patrol continued for some weeks, and at sundown a night guard was substituted. Nothing at all was proved against the colored people, bond or free. The wrath of the slaveholders was somewhat appeased by the capture of Nat Turner. The imprisoned were released. The slaves were sent to their masters, and the free were permitted to return to their ravaged homes. Visiting was strictly forbidden on the plantations. The slaves begged the privilege of again meeting at their little church in the woods, with their burying ground around it. It was built by the colored people, and they had no higher happiness than to meet there and sing hymns together, and pour out their hearts in spontaneous prayer. Their request was denied, and the church was demolished. They were permitted to attend the white churches, a certain portion of the galleries being appropriated to their use. There, when every body else had partaken of the communion, and the benediction had been pronounced, the minister said, "Come down, now, my colored friends." They obeyed the summons, and partook of the bread and wine, in commemoration of the meek and lowly Jesus, who said, "God is your Father, and all ye are brethren."

XIII.

THE CHURCH AND SLAVERY.

After the alarm caused by Nat Turner's insurrection had subsided, the slaveholders came to the conclusion that it would be well to give the slaves enough of religious instruction to keep them from murdering their masters. The Episcopal clergyman offered to hold a separate service on Sundays for their benefit. His colored members were very few, and also very respectable—a fact which I presume had some weight with him. The difficulty was to decide on a suitable place for them to worship. The Methodist and Baptist churches admitted them in the afternoon; but their carpets and cushions were not so costly as those at the Episcopal church. It was at last decided that they should meet at the house of a free colored man, who was a member.

I was invited to attend, because I could read. Sunday evening came, and, trusting to the cover of night, I ventured out. I rarely ventured out by daylight, for I always went with fear, expecting at every turn to encounter Dr. Flint, who was sure to turn me back, or order me to his office to inquire where I got my bonnet, or some other article of dress. When the Rev. Mr. Pike came, there were some twenty persons present. The reverend gentleman knelt in prayer, then seated himself, and requested all present, who could read, to open their books, while he gave out the portions he wished them to repeat or respond to.

His text was, "Servants, be obedient to them that are your masters according to the flesh, with fear and trembling, in singleness of your heart, as unto Christ."

Pious Mr. Pike brushed up his hair till it stood upright, and, in deep, solemn tones, began: "Hearken, ye servants! Give strict heed unto my words. You are rebellious sinners. Your hearts are filled with all manner of evil. 'Tis the devil who tempts you. God is angry with you, and will surely punish you, if you don't forsake your wicked ways. You that live in town are eye-servants behind your master's back. Instead of serving your masters faithfully, which is pleasing in the sight of your heavenly Master, you are idle, and shirk your work. God sees you. You tell lies. God hears you. Instead of being engaged in worshipping him, you are hidden away somewhere, feasting on your master's substance; tossing coffee-grounds with some wicked fortuneteller, or cutting cards with another old hag. Your masters may not find you out, but God sees you, and will punish you. O, the depravity of your hearts! When your master's work is done, are you quietly together, thinking of the goodness of God to such sinful creatures? No; you are quarrelling, and tying up little bags of roots to bury under the door-steps to poison each other with. God sees you. You men steal away to every grog shop to sell your master's corn, that you may buy rum to drink. God sees you. You sneak into the back streets, or among the bushes, to pitch coppers. Although your masters may not find you out, God sees you; and he will punish you. You must forsake your sinful ways, and be faithful servants. Obey your old master and your young master—your old mistress and your young mistress. If you disobey your earthly master, you offend your heavenly Master. You must obey God's commandments. When you go from here, don't stop at the corners of the streets to talk, but go directly home, and let your master and mistress see that you have come."

The benediction was pronounced. We went home, highly amused at brother Pike's gospel teaching, and we determined to hear him again. I went the next Sabbath evening, and heard pretty much a repetition of the last discourse. At the close of the meeting, Mr. Pike informed us that he found it very inconvenient to meet at the friend's house, and he should be glad to see us, every Sunday evening, at his own kitchen.

I went home with the feeling that I had heard the Rev-

erend Mr. Pike for the last time. Some of his members repaired to his house, and found that the kitchen sported two
tallow candles; the first time, I am sure, since its present oc-
cupant owned it, for the servants never had any thing but
pine knots. It was so long before the reverend gentleman descended from his comfortable parlor that the slaves left, and
went to enjoy a Methodist shout. They never seem so happy
as when shouting and singing at religious meetings. Many of
them are sincere, and nearer to the gate of heaven than sanc-
timonious Mr. Pike, and other long-faced Christians, who see
wounded Samaritans, and pass by on the other side.

The slaves generally compose their own songs and hymns;
and they do not trouble their heads much about the measure.
They often sing the following verses:

> "Old Satan is one busy ole man;
>   He rolls dem blocks all in my way;
>   But Jesus is my bosom friend;
>   He rolls dem blocks away.

> "If I had died when I was young,
>   Den how my stam'ring tongue would have sung;
>   But I am ole, and now I stand
>   A narrow chance for to tread dat heavenly land."

I well remember one occasion when I attended a Methodist
class meeting. I went with a burdened spirit, and happened to
sit next a poor, bereaved mother, whose heart was still heavier than mine. The class leader was the town constable—a
man who bought and sold slaves, who whipped his brethren
and sisters of the church at the public whipping post, in jail or
out of jail. He was ready to perform that Christian office any
where for fifty cents. This white-faced, black-hearted brother
came near us, and said to the stricken woman, "Sister, can't
you tell us how the Lord deals with your soul? Do you love
him as you did formerly?"

She rose to her feet, and said, in piteous tones, "My Lord
and Master, help me! My load is more than I can bear. God
has hid himself from me, and I am left in darkness and misery." Then, striking her breast, she continued, "I can't tell
you what is in here! They've got all my children. Last week

they took the last one. God only knows where they've sold her. They let me have her sixteen years, and then—— O! O! Pray for her brothers and sisters! I've got nothing to live for now. God make my time short!"

She sat down, quivering in every limb. I saw that constable class leader become crimson in the face with suppressed laughter, while he held up his handkerchief, that those who were weeping for the poor woman's calamity might not see his merriment. Then, with assumed gravity, he said to the bereaved mother, "Sister, pray to the Lord that every dispensation of his divine will may be sanctified to the good of your poor needy soul!"

The congregation struck up a hymn, and sung as though they were as free as the birds that warbled round us,—

> "Ole Satan thought he had a mighty aim;
> He missed my soul, and caught my sins.
> Cry Amen, cry Amen, cry Amen to God!

> "He took my sins upon his back;
> Went muttering and grumbling down to hell.
> Cry Amen, cry Amen, cry Amen to God!

> "Ole Satan's church is here below.
> Up to God's free church I hope to go.
> Cry Amen, cry Amen, cry Amen to God!"

Precious are such moments to the poor slaves. If you were to hear them at such times, you might think they were happy. But can that hour of singing and shouting sustain them through the dreary week, toiling without wages, under constant dread of the lash?

The Episcopal clergyman, who, ever since my earliest recollection, had been a sort of god among the slaveholders, concluded, as his family was large, that he must go where money was more abundant. A very different clergyman took his place. The change was very agreeable to the colored people, who said, "God has sent us a good man this time." They loved him, and their children followed him for a smile or a kind word. Even the slaveholders felt his influence. He brought to the rectory five slaves. His wife taught them to read and write, and to be useful to her and themselves. As soon as he was settled, he turned his attention to the needy slaves around him. He urged upon his parishioners the duty of having a meeting expressly for them every Sunday, with a sermon adapted to their comprehension. After much argument and importunity, it was finally agreed that they might occupy the gallery of the church on Sunday evenings. Many colored people, hitherto unaccustomed to attend church, now gladly went to hear the gospel preached. The sermons were simple, and they understood them. Moreover, it was the first time they had ever been addressed as human beings. It was not long before his white parishioners began to be dissatisfied. He was accused of preaching better sermons to the negroes than he did to them. He honestly confessed that he bestowed more pains upon those sermons than upon any others; for the slaves were reared in such ignorance that it was a difficult task to adapt himself to their comprehension. Dissensions arose in the parish. Some wanted he should preach to them in the evening, and to the slaves in the afternoon. In the midst of these disputings his wife died, after a very short illness. Her slaves gathered round her dying bed in great sorrow. She said, "I have tried to do you good and promote your happiness; and if I have failed, it has not been for want of interest in your welfare. Do not weep for me; but prepare for the new duties that lie before you. I leave you all free. May we meet in a better world." Her liberated slaves were sent away, with funds to establish them comfortably. The colored people will long bless the memory of that truly Christian woman. Soon after her death her husband preached his farewell sermon, and many tears were shed at his departure.

Several years after, he passed through our town and preached to his former congregation. In his afternoon sermon he addressed the colored people. "My friends," said he, "it affords me great happiness to have an opportunity of speaking to you again. For two years I have been striving to do something for the colored people of my own parish; but nothing is yet accomplished. I have not even preached a sermon to them. Try to live according to the word of God, my friends. Your skin is darker than mine; but God judges men by their hearts, not by the color of their skins." This was strange doctrine from a southern pulpit. It was very offensive to slaveholders. They said he and his wife had made fools of their slaves, and that he preached like a fool to the negroes.

I knew an old black man, whose piety and childlike trust in God were beautiful to witness. At fifty-three years old he joined the Baptist church. He had a most earnest desire to learn to read. He thought he should know how to serve God better if he could only read the Bible. He came to me, and begged me to teach him. He said he could not pay me, for he had no money; but he would bring me nice fruit when the season for it came. I asked him if he didn't know it was contrary to law; and that slaves were whipped and imprisoned for teaching each other to read. This brought the tears into his eyes. "Don't be troubled, uncle Fred," said I. "I have no thoughts of refusing to teach you. I only told you of the law, that you might know the danger, and be on your guard." He thought he could plan to come three times a week without its being suspected. I selected a quiet nook, where no intruder was likely to penetrate, and there I taught him his A, B, C. Considering his age, his progress was astonishing. As soon as he could spell in two syllables he wanted to spell out words in the Bible. The happy smile that illuminated his face put joy into my heart. After spelling out a few words, he paused, and said, "Honey, it 'pears when I can read dis good book I shall be nearer to God. White man is got all de sense. He can larn easy. It ain't easy for ole black man like me. I only wants to read dis book, dat I may know how to live; den I hab no fear 'bout dying."

I tried to encourage him by speaking of the rapid progress he had made. "Hab patience, child," he replied. "I larns slow."

I had no need of patience. His gratitude, and the happiness I imparted, were more than a recompense for all my trouble.

At the end of six months he had read through the New Testament, and could find any text in it. One day, when he had recited unusually well, I said, "Uncle Fred, how do you manage to get your lessons so well?"

"Lord bress you, chile," he replied. "You nebber gibs me a lesson dat I don't pray to God to help me to understan' what I spells and what I reads. And he *does* help me, chile. Bress his holy name!"

There are thousands, who, like good uncle Fred, are thirsting for the water of life; but the law forbids it, and the churches withhold it. They send the Bible to heathen abroad, and neglect the heathen at home. I am glad that missionaries go out to the dark corners of the earth; but I ask them not to overlook the dark corners at home. Talk to American slaveholders as you talk to savages in Africa. Tell *them* it is wrong to traffic in men. Tell them it is sinful to sell their own children, and atrocious to violate their own daughters. Tell them that all men are brethren, and that man has no right to shut out the light of knowledge from his brother. Tell them they are answerable to God for sealing up the Fountain of Life from souls that are thirsting for it.

There are men who would gladly undertake such missionary work as this; but, alas! their number is small. They are hated by the south, and would be driven from its soil, or dragged to prison to die, as others have been before them. The field is ripe for the harvest, and awaits the reapers. Perhaps the great grandchildren of uncle Fred may have freely imparted to them the divine treasures, which he sought by stealth, at the risk of the prison and the scourge.

Are doctors of divinity blind, or are they hypocrites? I suppose some are the one, and some the other; but I think if they felt the interest in the poor and the lowly, that they ought to feel, they would not be so *easily* blinded. A clergyman who goes to the south, for the first time, has usually some feeling, however vague, that slavery is wrong. The slaveholder suspects this, and plays his game accordingly. He makes himself as agreeable as possible; talks on theology, and other kindred topics. The reverend gentleman is asked to invoke a blessing on a table loaded with luxuries. After dinner he walks round the premises, and sees the beautiful groves and flowering vines, and the comfortable huts of favored household slaves. The southerner invites him to talk with these slaves. He asks them if they want to be free, and they say, "O, no, massa." This is sufficient to satisfy him. He comes home to publish a "South-Side View of Slavery," and to complain of the exaggerations of abolitionists. He assures people that he has been to the south, and seen slavery for himself; that it is a beautiful "patriarchal institution;" that the slaves don't want their freedom; that they have hallelujah meetings, and other religious privileges.

What does *he* know of the half-starved wretches toiling from dawn till dark on the plantations? of mothers shrieking for their children, torn from their arms by slave traders? of young girls dragged down into moral filth? of pools of blood around the whipping post? of hounds trained to tear human flesh? of men screwed into cotton gins to die? The slaveholder showed him none of these things, and the slaves dared not tell of them if he had asked them.

There is a great difference between Christianity and religion at the south. If a man goes to the communion table, and pays money into the treasury of the church, no matter if it be the price of blood, he is called religious. If a pastor has offspring by a woman not his wife, the church dismiss him, if she is a white woman; but if she is colored, it does not hinder his continuing to be their good shepherd.

When I was told that Dr. Flint had joined the Episcopal church, I was much surprised. I supposed that religion had a purifying effect on the character of men; but the worst persecutions I endured from him were after he was a communicant. The conversation of the doctor, the day after he had been confirmed, certainly gave *me* no indication that he had "renounced the devil and all his works." In answer to some of his usual talk, I reminded him that he had just joined the church. "Yes, Linda," said he. "It was proper for me to do so. I am getting in years, and my position in society requires it, and it puts an end to all the damned slang. You would do well to join the church, too, Linda."

"There are sinners enough in it already," rejoined I. "If I could be allowed to live like a Christian, I should be glad."

"You can do what I require; and if you are faithful to me, you will be as virtuous as my wife," he replied.

I answered that the Bible didn't say so.

His voice became hoarse with rage. "How dare you preach to me about your infernal Bible!" he exclaimed. "What right have you, who are my negro, to talk to me about what you would like, and what you wouldn't like? I am your master, and you shall obey me."

No wonder the slaves sing,—

"Ole Satan's church is here below;
Up to God's free church I hope to go."

XIV.

ANOTHER LINK TO LIFE.

I HAD not returned to my master's house since the birth of
my child. The old man raved to have me thus removed from
his immediate power; but his wife vowed, by all that was good
and great, she would kill me if I came back; and he did not
doubt her word. Sometimes he would stay away for a season.
Then he would come and renew the old threadbare discourse
about his forbearance and my ingratitude. He labored, most
unnecessarily, to convince me that I had lowered myself. The
venomous old reprobate had no need of descanting on that
theme. I felt humiliated enough. My unconscious babe was
the ever-present witness of my shame. I listened with silent
contempt when he talked about my having forfeited *his* good
opinion; but I shed bitter tears that I was no longer worthy
of being respected by the good and pure. Alas! slavery still
held me in its poisonous grasp. There was no chance for me
to be respectable. There was no prospect of being able to lead
a better life.

Sometimes, when my master found that I still refused to accept what he called his kind offers, he would threaten to sell
my child. "Perhaps that will humble you," said he.

Humble *me*! Was I not already in the dust? But his threat
lacerated my heart. I knew the law gave him power to fulfil
it; for slaveholders have been cunning enough to enact that
"the child shall follow the condition of the *mother*," not of
the *father*; thus taking care that licentiousness shall not interfere with avarice. This reflection made me clasp my innocent babe all the more firmly to my heart. Horrid visions
passed through my mind when I thought of his liability
to fall into the slave trader's hands. I wept over him, and
said, "O my child! perhaps they will leave you in some cold

cabin to die, and then throw you into a hole, as if you were a dog."

When Dr. Flint learned that I was again to be a mother, he was exasperated beyond measure. He rushed from the house, and returned with a pair of shears. I had a fine head of hair; and he often railed about my pride of arranging it nicely. He cut every hair close to my head, storming and swearing all the time. I replied to some of his abuse, and he struck me. Some months before, he had pitched me down stairs in a fit of passion; and the injury I received was so serious that I was unable to turn myself in bed for many days. He then said, "Linda, I swear by God I will never raise my hand against you again;" but I knew that he would forget his promise.

After he discovered my situation, he was like a restless spirit from the pit. He came every day; and I was subjected to such insults as no pen can describe. I would not describe them if I could; they were too low, too revolting. I tried to keep them from my grandmother's knowledge as much as I could. I knew she had enough to sadden her life, without having my troubles to bear. When she saw the doctor treat me with violence, and heard him utter oaths terrible enough to palsy a man's tongue, she could not always hold her peace. It was natural and motherlike that she should try to defend me; but it only made matters worse.

When they told me my new-born babe was a girl, my heart was heavier than it had ever been before. Slavery is terrible for men; but it is far more terrible for women. Superadded to the burden common to all, *they* have wrongs, and sufferings, and mortifications peculiarly their own.

Dr. Flint had sworn that he would make me suffer, to my last day, for this new crime against *him*, as he called it; and as long as he had me in his power he kept his word. On the fourth day after the birth of my babe, he entered my room suddenly, and commanded me to rise and bring my baby to him. The nurse who took care of me had gone out of the room to prepare some nourishment, and I was alone. There was no alternative. I rose, took up my babe, and crossed the room to where he sat. "Now stand there," said he, "till I tell you to go back!" My child bore a strong resemblance to her father, and to the deceased Mrs. Sands, her grandmother. He noticed this; and while I stood before him, trembling with weakness, he heaped upon me and my little one every vile epithet he could think of. Even the grandmother in her grave did not escape his curses. In the midst of his vituperations I fainted at his feet. This recalled him to his senses. He took the baby from my arms, laid it on the bed, dashed cold water in my face, took me up, and shook me violently, to restore my consciousness before any one entered the room. Just then my grandmother came in, and he hurried out of the house. I suffered in consequence of this treatment; but I begged my friends to let me die, rather than send for the doctor. There was nothing I dreaded so much as his presence. My life was spared; and I was glad for the sake of my little ones. Had it not been for these ties to life, I should have been glad to be released by death, though I had lived only nineteen years.

Always it gave me a pang that my children had no lawful claim to a name. Their father offered his; but, if I had wished to accept the offer, I dared not while my master lived. Moreover, I knew it would not be accepted at their baptism. A Christian name they were at least entitled to; and we resolved to call my boy for our dear good Benjamin, who had gone far away from us.

My grandmother belonged to the church; and she was very desirous of having the children christened. I knew Dr. Flint would forbid it, and I did not venture to attempt it. But chance favored me. He was called to visit a patient out of town, and was obliged to be absent during Sunday. "Now is the time," said my grandmother; "we will take the children to church, and have them christened."

When I entered the church, recollections of my mother came over me, and I felt subdued in spirit. There she had presented me for baptism, without any reason to feel ashamed. She had been married, and had such legal rights as slavery allows to a slave. The vows had at least been sacred to *her*, and she had never violated them. I was glad she was not alive, to know under what different circumstances her grandchildren were presented for baptism. Why had my lot been so different from my mother's? *Her* master had died when she was a child; and she remained with her mistress till she married. She was never in the power of any master; and thus she escaped one class of the evils that generally fall upon slaves.

When my baby was about to be christened, the former mistress of my father stepped up to me, and proposed to give it her Christian name. To this I added the surname of my father, who had himself no legal right to it; for my grandfather on the paternal side was a white gentleman. What tangled skeins are the genealogies of slavery! I loved my father; but it mortified me to be obliged to bestow his name on my children.

When we left the church, my father's old mistress invited me to go home with her. She clasped a gold chain round my baby's neck. I thanked her for this kindness; but I did not like the emblem. I wanted no chain to be fastened on my daughter, not even if its links were of gold. How earnestly I prayed that she might never feel the weight of slavery's chain, whose iron entereth into the soul!

XV.

CONTINUED PERSECUTIONS.

My children grew finely; and Dr. Flint would often say to me, with an exulting smile, "These brats will bring me a handsome sum of money one of these days."

I thought to myself that, God being my helper, they should never pass into his hands. It seemed to me I would rather see them killed than have them given up to his power. The money for the freedom of myself and my children could be obtained; but I derived no advantage from that circumstance. Dr. Flint loved money, but he loved power more. After much discussion, my friends resolved on making another trial. There was a slaveholder about to leave for Texas, and he was commissioned to buy me. He was to begin with nine hundred dollars, and go up to twelve. My master refused his offers. "Sir," said he, "she don't belong to me. She is my daughter's property, and I have no right to sell her. I mistrust that you come from her paramour. If so, you may tell him that he cannot buy her for any money; neither can he buy her children."

The doctor came to see me the next day, and my heart beat quicker as he entered. I never had seen the old man tread with so majestic a step. He seated himself and looked at me with withering scorn. My children had learned to be afraid of him. The little one would shut her eyes and hide her face on my shoulder whenever she saw him; and Benny, who was now nearly five years old, often inquired, "What makes that bad man come here so many times? Does he want to hurt us?" I would clasp the dear boy in my arms, trusting that he would be free before he was old enough to solve the problem. And now, as the doctor sat there so grim and silent, the child left his play and came and nestled up by me. At last my tormentor spoke. "So you are left in disgust, are you?" said he. "It is no more than I expected. You remember I told you years ago that you would be treated so. So he is tired of you? Ha! ha! ha! The virtuous madam don't like to hear about it, does she? Ha! ha! ha!" There was a sting in his calling me virtuous madam. I no longer had the power of answering him as I had formerly done. He continued: "So it seems you are trying to get up another intrigue. Your new paramour came to me, and offered to buy you; but you may be assured you will not succeed. You are mine; and you shall be mine for life. There lives no human being that can take you out of slavery. I would have done it; but you rejected my kind offer."

I told him I did not wish to get up any intrigue; that I had never seen the man who offered to buy me.

"Do you tell me I lie?" exclaimed he, dragging me from my chair. "Will you say again that you never saw that man?"

I answered, "I do say so."

He clinched my arm with a volley of oaths. Ben began to scream, and I told him to go to his grandmother.

"Don't you stir a step, you little wretch!" said he. The child drew nearer to me, and put his arms round me, as if he wanted to protect me. This was too much for my enraged master. He caught him up and hurled him across the room. I thought he was dead, and rushed towards him to take him up.

"Not yet!" exclaimed the doctor. "Let him lie there till he comes to."

"Let me go! Let me go!" I screamed, "or I will raise the

whole house." I struggled and got away; but he clinched me again. Somebody opened the door, and he released me. I picked up my insensible child, and when I turned my tormentor was gone. Anxiously I bent over the little form, so pale and still; and when the brown eyes at last opened, I don't know whether I was very happy.

All the doctor's former persecutions were renewed. He came morning, noon, and night. No jealous lover ever watched a rival more closely than he watched me and the unknown slaveholder, with whom he accused me of wishing to get up an intrigue. When my grandmother was out of the way he searched every room to find him.

In one of his visits, he happened to find a young girl, whom he had sold to a trader a few days previous. His statement was, that he sold her because she had been too familiar with the overseer. She had had a bitter life with him, and was glad to be sold. She had no mother, and no near ties. She had been torn from all her family years before. A few friends had entered into bonds for her safety, if the trader would allow her to spend with them the time that intervened between her sale and the gathering up of his human stock. Such a favor was rarely granted. It saved the trader the expense of board and jail fees, and though the amount was small, it was a weighty consideration in a slave-trader's mind.

Dr. Flint always had an aversion to meeting slaves after he had sold them. He ordered Rose out of the house; but he was no longer her master, and she took no notice of him. For once the crushed Rose was the conqueror. His gray eyes flashed angrily upon her; but that was the extent of his power. "How came this girl here?" he exclaimed. "What right had you to allow it, when you knew I had sold her?"

I answered "This is my grandmother's house, and Rose came to see her. I have no right to turn any body out of doors, that comes here for honest purposes."

He gave me the blow that would have fallen upon Rose if she had still been his slave. My grandmother's attention had been attracted by loud voices, and she entered in time to see a second blow dealt. She was not a woman to let such an outrage, in her own house, go unrebuked. The doctor undertook to explain that I had been insolent. Her indignant feelings rose higher and higher, and finally boiled over in words. "Get out of my house!" she exclaimed. "Go home, and take care of your wife and children, and you will have enough to do, without watching my family."

He threw the birth of my children in her face, and accused her of sanctioning the life I was leading. She told him I was living with her by compulsion of his wife; that he needn't accuse her, for he was the one to blame; he was the one who had caused all the trouble. She grew more and more excited as she went on. "I tell you what, Dr. Flint," said she, "you ain't got many more years to live, and you'd better be saying your prayers. It will take 'em all, and more too, to wash the dirt off your soul."

"Do you know whom you are talking to?" he exclaimed.

She replied, "Yes, I know very well who I am talking to."

He left the house in a great rage. I looked at my grandmother. Our eyes met. Their angry expression had passed away, but she looked sorrowful and weary—weary of incessant strife. I wondered that it did not lessen her love for me; but if it did she never showed it. She was always kind, always ready to sympathize with my troubles. There might have been peace and contentment in that humble home if it had not been for the demon Slavery.

The winter passed undisturbed by the doctor. The beautiful spring came; and when Nature resumes her loveliness, the human soul is apt to revive also. My drooping hopes came to life again with the flowers. I was dreaming of freedom again; more for my children's sake than my own. I planned and I planned. Obstacles hit against plans. There seemed no way of overcoming them; and yet I hoped.

Back came the wily doctor. I was not at home when he called. A friend had invited me to a small party, and to gratify her I went. To my great consternation, a messenger came in haste to say that Dr. Flint was at my grandmother's, and insisted on seeing me. They did not tell him where I was, or he would have come and raised a disturbance in my friend's house. They sent me a dark wrapper; I threw it on and hurried home. My speed did not save me; the doctor had gone away in anger. I dreaded the morning, but I could not delay it; it came, warm and bright. At an early hour the doctor came and asked me where I had been last night. I told him. He did not believe me, and sent to my friend's house to ascertain the facts. He came in the afternoon to assure me he was satisfied that I had spoken the truth. He seemed to be in a facetious mood, and I expected some jeers were coming. "I suppose you need some recreation," said he, "but I am surprised at your being there, among those negroes. It was not the place for *you*. Are you *allowed* to visit such people?"

I understood this covert fling at the white gentleman who was my friend; but I merely replied, "I went to visit my friends, and any company they keep is good enough for me."

He went on to say, "I have seen very little of you of late, but my interest in you is unchanged. When I said I would have no more mercy on you I was rash. I recall my words. Linda, you desire freedom for yourself and your children, and you can obtain it only through me. If you agree to what I am about to propose, you and they shall be free. There must be no communication of any kind between you and their father. I will procure a cottage, where you and the children can live together. Your labor shall be light, such as sewing for my family. Think what is offered you, Linda—a home and freedom! Let the past be forgotten. If I have been harsh with you at times, your wilfulness drove me to it. You know I exact obedience from my own children, and I consider you as yet a child."

He paused for an answer, but I remained silent.

"Why don't you speak?" said he. "What more do you wait for?"

"Nothing, sir."

"Then you accept my offer?"

"No, sir."

His anger was ready to break loose; but he succeeded in curbing it, and replied, "You have answered without thought. But I must let you know there are two sides to my proposition; if you reject the bright side, you will be obliged to take the dark one. You must either accept my offer, or you and your children shall be sent to your young master's plantation, there to remain till your young mistress is married; and your children shall fare like the rest of the negro children. I give you a week to consider of it."

He was shrewd; but I knew he was not to be trusted. I told him I was ready to give my answer now.

"I will not receive it now," he replied. "You act too much from impulse. Remember that you and your children can be free a week from to-day if you choose."

On what a monstrous chance hung the destiny of my children! I knew that my master's offer was a snare, and that if I entered it escape would be impossible. As for his promise, I knew him so well that I was sure if he gave me free papers, they would be so managed as to have no legal value. The alternative was inevitable. I resolved to go to the plantation. But then I thought how completely I should be in his power, and the prospect was apalling. Even if I should kneel before him, and implore him to spare me, for the sake of my children, I knew he would spurn me with his foot, and my weakness would be his triumph.

Before the week expired, I heard that young Mr. Flint was about to be married to a lady of his own stamp. I foresaw the position I should occupy in his establishment. I had once been sent to the plantation for punishment, and fear of the son had induced the father to recall me very soon. My mind was made up; I was resolved that I would foil my master and save my children, or I would perish in the attempt. I kept my plans to myself; I knew that friends would try to dissuade me from them, and I would not wound their feelings by rejecting their advice.

On the decisive day the doctor came, and said he hoped I had made a wise choice.

"I am ready to go to the plantation, sir," I replied.

"Have you thought how important your decision is to your children?" said he.

I told him I had.

"Very well. Go to the plantation, and my curse go with you," he replied. "Your boy shall be put to work, and he shall soon be sold; and your girl shall be raised for the purpose of selling well. Go your own ways!" He left the room with curses, not to be repeated.

As I stood rooted to the spot, my grandmother came and said, "Linda, child, what did you tell him?"

I answered that I was going to the plantation.

"*Must* you go?" said she. "Can't something be done to stop it?"

I told her it was useless to try; but she begged me not to give up. She said she would go to the doctor, and remind him how long and how faithfully she had served in the family, and how she had taken her own baby from her breast to nourish his wife. She would tell him I had been out of the family so long they would not miss me; that she would pay them for my time, and the money would procure a woman who had more strength for the situation than I had. I begged her not to go; but she persisted in saying, "He will listen to *me*, Linda." She went, and was treated as I expected. He coolly listened to what she said, but denied her request. He told her that what he did was for my good, that my feelings were entirely above my situation, and that on the plantation I would receive treatment that was suitable to my behavior.

My grandmother was much cast down. I had my secret hopes; but I must fight my battle alone. I had a woman's pride, and a mother's love for my children; and I resolved that out of the darkness of this hour a brighter dawn should rise for them. My master had power and law on his side; I had a determined will. There is might in each.

XVI.

SCENES AT THE PLANTATION.

Early the next morning I left my grandmother's with my youngest child. My boy was ill, and I left him behind. I had many sad thoughts as the old wagon jolted on. Hitherto, I had suffered alone; now, my little one was to be treated as a slave. As we drew near the great house, I thought of the time when I was formerly sent there out of revenge. I wondered for what purpose I was now sent. I could not tell. I resolved to obey orders so far as duty required; but within myself, I determined to make my stay as short as possible. Mr. Flint was waiting to receive us, and told me to follow him up stairs to receive orders for the day. My little Ellen was left below in the kitchen. It was a change for her, who had always been so carefully tended. My young master said she might amuse herself in the yard. This was kind of him, since the child was hateful to his sight. My task was to fit up the house for the reception of the bride. In the midst of sheets, tablecloths, towels, drapery, and carpeting, my head was as busy planning, as were my fingers with the needle. At noon I was allowed to go to Ellen. She had sobbed herself to sleep. I heard Mr. Flint say to a neighbor, "I've got her down here, and I'll soon take the town notions out of her head. My father is partly to blame for her nonsense. He ought to have broke her in long ago." The remark was made within my hearing, and it would have been quite as manly to have made it to my face. He *had* said things to my face which might, or might not, have surprised his neighbor if he had known of them. He was "a chip of the old block."

I resolved to give him no cause to accuse me of being too much of a lady, so far as work was concerned. I worked day and night, with wretchedness before me. When I lay down beside my child, I felt how much easier it would be to see her die than to see her master beat her about, as I daily saw him beat other little ones. The spirit of the mothers was so crushed by the lash, that they stood by, without courage to remonstrate. How much more must I suffer, before I should be "broke in" to that degree?

I wished to appear as contented as possible. Sometimes I had an opportunity to send a few lines home; and this brought up recollections that made it difficult, for a time, to seem calm and indifferent to my lot. Notwithstanding my efforts, I saw that Mr. Flint regarded me with a suspicious eye. Ellen broke down under the trials of her new life. Separated from me, with no one to look after her, she wandered about, and in a few days cried herself sick. One day, she sat under the window where I was at work, crying that weary cry which makes a mother's heart bleed. I was obliged to steel myself to bear it. After a while it ceased. I looked out, and she was gone. As it was near noon, I ventured to go down in search of her. The great house was raised two feet above the ground. I looked under it, and saw her about midway, fast asleep. I crept under and drew her out. As I held her in my arms, I thought how well it would be for her if she never waked up;

and I uttered my thought aloud. I was startled to hear some one say, "Did you speak to me?" I looked up, and saw Mr. Flint standing beside me. He said nothing further, but turned, frowning, away. That night he sent Ellen a biscuit and a cup of sweetened milk. This generosity surprised me. I learned afterwards, that in the afternoon he had killed a large snake, which crept from under the house; and I supposed that incident had prompted his unusual kindness.

The next morning the old cart was loaded with shingles for town. I put Ellen into it, and sent her to her grandmother. Mr. Flint said I ought to have asked his permission. I told him the child was sick, and required attention which I had no time to give. He let it pass; for he was aware that I had accomplished much work in a little time.

I had been three weeks on the plantation, when I planned a visit home. It must be at night, after every body was in bed. I was six miles from town, and the road was very dreary. I was to go with a young man, who, I knew, often stole to town to see his mother. One night, when all was quiet, we started. Fear gave speed to our steps, and we were not long in performing the journey. I arrived at my grandmother's. Her bed room was on the first floor, and the window was open, the weather being warm. I spoke to her and she awoke. She let me in and closed the window, lest some late passer-by should see me. A light was brought, and the whole household gathered round me, some smiling and some crying. I went to look at my children, and thanked God for their happy sleep. The tears fell as I leaned over them. As I moved to leave, Benny stirred. I turned back, and whispered, "Mother is here." After digging at his eyes with his little fist, they opened, and he sat up in bed, looking at me curiously. Having satisfied himself that it was I, he exclaimed, "O mother! you ain't dead, are you? They didn't cut off your head at the plantation, did they?"

My time was up too soon, and my guide was waiting for me. I laid Benny back in his bed, and dried his tears by a promise to come again soon. Rapidly we retraced our steps back to the plantation. About half way we were met by a company of four patrols. Luckily we heard their horse's hoofs before they came in sight, and we had time to hide behind a large tree. They passed, hallooing and shouting in a manner that indicated a recent carousal. How thankful we were that they had not their dogs with them! We hastened our footsteps, and when we arrived on the plantation we heard the sound of the hand-mill. The slaves were grinding their corn. We were safely in the house before the horn summoned them to their labor. I divided my little parcel of food with my guide, knowing that he had lost the chance of grinding his corn, and must toil all day in the field.

Mr. Flint often took an inspection of the house, to see that no one was idle. The entire management of the work was trusted to me, because he knew nothing about it; and rather than hire a superintendent he contented himself with my arrangements. He had often urged upon his father the necessity of having me at the plantation to take charge of his affairs, and make clothes for the slaves; but the old man knew him too well to consent to that arrangement.

When I had been working a month at the plantation, the great aunt of Mr. Flint came to make him a visit. This was the good old lady who paid fifty dollars for my grandmother, for the purpose of making her free, when she stood on the auction block. My grandmother loved this old lady, whom we all called Miss Fanny. She often came to take tea with us. On such occasions the table was spread with a snow-white cloth, and the china cups and silver spoons were taken from the old-fashioned buffet. There were hot muffins, tea rusks, and delicious sweetmeats. My grandmother kept two cows, and the fresh cream was Miss Fanny's delight. She invariably declared that it was the best in town. The old ladies had cosey times together. They would work and chat, and sometimes, while talking over old times, their spectacles would get dim with tears, and would have to be taken off and wiped. When Miss Fanny bade us good by, her bag was filled with grandmother's best cakes, and she was urged to come again soon.

There had been a time when Dr. Flint's wife came to take tea with us, and when her children were also sent to have a feast of "Aunt Marthy's" nice cooking. But after I became an object of her jealousy and spite, she was angry with grandmother for giving a shelter to me and my children. She would not even speak to her in the street. This wounded my grandmother's feelings, for she could not retain ill will against the woman whom she had nourished with her milk when a babe. The doctor's wife would gladly have prevented our intercourse with Miss Fanny if she could have done it, but fortunately she was not dependent on the bounty of the Flints. She had enough to be independent; and that is more than can ever be gained from charity, however lavish it may be.

Miss Fanny was endeared to me by many recollections, and I was rejoiced to see her at the plantation. The warmth of her large, loyal heart made the house seem pleasanter while she was in it. She staid a week, and I had many talks with her. She said her principal object in coming was to see how I was treated, and whether any thing could be done for me. She inquired whether she could help me in any way. I told her I believed not. She condoled with me in her own peculiar way; saying she wished that I and all my grandmother's family were at rest in our graves, for not until then should she feel any peace about us. The good old soul did not dream that I was planning to bestow peace upon her, with regard to myself and my children; not by death, but by securing our freedom

Again and again I had traversed those dreary twelve miles, to and from the town; and all the way, I was meditating upon some means of escape for myself and my children. My friends had made every effort that ingenuity could devise to effect our purchase, but all their plans had proved abortive. Dr. Flint was suspicious, and determined not to loosen his grasp upon us. I could have made my escape alone; but it was more for my helpless children than for myself that I longed for freedom. Though the boon would have been precious to me, above all price, I would not have taken it at the expense of leaving them in slavery. Every trial I endured, every sacrifice I made for their sakes, drew them closer to my heart, and gave me fresh courage to beat back the dark waves that rolled and rolled over me in a seemingly endless night of storms.

The six weeks were nearly completed, when Mr. Flint's bride was expected to take possession of her new home. The arrangements were all completed, and Mr. Flint said I had done well. He expected to leave home on Saturday, and return with his bride the following Wednesday. After receiving various orders from him, I ventured to ask permission to spend Sunday in town. It was granted; for which favor I was thankful. It was the first I had ever asked of him, and I intended it should be the last. It needed more than one night to accomplish the project I had in view; but the whole of Sunday would give me an opportunity. I spent the Sabbath with my grandmother. A calmer, more beautiful day never came down out of heaven. To me it was a day of conflicting emotions. Perhaps it was the last day I should ever spend under that dear, old sheltering roof! Perhaps these were the last talks I should ever have with the faithful old friend of my whole life! Perhaps it was the last time I and my children should be together! Well, better so, I thought, than that they should be slaves. I knew the doom that awaited my fair baby in slavery, and I determined to save her from it, or perish in the attempt. I went to make this vow at the graves of my poor parents, in the burying-ground of the slaves. "There the wicked cease from troubling, and there the weary be at rest. There the prisoners rest together; they hear not the voice of the oppressor; the servant is free from his master." I knelt by the graves of my parents, and thanked God, as I had often done before, that they had not lived to witness my trials, or to mourn over my sins. I had received my mother's blessing when she died; and in many an hour of tribulation I had seemed to hear her voice, sometimes chiding me, sometimes whispering loving words into my wounded heart. I have shed many and bitter tears, to think that when I am gone from my children they cannot remember me with such entire satisfaction as I remembered my mother.

The graveyard was in the woods, and twilight was coming on. Nothing broke the death-like stillness except the occasional twitter of a bird. My spirit was overawed by the solemnity of the scene. For more than ten years I had frequented this spot, but never had it seemed to me so sacred as now. A black stump, at the head of my mother's grave, was all that remained of a tree my father had planted. His grave was marked by a small wooden board, bearing his name, the letters of which were nearly obliterated. I knelt down and kissed them, and poured forth a prayer to God for guidance and support in the perilous step I was about to take. As I passed the wreck of the old meeting house, where, before Nat Turner's time, the slaves had been allowed to meet for worship, I seemed to hear my father's voice come from it, bidding me not to tarry till I reached freedom or the grave. I rushed on with reno- vated hopes. My trust in God had been strengthened by that prayer among the graves.

My plan was to conceal myself at the house of a friend, and remain there a few weeks till the search was over. My hope was that the doctor would get discouraged, and, for fear of losing my value, and also of subsequently finding my children among the missing, he would consent to sell us; and I knew somebody would buy us. I had done all in my power to make my children comfortable during the time I expected to be separated from them. I was packing my things, when grand- mother came into the room, and asked what I was doing. "I am putting my things in order," I replied. I tried to look and speak cheerfully; but her watchful eye detected something be- neath the surface. She drew me towards her, and asked me to sit down. She looked earnestly at me, and said, "Linda, do you want to kill your old grandmother? Do you mean to leave your little, helpless children? I am old now, and cannot do for your babies as I once did for you."

I replied, that if I went away, perhaps their father would be able to secure their freedom.

"Ah, my child," said she, "don't trust too much to him. Stand by your own children, and suffer with them till death. Nobody respects a mother who forsakes her children; and if you leave them, you will never have a happy moment. If you go, you will make me miserable the short time I have to live. You would be taken and brought back, and your sufferings would be dreadful. Remember poor Benjamin. Do give it up, Linda. Try to bear a little longer. Things may turn out better than we expect."

My courage failed me, in view of the sorrow I should bring on that faithful, loving old heart. I promised that I would try longer, and that I would take nothing out of her house with- out her knowledge.

Whenever the children climbed on my knee, or laid their heads on my lap, she would say, "Poor little souls! what would you do without a mother? She don't love you as I do." And she would hug them to her own bosom, as if to reproach me for my want of affection; but she knew all the while that I loved them better than my life. I slept with her that night, and it was the last time. The memory of it haunted me for many a year.

On Monday I returned to the plantation, and busied myself with preparations for the important day. Wednesday came. It was a beautiful day, and the faces of the slaves were as bright as the sunshine. The poor creatures were merry. They were expecting little presents from the bride, and hoping for better times under her administration. I had no such hopes for them. I knew that the young wives of slaveholders often thought their authority and importance would be best established and maintained by cruelty; and what I had heard of young Mrs. Flint gave me no reason to expect that her rule over them would be less severe than that of the master and overseer. Truly, the colored race are the most cheerful and forgiving people on the face of the earth. That their masters sleep in safety is owing to their superabundance of heart; and yet they look upon their sufferings with less pity than they would bestow on those of a horse or a dog.

I stood at the door with others to receive the bridegroom and bride. She was a handsome, delicate-looking girl, and her face flushed with emotion at sight of her new home. I thought it likely that visions of a happy future were rising before her. It made me sad; for I knew how soon clouds would come over her sunshine. She examined every part of the house, and told me she was delighted with the arrangements I had made. I was afraid old Mrs. Flint had tried to prejudice her against me, and I did my best to please her.

All passed off smoothly for me until dinner time arrived. I did not mind the embarrassment of waiting on a dinner party, for the first time in my life, half so much as I did the meeting with Dr. Flint and his wife, who would be among the guests. It was a mystery to me why Mrs. Flint had not made her appearance at the plantation during all the time I was putting the house in order. I had not met her, face to face, for five years, and I had no wish to see her now. She was a praying woman, and, doubtless, considered my present position a special answer to her prayers. Nothing could please her better than to see me humbled and trampled upon. I was just where she would have me—in the power of a hard, unprincipled master. She did not speak to me when she took her seat at table; but her satisfied, triumphant smile, when I handed her plate, was more eloquent than words. The old doctor was not so quiet in his demonstrations. He ordered me here and there, and spoke with peculiar emphasis when he said "your *mistress.*" I was drilled like a disgraced soldier. When all was over, and the last key turned, I sought my pillow, thankful that God had appointed a season of rest for the weary.

The next day my new mistress began her housekeeping. I was not exactly appointed maid of all work; but I was to do whatever I was told. Monday evening came. It was always a busy time. On that night the slaves received their weekly allowance of food. Three pounds of meat, a peck of corn, and perhaps a dozen herring were allowed to each man. Women received a pound and a half of meat, a peck of corn, and the same number of herring. Children over twelve years old had half the allowance of the women. The meat was cut and weighed by the foreman of the field hands, and piled on planks before the meat house. Then the second foreman went behind the building, and when the first foreman called out, "Who takes this piece of meat?" he answered by calling somebody's name. This method was resorted to as a means of preventing partiality in distributing the meat. The young mistress came out to see how things were done on her plantation, and she soon gave a specimen of her character. Among those in waiting for their allowance was a very old slave, who had faithfully served the Flint family through three generations. When he hobbled up to get his bit of meat, the mistress said he was too old to have any allowance; that when niggers were too old to work, they ought to be fed on grass. Poor old man! He suffered much before he found rest in the grave.

My mistress and I got along very well together. At the end of a week, old Mrs. Flint made us another visit, and was closeted a long time with her daughter-in-law. I had my suspicions what was the subject of the conference. The old doctor's wife had been informed that I could leave the plantation on one condition, and she was very desirous to keep me there. If she had trusted me, as I deserved to be trusted by her, she would have had no fears of my accepting that condition. When she entered her carriage to return home, she said to young Mrs. Flint, "Don't neglect to send for them as quick as possible." My heart was on the watch all the time, and I at once concluded that she spoke of my children. The doctor came the next day, and as I entered the room to spread the tea table, I heard him say, "Don't wait any longer. Send for them to-morrow." I saw through the plan. They thought my children's being there would fetter me to the spot, and that it was a good place to break us all in to abject submission to our lot as slaves. After the doctor left, a gentleman called, who had always manifested friendly feelings towards my grandmother and her family. Mr. Flint carried him over the plantation to show him the results of labor performed by men and women who were unpaid, miserably clothed, and half famished. The cotton crop was all they thought of. It was duly admired, and the gentleman returned with specimens to show his friends. I was ordered to carry water to wash his hands. As I did so, he said, "Linda, how do you like your new home?" I told him I liked it as well as I expected. He replied, "They don't think you are contented, and to-morrow they are going to bring your children to be with you. I am sorry for you, Linda. I hope they will treat you kindly." I hurried from the room, unable to thank him. My suspicions were correct. My children were to be brought to the plantation to be "broke in."

To this day I feel grateful to the gentleman who gave me this timely information. It nerved me to immediate action.

XVII.

THE FLIGHT.

MR. FLINT was hard pushed for house servants, and rather than lose me he had restrained his malice. I did my work faithfully, though not, of course, with a willing mind. They were evidently afraid I should leave them. Mr. Flint wished that I should sleep in the great house instead of the servants' quarters. His wife agreed to the proposition, but said I mustn't bring my bed into the house, because it would scatter feathers on her carpet. I knew when I went there that they would never think of such a thing as furnishing a bed of any kind for me and my little one. I therefore carried my own bed, and now I was forbidden to use it. I did as I was ordered. But now that I was certain my children were to be put in their power, in order to give them a stronger hold on me, I resolved to leave them that night. I remembered the grief this step would bring upon my dear old grandmother; and nothing less than the freedom of my children would have induced me to disregard her advice. I went about my evening work with trembling steps. Mr. Flint twice called from his chamber door to inquire why the house was not locked up. I replied that I had not done my work. "You have had time enough to do it," said he. "Take care how you answer me!"

I shut all the windows, locked all the doors, and went up to the third story, to wait till midnight. How long those hours seemed, and how fervently I prayed that God would not forsake me in this hour of utmost need! I was about to risk every thing on the throw of a die; and if I failed, O what would become of me and my poor children? They would be made to suffer for my fault.

At half past twelve I stole softly down stairs. I stopped on the second floor, thinking I heard a noise. I felt my way down into the parlor, and looked out of the window. The night was so intensely dark that I could see nothing. I raised the window very softly and jumped out. Large drops of rain were falling, and the darkness bewildered me. I dropped on my knees, and breathed a short prayer to God for guidance and protection. I groped my way to the road, and rushed towards the town with almost lightning speed. I arrived at my grandmother's house, but dared not see her. She would say, "Linda, you are killing me;" and I knew that would unnerve me. I tapped softly at the window of a room, occupied by a woman, who had lived in the house several years. I knew she was a faithful friend, and could be trusted with my secret. I tapped several times before she heard me. At last she raised the window, and I whispered, "Sally, I have run away. Let me in, quick." She opened the door softly, and said in low tones, "For God's sake, don't. Your grandmother is trying to buy you and de chillern. Mr. Sands was here last week. He tole her he was going away on business, but he wanted her to go ahead about buying you and de chillren, and he would help her all he could. Don't run away, Linda. Your grandmother is all bowed down wid trouble now."

I replied, "Sally, they are going to carry my children to the plantation to-morrow; and they will never sell them to any body so long as they have me in their power. Now, would you advise me to go back?"

"No, chile, no," answered she. "When dey finds you is gone, dey won't want de plague ob de chillern; but where is you going to hide? Dey knows ebery inch ob dis house."

I told her I had a hiding-place, and that was all it was best for her to know. I asked her to go into my room as soon as it was light, and take all my clothes out of my trunk, and pack them in hers; for I knew Mr. Flint and the constable would be there early to search my room. I feared the sight of my children would be too much for my full heart; but I could not go out into the uncertain future without one last look. I bent over the bed where lay my little Benny and baby Ellen. Poor little ones! fatherless and motherless! Memories of their father came over me. He wanted to be kind to them; but they were not all to him, as they were to my womanly heart. I knelt and prayed for the innocent little sleepers. I kissed them lightly, and turned away.

As I was about to open the street door, Sally laid her hand on my shoulder, and said, "Linda, is you gwine all alone? Let me call your uncle."

"No, Sally," I replied, "I want no one to be brought into trouble on my account."

I went forth into the darkness and rain. I ran on till I came to the house of the friend who was to conceal me.

Early the next morning Mr. Flint was at my grandmother's inquiring for me. She told him she had not seen me, and supposed I was at the plantation. He watched her face narrowly, and said, "Don't you know any thing about her running off?" She assured him that she did not. He went on to say, "Last night she ran off without the least provocation. We had treated her very kindly. My wife liked her. She will soon be found and brought back. Are her children with you?" When told that they were, he said, "I am very glad to hear that. If they are here, she cannot be far off. If I find out that any of my niggers have had any thing to do with this damned business, I'll give 'em five hundred lashes." As he started to go to his father's, he turned round and added, persuasively, "Let her be brought back, and she shall have her children to live with her."

The tidings made the old doctor rave and storm at a furious rate. It was a busy day for them. My grandmother's house was searched from top to bottom. As my trunk was empty, they concluded I had taken my clothes with me. Before ten o'clock every vessel northward bound was thoroughly examined, and the law against harboring fugitives was read to all on board. At night a watch was set over the town. Knowing how distressed my grandmother would be, I wanted to send her a message; but it could not be done. Every one who went in or out of her house was closely watched. The doctor said he would take my children, unless she became responsible for them; which of course she willingly did. The next day was spent in searching. Before night, the following advertisement was posted at every corner, and in every public place for miles round:—

"$300 REWARD! Ran away from the subscriber, an intelligent, bright, mulatto girl, named Linda, 21 years of age. Five feet four inches high. Dark eyes, and black hair inclined to curl; but it can be made straight. Has a decayed spot on a front tooth. She can read and write, and in all probability will try to get to the Free States. All persons are forbidden, under penalty of the law, to harbor or employ said slave. $150 will be given to whoever takes her in the state, and $300 if taken out of the state and delivered to me, or lodged in jail.

DR. FLINT."

XVIII.
MONTHS OF PERIL.

THE search for me was kept up with more perseverance than I had anticipated. I began to think that escape was impossible.

I was in great anxiety lest I should implicate the friend who harbored me. I knew the consequences would be frightful; and much as I dreaded being caught, even that seemed better than causing an innocent person to suffer for kindness to me. A week had passed in terrible suspense, when my pursuers came into such close vicinity that I concluded they had tracked me to my hiding-place. I flew out of the house, and concealed myself in a thicket of bushes. There I remained in an agony of fear for two hours. Suddenly, a reptile of some kind seized my leg. In my fright, I struck a blow which loosened its hold, but I could not tell whether I had killed it; it was so dark, I could not see what it was; I only knew it was something cold and slimy. The pain I felt soon indicated that the bite was poisonous. I was compelled to leave my place of concealment, and I groped my way back into the house. The pain had become intense, and my friend was startled by my look of anguish. I asked her to prepare a poultice of warm ashes and vinegar, and I applied it to my leg, which was already much swollen. The application gave me some relief, but the swelling did not abate. The dread of being disabled was greater than the physical pain I endured. My friend asked an old woman, who doctored among the slaves, what was good for the bite of a snake or a lizard. She told her to steep a dozen coppers in vinegar, over night, and apply the cankered vinegar to the inflamed part.*

I had succeeded in cautiously conveying some messages to my relatives. They were harshly threatened, and despairing of my having a chance to escape, they advised me to return to my master, ask his forgiveness, and let him make an example of me. But such counsel had no influence with me. When I started upon this hazardous undertaking, I had resolved that, come what would, there should be no turning back. "Give me liberty, or give me death," was my motto. When my friend contrived to make known to my relatives the painful situation I had been in for twenty-four hours, they said no more about

---

*The poison of a snake is a powerful acid, and is counteracted by powerful alkalies, such as potash, ammonia, &c. The Indians are accustomed to apply wet ashes, or plunge the limb into strong lie. White men, employed to lay out railroads in snaky places, often carry ammonia with them as an antidote.—EDITOR.

my going back to my master. Something must be done, and that speedily; but where to turn for help, they knew not. God in his mercy raised up "a friend in need."

Among the ladies who were acquainted with my grandmother, was one who had known her from childhood, and always been very friendly to her. She had also known my mother and her children, and felt interested for them. At this crisis of affairs she called to see my grandmother, as she not unfrequently did. She observed the sad and troubled expression of her face, and asked if she knew where Linda was, and whether she was safe. My grandmother shook her head, without answering. "Come, Aunt Martha," said the kind lady, "tell me all about it. Perhaps I can do something to help you." The husband of this lady held many slaves, and bought and sold slaves. She also held a number in her own name; but she treated them kindly, and would never allow any of them to be sold. She was unlike the majority of slaveholders' wives. My grandmother looked earnestly at her. Something in the expression of her face said "Trust me!" and she did trust her. She listened attentively to the details of my story, and sat thinking for a while. At last she said, "Aunt Martha, I pity you both. If you think there is any chance of Linda's getting to the Free States, I will conceal her for a time. But first you must solemnly promise that my name shall never be mentioned. If such a thing should become known, it would ruin me and my family. No one in my house must know of it, except the cook. She is so faithful that I would trust my own life with her; and I know she likes Linda. It is a great risk; but I trust no harm will come of it. Get word to Linda to be ready as soon as it is dark, before the patrols are out. I will send the housemaids on errands, and Betty shall go to meet Linda." The place where we were to meet was designated and agreed upon. My grandmother was unable to thank the lady for this noble deed; overcome by her emotions, she sank on her knees and sobbed like a child.

I received a message to leave my friend's house at such an hour, and go to a certain place where a friend would be waiting for me. As a matter of prudence no names were mentioned. I had no means of conjecturing who I was to meet, or where I was going. I did not like to move thus blindfolded, but I had no choice. It would not do for me to remain where I was. I disguised myself, summoned up courage to meet the worst, and went to the appointed place. My friend Betty was there; she was the last person I expected to see. We hurried along in silence. The pain in my leg was so intense that it seemed as if I should drop; but fear gave me strength. We reached the house and entered unobserved. Her first words were: "Honey, now you is safe. Dem devils ain't coming to search *dis* house. When I get you into missis' safe place, I will bring some nice hot supper. I specs you need it after all dis skeering." Betty's vocation led her to think eating the most important thing in life. She did not realize that my heart was too full for me to care much about supper.

The mistress came to meet us, and led me up stairs to a small room over her own sleeping apartment. "You will be safe here, Linda," said she; "I keep this room to store away things that are out of use. The girls are not accustomed to be sent to it, and they will not suspect any thing unless they hear some noise. I always keep it locked, and Betty shall take care of the key. But you must be very careful, for my sake as well as your own; and you must never tell my secret; for it would ruin me and my family. I will keep the girls busy in the morning, that Betty may have a chance to bring your breakfast; but it will not do for her to come to you again till night. I will come to see you sometimes. Keep up your courage. I hope this state of things will not last long." Betty came with the "nice hot supper," and the mistress hastened down stairs to keep things straight till she returned. How my heart overflowed with gratitude! Words choked in my throat; but I could have kissed the feet of my benefactress. For that deed of Christian womanhood, may God forever bless her!

I went to sleep that night with the feeling that I was for the present the most fortunate slave in town. Morning came and filled my little cell with light. I thanked the heavenly Father for this safe retreat. Opposite my window was a pile of feather beds. On the top of these I could lie perfectly concealed, and command a view of the street through which Dr. Flint passed to his office. Anxious as I was, I felt a gleam of satisfaction when I saw him. Thus far I had outwitted him, and I triumphed over it. Who can blame slaves for being cunning?

They are constantly compelled to resort to it. It is the only weapon of the weak and oppressed against the strength of their tyrants.

I was daily hoping to hear that my master had sold my children; for I knew who was on the watch to buy them. But Dr. Flint cared even more for revenge than he did for money. My brother William, and the good aunt who had served in his family twenty years, and my little Benny, and Ellen, who was a little over two years old, were thrust into jail, as a means of compelling my relatives to give some information about me. He swore my grandmother should never see one of them again till I was brought back. They kept these facts from me for several days. When I heard that my little ones were in a loathsome jail, my first impulse was to go to them. I was encountering dangers for the sake of freeing them, and must I be the cause of their death? The thought was agonizing. My benefactress tried to soothe me by telling me that my aunt would take good care of the children while they remained in jail. But it added to my pain to think that the good old aunt, who had always been so kind to her sister's orphan children, should be shut up in prison for no other crime than loving them. I suppose my friends feared a reckless movement on my part, knowing, as they did, that my life was bound up in my children. I received a note from my brother William. It was scarcely legible, and ran thus: "Wherever you are, dear sister, I beg of you not to come here. We are all much better off than you are. If you come, you will ruin us all. They would force you to tell where you had been, or they would kill you. Take the advice of your friends; if not for the sake of me and your children, at least for the sake of those you would ruin."

Poor William! He also must suffer for being my brother. I took his advice and kept quiet. My aunt was taken out of jail at the end of a month, because Mrs. Flint could not spare her any longer. She was tired of being her own housekeeper. It was quite too fatiguing to order her dinner and eat it too. My children remained in jail, where brother William did all he could for their comfort. Betty went to see them sometimes, and brought me tidings. She was not permitted to enter the jail; but William would hold them up to the grated window while she chatted with them. When she repeated their prattle, and told me how they wanted to see their ma, my tears would flow. Old Betty would exclaim, "Lors, chile! what's you crying 'bout? Dem young uns vil kill you dead. Don't be so chick'n hearted! If you does, you vil nebber git thro' dis world."

Good old soul! She had gone through the world childless. She had never had little ones to clasp their arms round her neck; she had never seen their soft eyes looking into hers; no sweet little voices had called her mother; she had never pressed her own infants to her heart, with the feeling that even in fetters there was something to live for. How could she realize my feelings? Betty's husband loved children dearly, and wondered why God had denied them to him. He expressed great sorrow when he came to Betty with the tidings that Ellen had been taken out of jail and carried to Dr. Flint's. She had the measles a short time before they carried her to jail, and the disease had left her eyes affected. The doctor had taken her home to attend to them. My children had always been afraid of the doctor and his wife. They had never been inside of their house. Poor little Ellen cried all day to be carried back to prison. The instincts of childhood are true. She knew she was loved in the jail. Her screams and sobs annoyed Mrs. Flint. Before night she called one of the slaves, and said, "Here, Bill, carry this brat back to the jail. I can't stand her noise. If she would be quiet I should like to keep the little minx. She would make a handy waiting-maid for my daughter by and by. But if she staid here, with her white face, I suppose I should either kill her or spoil her. I hope the doctor will sell them as far as wind and water can carry them. As for their mother, her ladyship will find out yet what she gets by running away. She hasn't so much feeling for her children as a cow has for its calf. If she had, she would have come back long ago, to get them out of jail, and save all this expense and trouble. The good-for-nothing hussy! When she is caught, she shall stay in jail, in irons, for one six months, and then be sold to a sugar plantation. I shall see her broke in yet. What do you stand there for, Bill? Why don't you go off with the brat? Mind, now, that you don't let any of the niggers speak to her in the street!"

When these remarks were reported to me, I smiled at Mrs.

Flint's saying that she should either kill my child or spoil her. I thought to myself there was very little danger of the latter. I have always considered it as one of God's special providences that Ellen screamed till she was carried back to jail.

That same night Dr. Flint was called to a patient, and did not return till near morning. Passing my grandmother's, he saw a light in the house, and thought to himself, "Perhaps this has something to do with Linda." He knocked, and the door was opened. "What calls you up so early?" said he. "I saw your light, and I thought I would just stop and tell you that I have found out where Linda is. I know where to put my hands on her, and I shall have her before twelve o'clock." When he had turned away, my grandmother and my uncle looked anxiously at each other. They did not know whether or not it was merely one of the doctor's tricks to frighten them. In their uncertainty, they thought it was best to have a message conveyed to my friend Betty. Unwilling to alarm her mistress, Betty resolved to dispose of me herself. She came to me, and told me to rise and dress quickly. We hurried down stairs, and across the yard, into the kitchen. She locked the door, and lifted up a plank in the floor. A buffalo skin and a bit of carpet were spread for me to lie on, and a quilt thrown over me. "Stay dar," said she, "till I sees if dey know 'bout you. Dey say dey vil put thar hans on you afore twelve o'-clock. If dey *did* know whar you are, dey won't know *now*. Dey'll be disapinted dis time. Dat's all I got to say. If dey comes rummagin 'mong *my* tings, dey'll get one bressed sarssin from dis 'ere nigger." In my shallow bed I had but just room enough to bring my hands to my face to keep the dust out of my eyes; for Betty walked over me twenty times in an hour, passing from the dresser to the fireplace. When she was alone, I could hear her pronouncing anathemas over Dr. Flint and all his tribe, every now and then saying, with a chuckling laugh, "Dis nigger's too cute for 'em dis time." When the housemaids were about, she had sly ways of drawing them out, that I might hear what they would say. She would repeat stories she had heard about my being in this, or that, or the other place. To which they would answer, that I was not fool enough to be staying round there; that I was in Philadelphia or New York before this time. When all were abed and asleep,

Betty raised the plank, and said, "Come out, chile; come out. Dey don't know nottin 'bout you. 'Twas only white folks' lies, to skeer de niggers."

Some days after this adventure I had a much worse fright. As I sat very still in my retreat above stairs, cheerful visions floated through my mind. I thought Dr. Flint would soon get discouraged, and would be willing to sell my children, when he lost all hopes of making them the means of my discovery. I knew who was ready to buy them. Suddenly I heard a voice that chilled my blood. The sound was too familiar to me, it had been too dreadful, for me not to recognize at once my old master. He was in the house, and I at once concluded he had come to seize me. I looked round in terror. There was no way of escape. The voice receded. I supposed the constable was with him, and they were searching the house. In my alarm I did not forget the trouble I was bringing on my generous benefactress. It seemed as if I were born to bring sorrow on all who befriended me, and that was the bitterest drop in the bitter cup of my life. After a while I heard approaching footsteps; the key was turned in my door. I braced myself against the wall to keep from falling. I ventured to look up, and there stood my kind benefactress alone. I was too much overcome to speak, and sunk down upon the floor.

"I thought you would hear your master's voice," she said; "and knowing you would be terrified, I came to tell you there is nothing to fear. You may even indulge in a laugh at the old gentleman's expense. He is so sure you are in New York, that he came to borrow five hundred dollars to go in pursuit of you. My sister had some money to loan on interest. He has obtained it, and proposes to start for New York to-night. So, for the present, you see you are safe. The doctor will merely lighten his pocket hunting after the bird he has left behind."

XIX.

THE CHILDREN SOLD.

THE doctor came back from New York, of course without accomplishing his purpose. He had expended considerable money, and was rather disheartened. My brother and the children had now been in jail two months, and that also was some expense. My friends thought it was a favorable time to work on his discouraged feelings. Mr. Sands sent a speculator to offer him nine hundred dollars for my brother William, and eight hundred for the two children. These were high prices, as slaves were then selling; but the offer was rejected. If it had been merely a question of money, the doctor would have sold any boy of Benny's age for two hundred dollars; but he could not bear to give up the power of revenge. But he was hard pressed for money, and he revolved the matter in his mind. He knew that if he could keep Ellen till she was fifteen, he could sell her for a high price; but I presume he reflected that she might die, or might be stolen away. At all events, he came to the conclusion that he had better accept the slave-trader's offer. Meeting him in the street, he inquired when he would leave town. "To-day, at ten o'clock," he replied. "Ah, do you go so soon?" said the doctor; "I have been reflecting upon your proposition, and I have concluded to let you have the three negroes if you will say nineteen hundred dollars." After some parley, the trader agreed to his terms. He wanted the bill of sale drawn up and signed immediately, as he had a great deal to attend to during the short time he remained in town. The doctor went to the jail and told William he would take him back into his service if he would promise to behave himself; but he replied that he would rather be sold. "And you *shall* be sold, you ungrateful rascal!" exclaimed the doctor. In less than an hour the money was paid, the papers were signed, sealed, and delivered, and my brother and children were in the hands of the trader.

It was a hurried transaction; and after it was over, the doctor's characteristic caution returned. He went back to the speculator, and said, "Sir, I have come to lay you under obligations of a thousand dollars not to sell any of those negroes in this state." "You come too late," replied the trader; "our bargain is closed." He had, in fact, already sold them to Mr. Sands, but he did not mention it. The doctor required him to put irons on "that rascal, Bill," and to pass through the back streets when he took his gang out of town. The trader was privately instructed to concede to his wishes. My good old aunt went to the jail to bid the children good by, supposing them to be the speculator's property, and that she should never see them again. As she held Benny in her lap, he said, "Aunt Nancy, I want to show you something." He led her to the door and showed her a long row of marks, saying, "Uncle Will taught me to count. I have made a mark for every day I have been here, and it is sixty days. It is a long time; and the speculator is going to take me and Ellen away. He's a bad man. It's wrong for him to take grandmother's children. I want to go to my mother."

My grandmother was told that the children would be restored to her, but she was requested to act as if they were really to be sent away. Accordingly, she made up a bundle of clothes and went to the jail. When she arrived, she found William handcuffed among the gang, and the children in the trader's cart. The scene seemed too much like reality. She was afraid there might have been some deception or mistake. She fainted, and was carried home.

When the wagon stopped at the hotel, several gentlemen came out and proposed to purchase William, but the trader refused their offers, without stating that he was already sold. And now came the trying hour for that drove of human beings, driven away like cattle, to be sold they knew not where. Husbands were torn from wives, parents from children, never to look upon each other again this side the grave. There was wringing of hands and cries of despair.

Dr. Flint had the supreme satisfaction of seeing the wagon leave town, and Mrs. Flint had the gratification of supposing that my children were going "as far as wind and water would carry them." According to agreement, my uncle followed the wagon some miles, until they came to an old farm house. There the trader took the irons from William, and as he did so, he said, "You are a damned clever fellow. I should like to own you myself. Them gentlemen that wanted to buy you said you was a bright, honest chap, and I must git you a good home. I guess your old master will swear to-morrow, and call himself an old fool for selling the children. I reckon he'll never git their mammy back again. I expect she's made tracks for the north. Good by, old boy. Remember, I have done you a good turn. You must thank me by coaxing all the pretty gals to go with me next fall. That's going to be my last trip. This trading in niggers is a bad business for a fellow that's got any heart. Move on, you fellows!" And the gang went on, God alone knows where.

Much as I despise and detest the class of slave-traders, whom I regard as the vilest wretches on earth, I must do this man the justice to say that he seemed to have some feeling. He took a fancy to William in the jail, and wanted to buy him. When he heard the story of my children, he was willing to aid them in getting out of Dr. Flint's power, even without charging the customary fee.

My uncle procured a wagon and carried William and the children back to town. Great was the joy in my grandmother's house! The curtains were closed, and the candles lighted. The happy grandmother cuddled the little ones to her bosom. They hugged her, and kissed her, and clapped their hands, and shouted. She knelt down and poured forth one of her heartfelt prayers of thanksgiving to God. The father was present for a while; and though such a "parental relation" as existed between him and my children takes slight hold of the hearts or consciences of slaveholders, it must be that he experienced some moments of pure joy in witnessing the happiness he had imparted.

I had no share in the rejoicings of that evening. The events of the day had not come to my knowledge. And now I will tell you something that happened to me; though you will, perhaps, think it illustrates the superstition of slaves. I sat in my usual place on the floor near the window, where I could hear much that was said in the street without being seen. The family had retired for the night, and all was still. I sat there thinking of my children, when I heard a low strain of music. A band of serenaders were under the window, playing "Home, sweet home." I listened till the sounds did not seem like music, but like the moaning of children. It seemed as if my heart would burst. I rose from my sitting posture, and knelt. A streak of moonlight was on the floor before me, and in the midst of it appeared the forms of my two children. They vanished; but I had seen them distinctly. Some will call it a dream, others a vision. I know not how to account for it, but it made a strong impression on my mind, and I felt certain something had happened to my little ones.

I had not seen Betty since morning. Now I heard her softly turning the key. As soon as she entered, I clung to her, and begged her to let me know whether my children were dead, or whether they were sold; for I had seen their spirits in my room, and I was sure something had happened to them. "Lor, chile," said she, putting her arms round me, "you's got de high-sterics. I'll sleep wid you to-night, 'cause you'll make a noise, and ruin missis. Something has stirred you up mightily. When you is done cryin, I'll talk wid you. De chillern is well, and mighty happy. I seed 'em myself. Does dat satisfy you? Dar, chile, be still! Somebody vill hear you." I tried to obey her. She lay down, and was soon sound asleep; but no sleep would come to my eyelids.

At dawn, Betty was up and off to the kitchen. The hours passed on, and the vision of the night kept constantly recurring to my thoughts. After a while I heard the voices of two women in the entry. In one of them I recognized the housemaid. The other said to her, "Did you know Linda Brent's children was sold to the speculator yesterday. They say ole massa Flint was mighty glad to see 'em drove out of town; but they say they've come back agin. I 'spect it's all their daddy's doings. They say he's bought William too. Lor! how it will take hold of ole massa Flint! I'm going roun' to aunt Marthy's to see 'bout it."

I bit my lips till the blood came to keep from crying out. Were my children with their grandmother, or had the speculator carried them off? The suspense was dreadful. Would Betty *never* come, and tell me the truth about it? At last she came, and I eagerly repeated what I had overheard. Her face was one broad, bright smile. "Lor, you foolish ting!" said she. "I'se gwine to tell you all 'bout it. De gals is eating thar breakfast, and missus tole me to let her tell you; but, poor creeter! t'aint right to keep you waitin', and I'se gwine to tell you. Brudder, chillern, all is bought by de daddy! I'se laugh more dan nuff, tinking 'bout ole massa Flint. Lor, how he *vill* swar! He's got ketched dis time, any how; but I must be getting out o' dis, or dem gals vill come and ketch *me*."

Betty went off laughing; and I said to myself, "Can it be true that my children are free? I have not suffered for them in vain. Thank God!"

Great surprise was expressed when it was known that my children had returned to their grandmother's. The news spread through the town, and many a kind word was bestowed on the little ones.

Dr. Flint went to my grandmother's to ascertain who was the owner of my children, and she informed him. "I expected as much," said he. "I am glad to hear it. I have had news from Linda lately, and I shall soon have her. You need never expect to see *her* free. She shall be my slave as long as I live, and when I am dead she shall be the slave of my children. If I ever find out that you or Phillip had any thing to do with her running off I'll kill him. And if I meet William in the street, and he presumes to look at me, I'll flog him within an inch of his life. Keep those brats out of my sight!"

As he turned to leave, my grandmother said something to remind him of his own doings. He looked back upon her, as if he would have been glad to strike her to the ground.

I had my season of joy and thanksgiving. It was the first time since my childhood that I had experienced any real happiness. I heard of the old doctor's threats, but they no longer had the same power to trouble me. The darkest cloud that hung over my life had rolled away. Whatever slavery might do to me, it could not shackle my children. If I fell a sacrifice, my little ones were saved. It was well for me that my simple heart believed all that had been promised for their welfare. It is always better to trust than to doubt.

XX.

NEW PERILS.

THE doctor, more exasperated than ever, again tried to revenge himself on my relatives. He arrested uncle Phillip on the charge of having aided my flight. He was carried before a court, and swore truly that he knew nothing of my intention to escape, and that he had not seen me since I left my master's plantation. The doctor then demanded that he should give bail for five hundred dollars that he would have nothing to do with me. Several gentlemen offered to be security for him; but Mr. Sands told him he had better go back to jail, and he would see that he came out without giving bail.

The news of his arrest was carried to my grandmother, who conveyed it to Betty. In the kindness of her heart, she again stowed me away under the floor; and as she walked back and forth, in the performance of her culinary duties, she talked apparently to herself, but with the intention that I should hear what was going on. I hoped that my uncle's imprisonment would last but few days; still I was anxious. I thought it likely Dr. Flint would do his utmost to taunt and insult him, and I was afraid my uncle might lose control of himself, and retort in some way that would be construed into a punishable offence; and I was well aware that in court his word would not be taken against any white man's. The search for me was renewed. Something had excited suspicions that I was in the vicinity. They searched the house I was in. I heard their steps and their voices. At night, when all were asleep, Betty came to release me from my place of confinement. The fright I had undergone, the constrained posture, and the dampness of the ground, made me ill for several days. My uncle was soon after taken out of prison; but the movements of all my relatives, and of all our friends, were very closely watched.

We all saw that I could not remain where I was much longer. I had already staid longer than was intended, and I knew my presence must be a source of perpetual anxiety to my kind benefactress. During this time, my friends had laid many plans for my escape, but the extreme vigilance of my persecutors made it impossible to carry them into effect.

One morning I was much startled by hearing somebody trying to get into my room. Several keys were tried, but none fitted. I instantly conjectured it was one of the housemaids; and I concluded she must either have heard some noise in the room, or have noticed the entrance of Betty. When my friend came, at her usual time, I told her what had happened. "I knows who it was," said she. "'Pend upon it, 'twas dat Jenny. Dat nigger allers got de debble in her." I suggested that she might have seen or heard something that excited her curiosity.

"Tut! tut! chile!" exclaimed Betty, "she ain't seen notin', nor hearn notin'. She only 'spects someting. Dat's all. She wants to fine out who hab cut and make my gownd. But she won't nebber know. Dat's sartin. I'll git missis to fix her."

I reflected a moment, and said, "Betty, I must leave here to-night."

"Do as you tink best, poor chile," she replied. "I'se mighty 'fraid dat 'ere nigger vill pop on you some time."

She reported the incident to her mistress, and received orders to keep Jenny busy in the kitchen till she could see my uncle Phillip. He told her he would send a friend for me that very evening. She told him she hoped I was going to the north, for it was very dangerous for me to remain any where in the vicinity. Alas, it was not an easy thing, for one in my situation, to go to the north. In order to leave the coast quite clear for me, she went into the country to spend the day with her brother, and took Jenny with her. She was afraid to come and bid me good by, but she left a kind message with Betty. I heard her carriage roll from the door, and I never again saw her who had so generously befriended the poor, trembling fugitive! Though she was a slaveholder, to this day my heart blesses her!

I had not the slightest idea where I was going. Betty brought me a suit of sailor's clothes,—jacket, trowsers, and tarpaulin hat. She gave me a small bundle, saying I might need it where I was going. In cheery tones, she exclaimed, "I'se *so* glad you is gwine to free parts! Don't forget ole Betty. P'raps I'll come 'long by and by."

I tried to tell her how grateful I felt for all her kindness, but she interrupted me. "I don't want no tanks, honey. I'se glad I could help you, and I hope de good Lord vill open de path for you. I'se gwine wid you to de lower gate. Put your hands in your pockets, and walk ricketty, like de sailors."

I performed to her satisfaction. At the gate I found Peter, a young colored man, waiting for me. I had known him for years. He had been an apprentice to my father, and had always borne a good character. I was not afraid to trust to him. Betty bade me a hurried good by, and we walked off. "Take courage, Linda," said my friend Peter. "I've got a dagger, and no man shall take you from me, unless he passes over my dead body."

It was a long time since I had taken a walk out of doors, and the fresh air revived me. It was also pleasant to hear a human voice speaking to me above a whisper. I passed several people whom I knew, but they did not recognize me in my disguise. I prayed internally that, for Peter's sake, as well as my own, nothing might occur to bring out his dagger. We walked on till we came to the wharf. My aunt Nancy's husband was a seafaring man, and it had been deemed necessary to let him into our secret. He took me into his boat, rowed out to a vessel not far distant, and hoisted me on board. We three were the only occupants of the vessel. I now ventured to ask what they proposed to do with me. They said I was to remain on board till near dawn, and then they would hide me in Snaky Swamp, till my uncle Phillip had prepared a place of concealment for me. If the vessel had been bound north, it would have been of no avail to me, for it would certainly have been searched. About four o'clock, we were again seated in the boat, and rowed three miles to the swamp. My fear of snakes had been increased by the venomous bite I had received, and I dreaded to enter this hiding-place. But I was in no situation to choose, and I gratefully accepted the best that my poor, persecuted friends could do for me.

Peter landed first, and with a large knife cut a path through bamboos and briers of all descriptions. He came back, took me in his arms, and carried me to a seat made among the bamboos. Before we reached it, we were covered with hundreds of mosquitos. In an hour's time they had so poisoned my flesh that I was a pitiful sight to behold. As the light increased, I saw snake after snake crawling round us. I had been accustomed to the sight of snakes all my life, but these were larger than any I had ever seen. To this day I shudder when I remember that morning. As evening approached, the number of snakes increased so much that we were continually obliged to thrash them with sticks to keep them from crawling over us. The bamboos were so high and so thick that it was impossible to see beyond a very short distance. Just before it became dark we procured a seat nearer to the entrance of the swamp, being fearful of losing our way back to the boat. It was not long before we heard the paddle of oars, and the low whistle, which had been agreed upon as a signal. We made haste to enter the boat, and were rowed back to the vessel. I passed a wretched night; for the heat of the swamp, the mosquitos, and the constant terror of snakes, had brought on a burning fever. I had just dropped asleep, when they came and told me it was time to go back to that horrid swamp. I could scarcely summon courage to rise. But even those large, venomous snakes were less dreadful to my imagination than the white men in that community called civilized. This time Peter took a quantity of tobacco to burn, to keep off the mosquitos. It produced the desired effect on them, but gave me nausea and severe headache. At dark we returned to the vessel. I had been so sick during the day, that Peter declared I should go home that night, if the devil himself was on patrol. They told me a place of concealment had been provided for me at my grandmother's. I could not imagine how it was possible to hide me in her house, every nook and corner of which was known to the Flint family. They told me to wait and see. We were rowed ashore, and went boldly through the streets, to my grandmother's. I wore my sailor's clothes, and had blackened my face with charcoal. I passed several people whom I knew. The father of my children came so near that I brushed against his arm; but he had no idea who it was.

"You must make the most of this walk," said my friend Peter, "for you may not have another very soon."

I thought his voice sounded sad. It was kind of him to conceal from me what a dismal hole was to be my home for a long, long time.

XXI.

THE LOOPHOLE OF RETREAT.

A SMALL shed had been added to my grandmother's house years ago. Some boards were laid across the joists at the top, and between these boards and the roof was a very small garret, never occupied by any thing but rats and mice. It was a pent roof, covered with nothing but shingles, according to the southern custom for such buildings. The garret was only nine feet long and seven wide. The highest part was three feet high, and sloped down abruptly to the loose board floor. There was no admission for either light or air. My uncle Phillip, who was a carpenter, had very skilfully made a concealed trap-door, which communicated with the storeroom. He had been doing this while I was waiting in the swamp. The storeroom opened upon a piazza. To this hole I was conveyed as soon as I entered the house. The air was stifling; the darkness total. A bed had been spread on the floor. I could sleep quite comfortably on one side; but the slope was so sudden that I could not turn on the other without hitting the roof. The rats and mice ran over my bed; but I was weary, and I slept such sleep as the wretched may, when a tempest has passed over them. Morning came. I knew it only by the noises I heard; for in my small den day and night were all the same. I suffered for air even more than for light. But I was not comfortless. I heard the voices of my children. There was joy and there was sadness in the sound. It made my tears flow. How I longed to speak to them! I was eager to look on their faces; but there was no hole, no crack, through which I could peep. This continued darkness was oppressive. It seemed horrible to sit or lie in a cramped position day after day, without one gleam of light. Yet I would have chosen this, rather than my lot as a slave, though white people considered it an easy one; and it was so compared with the fate of others. I was never cruelly over-worked; I was never lacerated with the whip from head to foot; I was never so beaten and bruised that I could not turn from one side to the other; I never had my heel-strings cut to prevent my running away; I was never chained to a log and forced to drag it about, while I toiled in the fields from morning till night; I was never branded with hot iron, or torn by bloodhounds. On the contrary, I had always been kindly treated, and tenderly cared for, until I came into the hands of Dr. Flint. I had never wished for freedom till then. But though my life in slavery was comparatively devoid of hardships, God pity the woman who is compelled to lead such a life!

My food was passed up to me through the trap-door my uncle had contrived; and my grandmother, my uncle Phillip, and aunt Nancy would seize such opportunities as they could, to mount up there and chat with me at the opening. But of course this was not safe in the daytime. It must all be done in darkness. It was impossible for me to move in an erect position, but I crawled about my den for exercise. One day I hit my head against something, and found it was a gimlet. My uncle had left it sticking there when he made the trap-door. I was as rejoiced as Robinson Crusoe could have been at finding such a treasure. It put a lucky thought into my head. I said to myself, "Now I will have some light. Now I will see my children." I did not dare to begin my work during the daytime, for fear of attracting attention. But I groped round; and having found the side next the street, where I could frequently see my children, I stuck the gimlet in and waited for evening. I bored three rows of holes, one above another; then I bored out the interstices between. I thus succeeded in making one hole about an inch long and an inch broad. I sat by it till late into the night, to enjoy the little whiff of air that floated in. In the morning I watched for my children. The first person I saw in the street was Dr. Flint. I had a shuddering, superstitious feeling that it was a bad omen. Several familiar faces passed by. At last I heard the merry laugh of children, and presently two sweet little faces were looking up at me, as though they knew I was there, and were conscious of the joy they imparted. How I longed to *tell* them I was there!

My condition was now a little improved. But for weeks I was tormented by hundreds of little red insects, fine as a needle's point, that pierced through my skin, and produced an intolerable burning. The good grandmother gave me herb teas and cooling medicines, and finally I got rid of them. The heat of my den was intense, for nothing but thin shingles protected me from the scorching summer's sun. But I had my consolations. Through my peeping-hole I could watch the children, and when they were near enough, I could hear their talk. Aunt Nancy brought me all the news she could hear at Dr. Flint's. From her I learned that the doctor had written to New York to a colored woman, who had been born and raised in our neighborhood, and had breathed his contaminating atmosphere. He offered her a reward if she could find out any thing about me. I know not what was the nature of her reply; but he soon after started for New York in haste, saying to his family that he had business of importance to transact. I peeped at him as he passed on his way to the steamboat. It was a satisfaction to have miles of land and water between us, even for a little while; and it was a still greater satisfaction to know that he believed me to be in the Free States. My little den seemed less dreary than it had done. He returned, as he did from his former journey to New York, without obtaining any satisfactory information. When he passed our house next morning, Benny was standing at the gate. He had heard them say that he had gone to find me, and he called out, "Dr. Flint, did you bring my mother home? I want to see her." The doctor stamped his foot at him in a rage, and exclaimed, "Get out of the way, you little damned rascal! If you don't, I'll cut off your head."

Benny ran terrified into the house, saying, "You can't put me in jail again. I don't belong to you now." It was well that the wind carried the words away from the doctor's ear. I told my grandmother of it, when we had our next conference at the trap-door; and begged of her not to allow the children to be impertinent to the irascible old man.

Autumn came, with a pleasant abatement of heat. My eyes had become accustomed to the dim light, and by holding my book or work in a certain position near the aperture I contrived to read and sew. That was a great relief to the tedious monotony of my life. But when winter came, the cold penetrated through the thin shingle roof, and I was dreadfully chilled. The winters there are not so long, or so severe, as in northern latitudes; but the houses are not built to shelter from cold, and my little den was peculiarly comfortless. The kind grandmother brought me bed-clothes and warm drinks. Often I was obliged to lie in bed all day to keep comfortable; but with all my precautions, my shoulders and feet were frostbitten. O, those long, gloomy days, with no object for my eye to rest upon, and no thoughts to occupy my mind, except the dreary past and the uncertain future! I was thankful when there came a day sufficiently mild for me to wrap myself up and sit at the loophole to watch the passers by. Southerners have the habit of stopping and talking in the streets, and I heard many conversations not intended to meet my ears. I heard slave-hunters planning how to catch some poor fugitive. Several times I heard allusions to Dr. Flint, myself, and the history of my children, who, perhaps, were playing near the gate. One would say, "I wouldn't move my little finger to catch her, as old Flint's property." Another would say, "I'll catch *any* nigger for the reward. A man ought to have what belongs to him, if he *is* a damned brute." The opinion was often expressed that I was in the Free States. Very rarely did any one suggest that I might be in the vicinity. Had the least suspicion rested on my grandmother's house, it would have been burned to the ground. But it was the last place they thought of. Yet there was no place, where slavery existed, that could have afforded me so good a place of concealment.

Dr. Flint and his family repeatedly tried to coax and bribe my children to tell something they had heard said about me. One day the doctor took them into a shop, and offered them some bright little silver pieces and gay handkerchiefs if they would tell where their mother was. Ellen shrank away from him, and would not speak; but Benny spoke up, and said, "Dr. Flint, I don't know where my mother is. I guess she's in New York; and when you go there again, I wish you'd ask her to come home, for I want to see her; but if you put her in jail, or tell her you'll cut her head off, I'll tell her to go right back."

XXII.

CHRISTMAS FESTIVITIES.

Christmas was approaching. Grandmother brought me materials, and I busied myself making some new garments and little playthings for my children. Were it not that hiring day is near at hand, and many families are fearfully looking forward to the probability of separation in a few days, Christmas might be a happy season for the poor slaves. Even slave mothers try to gladden the hearts of their little ones on that occasion. Benny and Ellen had their Christmas stockings filled. Their imprisoned mother could not have the privilege of witnessing their surprise and joy. But I had the pleasure of peeping at them as they went into the street with their new suits on. I heard Benny ask a little playmate whether Santa Claus brought him any thing. "Yes," replied the boy; "but Santa Claus ain't a real man. It's the children's mothers that put things into the stockings." "No, that can't be," replied Benny, "for Santa Claus brought Ellen and me these new clothes, and my mother has been gone this long time."

How I longed to tell him that his mother made those garments, and that many a tear fell on them while she worked!

Every child rises early on Christmas morning to see the Johnkannaus. Without them, Christmas would be shorn of its greatest attraction. They consist of companies of slaves from the plantations, generally of the lower class. Two athletic men, in calico wrappers, have a net thrown over them, covered with all manner of bright-colored stripes. Cows' tails are fastened to their backs, and their heads are decorated with horns. A box, covered with sheepskin, is called the gumbo box. A dozen beat on this, while others strike triangles and jawbones, to which bands of dancers keep time. For a month previous they are composing songs, which are sung on this occasion. These companies, of a hundred each, turn out early in the morning, and are allowed to go round till twelve o'clock, begging for contributions. Not a door is left unvisited where there is the least chance of obtaining a penny or a glass of rum. They do not drink while they are out, but carry the rum home in jugs, to have a carousal. These Christmas donations frequently amount to twenty or thirty dollars. It is seldom that any white man or child refuses to give them a trifle. If he does, they regale his ears with the following song:—

> "Poor massa, so dey say;
> Down in de heel, so dey say;
> Got no money, so dey say;
> Not one shillin, so dey say;
> God A'mighty bress you, so dey say."

Christmas is a day of feasting, both with white and colored people. Slaves, who are lucky enough to have a few shillings, are sure to spend them for good eating; and many a turkey and pig is captured, without saying, "By your leave, sir." Those who cannot obtain these, cook a 'possum, or a raccoon, from which savory dishes can be made. My grandmother raised poultry and pigs for sale; and it was her established custom to have both a turkey and a pig roasted for Christmas dinner.

On this occasion, I was warned to keep extremely quiet, because two guests had been invited. One was the town constable, and the other was a free colored man, who tried to pass himself off for white, and who was always ready to do any mean work for the sake of currying favor with white people. My grandmother had a motive for inviting them. She managed to take them all over the house. All the rooms on the lower floor were thrown open for them to pass in and out; and after dinner, they were invited up stairs to look at a fine mocking bird my uncle had just brought home. There, too, the rooms were all thrown open, that they might look in. When I heard them talking on the piazza, my heart almost stood still. I knew this colored man had spent many nights hunting for me. Every body knew he had the blood of a slave father in his veins; but for the sake of passing himself off for white, he was ready to kiss the slaveholders' feet. How I despised him! As for the constable, he wore no false colors. The duties of his office were despicable, but he was superior to his companion, inasmuch as he did not pretend to be what he was not. Any white man, who could raise money enough to buy a slave, would have considered himself degraded by being a constable; but the office enabled its possessor to exercise authority. If he found any slave out after nine o'clock, he could whip him as much as he liked; and that was a privilege to be coveted. When the guests were ready to depart, my grandmother gave each of them some of her nice pudding, as a present for their wives. Through my peep-hole I saw them go out of the gate, and I was glad when it closed after them. So passed the first Christmas in my den.

XXIII.

STILL IN PRISON.

When spring returned, and I took in the little patch of green the aperture commanded, I asked myself how many more summers and winters I must be condemned to spend thus. I longed to draw in a plentiful draught of fresh air, to stretch my cramped limbs, to have room to stand erect, to feel the earth under my feet again. My relatives were constantly on the lookout for a chance of escape; but none offered that seemed practicable, and even tolerably safe. The hot summer came again, and made the turpentine drop from the thin roof over my head.

During the long nights I was restless for want of air, and I had no room to toss and turn. There was but one compensation; the atmosphere was so stifled that even mosquitos would not condescend to buzz in it. With all my detestation of Dr. Flint, I could hardly wish him a worse punishment, either in this world or that which is to come, than to suffer what I suffered in one single summer. Yet the laws allowed *him* to be out in the free air, while I, guiltless of crime, was pent up here, as the only means of avoiding the cruelties the laws allowed him to inflict upon me! I don't know what kept life within me. Again and again, I thought I should die before long; but I saw the leaves of another autumn whirl through the air, and felt the touch of another winter. In summer the most terrible thunder storms were acceptable, for the rain came through the roof, and I rolled up my bed that it might cool the hot boards under it. Later in the season, storms sometimes wet my clothes through and through, and that was not comfortable when the air grew chilly. Moderate storms I could keep out by filling the chinks with oakum.

But uncomfortable as my situation was, I had glimpses of things out of doors, which made me thankful for my wretched hiding-place. One day I saw a slave pass our gate, muttering, "It's his own, and he can kill it if he will." My grandmother told me that woman's history. Her mistress had that day seen her baby for the first time, and in the lineaments of its fair face she saw a likeness to her husband. She turned the bondwoman and her child out of doors, and forbade her ever to return. The slave went to her master, and told him what had happened. He promised to talk with her mistress, and make it all right. The next day she and her baby were sold to a Georgia trader.

Another time I saw a woman rush wildly by, pursued by

two men. She was a slave, the wet nurse of her mistress's children. For some trifling offence her mistress ordered her to be stripped and whipped. To escape the degradation and the torture, she rushed to the river, jumped in, and ended her wrongs in death.

Senator Brown, of Mississippi, could not be ignorant of many such facts as these, for they are of frequent occurrence in every Southern State. Yet he stood up in the Congress of the United States, and declared that slavery was "a great moral, social, and political blessing; a blessing to the master, and a blessing to the slave!"

I suffered much more during the second winter than I did during the first. My limbs were benumbed by inaction, and the cold filled them with cramp. I had a very painful sensation of coldness in my head; even my face and tongue stiffened, and I lost the power of speech. Of course it was impossible, under the circumstances, to summon any physician. My brother William came and did all he could for me. Uncle Phillip also watched tenderly over me; and poor grandmother crept up and down to inquire whether there were any signs of returning life. I was restored to consciousness by the dashing of cold water in my face, and found myself leaning against my brother's arm, while he bent over me with streaming eyes. He afterwards told me he thought I was dying, for I had been in an unconscious state sixteen hours. I next became delirious, and was in great danger of betraying myself and my friends. To prevent this, they stupefied me with drugs. I remained in bed six weeks, weary in body and sick at heart. How to get medical advice was the question. William finally went to a Thompsonian doctor, and described himself as having all my pains and aches. He returned with herbs, roots, and ointment. He was especially charged to rub on the ointment by a fire; but how could a fire be made in my little den? Charcoal in a furnace was tried, but there was no outlet for the gas, and it nearly cost me my life. Afterwards coals, already kindled, were brought up in an iron pan, and placed on bricks. I was so weak, and it was so long since I had enjoyed the warmth of a fire, that those few coals actually made me weep. I think the medicines did me some good; but my recovery was very slow. Dark thoughts passed through my mind as I lay there day after day. I tried to be thankful for my little cell, dismal as it was, and even to love it, as part of the price I had paid for the redemption of my children. Sometimes I thought God was a compassionate Father, who would forgive my sins for the sake of my sufferings. At other times, it seemed to me there was no justice or mercy in the divine government. I asked why the curse of slavery was permitted to exist, and why I had been so persecuted and wronged from youth upward. These things took the shape of mystery, which is to this day not so clear to my soul as I trust it will be hereafter.

In the midst of my illness, grandmother broke down under the weight of anxiety and toil. The idea of losing her, who had always been my best friend and a mother to my children, was the sorest trial I had yet had. O, how earnestly I prayed that she might recover! How hard it seemed, that I could not tend upon her, who had so long and so tenderly watched over me!

One day the screams of a child nerved me with strength to crawl to my peeping-hole, and I saw my son covered with blood. A fierce dog, usually kept chained, had seized and bitten him. A doctor was sent for, and I heard the groans and screams of my child while the wounds were being sewed up. O, what torture to a mother's heart, to listen to this and be unable to go to him!

But childhood is like a day in spring, alternately shower and sunshine. Before night Benny was bright and lively, threatening the destruction of the dog; and great was his delight when the doctor told him the next day that the dog had bitten another boy and been shot. Benny recovered from his wounds; but it was long before he could walk.

When my grandmother's illness became known, many ladies, who were her customers, called to bring her some little comforts, and to inquire whether she had every thing she wanted. Aunt Nancy one night asked permission to watch with her sick mother, and Mrs. Flint replied, "I don't see any need of your going. I can't spare you." But when she found other ladies in the neighborhood were so attentive, not wishing to be outdone in Christian charity, she also sallied forth, in magnificent condescension, and stood by the bedside of her who had loved her in her infancy, and who had been repaid by such grievous wrongs. She seemed surprised to find her so ill, and scolded uncle Phillip for not sending for Dr. Flint. She herself sent for him immediately, and he came. Secure as I was in my retreat, I should have been terrified if I had known he was so near me. He pronounced my grandmother in a very critical situation, and said if her attending physician wished it, he would visit her. Nobody wished to have him coming to the house at all hours, and we were not disposed to give him a chance to make out a long bill.

As Mrs. Flint went out, Sally told her the reason Benny was lame was, that a dog had bitten him. "I'm glad of it," replied she. "I wish he had killed him. It would be good news to send to his mother. *Her* day will come. The dogs will grab *her* yet." With these Christian words she and her husband departed, and, to my great satisfaction, returned no more.

I heard from uncle Phillip, with feelings of unspeakable joy and gratitude, that the crisis was passed and grandmother would live. I could now say from my heart, "God is merciful. He has spared me the anguish of feeling that I caused her death."

XXIV.

THE CANDIDATE FOR CONGRESS.

THE summer had nearly ended, when Dr. Flint made a third visit to New York, in search of me. Two candidates were running for Congress, and he returned in season to vote. The father of my children was the Whig candidate. The doctor had hitherto been a stanch Whig; but now he exerted all his energies for the defeat of Mr. Sands. He invited large parties of men to dine in the shade of his trees, and supplied them with plenty of rum and brandy. If any poor fellow drowned his wits in the bowl, and, in the openness of his convivial heart, proclaimed that he did not mean to vote the Democratic ticket, he was shoved into the street without ceremony.

The doctor expended his liquor in vain. Mr. Sands was elected; an event which occasioned me some anxious thoughts. He had not emancipated my children, and if he should die they would be at the mercy of his heirs. Two little voices, that frequently met my ear, seemed to plead with me not to let their father depart without striving to make their freedom secure. Years had passed since I had spoken to him. I had not even seen him since the night I passed him, unrecognized, in my disguise of a sailor. I supposed he would call before he left, to say something to my grandmother concerning the children, and I resolved what course to take.

The day before his departure for Washington I made arrangements, towards evening, to get from my hiding-place into the storeroom below. I found myself so stiff and clumsy that it was with great difficulty I could hitch from one resting place to another. When I reached the storeroom my ankles gave way under me, and I sank exhausted on the floor. It seemed as if I could never use my limbs again. But the purpose I had in view roused all the strength I had. I crawled on my hands and knees to the window, and, screened behind a barrel, I waited for his coming. The clock struck nine, and I knew the steamboat would leave between ten and eleven. My hopes were failing. But presently I heard his voice, saying to some one, "Wait for me a moment. I wish to see aunt Martha." When he came out, as he passed the window, I said, "Stop one moment, and let me speak for my children." He started, hesitated, and then passed on, and went out of the gate. I closed the shutter I had partially opened, and sank down behind the barrel. I had suffered much; but seldom had I experienced a keener pang than I then felt. Had my children, then, become of so little consequence to him? And had he so little feeling for their wretched mother that he would not listen a moment while she pleaded for them? Painful memories were so busy within me, that I forgot I had not hooked the shutter, till I heard some one opening it. I looked up. He had come back. "Who called me?" said he, in a low tone. "I did," I replied. "Oh, Linda," said he, "I knew your voice; but I was afraid to answer, lest my friend should hear me. Why do you come here? Is it possible you risk yourself in this house? They are mad to allow it. I shall expect to hear that you are all ruined." I did not wish to implicate him, by letting him know my place of concealment; so I merely said, "I thought you would come to bid grandmother good by, and so I came here to speak a few words to you about emancipating my children. Many changes may take place during the six months you are gone to Washington, and it does not seem right for you to expose them to the risk of such changes. I want nothing for myself; all I ask is, that you will free my children, or authorize some friend to do it, before you go."

He promised he would do it, and also expressed a readiness to make any arrangements whereby I could be purchased.

I heard footsteps approaching, and closed the shutter hastily. I wanted to crawl back to my den, without letting the family know what I had done; for I knew they would deem it very imprudent. But he stepped back into the house, to tell my grandmother that he had spoken with me at the storeroom window, and to beg of her not to allow me to remain in the house over night. He said it was the height of madness for me to be there; that we should certainly all be ruined. Luckily, he was in too much of a hurry to wait for a reply, or the dear old woman would surely have told him all.

I tried to go back to my den, but found it more difficult to go up than I had to come down. Now that my mission was fulfilled, the little strength that had supported me through it was gone, and I sank helpless on the floor. My grandmother, alarmed at the risk I had run, came into the storeroom in the dark, and locked the door behind her. "Linda," she whispered, "where are you?"

"I am here by the window," I replied. "I *couldn't* have him go away without emancipating the children. Who knows what may happen?"

"Come, come, child," said she, "it won't do for you to stay here another minute. You've done wrong; but I can't blame you, poor thing!"

I told her I could not return without assistance, and she must call my uncle. Uncle Phillip came, and pity prevented him from scolding me. He carried me back to my dungeon, laid me tenderly on the bed, gave me some medicine, and asked me if there was any thing more he could do. Then he went away, and I was left with my own thoughts—starless as the midnight darkness around me.

My friends feared I should become a cripple for life; and I was so weary of my long imprisonment that, had it not been for the hope of serving my children, I should have been thankful to die; but, for their sakes, I was willing to bear on.

XXV.

COMPETITION IN CUNNING.

DR. FLINT had not given me up. Every now and then he would say to my grandmother that I would yet come back, and voluntarily surrender myself; and that when I did, I could be purchased by my relatives, or any one who wished to buy me. I knew his cunning nature too well not to perceive that this was a trap laid for me; and so all my friends understood it. I resolved to match my cunning against his cunning. In order to make him believe that I was in New York, I resolved to write him a letter dated from that place. I sent for my friend Peter, and asked him if he knew any trustworthy seafaring person, who would carry such a letter to New York, and put it in the post office there. He said he knew one that he would trust with his own life to the ends of the world. I reminded him that it was a hazardous thing for him to undertake. He said he knew it, but he was willing to do any thing to help me. I expressed a wish for a New York paper, to ascertain the names of some of the streets. He run his hand into his pocket, and said, "Here is half a one, that was round a cap I bought of a pedler yesterday." I told him the letter would be ready the next evening. He bade me good by, adding, "Keep up your spirits, Linda; brighter days will come by and by."

My uncle Phillip kept watch over the gate until our brief interview was over. Early the next morning, I seated myself near the little aperture to examine the newspaper. It was a piece of the New York Herald; and, for once, the paper that systematically abuses the colored people, was made to render them a service. Having obtained what information I wanted concerning streets and numbers, I wrote two letters, one to my grandmother, the other to Dr. Flint. I reminded him how he, a gray-headed man, had treated a helpless child, who had been placed in his power, and what years of misery he had brought upon her. To my grandmother, I expressed a wish to have my children sent to me at the north, where I could teach them to respect themselves, and set them a virtuous example; which a slave mother was not allowed to do at the south. I asked her to direct her answer to a certain street in Boston, as I did not live in New York, though I went there sometimes. I dated these letters ahead, to allow for the time it would take to carry them, and sent a memorandum of the date to the messenger. When my friend came for the letters, I said, "God bless and reward you, Peter, for this disinterested kindness. Pray be careful. If you are detected, both you and I will have to suffer dreadfully. I have not a relative who would dare to do it for me." He replied, "You may trust to me, Linda. I don't forget that your father was my best friend, and I will be a friend to his children so long as God lets me live."

It was necessary to tell my grandmother what I had done, in order that she might be ready for the letter, and prepared to hear what Dr. Flint might say about my being at the north. She was sadly troubled. She felt sure mischief would come of it. I also told my plan to aunt Nancy, in order that she might report to us what was said at Dr. Flint's house. I whispered it to her through a crack, and she whispered back, "I hope it will succeed. I shan't mind being a slave all *my* life, if I can only see you and the children free."

I had directed that my letters should be put into the New York post office on the 20th of the month. On the evening of the 24th my aunt came to say that Dr. Flint and his wife had been talking in a low voice about a letter he had received, and that when he went to his office he promised to bring it when he came to tea. So I concluded I should hear my letter read the next morning. I told my grandmother Dr. Flint would be sure to come, and asked her to have him sit near a certain door, and leave it open, that I might hear what he said. The next morning I took my station within sound of that door, and remained motionless as a statue. It was not long before I heard the gate slam, and the well-known footsteps enter the house. He seated himself in the chair that was placed for him, and said, "Well, Martha, I've brought you a letter from Linda. She has sent me a letter, also. I know exactly where to find her; but I don't choose to go to Boston for her. I had

rather she would come back of her own accord, in a respectable manner. Her uncle Phillip is the best person to go
for her. With *him*, she would feel perfectly free to act. I am
willing to pay his expenses going and returning. She shall be
sold to her friends. Her children are free; at least I suppose
they are; and when you obtain her freedom, you'll make a
happy family. I suppose, Martha, you have no objection to my
reading to you the letter Linda has written to you."

He broke the seal, and I heard him read it. The old villain!
He had suppressed the letter I wrote to grandmother, and
prepared a substitute of his own, the purport of which was as
follows:—

> "Dear Grandmother: I have long wanted to write to
> you; but the disgraceful manner in which I left you and
> my children made me ashamed to do it. If you knew
> how much I have suffered since I ran away, you would
> pity and forgive me. I have purchased freedom at a dear
> rate. If any arrangement could be made for me to return
> to the south without being a slave, I would gladly come.
> If not, I beg of you to send my children to the north. I
> cannot live any longer without them. Let me know in
> time, and I will meet them in New York or Philadelphia,
> whichever place best suits my uncle's convenience. Write
> as soon as possible to your unhappy daughter,
>
> LINDA."

"It is very much as I expected it would be," said the old
hypocrite, rising to go. "You see the foolish girl has repented
of her rashness, and wants to return. We must help her to do
it, Martha. Talk with Phillip about it. If he will go for her, she
will trust to him, and come back. I should like an answer to-
morrow. Good morning, Martha."

As he stepped out on the piazza, he stumbled over my little girl. "Ah, Ellen, is that you?" he said, in his most gracious
manner. "I didn't see you. How do you do?"

"Pretty well, sir," she replied. "I heard you tell grandmother that my mother is coming home. I want to see her."

"Yes, Ellen, I am going to bring her home very soon,"
rejoined he; "and you shall see her as much as you like, you
little curly-headed nigger."

This was as good as a comedy to me, who had heard it all; but grandmother was frightened and distressed, because the doctor wanted my uncle to go for me.

The next evening Dr. Flint called to talk the matter over. My uncle told him that from what he had heard of Massachusetts, he judged he should be mobbed if he went there after a runaway slave. "All stuff and nonsense, Phillip!" replied the doctor. "Do you suppose I want you to kick up a row in Boston? The business can all be done quietly. Linda writes that she wants to come back. You are her relative, and she would trust *you*. The case would be different if I went. She might object to coming with *me*; and the damned abolitionists, if they knew I was her master, would not believe me, if I told them she had begged to go back. They would get up a row; and I should not like to see Linda dragged through the streets like a common negro. She has been very ungrateful to me for all my kindness; but I forgive her, and want to act the part of a friend towards her. I have no wish to hold her as my slave. Her friends can buy her as soon as she arrives here."

Finding that his arguments failed to convince my uncle, the doctor "let the cat out of the bag," by saying that he had written to the mayor of Boston, to ascertain whether there was a person of my description at the street and number from which my letter was dated. He had omitted this date in the letter he had made up to read to my grandmother. If I had dated from New York, the old man would probably have made another journey to that city. But even in that dark region, where knowledge is so carefully excluded from the slave, I had heard enough about Massachusetts to come to the conclusion that slaveholders did not consider it a comfortable place to go to in search of a runaway. That was before the Fugitive Slave Law was passed; before Massachusetts had consented to become a "nigger hunter" for the south.

My grandmother, who had become skittish by seeing her family always in danger, came to me with a very distressed countenance, and said, "What will you do if the mayor of Boston sends him word that you haven't been there? Then he will suspect the letter was a trick; and maybe he'll find out something about it, and we shall all get into trouble. O Linda, I wish you had never sent the letters."

"Don't worry yourself, grandmother," said I. "The mayor of Boston won't trouble himself to hunt niggers for Dr. Flint. The letters will do good in the end. I shall get out of this dark hole some time or other."

"I hope you will, child," replied the good, patient old friend. "You have been here a long time; almost five years; but whenever you do go, it will break your old grandmother's heart. I should be expecting every day to hear that you were brought back in irons and put in jail. God help you, poor child! Let us be thankful that some time or other we shall go 'where the wicked cease from troubling, and the weary are at rest.'" My heart responded, Amen.

The fact that Dr. Flint had written to the mayor of Boston convinced me that he believed my letter to be genuine, and of course that he had no suspicion of my being any where in the vicinity. It was a great object to keep up this delusion, for it made me and my friends feel less anxious, and it would be very convenient whenever there was a chance to escape. I resolved, therefore, to continue to write letters from the north from time to time.

Two or three weeks passed, and as no news came from the mayor of Boston, grandmother began to listen to my entreaty to be allowed to leave my cell, sometimes, and exercise my limbs to prevent my becoming a cripple. I was allowed to slip down into the small storeroom, early in the morning, and remain there a little while. The room was all filled up with barrels, except a small open space under my trap-door. This faced the door, the upper part of which was of glass, and purposely left uncurtained, that the curious might look in. The air of this place was close; but it was so much better than the atmosphere of my cell, that I dreaded to return. I came down as soon as it was light, and remained till eight o'clock, when people began to be about, and there was danger that some one might come on the piazza. I had tried various applications to bring warmth and feeling into my limbs, but without avail. They were so numb and stiff that it was a painful effort to move; and had my enemies come upon me during the first mornings I tried to exercise them a little in the small unoccupied space of the storeroom, it would have been impossible for me to have escaped.

XXVI.

IMPORTANT ERA IN MY BROTHER'S LIFE.

I MISSED the company and kind attentions of my brother William, who had gone to Washington with his master, Mr. Sands. We received several letters from him, written without any allusion to me, but expressed in such a manner that I knew he did not forget me. I disguised my hand, and wrote to him in the same manner. It was a long session; and when it closed, William wrote to inform us that Mr. Sands was going to the north, to be gone some time, and that he was to accompany him. I knew that his master had promised to give him his freedom, but no time had been specified. Would William trust to a slave's chances? I remembered how we used to talk together, in our young days, about obtaining our freedom, and I thought it very doubtful whether he would come back to us.

Grandmother received a letter from Mr. Sands, saying that William had proved a most faithful servant, and he would also say a valued friend; that no mother had ever trained a better boy. He said he had travelled through the Northern States and Canada; and though the abolitionists had tried to decoy him away, they had never succeeded. He ended by saying they should be at home shortly.

We expected letters from William, describing the novelties of his journey, but none came. In time, it was reported that Mr. Sands would return late in the autumn, accompanied by a bride. Still no letters from William. I felt almost sure I should never see him again on southern soil; but had he no word of comfort to send to his friends at home? to the poor captive in her dungeon? My thoughts wandered through the dark past, and over the uncertain future. Alone in my cell, where no eye but God's could see me, I wept bitter tears. How earnestly I prayed to him to restore me to my children, and enable me to be a useful woman and a good mother!

At last the day arrived for the return of the travellers. Grandmother had made loving preparations to welcome her absent boy back to the old hearthstone. When the dinner table was laid, William's plate occupied its old place. The stage coach went by empty. My grandmother waited dinner.

She thought perhaps he was necessarily detained by his master. In my prison I listened anxiously, expecting every moment to hear my dear brother's voice and step. In the course of the afternoon a lad was sent by Mr. Sands to tell grandmother that William did not return with him; that the abolitionists had decoyed him away. But he begged her not to feel troubled about it, for he felt confident she would see William in a few days. As soon as he had time to reflect he would come back, for he could never expect to be so well off at the north as he had been with him.

If you had seen the tears, and heard the sobs, you would have thought the messenger had brought tidings of death instead of freedom. Poor old grandmother felt that she should never see her darling boy again. And I was selfish. I thought more of what I had lost, than of what my brother had gained. A new anxiety began to trouble me. Mr. Sands had expended a good deal of money, and would naturally feel irritated by the loss he had incurred. I greatly feared this might injure the prospects of my children, who were now becoming valuable property. I longed to have their emancipation made certain. The more so, because their master and father was now married. I was too familiar with slavery not to know that promises made to slaves, though with kind intentions, and sincere at the time, depend upon many contingencies for their fulfilment.

Much as I wished William to be free, the step he had taken made me sad and anxious. The following Sabbath was calm and clear; so beautiful that it seemed like a Sabbath in the eternal world. My grandmother brought the children out on the piazza, that I might hear their voices. She thought it would comfort me in my despondency; and it did. They chatted merrily, as only children can. Benny said, "Grandmother, do you think uncle Will has gone for good? Won't he ever come back again? May be he'll find mother. If he does, *won't* she be glad to see him! Why don't you and uncle Phillip, and all of us, go and live where mother is? I should like it; wouldn't you, Ellen?"

"Yes, I should like it," replied Ellen; "but how could we find her? Do you know the place, grandmother? I don't remember how mother looked—do you, Benny?"

Benny was just beginning to describe me when they were interrupted by an old slave woman, a near neighbor, named Aggie. This poor creature had witnessed the sale of her children, and seen them carried off to parts unknown, without any hopes of ever hearing from them again. She saw that my grandmother had been weeping, and she said, in a sympathizing tone, "What's the matter, aunt Marthy?"

"O Aggie," she replied, "it seems as if I shouldn't have any of my children or grandchildren left to hand me a drink when I'm dying, and lay my old body in the ground. My boy didn't come back with Mr. Sands. He staid at the north."

Poor old Aggie clapped her hands for joy. "Is *dat* what you's crying fur?" she exclaimed. "Git down on your knees and bress de Lord! I don't know whar my poor chillern is, and I nebber 'spect to know. You don't know whar poor Linda's gone to; but you *do* know whar her brudder is. He's in free parts; and dat's de right place. Don't murmur at de Lord's doings, but git down on your knees and tank him for his goodness."

My selfishness was rebuked by what poor Aggie said. She rejoiced over the escape of one who was merely her fellow-bondman, while his own sister was only thinking what his good fortune might cost her children. I knelt and prayed God to forgive me; and I thanked him from my heart, that one of my family was saved from the grasp of slavery.

It was not long before we received a letter from William. He wrote that Mr. Sands had always treated him kindly, and that he had tried to do his duty to him faithfully. But ever since he was a boy, he had longed to be free; and he had already gone through enough to convince him he had better not lose the chance that offered. He concluded by saying, "Don't worry about me, dear grandmother. I shall think of you always; and it will spur me on to work hard and try to do right. When I have earned money enough to give you a home, perhaps you will come to the north, and we can all live happy together."

Mr. Sands told my uncle Phillip the particulars about William's leaving him. He said, "I trusted him as if he were my own brother, and treated him as kindly. The abolitionists talked to him in several places; but I had no idea they could tempt him. However, I don't blame William. He's young and inconsiderate, and those Northern rascals decoyed him. I must confess the scamp was very bold about it. I met him coming down the steps of the Astor House with his trunk on his shoulder, and I asked him where he was going. He said he was going to change his old trunk. I told him it was rather shabby, and asked if he didn't need some money. He said, No, thanked me, and went off. He did not return so soon as I expected; but I waited patiently. At last I went to see if our trunks were packed, ready for our journey. I found them locked, and a sealed note on the table informed me where I could find the keys. The fellow even tried to be religious. He wrote that he hoped God would always bless me, and reward me for my kindness; that he was not unwilling to serve me; but he wanted to be a free man; and that if I thought he did wrong, he hoped I would forgive him. I intended to give him his freedom in five years. He might have trusted me. He has shown himself ungrateful; but I shall not go for him, or send for him. I feel confident that he will soon return to me."

I afterwards heard an account of the affair from William himself. He had not been urged away by abolitionists. He needed no information they could give him about slavery to stimulate his desire for freedom. He looked at his hands, and remembered that they were once in irons. What security had he that they would not be so again? Mr. Sands was kind to him; but he might indefinitely postpone the promise he had made to give him his freedom. He might come under pecuniary embarrassments, and his property be seized by creditors; or he might die, without making any arrangements in his favor. He had too often known such accidents to happen to slaves who had kind masters, and he wisely resolved to make sure of the present opportunity to own himself. He was scrupulous about taking any money from his master on false pretences; so he sold his best clothes to pay for his passage to Boston. The slaveholders pronounced him a base, ungrateful wretch, for thus requiting his master's indulgence. What would *they* have done under similar circumstances?

When Dr. Flint's family heard that William had deserted Mr. Sands, they chuckled greatly over the news. Mrs. Flint made her usual manifestations of Christian feeling, by saying,

"I'm glad of it. I hope he'll never get him again. I like to see people paid back in their own coin. I reckon Linda's children will have to pay for it. I should be glad to see them in the speculator's hands again, for I'm tired of seeing those little niggers march about the streets."

XXVII.
NEW DESTINATION FOR THE CHILDREN.

MRS. FLINT proclaimed her intention of informing Mrs. Sands who was the father of my children. She likewise proposed to tell her what an artful devil I was; that I had made a great deal of trouble in her family; that when Mr. Sands was at the north, she didn't doubt I had followed him in disguise, and persuaded William to run away. She had some reason to entertain such an idea; for I had written from the north, from time to time, and I dated my letters from various places. Many of them fell into Dr. Flint's hands, as I expected they would; and he must have come to the conclusion that I travelled about a good deal. He kept a close watch over my children, thinking they would eventually lead to my detection.

A new and unexpected trial was in store for me. One day, when Mr. Sands and his wife were walking in the street, they met Benny. The lady took a fancy to him, and exclaimed, "What a pretty little negro! Whom does he belong to?"

Benny did not hear the answer; but he came home very indignant with the stranger lady, because she had called him a negro. A few days afterwards, Mr. Sands called on my grandmother, and told her he wanted her to take the children to his house. He said he had informed his wife of his relation to them, and told her they were motherless; and she wanted to see them.

When he had gone, my grandmother came and asked what I would do. The question seemed a mockery. What *could* I do? They were Mr. Sands's slaves, and their mother was a slave, whom he had represented to be dead. Perhaps he thought I was. I was too much pained and puzzled to come to any decision; and the children were carried without my knowledge.

Mrs. Sands had a sister from Illinois staying with her. This lady, who had no children of her own, was so much pleased with Ellen, that she offered to adopt her, and bring her up as she would a daughter. Mrs. Sands wanted to take Benjamin. When grandmother reported this to me, I was tried almost beyond endurance. Was this all I was to gain by what I had suffered for the sake of having my children free? True, the prospect *seemed* fair; but I knew too well how lightly slave-holders held such "parental relations." If pecuniary troubles should come, or if the new wife required more money than could conveniently be spared, my children might be thought of as a convenient means of raising funds. I had no trust in thee, O Slavery! Never should I know peace till my children were emancipated with all due formalities of law.

I was too proud to ask Mr. Sands to do any thing for my own benefit; but I could bring myself to become a supplicant for my children. I resolved to remind him of the promise he had made me, and to throw myself upon his honor for the performance of it. I persuaded my grandmother to go to him, and tell him I was not dead, and that I earnestly entreated him to keep the promise he had made me; that I had heard of the recent proposals concerning my children, and did not feel easy to accept them; that he had promised to emancipate them, and it was time for him to redeem his pledge. I knew there was some risk in thus betraying that I was in the vicinity; but what will not a mother do for her children? He received the message with surprise, and said, "The children are free. I have never intended to claim them as slaves. Linda may decide their fate. In my opinion, they had better be sent to the north. I don't think they are quite safe here. Dr. Flint boasts that they are still in his power. He says they were his daughter's property, and as she was not of age when they were sold, the contract is not legally binding."

So, then, after all I had endured for their sakes, my poor children were between two fires; between my old master and their new master! And I was powerless. There was no protecting arm of the law for me to invoke. Mr. Sands proposed that Ellen should go, for the present, to some of his relatives, who had removed to Brooklyn, Long Island. It was promised that she should be well taken care of, and sent to school. I consented to it, as the best arrangement I could make for her. My grandmother, of course, negotiated it all; and Mrs. Sands knew of no other person in the transaction. She proposed that they should take Ellen with them to Washington, and keep her till they had a good chance of sending her, with friends, to Brooklyn. She had an infant daughter. I had had a glimpse of it, as the nurse passed with it in her arms. It was not a pleasant thought to me, that the bondwoman's child should tend her free-born sister; but there was no alternative. Ellen was made ready for the journey. O, how it tried my heart to send her away, so young, alone, among strangers! Without a mother's love to shelter her from the storms of life; almost without memory of a mother! I doubted whether she and Benny would have for me the natural affection that children feel for a parent. I thought to myself that I might perhaps never see my daughter again, and I had a great desire that she should look upon me, before she went, that she might take my image with her in her memory. It seemed to me cruel to have her brought to my dungeon. It was sorrow enough for her young heart to know that her mother was a victim of slavery, without seeing the wretched hiding-place to which it had driven her. I begged permission to pass the last night in one of the open chambers, with my little girl. They thought I was crazy to think of trusting such a young child with my perilous secret. I told them I had watched her character, and I felt sure she would not betray me; that I was determined to have an interview, and if they would not facilitate it, I would take my own way to obtain it. They remonstrated against the rashness of such a proceeding; but finding they could not change my purpose, they yielded. I slipped through the trap-door into the storeroom, and my uncle kept watch at the gate, while I passed into the piazza and went up stairs, to the room I used to occupy. It was more than five years since I had seen it; and how the memories crowded on me! There I had taken shelter when my mistress drove me from her house; there came my old tyrant, to mock, insult, and curse me; there my children were first laid in my arms; there I had watched over them, each day with a deeper and sadder love; there I had knelt to God, in anguish of heart, to forgive the wrong I had done. How vividly it all came back! And after this long, gloomy interval, I stood there such a wreck!

In the midst of these meditations, I heard footsteps on the stairs. The door opened, and my uncle Phillip came in, leading Ellen by the hand. I put my arms round her, and said, "Ellen, my dear child, I am your mother." She drew back a little, and looked at me; then, with sweet confidence, she laid her cheek against mine, and I folded her to the heart that had been so long desolated. She was the first to speak. Raising her head, she said, inquiringly, "You really *are* my mother?" I told her I really was; that during all the long time she had not seen me, I had loved her most tenderly; and that now she was going away, I wanted to see her and talk with her, that she might remember me. With a sob in her voice, she said, "I'm glad you've come to see me; but why didn't you ever come before? Benny and I have wanted so much to see you! He remembers you, and sometimes he tells me about you. Why didn't you come home when Dr. Flint went to bring you?"

I answered, "I couldn't come before, dear. But now that I am with you, tell me whether you like to go away." "I don't know," said she, crying. "Grandmother says I ought not to cry; that I am going to a good place, where I can learn to read and write, and that by and by I can write her a letter. But I shan't have Benny, or grandmother, or uncle Phillip, or any body to love me. Can't you go with me? O, *do* go, dear mother!"

I told her I couldn't go now; but sometime I would come to her, and then she and Benny and I would live together, and have happy times. She wanted to run and bring Benny to see me now. I told her he was going to the north, before long, with uncle Phillip, and then I would come to see him before he went away. I asked if she would like to have me stay all night and sleep with her. "O, yes," she replied. Then, turning to her uncle, she said, pleadingly, "*May* I stay? Please, uncle! She is my own mother." He laid his hand on her head, and said, solemnly, "Ellen, this is the secret you have promised grandmother never to tell. If you ever speak of it to any body, they will never let you see your grandmother again, and your mother can never come to Brooklyn." "Uncle," she replied, "I will never tell." He told her she might stay with me; and when he had gone, I took her in my arms and told her I was a slave, and that was the reason she must never say she had seen me. I exhorted her to be a good child, to try to please the people where she was going, and that God would raise her up friends. I told her to say her prayers, and remember always to pray for her poor mother, and that God would permit us to meet again. She wept, and I did not check her tears. Perhaps she would never again have a chance to pour her tears into a mother's bosom. All night she nestled in my arms, and I had no inclination to slumber. The moments were too precious to lose any of them. Once, when I thought she was asleep, I kissed her forehead softly, and she said, "I am not asleep, dear mother."

Before dawn they came to take me back to my den. I drew aside the window curtain, to take a last look of my child. The moonlight shone on her face, and I bent over her, as I had done years before, that wretched night when I ran away. I hugged her close to my throbbing heart; and tears, too sad for such young eyes to shed, flowed down her cheeks, as she gave her last kiss, and whispered in my ear, "Mother, I will never tell." And she never did.

When I got back to my den, I threw myself on the bed and wept there alone in the darkness. It seemed as if my heart would burst. When the time for Ellen's departure drew nigh, I could hear neighbors and friends saying to her, "Good by, Ellen. I hope your poor mother will find you out. *Won't* you be glad to see her!" She replied, "Yes, ma'am;" and they little dreamed of the weighty secret that weighed down her young heart. She was an affectionate child, but naturally very reserved, except with those she loved, and I felt secure that my secret would be safe with her. I heard the gate close after her, with such feelings as only a slave mother can experience. During the day my meditations were very sad. Sometimes I feared I had been very selfish not to give up all claim to her, and let her go to Illinois, to be adopted by Mrs. Sands's sister. It was my experience of slavery that decided me against it. I feared that circumstances might arise that would cause her to be sent back. I felt confident that I should go to New York myself; and then I should be able to watch over her, and in some degree protect her.

Dr. Flint's family knew nothing of the proposed arrangement till after Ellen was gone, and the news displeased them greatly. Mrs. Flint called on Mrs. Sands's sister to inquire into the matter. She expressed her opinion very freely as to the respect Mr. Sands showed for his wife, and for his own character, in acknowledging those "young niggers." And as for sending Ellen away, she pronounced it to be just as much stealing as it would be for him to come and take a piece of furniture out of her parlor. She said her daughter was not of age to sign the bill of sale, and the children were her property; and when she became of age, or was married, she could take them, wherever she could lay hands on them.

Miss Emily Flint, the little girl to whom I had been bequeathed, was now in her sixteenth year. Her mother considered it all right and honorable for her, or her future husband, to steal my children; but she did not understand how any body could hold up their heads in respectable society, after they had purchased their own children, as Mr. Sands had done. Dr. Flint said very little. Perhaps he thought that Benny would be less likely to be sent away if he kept quiet. One of my letters, that fell into his hands, was dated from Canada; and he seldom spoke of me now. This state of things enabled me to slip down into the storeroom more frequently, where I could stand upright, and move my limbs more freely.

Days, weeks, and months passed, and there came no news of Ellen. I sent a letter to Brooklyn, written in my grandmother's name, to inquire whether she had arrived there. Answer was returned that she had not. I wrote to her in Washington; but no notice was taken of it. There was one person there, who ought to have had some sympathy with the anxiety of the child's friends at home; but the links of such relations as he had formed with me, are easily broken and cast away as rubbish. Yet how protectingly and persuasively he once talked to the poor, helpless slave girl! And how entirely I trusted him! But now suspicions darkened my mind. Was my child dead, or had they deceived me, and sold her?

If the secret memoirs of many members of Congress should be published, curious details would be unfolded. I once saw a letter from a member of Congress to a slave, who was the mother of six of his children. He wrote to request that she would send her children away from the great house before his return, as he expected to be accompanied by friends. The woman could not read, and was obliged to employ another to read the letter. The existence of the colored children did not trouble this gentleman, it was only the fear that friends might recognize in their features a resemblance to him.

At the end of six months, a letter came to my grandmother, from Brooklyn. It was written by a young lady in the family, and announced that Ellen had just arrived. It contained the following message from her: "I do try to do just as you told me to, and I pray for you every night and morning." I understood that these words were meant for me; and they were a balsam to my heart. The writer closed her letter by saying, "Ellen is a nice little girl, and we shall like to have her with us. My cousin, Mr. Sands, has given her to me, to be my little waiting maid. I shall send her to school, and I hope some day she will write to you herself." This letter perplexed and troubled me. Had my child's father merely placed her there till she was old enough to support herself? Or had he given her to his cousin, as a piece of property? If the last idea was correct, his cousin might return to the south at any time, and hold Ellen as a slave. I tried to put away from me the painful thought that such a foul wrong could have been done to us. I said to myself, "Surely there must be *some* justice in man;" then I remembered, with a sigh, how slavery perverted all the natural feelings of the human heart. It gave me a pang to look on my light-hearted boy. He believed himself free; and to have him brought under the yoke of slavery, would be more than I could bear. How I longed to have him safely out of the reach of its power!

XXVIII.

AUNT NANCY.

I HAVE mentioned my great-aunt, who was a slave in Dr. Flint's family, and who had been my refuge during the shameful persecutions I suffered from him. This aunt had been married at twenty years of age; that is, as far as slaves *can* marry.

She had the consent of her master and mistress, and a clergy-man performed the ceremony. But it was a mere form, without any legal value. Her master or mistress could annul it any day they pleased. She had always slept on the floor in the entry, near Mrs. Flint's chamber door, that she might be within call. When she was married, she was told she might have the use of a small room in an out-house. Her mother and her husband furnished it. He was a seafaring man, and was allowed to sleep there when he was at home. But on the wedding evening, the bride was ordered to her old post on the entry floor.

Mrs. Flint, at that time, had no children; but she was expecting to be a mother, and if she should want a drink of water in the night, what could she do without her slave to bring it? So my aunt was compelled to lie at her door, until one midnight she was forced to leave, to give premature birth to a child. In a fortnight she was required to resume her place on the entry floor, because Mrs. Flint's babe needed her attentions. She kept her station there through summer and winter, until she had given premature birth to six children; and all the while she was employed as night-nurse to Mrs. Flint's children. Finally, toiling all day, and being deprived of rest at night, completely broke down her constitution, and Dr. Flint declared it was impossible she could ever become the mother of a living child. The fear of losing so valuable a servant by death, now induced them to allow her to sleep in her little room in the out-house, except when there was sickness in the family. She afterwards had two feeble babes, one of whom died in a few days, and the other in four weeks. I well remember her patient sorrow as she held the last dead baby in her arms. "I wish it could have lived," she said; "it is not the will of God that any of my children should live. But I will try to be fit to meet their little spirits in heaven."

Aunt Nancy was housekeeper and waiting-maid in Dr. Flint's family. Indeed, she was the *factotum* of the household. Nothing went on well without her. She was my mother's twin sister, and, as far as was in her power, she supplied a mother's place to us orphans. I slept with her all the time I lived in my old master's house, and the bond between us was very strong. When my friends tried to discourage me from running away, she always encouraged me. When they thought I had better return and ask my master's pardon, because there was no possibility of escape, she sent me word never to yield. She said if I persevered I might, perhaps, gain the freedom of my children; and even if I perished in doing it, that was better than to leave them to groan under the same persecutions that had blighted my own life. After I was shut up in my dark cell, she stole away, whenever she could, to bring me the news and say something cheering. How often did I kneel down to listen to her words of consolation, whispered through a crack! "I am old, and have not long to live," she used to say; "and I could die happy if I could only see you and the children free. You must pray to God, Linda, as I do for you, that he will lead you out of this darkness." I would beg her not to worry herself on my account; that there was an end of all suffering sooner or later, and that whether I lived in chains or in freedom, I should always remember her as the good friend who had been the comfort of my life. A word from her always strengthened me; and not me only. The whole family relied upon her judgment, and were guided by her advice.

I had been in my cell six years when my grandmother was summoned to the bedside of this, her last remaining daughter. She was very ill, and they said she would die. Grandmother had not entered Dr. Flint's house for several years. They had treated her cruelly, but she thought nothing of that now. She was grateful for permission to watch by the deathbed of her child. They had always been devoted to each other; and now they sat looking into each other's eyes, longing to speak of the secret that had weighed so much on the hearts of both. My aunt had been stricken with paralysis. She lived but two days, and the last day she was speechless. Before she lost the power of utterance, she told her mother not to grieve if she could not speak to her; that she would try to hold up her hand, to let her know that all was well with her. Even the hard-hearted doctor was a little softened when he saw the dying woman try to smile on the aged mother, who was kneeling by her side. His eyes moistened for a moment, as he said she had always been a faithful servant, and they should never be able to supply her place. Mrs. Flint took to her bed, quite overcome by the shock. While my grandmother sat alone with the dead, the doctor came in, leading his youngest son, who had always been a great pet with aunt Nancy, and was much attached to her. "Martha," said he, "aunt Nancy loved this child, and when he comes where you are, I hope you will be kind to him, for her sake." She replied, "Your wife was my foster-child, Dr. Flint, the foster-sister of my poor Nancy, and you little know me if you think I can feel any thing but good will for her children."

"I wish the past could be forgotten, and that we might never think of it," said he; "and that Linda would come to supply her aunt's place. She would be worth more to us than all the money that could be paid for her. I wish it for your sake also, Martha. Now that Nancy is taken away from you, she would be a great comfort to your old age."

He knew he was touching a tender chord. Almost choking with grief, my grandmother replied, "It was not I that drove Linda away. My grandchildren are gone; and of my nine children only one is left. God help me!"

To me, the death of this kind relative was an inexpressible sorrow. I knew that she had been slowly murdered; and I felt that my troubles had helped to finish the work. After I heard of her illness, I listened constantly to hear what news was brought from the great house; and the thought that I could not go to her made me utterly miserable. At last, as uncle Phillip came into the house, I heard some one inquire, "How is she?" and he answered, "She is dead." My little cell seemed whirling round, and I knew nothing more till I opened my eyes and found uncle Phillip bending over me. I had no need to ask any questions. He whispered, "Linda, she died happy." I could not weep. My fixed gaze troubled him. "Don't look *so*," he said. "Don't add to my poor mother's trouble. Remember how much she has to bear, and that we ought to do all we can to comfort her." Ah, yes, that blessed old grandmother, who for seventy-three years had borne the pelting storms of a slave-mother's life. She did indeed need consolation!

Mrs. Flint had rendered her poor foster-sister childless, apparently without any compunction; and with cruel selfishness had ruined her health by years of incessant, unrequited toil, and broken rest. But now she became very sentimental. I suppose she thought it would be a beautiful illustration of the attachment existing between slaveholder and slave, if the body of her old worn-out servant was buried at her feet. She sent for the clergyman and asked if he had any objection to burying aunt Nancy in the doctor's family burial-place. No colored person had ever been allowed interment in the white people's burying-ground, and the minister knew that all the deceased of our family reposed together in the old graveyard of the slaves. He therefore replied, "I have no objection to complying with your wish; but perhaps aunt Nancy's *mother* may have some choice as to where her remains shall be deposited."

It had never occurred to Mrs. Flint that slaves could have any feelings. When my grandmother was consulted, she at once said she wanted Nancy to lie with all the rest of her family, and where her own old body would be buried. Mrs. Flint graciously complied with her wish, though she said it was painful to her to have Nancy buried away from *her*. She might have added with touching pathos, "I was so long *used* to sleep with her lying near me, on the entry floor."

My uncle Phillip asked permission to bury his sister at his own expense; and slaveholders are always ready to grant *such* favors to slaves and their relatives. The arrangements were very plain, but perfectly respectable. She was buried on the Sabbath, and Mrs. Flint's minister read the funeral service. There was a large concourse of colored people, bond and free, and a few white persons who had always been friendly to our family. Dr. Flint's carriage was in the procession; and when the body was deposited in its humble resting place, the mistress dropped a tear, and returned to her carriage, probably thinking she had performed her duty nobly.

It was talked of by the slaves as a mighty grand funeral. Northern travellers, passing through the place, might have described this tribute of respect to the humble dead as a beautiful feature in the "patriarchal institution;" a touching proof of the attachment between slaveholders and their servants; and tender-hearted Mrs. Flint would have confirmed this impression, with handkerchief at her eyes. *We* could have told them a different story. We could have given them a chapter of wrongs and sufferings, that would have touched their hearts, if they *had* any hearts to feel for the colored people. We could have told them how the poor old slave-mother had toiled, year after year, to earn eight hundred dollars to buy her son Phillip's right to his own earnings; and how that same Phillip paid the expenses of the funeral, which they regarded as doing so much credit to the master. We could also have told them of a poor, blighted young creature, shut up in a living grave for years, to avoid the tortures that would be inflicted on her, if she ventured to come out and look on the face of her departed friend.

All this, and much more, I thought of, as I sat at my loop-hole, waiting for the family to return from the grave; sometimes weeping, sometimes falling asleep, dreaming strange dreams of the dead and the living.

It was sad to witness the grief of my bereaved grandmother. She had always been strong to bear, and now, as ever, religious faith supported her. But her dark life had become still darker, and age and trouble were leaving deep traces on her withered face. She had four places to knock for me to come to the trap-door, and each place had a different meaning. She now came oftener than she had done, and talked to me of her dead daughter, while tears trickled slowly down her furrowed cheeks. I said all I could to comfort her; but it was a sad reflection, that instead of being able to help her, I was a constant source of anxiety and trouble. The poor old back was fitted to its burden. It bent under it, but did not break.

XXIX.

PREPARATIONS FOR ESCAPE.

I HARDLY expect that the reader will credit me, when I affirm that I lived in that little dismal hole, almost deprived of light and air, and with no space to move my limbs, for nearly seven years. But it is a fact; and to me a sad one, even now; for my body still suffers from the effects of that long imprisonment, to say nothing of my soul. Members of my family, now living in New York and Boston, can testify to the truth of what I say.

Countless were the nights that I sat late at the little loophole scarcely large enough to give me a glimpse of one twin-kling star. There, I heard the patrols and slave-hunters con-ferring together about the capture of runaways, well knowing how rejoiced they would be to catch me.

Season after season, year after year, I peeped at my chil-dren's faces, and heard their sweet voices, with a heart yearn-ing all the while to say, "Your mother is here." Sometimes it appeared to me as if ages had rolled away since I entered upon that gloomy, monotonous existence. At times, I was stupefied and listless; at other times I became very impatient to know when these dark years would end, and I should again be allowed to feel the sunshine, and breathe the pure air.

After Ellen left us, this feeling increased. Mr. Sands had agreed that Benny might go to the north whenever his uncle Phillip could go with him; and I was anxious to be there also, to watch over my children, and protect them so far as I was able. Moreover, I was likely to be drowned out of my den, if I remained much longer; for the slight roof was getting badly out of repair, and uncle Phillip was afraid to remove the shin-gles, lest some one should get a glimpse of me. When storms occurred in the night, they spread mats and bits of carpet, which in the morning appeared to have been laid out to dry; but to cover the roof in the daytime might have attracted at-tention. Consequently, my clothes and bedding were often drenched; a process by which the pains and aches in my cramped and stiffened limbs were greatly increased. I revolved various plans of escape in my mind, which I sometimes im-parted to my grandmother, when she came to whisper with me at the trap-door. The kind-hearted old woman had an in-tense sympathy for runaways. She had known too much of the cruelties inflicted on those who were captured. Her mem-ory always flew back at once to the sufferings of her bright and handsome son, Benjamin, the youngest and dearest of her flock. So, whenever I alluded to the subject, she would groan out, "O, don't think of it, child. You'll break my heart." I had no good old aunt Nancy now to encourage me; but my brother William and my children were continually beckoning me to the north.

And now I must go back a few months in my story. I have stated that the first of January was the time for selling slaves, or leasing them out to new masters. If time were counted by heart-throbs, the poor slaves might reckon years of suffering during that festival so joyous to the free. On the New Year's day preceding my aunt's death, one of my friends, named Fanny, was to be sold at auction, to pay her master's debts. My thoughts were with her during all the day, and at night I anxiously inquired what had been her fate. I was told that she had been sold to one master, and her four little girls to another master, far distant; that she had escaped from her purchaser, and was not to be found. Her mother was the old Aggie I have spoken of. She lived in a small tenement belonging to my grandmother, and built on the same lot with her own house. Her dwelling was searched and watched, and that brought the patrols so near me that I was obliged to keep very close in my den. The hunters were somehow eluded; and not long afterwards Benny accidentally caught sight of Fanny in her mother's hut. He told his grandmother, who charged him never to speak of it, explaining to him the frightful consequences; and he never betrayed the trust. Aggie little dreamed that my grandmother knew where her daughter was concealed, and that the stooping form of her old neighbor was bending under a similar burden of anxiety and fear; but these dangerous secrets deepened the sympathy between the two old persecuted mothers.

My friend Fanny and I remained many weeks hidden within call of each other; but she was unconscious of the fact. I longed to have her share my den, which seemed a more secure retreat than her own; but I had brought so much trouble on my grandmother, that it seemed wrong to ask her to incur greater risks. My restlessness increased. I had lived too long in bodily pain and anguish of spirit. Always I was in dread that by some accident, or some contrivance, slavery would succeed in snatching my children from me. This thought drove me nearly frantic, and I determined to steer for the North Star at all hazards. At this crisis, Providence opened an unexpected way for me to escape. My friend Peter came one evening, and asked to speak with me. "Your day has come, Linda," said he. "I have found a chance for you to go to the Free States. You have a fortnight to decide." The news seemed too good to be true; but Peter explained his arrangements, and told me all that was necessary was for me to say I would go. I was going to answer him with a joyful yes, when the thought of Benny came to my mind. I told him the temptation was exceedingly strong, but I was terribly afraid of Dr. Flint's alleged power over my child, and that I could not go and leave him behind. Peter remonstrated earnestly. He said such a good chance might never occur again; that Benny was free, and could be sent to me; and that for the sake of my children's welfare I ought not to hesitate a moment. I told him I would consult with uncle Phillip. My uncle rejoiced in the plan, and bade me go by all means. He promised, if his life was spared, that he would either bring or send my son to me as soon as I reached a place of safety. I resolved to go, but thought nothing had better be said to my grandmother till very near the time of departure. But my uncle thought she would feel it more keenly if I left her so suddenly. "I will reason with her," said he, "and convince her how necessary it is, not only for your sake, but for hers also. You cannot be blind to the fact that she is sinking under her burdens." I was not blind to it. I knew that my concealment was an ever-present source of anxiety, and that the older she grew the more nervously fearful she was of discovery. My uncle talked with her, and finally succeeded in persuading her that it was absolutely necessary for me to seize the chance so unexpectedly offered.

The anticipation of being a free woman proved almost too much for my weak frame. The excitement stimulated me, and at the same time bewildered me. I made busy preparations for my journey, and for my son to follow me. I resolved to have an interview with him before I went, that I might give him cautions and advice, and tell him how anxiously I should be waiting for him at the north. Grandmother stole up to me as often as possible to whisper words of counsel. She insisted upon my writing to Dr. Flint, as soon as I arrived in the Free States, and asking him to sell me to her. She said she would sacrifice her house, and all she had in the world, for the sake of having me safe with my children in any part of the world. If she could only live to know *that* she could die in peace. I promised the dear old faithful friend that I would write to her as soon as I arrived, and put the letter in a safe way to reach her; but in my own mind I resolved that not another cent of her hard earnings should be spent to pay rapacious slaveholders for what they called their property. And even if I had not been unwilling to buy what I had already a right to possess, common humanity would have prevented me from accepting the generous offer, at the expense of turning my aged relative out of house and home, when she was trembling on the brink of the grave.

I was to escape in a vessel; but I forbear to mention any further particulars. I was in readiness, but the vessel was unexpectedly detained several days. Meantime, news came to town of a most horrible murder committed on a fugitive slave, named James. Charity, the mother of this unfortunate young man, had been an old acquaintance of ours. I have told the shocking particulars of his death, in my description of some of the neighboring slaveholders. My grandmother, always nervously sensitive about runaways, was terribly frightened. She felt sure that a similar fate awaited me, if I did not desist from my enterprise. She sobbed, and groaned, and entreated me not to go. Her excessive fear was somewhat contagious, and my heart was not proof against her extreme agony. I was grievously disappointed, but I promised to relinquish my project.

When my friend Peter was apprised of this, he was both disappointed and vexed. He said, that judging from our past experience, it would be a long time before I had such another chance to throw away. I told him it need not be thrown away; that I had a friend concealed near by, who would be glad enough to take the place that had been provided for me. I told him about poor Fanny, and tho kind-hearted, noble fellow, who never turned his back upon any body in distress, white or black, expressed his readiness to help her. Aggie was much surprised when she found that we knew her secret. She was rejoiced to hear of such a chance for Fanny, and arrangements were made for her to go on board the vessel the next night. They both supposed that I had long been at the north, therefore my name was not mentioned in the transaction. Fanny was carried on board at the appointed time, and stowed away in a very small cabin. This accommodation had been purchased at a price that would pay for a voyage to England. But when one proposes to go to fine old England, they stop to calculate whether they can afford the cost of the pleasure; while in making a bargain to escape from slavery, the trembling victim is ready to say, "Take all I have, only don't betray me!"

The next morning I peeped through my loophole, and saw that it was dark and cloudy. At night I received news that the wind was ahead, and the vessel had not sailed. I was exceedingly anxious about Fanny, and Peter too, who was running a tremendous risk at my instigation. Next day the wind and weather remained the same. Poor Fanny had been half dead with fright when they carried her on board, and I could readily imagine how she must be suffering now. Grandmother came often to my den, to say how thankful she was I did not go. On the third morning she rapped for me to come down to the storeroom. The poor old sufferer was breaking down under her weight of trouble. She was easily flurried now. I found her in a nervous, excited state, but I was not aware that she had forgotten to lock the door behind her, as usual. She was exceedingly worried about the detention of the vessel. She was afraid all would be discovered, and then Fanny, and Peter, and I, would all be tortured to death, and Phillip would be utterly ruined, and her house would be torn down. Poor Peter! If he should die such a horrible death as the poor slave James had lately done, and all for his kindness in trying to help me, how dreadful it would be for us all! Alas, the thought was familiar to me, and had sent many a sharp pang through my heart. I tried to suppress my own anxiety, and speak soothingly to her. She brought in some allusion to aunt Nancy, the dear daughter she had recently buried, and then she lost all control of herself. As she stood there, trembling and sobbing, a voice from the piazza called out, "Whar is you, aunt Marthy?" Grandmother was startled, and in her agitation opened the door, without thinking of me. In stepped Jenny, the mischievous housemaid, who had tried to enter my room, when I was concealed in the house of my white benefactress. "I's bin huntin ebery whar for you, aunt Marthy," said she. "My missis wants you to send her some crackers." I had slunk down behind a barrel, which entirely screened me, but I imagined that Jenny was looking directly at the spot, and my

heart beat violently. My grandmother immediately thought
what she had done, and went out quickly with Jenny to count
the crackers locking the door after her. She returned to me, in
a few minutes, the perfect picture of despair. "Poor child!"
she exclaimed, "my carelessness has ruined you. The boat
ain't gone yet. Get ready immediately, and go with Fanny. I
ain't got another word to say against it now; for there's no
telling what may happen this day."

Uncle Phillip was sent for, and he agreed with his mother
in thinking that Jenny would inform Dr. Flint in less than
twenty-four hours. He advised getting me on board the boat,
if possible; if not, I had better keep very still in my den, where
they could not find me without tearing the house down. He
said it would not do for him to move in the matter, because
suspicion would be immediately excited; but he promised to
communicate with Peter. I felt reluctant to apply to him
again, having implicated him too much already; but there
seemed to be no alternative. Vexed as Peter had been by my
indecision, he was true to his generous nature, and said at
once that he would do his best to help me, trusting I should
show myself a stronger woman this time.

He immediately proceeded to the wharf, and found that
the wind had shifted, and the vessel was slowly beating down
stream. On some pretext of urgent necessity, he offered two
boatmen a dollar apiece to catch up with her. He was of
lighter complexion than the boatmen he hired, and when the
captain saw them coming so rapidly, he thought officers were
pursuing his vessel in search of the runaway slave he had on
board. They hoisted sails, but the boat gained upon them,
and the indefatigable Peter sprang on board.

The captain at once recognized him. Peter asked him to go
below, to speak about a bad bill he had given him. When he
told his errand, the captain replied, "Why, the woman's here
already; and I've put her where you or the devil would have a
tough job to find her."

"But it is another woman I want to bring," said Peter. "*She*
is in great distress, too, and you shall be paid any thing within
reason, if you'll stop and take her."

"What's her name?" inquired the captain.

"Linda," he replied.

"That's the name of the woman already here," rejoined the captain. "By George! I believe you mean to betray me."

"O!" exclaimed Peter, "God knows I wouldn't harm a hair of your head. I am too grateful to you. But there really *is* another woman in great danger. Do have the humanity to stop and take her!"

After a while they came to an understanding. Fanny, not dreaming I was any where about in that region, had assumed my name, though she called herself Johnson. "Linda is a common name," said Peter, "and the woman I want to bring is Linda Brent."

The captain agreed to wait at a certain place till evening, being handsomely paid for his detention.

Of course, the day was an anxious one for us all. But we concluded that if Jenny had seen me, she would be too wise to let her mistress know of it; and that she probably would not get a chance to see Dr. Flint's family till evening, for I knew very well what were the rules in that household. I afterwards believed that she did not see me; for nothing ever came of it, and she was one of those base characters that would have jumped to betray a suffering fellow being for the sake of thirty pieces of silver.

I made all my arrangements to go on board as soon as it was dusk. The intervening time I resolved to spend with my son. I had not spoken to him for seven years, though I had been under the same roof, and seen him every day, when I was well enough to sit at the loophole. I did not dare to venture beyond the storeroom; so they brought him there, and locked us up together, in a place concealed from the piazza door. It was an agitating interview for both of us. After we had talked and wept together for a little while, he said, "Mother, I'm glad you're going away. I wish I could go with you. I knew you was here; and I have been *so* afraid they would come and catch you!"

I was greatly surprised, and asked him how he had found it out.

He replied, "I was standing under the eaves, one day, before Ellen went away, and I heard somebody cough up over the wood shed. I don't know what made me think it was you, but I did think so. I missed Ellen, the night before she went away; and grandmother brought her back into the room in the night; and I thought maybe she'd been to see *you*, before she went, for I heard grandmother whisper to her, 'Now go to sleep; and remember never to tell.' "

I asked him if he ever mentioned his suspicions to his sister. He said he never did; but after he heard the cough, if he saw her playing with other children on that side of the house, he always tried to coax her round to the other side, for fear they would hear me cough, too. He said he had kept a close look-out for Dr. Flint, and if he saw him speak to a constable, or a patrol, he always told grandmother. I now recollected that I had seen him manifest uneasiness, when people were on that side of the house, and I had at the time been puzzled to conjecture a motive for his actions. Such prudence may seem extraordinary in a boy of twelve years, but slaves, being surrounded by mysteries, deceptions, and dangers, early learn to be suspicious and watchful, and prematurely cautious and cunning. He had never asked a question of grandmother, or uncle Phillip, and I had often heard him chime in with other children, when they spoke of my being at the north.

I told him I was now really going to the Free States, and if he was a good, honest boy, and a loving child to his dear old grandmother, the Lord would bless him, and bring him to me, and we and Ellen would live together. He began to tell me that grandmother had not eaten any thing all day. While he was speaking, the door was unlocked, and she came in with a small bag of money, which she wanted me to take. I begged her to keep a part of it, at least, to pay for Benny's being sent to the north; but she insisted, while her tears were falling fast, that I should take the whole. "You may be sick among strangers," she said, "and they would send you to the poorhouse to die." Ah, that good grandmother!

For the last time I went up to my nook. Its desolate appearance no longer chilled me, for the light of hope had risen in my soul. Yet, even with the blessed prospect of freedom before me, I felt very sad at leaving forever that old homestead, where I had been sheltered so long by the dear old grandmother; where I had dreamed my first young dream of love; and where, after that had faded away, my children came to twine themselves so closely round my desolate heart. As the hour approached for me to leave, I again descended to the storeroom. My grandmother and Benny were there. She took me by the hand, and said, "Linda, let us pray." We knelt down together, with my child pressed to my heart, and my other arm round the faithful, loving old friend I was about to leave forever. On no other occasion has it ever been my lot to listen to so fervent a supplication for mercy and protection. It thrilled through my heart, and inspired me with trust in God.

Peter was waiting for me in the street. I was soon by his side, faint in body, but strong of purpose. I did not look back upon the old place, though I felt that I should never see it again.

XXX.

NORTHWARD BOUND.

I NEVER could tell how we reached the wharf. My brain was all of a whirl, and my limbs tottered under me. At an appointed place we met my uncle Phillip, who had started before us on a different route, that he might reach the wharf first, and give us timely warning if there was any danger. A row-boat was in readiness. As I was about to step in, I felt something pull me gently, and turning round I saw Benny, looking pale and anxious. He whispered in my ear, "I've been peeping into the doctor's window, and he's at home. Good by, mother. Don't cry; I'll come." He hastened away. I clasped the hand of my good uncle, to whom I owed so much, and of Peter, the brave, generous friend who had volunteered to run such terrible risks to secure my safety. To this day I remember how his bright face beamed with joy, when he told me he had discovered a safe method for me to escape. Yet that intelligent, enterprising, noble-hearted man was a chattel! liable, by the laws of a country that calls itself civilized, to be sold with horses and pigs! We parted in silence. Our hearts were all too full for words!

Swiftly the boat glided over the water. After a while, one of the sailors said, "Don't be down-hearted, madam. We will take you safely to your husband, in ——." At first I could not imagine what he meant; but I had presence of mind to think that it probably referred to something the captain had told him; so I thanked him, and said I hoped we should have pleasant weather.

When I entered the vessel the captain came forward to meet me. He was an elderly man, with a pleasant countenance. He showed me to a little box of a cabin, where sat my friend Fanny. She started as if she had seen a spectre. She gazed on me in utter astonishment, and exclaimed, "Linda, can this be *you*? or is it your ghost?" When we were locked in each other's arms, my overwrought feelings could no longer be restrained. My sobs reached the ears of the captain, who came and very kindly reminded us, that for his safety, as well as our own, it would be prudent for us not to attract any attention. He said that when there was a sail in sight he wished us to keep below; but at other times, he had no objection to our being on deck. He assured us that he would keep a good lookout, and if we acted prudently, he thought we should be in no danger. He had represented us as women going to meet our husbands in ——. We thanked him, and promised to observe carefully all the directions he gave us.

Fanny and I now talked by ourselves, low and quietly, in our little cabin. She told me of the sufferings she had gone through in making her escape, and of her terrors while she was concealed in her mother's house. Above all, she dwelt on the agony of separation from all her children on that dreadful auction day. She could scarcely credit me, when I told her of the place where I had passed nearly seven years. "We have the same sorrows," said I. "No," replied she, "you are going to see your children soon, and there is no hope that I shall ever even hear from mine."

The vessel was soon under way, but we made slow progress. The wind was against us. I should not have cared for this, if we had been out of sight of the town; but until there were miles of water between us and our enemies, we were filled with constant apprehensions that the constables would come on board. Neither could I feel quite at ease with the captain and his men. I was an entire stranger to that class of people, and I had heard that sailors were rough, and sometimes cruel. We were so completely in their power, that if they were bad men, our situation would be dreadful. Now that the captain was paid for our passage, might he not be tempted to make more money by giving us up to those who claimed us as property? I was naturally of a confiding disposition, but slavery had made me suspicious of every body. Fanny did not share my distrust of the captain or his men. She said she was afraid at first, but she had been on board three days while the vessel lay in the dock, and nobody had betrayed her, or treated her otherwise than kindly.

The captain soon came to advise us to go on deck for fresh air. His friendly and respectful manner, combined with Fanny's testimony, reassured me, and we went with him. He placed us in a comfortable seat, and occasionally entered into conversation. He told us he was a Southerner by birth, and had spent the greater part of his life in the Slave States, and that he had recently lost a brother who traded in slaves. "But," said he, "it is a pitiable and degrading business, and I always felt ashamed to acknowledge my brother in connection with it." As we passed Snaky Swamp, he pointed to it, and said, "There is a slave territory that defies all the laws." I thought of the terrible days I had spent there, and though it was not called Dismal Swamp, it made me feel very dismal as I looked at it.

I shall never forget that night. The balmy air of spring was so refreshing! And how shall I describe my sensations when we were fairly sailing on Chesapeake Bay? O, the beautiful sunshine! the exhilarating breeze! and I could enjoy them without fear or restraint. I had never realized what grand things air and sunlight are till I had been deprived of them.

Ten days after we left land we were approaching Philadelphia. The captain said we should arrive there in the night, but he thought we had better wait till morning, and go on shore in broad daylight, as the best way to avoid suspicion.

I replied, "You know best. But will you stay on board and protect us?"

He saw that I was suspicious, and he said he was sorry, now that he had brought us to the end of our voyage, to find I had so little confidence in him. Ah, if he had ever been a slave he would have known how difficult it was to trust a white man. He assured us that we might sleep through the night

without fear; that he would take care we were not left unprotected. Be it said to the honor of this captain, Southerner as
he was, that if Fanny and I had been white ladies, and our
passage lawfully engaged, he could not have treated us more
respectfully. My intelligent friend, Peter, had rightly estimated
the character of the man to whose honor he had intrusted us.

The next morning I was on deck as soon as the day
dawned. I called Fanny to see the sun rise, for the first time in
our lives, on free soil; for such I *then* believed it to be. We
watched the reddening sky, and saw the great orb come up
slowly out of the water, as it seemed. Soon the waves began
to sparkle, and every thing caught the beautiful glow. Before
us lay the city of strangers. We looked at each other, and the
eyes of both were moistened with tears. We had escaped from
slavery, and we supposed ourselves to be safe from the
hunters. But we were alone in the world, and we had left dear
ties behind us; ties cruelly sundered by the demon Slavery.

XXXI.

INCIDENTS IN PHILADELPHIA.

I HAD heard that the poor slave had many friends at the
north. I trusted we should find some of them. Meantime, we
would take it for granted that all were friends, till they proved
to the contrary. I sought out the kind captain, thanked him
for his attentions, and told him I should never cease to be
grateful for the service he had rendered us. I gave him a message to the friends I had left at home, and he promised to deliver it. We were placed in a row-boat, and in about fifteen
minutes were landed on a wood wharf in Philadelphia. As I
stood looking round, the friendly captain touched me on the
shoulder, and said, "There is a respectable-looking colored
man behind you. I will speak to him about the New York
trains, and tell him you wish to go directly on." I thanked
him, and asked him to direct me to some shops where I could
buy gloves and veils. He did so, and said he would talk with
the colored man till I returned. I made what haste I could.
Constant exercise on board the vessel, and frequent rubbing

with salt water, had nearly restored the use of my limbs. The noise of the great city confused me, but I found the shops, and bought some double veils and gloves for Fanny and myself. The shopman told me they were so many levies. I had never heard the word before, but I did not tell him so. I thought if he knew I was a stranger he might ask me where I came from. I gave him a gold piece, and when he returned the change, I counted it, and found out how much a levy was. I made my way back to the wharf, where the captain introduced me to the colored man, as the Rev. Jeremiah Durham, minister of Bethel church. He took me by the hand, as if I had been an old friend. He told us we were too late for the morning cars to New York, and must wait until the evening, or the next morning. He invited me to go home with him, assuring me that his wife would give me a cordial welcome; and for my friend he would provide a home with one of his neighbors. I thanked him for so much kindness to strangers, and told him if I must be detained, I should like to hunt up some people who formerly went from our part of the country. Mr. Durham insisted that I should dine with him, and then he would assist me in finding my friends. The sailors came to bid us good by. I shook their hardy hands, with tears in my eyes. They had all been kind to us, and they had rendered us a greater service than they could possibly conceive of.

I had never seen so large a city, or been in contact with so many people in the streets. It seemed as if those who passed looked at us with an expression of curiosity. My face was so blistered and peeled, by sitting on deck, in wind and sunshine, that I thought they could not easily decide to what nation I belonged.

Mrs. Durham met me with a kindly welcome, without asking any questions. I was tired, and her friendly manner was a sweet refreshment. God bless her! I was sure that she had comforted other weary hearts, before I received her sympathy. She was surrounded by her husband and children, in a home made sacred by protecting laws. I thought of my own children, and sighed.

After dinner Mr. Durham went with me in quest of the friends I had spoken of. They went from my native town, and I anticipated much pleasure in looking on familiar faces. They were not at home, and we retraced our steps through streets delightfully clean. On the way, Mr. Durham observed that I had spoken to him of a daughter I expected to meet; that he was surprised, for I looked so young he had taken me for a single woman. He was approaching a subject on which I was extremely sensitive. He would ask about my husband next, I thought, and if I answered him truly, what would he think of me? I told him I had two children, one in New York the other at the south. He asked some further questions, and I frankly told him some of the most important events of my life. It was painful for me to do it; but I would not deceive him. If he was desirous of being my friend, I thought he ought to know how far I was worthy of it. "Excuse me, if I have tried your feelings," said he. "I did not question you from idle curiosity. I wanted to understand your situation, in order to know whether I could be of any service to you, or your little girl. Your straight-forward answers do you credit; but don't answer every body so openly. It might give some heartless people a pretext for treating you with contempt."

That word *contempt* burned me like coals of fire. I replied, "God alone knows how I have suffered; and He, I trust, will forgive me. If I am permitted to have my children, I intend to be a good mother, and to live in such a manner that people cannot treat me with contempt."

"I respect your sentiments," said he. "Place your trust in God, and be governed by good principles, and you will not fail to find friends."

When we reached home, I went to my room, glad to shut out the world for a while. The words he had spoken made an indelible impression upon me. They brought up great shadows from the mournful past. In the midst of my meditations I was startled by a knock at the door. Mrs. Durham entered, her face all beaming with kindness, to say that there was an anti-slavery friend down stairs, who would like to see me. I overcame my dread of encountering strangers, and went with her. Many questions were asked concerning my experiences, and my escape from slavery; but I observed how careful they all were not to say any thing that might wound my feelings. How gratifying this was, can be fully understood only by those who have been accustomed to be treated as if they were

not included within the pale of human beings. The anti-slavery friend had come to inquire into my plans, and to offer assistance, if needed. Fanny was comfortably established, for the
present, with a friend of Mr. Durham. The Anti-Slavery Society agreed to pay her expenses to New York. The same was
offered to me, but I declined to accept it; telling them that
my grandmother had given me sufficient to pay my expenses
to the end of my journey. We were urged to remain in
Philadelphia a few days, until some suitable escort could be
found for us. I gladly accepted the proposition, for I had a
dread of meeting slaveholders, and some dread also of railroads. I had never entered a railroad car in my life, and it
seemed to me quite an important event.

That night I sought my pillow with feelings I had never
carried to it before. I verily believed myself to be a free
woman. I was wakeful for a long time, and I had no sooner
fallen asleep, than I was roused by fire-bells. I jumped up, and
hurried on my clothes. Where I came from, every body hastened to dress themselves on such occasions. The white people thought a great fire might be used as a good opportunity
for insurrection, and that it was best to be in readiness; and
the colored people were ordered out to labor in extinguishing
the flames. There was but one engine in our town, and colored women and children were often required to drag it to
the river's edge, and fill it. Mrs. Durham's daughter slept in
the same room with me, and seeing that she slept through all
the din, I thought it was my duty to wake her. "What's the
matter?" said she, rubbing her eyes.

"They're screaming fire in the streets, and the bells are
ringing," I replied.

"What of that?" said she, drowsily. "We are used to it. We
never get up, without the fire is very near. What good would
it do?"

I was quite surprised that it was not necessary for us to go
and help fill the engine. I was an ignorant child, just beginning to learn how things went on in great cities.

At daylight, I heard women crying fresh fish, berries,
radishes, and various other things. All this was new to me. I
dressed myself at an early hour, and sat at the window to
watch that unknown tide of life. Philadelphia seemed to me a

wonderfully great place. At the breakfast table, my idea of
going out to drag the engine was laughed over, and I joined
in the mirth.

I went to see Fanny, and found her so well contented
among her new friends that she was in no haste to leave. I
was also very happy with my kind hostess. She had had advantages for education, and was vastly my superior. Every
day, almost every hour, I was adding to my little stock of
knowledge. She took me out to see the city as much as she
deemed prudent. One day she took me to an artist's room,
and showed me the portraits of some of her children. I had
never seen any paintings of colored people before, and they
seemed to me beautiful.

At the end of five days, one of Mrs. Durham's friends offered to accompany us to New York the following morning.
As I held the hand of my good hostess in a parting clasp, I
longed to know whether her husband had repeated to her
what I had told him. I supposed he had, but she never made
any allusion to it. I presume it was the delicate silence of
womanly sympathy.

When Mr. Durham handed us our tickets, he said, "I am
afraid you will have a disagreeable ride; but I could not procure tickets for the first class cars."

Supposing I had not given him money enough, I offered
more. "O, no," said he, "they could not be had for any
money. They don't allow colored people to go in the first-
class cars."

This was the first chill to my enthusiasm about the Free
States. Colored people were allowed to ride in a filthy box,
behind white people, at the south, but there they were not required to pay for the privilege. It made me sad to find how
the north aped the customs of slavery.

We were stowed away in a large, rough car, with windows
on each side, too high for us to look out without standing up.
It was crowded with people, apparently of all nations. There
were plenty of beds and cradles, containing screaming and
kicking babies. Every other man had a cigar or pipe in his
mouth, and jugs of whiskey were handed round freely. The
fumes of the whiskey and the dense tobacco smoke were sick-
ening to my senses, and my mind was equally nauseated by

the coarse jokes and ribald songs around me. It was a very disagreeable ride. Since that time there has been some improvement in these matters.

XXXII.

THE MEETING OF MOTHER AND DAUGHTER.

WHEN we arrived in New York, I was half crazed by the crowd of coachmen calling out, "Carriage, ma'am?" We bargained with one to take us to Sullivan Street for twelve shillings. A burly Irishman stepped up and said, "I'll tak' ye for sax shillings." The reduction of half the price was an object to us, and we asked if he could take us right away. "Troth an I will, ladies," he replied. I noticed that the hackmen smiled at each other, and I inquired whether his conveyance was decent. "Yes, it's dacent it is, marm. Devil a bit would I be after takin' ladies in a cab that was not dacent." We gave him our checks. He went for the baggage, and soon reappeared, saying, "This way, if you plase, ladies." We followed, and found our trunks on a truck, and we were invited to take our seats on them. We told him that was not what we bargained for, and he must take the trunks off. He swore they should not be touched till we had paid him six shillings. In our situation it was not prudent to attract attention, and I was about to pay him what he required, when a man near by shook his head for me not to do it. After a great ado we got rid of the Irishman, and had our trunks fastened on a hack. We had been recommended to a boarding-house in Sullivan Street, and thither we drove. There Fanny and I separated. The Anti-Slavery Society provided a home for her, and I afterwards heard of her in prosperous circumstances. I sent for an old friend from my part of the country, who had for some time been doing business in New York. He came immediately. I told him I wanted to go to my daughter, and asked him to aid me in procuring an interview.

I cautioned him not to let it be known to the family that I

had just arrived from the south, because they supposed I had been at the north seven years. He told me there was a colored woman in Brooklyn who came from the same town I did, and I had better go to her house, and have my daughter meet me there. I accepted the proposition thankfully, and he agreed to escort me to Brooklyn. We crossed Fulton ferry, went up Myrtle Avenue, and stopped at the house he designated. I was just about to enter, when two girls passed. My friend called my attention to them. I turned, and recognized in the eldest, Sarah, the daughter of a woman who used to live with my grandmother, but who had left the south years ago. Surprised and rejoiced at this unexpected meeting, I threw my arms round her, and inquired concerning her mother.

"You take no notice of the other girl," said my friend. I turned, and there stood my Ellen! I pressed her to my heart, then held her away from me to take a look at her. She had changed a good deal in the two years since I parted from her. Signs of neglect could be discerned by eyes less observing than a mother's. My friend invited us all to go into the house; but Ellen said she had been sent on an errand, which she would do as quickly as possible, and go home and ask Mrs. Hobbs to let her come and see me. It was agreed that I should send for her the next day. Her companion, Sarah, hastened to tell her mother of my arrival. When I entered the house, I found the mistress of it absent, and I waited for her return. Before I saw her, I heard her saying, "Where is Linda Brent? I used to know her father and mother." Soon Sarah came with her mother. So there was quite a company of us, all from my grandmother's neighborhood. These friends gathered round me and questioned me eagerly. They laughed, they cried, and they shouted. They thanked God that I had got away from my persecutors and was safe on Long Island. It was a day of great excitement. How different from the silent days I had passed in my dreary den!

The next morning was Sunday. My first waking thoughts were occupied with the note I was to send to Mrs. Hobbs, the lady with whom Ellen lived. That I had recently come into that vicinity was evident; otherwise I should have sooner inquired for my daughter. It would not do to let them know I had just arrived from the south, for that would involve the suspicion of my having been harbored there, and might bring trouble, if not ruin, on several people.

I like a straightforward course, and am always reluctant to resort to subterfuges. So far as my ways have been crooked, I charge them all upon slavery. It was that system of violence and wrong which now left me no alternative but to enact a falsehood. I began my note by stating that I had recently arrived from Canada, and was very desirous to have my daughter come to see me. She came and brought a message from Mrs. Hobbs, inviting me to her house, and assuring me that I need not have any fears. The conversation I had with my child did not leave my mind at ease. When I asked if she was well treated, she answered yes; but there was no heartiness in the tone, and it seemed to me that she said it from an unwillingness to have me troubled on her account. Before she left me, she asked very earnestly, "Mother, when will you take me to live with you?" It made me sad to think that I could not give her a home till I went to work and earned the means; and that might take me a long time. When she was placed with Mrs. Hobbs, the agreement was that she should be sent to school. She had been there two years, and was now nine years old, and she scarcely knew her letters. There was no excuse for this, for there were good public schools in Brooklyn, to which she could have been sent without expense.

She staid with me till dark, and I went home with her. I was received in a friendly manner by the family, and all agreed in saying that Ellen was a useful, good girl. Mrs. Hobbs looked me coolly in the face, and said, "I suppose you know that my cousin, Mr. Sands, has *given* her to my eldest daughter. She will make a nice waiting-maid for her when she grows up." I did not answer a word. How *could* she, who knew by experience the strength of a mother's love, and who was perfectly aware of the relation Mr. Sands bore to my children,—how *could* she look me in the face, while she thrust such a dagger into my heart?

I was no longer surprised that they had kept her in such a state of ignorance. Mr. Hobbs had formerly been wealthy, but he had failed, and afterwards obtained a subordinate situation in the Custom House. Perhaps they expected to return to the south some day; and Ellen's knowledge was quite sufficient for a slave's condition. I was impatient to go to work and earn money, that I might change the uncertain position of my children. Mr. Sands had not kept his promise to emancipate them. I had also been deceived about Ellen. What security had I with regard to Benjamin? I felt that I had none.

I returned to my friend's house in an uneasy state of mind. In order to protect my children, it was necessary that I should own myself. I called myself free, and sometimes felt so; but I knew I was insecure. I sat down that night and wrote a civil letter to Dr. Flint, asking him to state the lowest terms on which he would sell me; and as I belonged by law to his daughter, I wrote to her also, making a similar request.

Since my arrival at the north I had not been unmindful of my dear brother William. I had made diligent inquiries for him, and having heard of him in Boston, I went thither. When I arrived there, I found he had gone to New Bedford. I wrote to that place, and was informed he had gone on a whaling voyage, and would not return for some months. I went back to New York to get employment near Ellen. I received an answer from Dr. Flint, which gave me no encouragement. He advised me to return and submit myself to my rightful owners, and then any request I might make would be granted. I lent this letter to a friend, who lost it; otherwise I would present a copy to my readers.

XXXIII.

A HOME FOUND.

My greatest anxiety now was to obtain employment. My health was greatly improved, though my limbs continued to trouble me with swelling whenever I walked much. The greatest difficulty in my way was, that those who employed strangers required a recommendation; and in my peculiar position, I could, of course, obtain no certificates from the families I had so faithfully served.

One day an acquaintance told me of a lady who wanted a nurse for her babe, and I immediately applied for the situation. The lady told me she preferred to have one who had been a mother, and accustomed to the care of infants. I told her I had nursed two babes of my own. She asked me many questions, but, to my great relief, did not require a recommendation from my former employers. She told me she was an English woman, and that was a pleasant circumstance to me, because I had heard they had less prejudice against color than Americans entertained. It was agreed that we should try each other for a week. The trial proved satisfactory to both parties, and I was engaged for a month.

The heavenly Father had been most merciful to me in leading me to this place. Mrs. Bruce was a kind and gentle lady, and proved a true and sympathizing friend. Before the stipulated month expired, the necessity of passing up and down stairs frequently, caused my limbs to swell so painfully, that I became unable to perform my duties. Many ladies would have thoughtlessly discharged me; but Mrs. Bruce made arrangements to save me steps, and employed a physician to attend upon me. I had not yet told her that I was a fugitive slave. She noticed that I was often sad, and kindly inquired the cause. I spoke of being separated from my children, and from relatives who were dear to me; but I did not mention the constant feeling of insecurity which oppressed my spirits. I longed for some one to confide in; but I had been so deceived by white people, that I had lost all confidence in them. If they spoke kind words to me, I thought it was for some selfish purpose. I had entered this family with the distrustful feelings I had brought with me out of slavery; but ere six months had passed, I found that the gentle deportment of Mrs. Bruce and the smiles of her lovely babe were thawing my chilled heart. My narrow mind also began to expand under the influences of her intelligent conversation, and the opportunities for reading, which were gladly allowed me whenever I had leisure from my duties. I gradually became more energetic and more cheerful.

The old feeling of insecurity, especially with regard to my children, often threw its dark shadow across my sunshine. Mrs. Bruce offered me a home for Ellen; but pleasant as it would have been, I did not dare to accept it, for fear of offending the Hobbs family. Their knowledge of my precarious situation placed me in their power; and I felt that it was important for me to keep on the right side of them, till, by dint of labor and economy, I could make a home for my children. I was far from feeling satisfied with Ellen's situation. She was not well cared for. She sometimes came to New York to visit me; but she generally brought a request from Mrs. Hobbs that I would buy her a pair of shoes, or some article of clothing. This was accompanied by a promise of payment when Mr. Hobbs's salary at the Custom House became due; but some how or other the pay-day never came. Thus many dollars of my earnings were expended to keep my child comfortably clothed. That, however, was a slight trouble, compared with the fear that their pecuniary embarrassments might induce them to sell my precious young daughter. I knew they were in constant communication with Southerners, and had frequent opportunities to do it. I have stated that when Dr. Flint put Ellen in jail, at two years old, she had an inflammation of the eyes, occasioned by measles. This disease still troubled her; and kind Mrs. Bruce proposed that she should come to New York for a while, to be under the care of Dr. Elliott, a well known oculist. It did not occur to me that there was any thing improper in a mother's making such a request; but Mrs. Hobbs was very angry, and refused to let her go. Situated as I was, it was not politic to insist upon it. I made no complaint, but I longed to be entirely free to act a mother's part towards my children. The next time I went over to Brooklyn, Mrs. Hobbs, as if to apologize for her anger, told me she had employed her own physician to attend to Ellen's eyes, and that she had refused my request because she did not consider it safe to trust her in New York. I accepted the explanation in silence; but she had told me that my child *belonged* to her daughter, and I suspected that her real motive was a fear of my conveying her property away from her. Perhaps I did her injustice; but my knowledge of Southerners made it difficult for me to feel otherwise.

Sweet and bitter were mixed in the cup of my life, and I was thankful that it had ceased to be entirely bitter. I loved Mrs. Bruce's babe. When it laughed and crowed in my face, and twined its little tender arms confidingly about my neck, it made me think of the time when Benny and Ellen were babies, and my wounded heart was soothed. One bright morning, as I stood at the window, tossing baby in my arms, my attention was attracted by a young man in sailor's dress, who was closely observing every house as he passed. I looked at him earnestly. Could it be my brother William? It *must* be he—and yet, how changed! I placed the baby safely, flew down stairs, opened the front door, beckoned to the sailor, and in less than a minute I was clasped in my brother's arms. How much we had to tell each other! How we laughed, and how we cried, over each other's adventures! I took him to Brooklyn, and again saw him with Ellen, the dear child whom he had loved and tended so carefully, while I was shut up in my miserable den. He staid in New York a week. His old feelings of affection for me and Ellen were as lively as ever. There are no bonds so strong as those which are formed by suffering together.

XXXIV.

THE OLD ENEMY AGAIN.

My young mistress, Miss Emily Flint, did not return any answer to my letter requesting her to consent to my being sold. But after a while, I received a reply, which purported to be written by her younger brother. In order rightly to enjoy the contents of this letter, the reader must bear in mind that the Flint family supposed I had been at the north many years. They had no idea that I knew of the doctor's three excursions to New York in search of me; that I had heard his voice, when he came to borrow five hundred dollars for that purpose; and that I had seen him pass on his way to the steamboat. Neither were they aware that all the particulars of aunt Nancy's death and burial were conveyed to me at the time they occurred. I have kept the letter, of which I herewith subjoin a copy:—

"Your letter to sister was received a few days ago. I gather from it that you are desirous of returning to your native place, among your friends and relatives. We were all gratified with the contents of your letter; and let me assure you that if any members of the family have had any feeling of resentment towards you, they feel it no longer. We all sympathize with you in your unfortunate condition, and are ready to do all in our power to make you contented and happy. It is difficult for you to return home as a free person. If you were purchased by your grandmother, it is doubtful whether you would be permitted to remain, although it would be lawful for you to do so. If a servant should be allowed to purchase herself, after absenting herself so long from her owners, and return free, it would have an injurious effect. From your letter, I think your situation must be hard and uncomfortable. Come home. You have it in your power to be reinstated in our affections. We would receive you with open arms and tears of joy. You need not apprehend any unkind treatment, as we have not put ourselves to any trouble or expense to get you. Had we done so, perhaps we should feel otherwise. You know my sister was always attached to you, and that you were never treated as a slave. You were never put to hard work, nor exposed to field labor. On the contrary, you were taken into the house, and treated as one of us, and almost as free; and we, at least, felt that you were above disgracing yourself by running away. Believing you may be induced to come home voluntarily has induced me to write for my sister. The family will be rejoiced to see you; and your poor old grandmother expressed a great desire to have you come, when she heard your letter read. In her old age she needs the consolation of having her children round her. Doubtless you have heard of the death of your aunt. She was a faithful servant, and a faithful member of the Episcopal church. In her Christian life she taught us how to live—and, O, too high the price of knowledge, she taught us how to die! Could you have seen us round her death bed, with her mother, all mingling our tears in one common stream, you would have thought the same heartfelt tie existed between a master and his servant, as between a mother and her child. But this subject is too painful to dwell upon. I must bring my letter to a close. If you are contented to stay away from your old grandmother, your child, and the friends who love you, stay where you are. We shall never trouble ourselves to apprehend you. But should you prefer to come home, we will do all that we can to make you happy. If you do not wish to remain in the family, I know that father, by our persuasion, will be induced to let you be purchased by any person you may choose in our community. You will please answer this as soon as possible, and let us know your decision. Sister sends much love to you. In the mean time believe me your sincere friend and well wisher."

This letter was signed by Emily's brother, who was as yet a mere lad. I knew, by the style, that it was not written by a person of his age, and though the writing was disguised, I had been made too unhappy by it, in former years, not to recognize at once the hand of Dr. Flint. O, the hypocrisy of slaveholders! Did the old fox suppose I was goose enough to go into such a trap? Verily, he relied too much on "the stupidity of the African race." I did not return the family of Flints any thanks for their cordial invitation—a remissness for which I was, no doubt, charged with base ingratitude.

Not long afterwards I received a letter from one of my friends at the south, informing me that Dr. Flint was about to visit the north. The letter had been delayed, and I supposed he might be already on the way. Mrs. Bruce did not know I was a fugitive. I told her that important business called me to Boston, where my brother then was, and asked permission to bring a friend to supply my place as nurse, for a fortnight. I started on my journey immediately; and as soon as I arrived, I wrote to my grandmother that if Benny came, he must be sent to Boston. I knew she was only waiting for a good chance to send him north, and, fortunately, she had the legal power to do so, without asking leave of any body. She was a free woman; and when my children were purchased, Mr. Sands preferred to have the bill of sale drawn up in her name. It was conjectured that he advanced the money, but it was not known. At the south, a gentleman may have a shoal of colored children without any disgrace; but if he is known to purchase them, with the view of setting them free, the example is thought to be dangerous to their "peculiar institution," and he becomes unpopular.

There was a good opportunity to send Benny in a vessel coming directly to New York. He was put on board with a letter to a friend, who was requested to see him off to Boston. Early one morning, there was a loud rap at my door, and in rushed

Benjamin, all out of breath. "O mother!" he exclaimed, "here I am! I run all the way; and I come all alone. How d'you do?"

O reader, can you imagine my joy? No, you cannot, unless you have been a slave mother. Benjamin rattled away as fast as his tongue could go. "Mother, why don't you bring Ellen here? I went over to Brooklyn to see her, and she felt very bad when I bid her good by. She said, 'O Ben, I wish I was going too.' I thought she'd know ever so much; but she don't know so much as I do; for I can read, and she can't. And, mother, I lost all my clothes coming. What can I do to get some more? I 'spose free boys can get along here at the north as well as white boys."

I did not like to tell the sanguine, happy little fellow how much he was mistaken. I took him to a tailor, and procured a change of clothes. The rest of the day was spent in mutual asking and answering of questions, with the wish constantly repeated that the good old grandmother was with us, and frequent injunctions from Benny to write to her immediately, and be sure to tell her every thing about his voyage, and his journey to Boston.

Dr. Flint made his visit to New York, and made every exertion to call upon me, and invite me to return with him; but not being able to ascertain where I was, his hospitable intentions were frustrated, and the affectionate family, who were waiting for me with "open arms," were doomed to disappointment.

As soon as I knew he was safely at home, I placed Benjamin in the care of my brother William, and returned to Mrs. Bruce. There I remained through the winter and spring, endeavoring to perform my duties faithfully, and finding a good degree of happiness in the attractions of baby Mary, the considerate kindness of her excellent mother, and occasional interviews with my darling daughter.

But when summer came, the old feeling of insecurity haunted me. It was necessary for me to take little Mary out daily, for exercise and fresh air, and the city was swarming with Southerners, some of whom might recognize me. Hot weather brings out snakes and slaveholders, and I like one class of the venomous creatures as little as I do the other. What a comfort it is, to be free to *say* so!

XXXV.

PREJUDICE AGAINST COLOR.

IT was a relief to my mind to see preparations for leaving the city. We went to Albany in the steamboat Knickerbocker. When the gong sounded for tea, Mrs. Bruce said, "Linda, it is late, and you and baby had better come to the table with me." I replied, "I know it is time baby had her supper, but I had rather not go with you, if you please. I am afraid of being insulted." "O no, not if you are with *me*," she said. I saw several white nurses go with their ladies, and I ventured to do the same. We were at the extreme end of the table. I was no sooner seated, than a gruff voice said, "Get up! You know you are not allowed to sit here." I looked up, and, to my astonishment and indignation, saw that the speaker was a colored man. If his office required him to enforce the by-laws of the boat, he might, at least, have done it politely. I replied, "I shall not get up, unless the captain comes and takes me up." No cup of tea was offered me, but Mrs. Bruce handed me hers and called for another. I looked to see whether the other nurses were treated in a similar manner. They were all properly waited on.

Next morning, when we stopped at Troy for breakfast, every body was making a rush for the table. Mrs. Bruce said, "Take my arm, Linda, and we'll go in together." The landlord heard her, and said, "Madam, will you allow your nurse and baby to take breakfast with my family?" I knew this was to be attributed to my complexion; but he spoke courteously, and therefore I did not mind it.

At Saratoga we found the United States Hotel crowded, and Mr. Bruce took one of the cottages belonging to the hotel. I had thought, with gladness, of going to the quiet of the country, where I should meet few people, but here I found myself in the midst of a swarm of Southerners. I looked round me with fear and trembling, dreading to see some one who would recognize me. I was rejoiced to find that we were to stay but a short time.

We soon returned to New York, to make arrangements for spending the remainder of the summer at Rockaway. While the laundress was putting the clothes in order, I took an op-

portunity to go over to Brooklyn to see Ellen. I met her
going to a grocery store, and the first words she said, were,
"O, mother, don't go to Mrs. Hobbs's. Her brother, Mr.
Thorne, has come from the south, and may be he'll tell where
you are." I accepted the warning. I told her I was going away
with Mrs. Bruce the next day, and would try to see her when
I came back.

Being in servitude to the Anglo-Saxon race, I was not put
into a "Jim Crow car," on our way to Rockaway, neither was
I invited to ride through the streets on the top of trunks in a
truck; but every where I found the same manifestations of
that cruel prejudice, which so discourages the feelings, and represses the energies of the colored people. We reached Rockaway before dark, and put up at the Pavilion— a large hotel,
beautifully situated by the sea-side—a great resort of the fashionable world. Thirty or forty nurses were there, of a great variety of nations. Some of the ladies had colored waiting-maids
and coachmen, but I was the only nurse tinged with the
blood of Africa. When the tea bell rang, I took little Mary and
followed the other nurses. Supper was served in a long hall. A
young man, who had the ordering of things, took the circuit
of the table two or three times, and finally pointed me to a
seat at the lower end of it. As there was but one chair, I sat
down and took the child in my lap. Whereupon the young
man came to me and said, in the blandest manner possible,
"Will you please to seat the little girl in the chair, and stand
behind it and feed her? After they have done, you will be
shown to the kitchen, where you will have a good supper."

This was the climax! I found it hard to preserve my self-
control, when I looked round, and saw women who were
nurses, as I was, and only one shade lighter in complexion,
eyeing me with a defiant look, as if my presence were a contamination. However, I said nothing. I quietly took the child
in my arms, went to our room, and refused to go to the table
again. Mr. Bruce ordered meals to be sent to the room for little Mary and I. This answered for a few days; but the waiters
of the establishment were white, and they soon began to
complain, saying they were not hired to wait on negroes. The
landlord requested Mr. Bruce to send me down to my meals,
because his servants rebelled against bringing them up, and

the colored servants of other boarders were dissatisfied because all were not treated alike.

My answer was that the colored servants ought to be dissatisfied with *themselves*, for not having too much self-respect to submit to such treatment; that there was no difference in the price of board for colored and white servants, and there was no justification for difference of treatment. I staid a month after this, and finding I was resolved to stand up for my rights, they concluded to treat me well. Let every colored man and woman do this, and eventually we shall cease to be trampled under foot by our oppressors.

XXXVI.

THE HAIRBREADTH ESCAPE.

AFTER we returned to New York, I took the earliest opportunity to go and see Ellen. I asked to have her called down stairs; for I supposed Mrs. Hobbs's southern brother might still be there, and I was desirous to avoid seeing him, if possible. But Mrs. Hobbs came to the kitchen, and insisted on my going up stairs. "My brother wants to see you," said she, "and he is sorry you seem to shun him. He knows you are living in New York. He told me to say to you that he owes thanks to good old aunt Martha for too many little acts of kindness for him to be base enough to betray her grandchild."

This Mr. Thorne had become poor and reckless long before he left the south, and such persons had much rather go to one of the faithful old slaves to borrow a dollar, or get a good dinner, than to go to one whom they consider an equal. It was such acts of kindness as these for which he professed to feel grateful to my grandmother. I wished he had kept at a distance, but as he was here, and knew where I was, I concluded there was nothing to be gained by trying to avoid him; on the contrary, it might be the means of exciting his ill will. I followed his sister up stairs. He met me in a very friendly manner, congratulated me on my escape from slavery, and hoped I had a good place, where I felt happy.

I continued to visit Ellen as often as I could. She, good thoughtful child, never forgot my hazardous situation, but always kept a vigilant lookout for my safety. She never made any complaint about her own inconveniences and troubles; but a mother's observing eye easily perceived that she was not happy. On the occasion of one of my visits I found her unusually serious. When I asked her what was the matter, she said nothing was the matter. But I insisted upon knowing what made her look so very grave. Finally, I ascertained that she felt troubled about the dissipation that was continually going on in the house. She was sent to the store very often for rum and brandy, and she felt ashamed to ask for it so often; and Mr. Hobbs and Mr. Thorne drank a great deal, and their hands trembled so that they had to call her to pour out the liquor for them. "But for all that," said she, "Mr. Hobbs is good to me, and I can't help liking him. I feel sorry for him." I tried to comfort her, by telling her that I had laid up a hundred dollars, and that before long I hoped to be able to give her and Benjamin a home, and send them to school. She was always desirous not to add to my troubles more than she could help, and I did not discover till years afterwards that Mr. Thorne's intemperance was not the only annoyance she suffered from him. Though he professed too much gratitude to my grandmother to injure any of her descendants, he had poured vile language into the ears of her innocent great-grandchild.

I usually went to Brooklyn to spend Sunday afternoon. One Sunday, I found Ellen anxiously waiting for me near the house. "O, mother," said she, "I've been waiting for you this long time. I'm afraid Mr. Thorne has written to tell Dr. Flint where you are. Make haste and come in. Mrs. Hobbs will tell you all about it!"

The story was soon told. While the children were playing in the grape-vine arbor, the day before, Mr. Thorne came out with a letter in his hand, which he tore up and scattered about. Ellen was sweeping the yard at the time, and having her mind full of suspicions of him, she picked up the pieces and carried them to the children, saying, "I wonder who Mr. Thorne has been writing to."

"I'm sure I don't know, and don't care," replied the oldest of the children; "and I don't see how it concerns you."

"But it does concern me," replied Ellen; "for I'm afraid he's been writing to the south about my mother."

They laughed at her, and called her a silly thing, but good-naturedly put the fragments of writing together, in order to read them to her. They were no sooner arranged, than the little girl exclaimed, "I declare, Ellen, I believe you are right."

The contents of Mr. Thorne's letter, as nearly as I can remember, were as follows: "I have seen your slave, Linda, and conversed with her. She can be taken very easily, if you manage prudently. There are enough of us here to swear to her identity as your property. I am a patriot, a lover of my country, and I do this as an act of justice to the laws." He concluded by informing the doctor of the street and number where I lived. The children carried the pieces to Mrs. Hobbs, who immediately went to her brother's room for an explanation. He was not to be found. The servants said they saw him go out with a letter in his hand, and they supposed he had gone to the post office. The natural inference was, that he had sent to Dr. Flint a copy of those fragments. When he returned, his sister accused him of it, and he did not deny the charge. He went immediately to his room, and the next morning he was missing. He had gone over to New York, before any of the family were astir.

It was evident that I had no time to lose; and I hastened back to the city with a heavy heart. Again I was to be torn from a comfortable home, and all my plans for the welfare of my children were to be frustrated by that demon Slavery! I now regretted that I never told Mrs. Bruce my story. I had not concealed it merely on account of being a fugitive; that would have made her anxious, but it would have excited sympathy in her kind heart. I valued her good opinion, and I was afraid of losing it, if I told her all the particulars of my sad story. But now I felt that it was necessary for her to know how I was situated. I had once left her abruptly, without explaining the reason, and it would not be proper to do it again. I went home resolved to tell her in the morning. But the sadness of my face attracted her attention, and, in answer to her kind inquiries, I poured out my full heart to her, before bed time. She listened with true womanly sympathy, and told me she would do all she could to protect me. How my heart blessed her!

Early the next morning, Judge Vanderpool and Lawyer Hopper were consulted. They said I had better leave the city at once, as the risk would be great if the case came to trial. Mrs. Bruce took me in a carriage to the house of one of her friends, where she assured me I should be safe until my brother could arrive, which would be in a few days. In the interval my thoughts were much occupied with Ellen. She was mine by birth, and she was also mine by Southern law, since my grandmother held the bill of sale that made her so. I did not feel that she was safe unless I had her with me. Mrs. Hobbs, who felt badly about her brother's treachery, yielded to my entreaties, on condition that she should return in ten days. I avoided making any promise. She came to me clad in very thin garments, all outgrown, and with a school satchel on her arm, containing a few articles. It was late in October, and I knew the child must suffer; and not daring to go out in the streets to purchase any thing, I took off my own flannel skirt and converted it into one for her. Kind Mrs. Bruce came to bid me good by, and when she saw that I had taken off my clothing for my child, the tears came to her eyes. She said, "Wait for me, Linda," and went out. She soon returned with a nice warm shawl and hood for Ellen. Truly, of such souls as hers are the kingdom of heaven.

My brother reached New York on Wednesday. Lawyer Hopper advised us to go to Boston by the Stonington route, as there was less Southern travel in that direction. Mrs. Bruce directed her servants to tell all inquirers that I formerly lived there, but had gone from the city.

We reached the steamboat Rhode Island in safety. That boat employed colored hands, but I knew that colored passengers were not admitted to the cabin. I was very desirous for the seclusion of the cabin, not only on account of exposure to the night air, but also to avoid observation. Lawyer Hopper was waiting on board for us. He spoke to the stewardess, and asked, as a particular favor, that she would treat us well. He said to me, "Go and speak to the captain yourself by and by. Take your little girl with you, and I am sure that he will not let her sleep on deck." With these kind words and a shake of the hand he departed.

The boat was soon on her way, bearing me rapidly from the friendly home where I had hoped to find security and rest. My brother had left me to purchase the tickets, thinking that I might have better success than he would. When the stewardess came to me, I paid what she asked, and she gave me three tickets with clipped corners. In the most unsophisticated manner I said, "You have made a mistake; I asked you for cabin tickets. I cannot possibly consent to sleep on deck with my little daughter." She assured me there was no mistake. She said on some of the routes colored people were allowed to sleep in the cabin, but not on this route, which was much travelled by the wealthy. I asked her to show me to the captain's office, and she said she would after tea. When the time came, I took Ellen by the hand and went to the captain, politely requesting him to change our tickets, as we should be very uncomfortable on deck. He said it was contrary to their custom, but he would see that we had berths below; he would also try to obtain comfortable seats for us in the cars; of that he was not certain, but he would speak to the conductor about it, when the boat arrived. I thanked him, and returned to the ladies' cabin. He came afterwards and told me that the conductor of the cars was on board, that he had spoken to him, and he had promised to take care of us. I was very much surprised at receiving so much kindness. I don't know whether the pleasing face of my little girl had won his heart, or whether the stewardess inferred from Lawyer Hopper's manner that I was a fugitive, and had pleaded with him in my behalf.

When the boat arrived at Stonington, the conductor kept his promise, and showed us to seats in the first car, nearest the engine. He asked us to take seats next the door, but as he passed through, we ventured to move on toward the other end of the car. No incivility was offered us, and we reached Boston in safety.

The day after my arrival was one of the happiest of my life. I felt as if I was beyond the reach of the bloodhounds; and, for the first time during many years, I had both my children together with me. They greatly enjoyed their reunion, and laughed and chatted merrily. I watched them with a swelling heart. Their every motion delighted me.

I could not feel safe in New York, and I accepted the offer of a friend, that we should share expenses and keep house together. I represented to Mrs. Hobbs that Ellen must have some schooling, and must remain with me for that purpose. She felt ashamed of being unable to read or spell at her age, so instead of sending her to school with Benny, I instructed her myself till she was fitted to enter an intermediate school. The winter passed pleasantly, while I was busy with my needle, and my children with their books.

XXXVII.

A VISIT TO ENGLAND.

In the spring, sad news came to me. Mrs. Bruce was dead. Never again, in this world, should I see her gentle face, or hear her sympathizing voice. I had lost an excellent friend, and little Mary had lost a tender mother. Mr. Bruce wished the child to visit some of her mother's relatives in England, and he was desirous that I should take charge of her. The little motherless one was accustomed to me, and attached to me, and I thought she would be happier in my care than in that of a stranger. I could also earn more in this way than I could by my needle. So I put Benny to a trade, and left Ellen to remain in the house with my friend and go to school.

We sailed from New York, and arrived in Liverpool after a pleasant voyage of twelve days. We proceeded directly to London, and took lodgings at the Adelaide Hotel. The supper seemed to me less luxurious than those I had seen in American hotels; but my situation was indescribably more pleasant. For the first time in my life I was in a place where I was treated according to my deportment, without reference to my complexion. I felt as if a great millstone had been lifted from my breast. Ensconced in a pleasant room, with my dear little charge, I laid my head on my pillow, for the first time, with the delightful consciousness of pure, unadulterated freedom.

As I had constant care of the child, I had little opportunity to see the wonders of that great city; but I watched the tide of life that flowed through the streets, and found it a strange contrast to the stagnation in our Southern towns. Mr. Bruce took his little daughter to spend some days with friends in Oxford Crescent, and of course it was necessary for me to accompany her. I had heard much of the systematic method of English education, and I was very desirous that my dear Mary should steer straight in the midst of so much propriety. I closely observed her little playmates and their nurses, being ready to take any lessons in the science of good management. The children were more rosy than American children, but I did not see that they differed materially in other respects. They were like all children—sometimes docile and sometimes wayward.

We next went to Steventon, in Berkshire. It was a small town, said to be the poorest in the county. I saw men working in the fields for six shillings, and seven shillings, a week, and women for sixpence, and sevenpence, a day, out of which they boarded themselves. Of course they lived in the most primitive manner; it could not be otherwise, where a woman's wages for an entire day were not sufficient to buy a pound of meat. They paid very low rents, and their clothes were made of the cheapest fabrics, though much better than could have been procured in the United States for the same money. I had heard much about the oppression of the poor in Europe. The people I saw around me were, many of them, among the poorest poor. But when I visited them in their little thatched cottages, I felt that the condition of even the meanest and most ignorant among them was vastly superior to the condition of the most favored slaves in America. They labored hard; but they were not ordered out to toil while the stars were in the sky, and driven and slashed by an overseer, through heat and cold, till the stars shone out again. Their homes were very humble; but they were protected by law. No insolent patrols could come, in the dead of night, and flog them at their pleasure. The father, when he closed his cottage door, felt safe with his family around him. No master or overseer could come and take from him his wife, or his daughter. They must separate to earn their living; but the parents knew where their children were going, and could communicate with them by letters. The relations of husband and wife, parent and child, were too sacred for the richest noble in the land to violate with impunity. Much was being done to enlighten these poor people. Schools were established among them, and benevolent societies were active in efforts to ameliorate their condition. There was no law forbidding them to learn to read and write; and if they helped each other in spelling out the Bible, they were in no danger of thirty-nine lashes, as was the case with myself and poor, pious, old uncle Fred. I repeat that the most ignorant and the most destitute of these peasants was a thousand fold better off than the most pampered American slave.

I do not deny that the poor are oppressed in Europe. I am not disposed to paint their condition so rose-colored as the Hon. Miss Murray paints the condition of the slaves in the United States. A small portion of *my* experience would enable her to read her own pages with anointed eyes. If she were to lay aside her title, and, instead of visiting among the fashionable, become domesticated, as a poor governess, on some plantation in Louisiana or Alabama, she would see and hear things that would make her tell quite a different story.

My visit to England is a memorable event in my life, from the fact of my having there received strong religious impressions. The contemptuous manner in which the communion had been administered to colored people, in my native place; the church membership of Dr. Flint, and others like him; and the buying and selling of slaves, by professed ministers of the gospel, had given me a prejudice against the Episcopal church. The whole service seemed to me a mockery and a sham. But my home in Steventon was in the family of a clergyman, who was a true disciple of Jesus. The beauty of his daily life inspired me with faith in the genuineness of Christian professions. Grace entered my heart, and I knelt at the communion table, I trust, in true humility of soul.

I remained abroad ten months, which was much longer than I had anticipated. During all that time, I never saw the slightest symptom of prejudice against color. Indeed, I entirely forgot it, till the time came for us to return to America.

XXXVIII.
RENEWED INVITATIONS TO GO SOUTH.

WE had a tedious winter passage, and from the distance spectres seemed to rise up on the shores of the United States. It is a sad feeling to be afraid of one's native country. We arrived in New York safely, and I hastened to Boston to look after my children. I found Ellen well, and improving at her school; but Benny was not there to welcome me. He had been left at a good place to learn a trade, and for several months every thing worked well. He was liked by the master, and was a favorite with his fellow-apprentices; but one day they accidentally discovered a fact they had never before suspected—that he was colored! This at once transformed him into a different being. Some of the apprentices were Americans, others American-born Irish; and it was offensive to their dignity to have a "nigger" among them, after they had been told that he *was* a "nigger." They began by treating him with silent scorn, and finding that he returned the same, they resorted to insults and abuse. He was too spirited a boy to stand that, and he went off. Being desirous to do something to support himself, and having no one to advise him, he shipped for a whaling voyage. When I received these tidings I shed many tears, and bitterly reproached myself for having left him so long. But I had done it for the best, and now all I could do was to pray to the heavenly Father to guide and protect him.

Not long after my return, I received the following letter from Miss Emily Flint, now Mrs. Dodge:—

"In this you will recognize the hand of your friend and mistress. Having heard that you had gone with a family to Europe, I have waited to hear of your return to write to you. I should have answered the letter you wrote to me long since, but as I could not then act independently of my father, I knew there could be nothing done satisfactory to you. There were persons here who were willing to buy you and run the risk of getting you. To this I would not consent. I have always been attached to you, and would not like to see you the slave of another, or have unkind treatment. I am married now, and can protect you. My husband expects to move to Virginia this spring, where we think of settling. I am very anxious that you should come and live with me. If you are not willing to come, you may purchase yourself; but I should prefer having you live with me. If you come, you may, if you like, spend a month with your grandmother and friends, then come to me in Norfolk, Virginia. Think this over, and write as soon as possible, and let me know the conclusion. Hoping that your children are well, I remain your friend and mistress."

Of course I did not write to return thanks for this cordial invitation. I felt insulted to be thought stupid enough to be caught by such professions.

" 'Come up into my parlor,' said the spider to the fly;
 ''Tis the prettiest little parlor that ever you did spy.' "

It was plain that Dr. Flint's family were apprised of my movements, since they knew of my voyage to Europe. I expected to have further trouble from them; but having eluded them thus far, I hoped to be as successful in future. The money I had earned, I was desirous to devote to the education of my children, and to secure a home for them. It seemed not only hard, but unjust, to pay for myself. I could not possibly regard myself as a piece of property. Moreover, I had worked many years without wages, and during that time had been obliged to depend on my grandmother for many comforts in food and clothing. My children certainly belonged to me; but though Dr. Flint had incurred no expense for their support, he had received a large sum of money for them. I knew the law would decide that I was his property, and would probably still give his daughter a claim to my children; but I regarded such laws as the regulations of robbers, who had no rights that I was bound to respect.

The Fugitive Slave Law had not then passed. The judges of Massachusetts had not then stooped under chains to enter her courts of justice, so called. I knew my old master was rather skittish of Massachusetts. I relied on her love of freedom, and felt safe on her soil. I am now aware that I honored the old Commonwealth beyond her deserts.

XXXIX.

THE CONFESSION.

For two years my daughter and I supported ourselves comfortably in Boston. At the end of that time, my brother William offered to send Ellen to a boarding school. It required a great effort for me to consent to part with her, for I had few near ties, and it was her presence that made my two little rooms seem home-like. But my judgment prevailed over my selfish feelings. I made preparations for her departure. During the two years we had lived together I had often resolved to tell her something about her father; but I had never been able to muster sufficient courage. I had a shrinking dread of diminishing my child's love. I knew she must have curiosity on the subject, but she had never asked a question. She was always very careful not to say any thing to remind me of my troubles. Now that she was going from me, I thought if I should die before she returned, she might hear my story from some one who did not understand the palliating circumstances; and that if she were entirely ignorant on the subject, her sensitive nature might receive a rude shock.

When we retired for the night, she said, "Mother, it is very hard to leave you alone. I am almost sorry I am going, though I do want to improve myself. But you will write to me often; won't you, mother?"

I did not throw my arms round her. I did not answer her. But in a calm, solemn way, for it cost me great effort, I said, "Listen to me, Ellen; I have something to tell you!" I recounted my early sufferings in slavery, and told her how nearly they had crushed me. I began to tell her how they had driven me into a great sin, when she clasped me in her arms, and exclaimed, "O, don't, mother! Please don't tell me any more."

I said, "But, my child, I want you to know about your father."

"I know all about it, mother," she replied; "I am nothing to my father, and he is nothing to me. All my love is for you. I was with him five months in Washington, and he never cared for me. He never spoke to me as he did to his little Fanny. I knew all the time he was my father, for Fanny's nurse told me so; but she said I must never tell any body, and I never did. I used to wish he would take me in his arms and kiss me, as he did Fanny; or that he would sometimes smile at me, as he did at her. I thought if he was my own father, he ought to love me. I was a little girl then, and didn't know any better. But now I never think any thing about my father. All my love is for you." She hugged me closer as she spoke, and I thanked God that the knowledge I had so much dreaded to impart had not diminished the affection of my child. I had not the slightest idea she knew that portion of my history. If I had, I should have spoken to her long before; for my pent-up feelings had often longed to pour themselves out to some one I could trust. But I loved the dear girl better for the delicacy she had manifested towards her unfortunate mother.

The next morning, she and her uncle started on their journey to the village in New York, where she was to be placed at school. It seemed as if all the sunshine had gone away. My little room was dreadfully lonely. I was thankful when a message came from a lady, accustomed to employ me, requesting me to come and sew in her family for several weeks. On my return, I found a letter from brother William. He thought of opening an anti-slavery reading room in Rochester, and combining with it the sale of some books and stationery; and he wanted me to unite with him. We tried it, but it was not successful. We found warm anti-slavery friends there, but the feeling was not general enough to support such an establishment. I passed nearly a year in the family of Isaac and Amy Post, practical believers in the Christian doctrine of human brotherhood. They measured a man's worth by his character, not by his complexion. The memory of those beloved and honored friends will remain with me to my latest hour.

XL.

THE FUGITIVE SLAVE LAW.

My brother, being disappointed in his project, concluded to go to California; and it was agreed that Benjamin should go with him. Ellen liked her school; and was a great favorite there. They did not know her history, and she did not tell it, because she had no desire to make capital out of their sympathy. But when it was accidentally discovered that her mother was a fugitive slave, every method was used to increase her advantages and diminish her expenses.

I was alone again. It was necessary for me to be earning money, and I preferred that it should be among those who knew me. On my return from Rochester, I called at the house of Mr. Bruce, to see Mary, the darling little babe that had thawed my heart, when it was freezing into a cheerless distrust of all my fellow-beings. She was growing a tall girl now, but I loved her always. Mr. Bruce had married again, and it was proposed that I should become nurse to a new infant. I had but one hesitation, and that was my feeling of insecurity in New York, now greatly increased by the passage of the Fugitive Slave Law. However, I resolved to try the experiment. I was again fortunate in my employer. The new Mrs. Bruce was an American, brought up under aristocratic influences, and still living in the midst of them; but if she had any prejudice against color, I was never made aware of it; and as for the system of slavery, she had a most hearty dislike of it. No sophistry of Southerners could blind her to its enormity. She was a person of excellent principles and a noble heart. To me, from that hour to the present, she has been a true and sympathizing friend. Blessings be with her and hers!

About the time that I reëntered the Bruce family, an event occurred of disastrous import to the colored people. The slave Hamlin, the first fugitive that came under the new law, was given up by the bloodhounds of the north to the bloodhounds of the south. It was the beginning of a reign of terror to the colored population. The great city rushed on in its whirl of excitement, taking no note of the "short and simple annals of the poor." But while fashionables were listening to the thrilling voice of Jenny Lind in Metropolitan Hall, the thrilling voices of poor hunted colored people went up, in an agony of supplication, to the Lord, from Zion's church. Many families, who had lived in the city for twenty years, fled from it now. Many a poor washerwoman, who, by hard labor, had made herself a comfortable home, was obliged to sacrifice her furniture, bid a hurried farewell to friends, and seek her fortune among strangers in Canada. Many a wife discovered a secret she had never known before—that her husband was a fugitive, and must leave her to insure his own safety. Worse still, many a husband discovered that his wife had fled from slavery years ago, and as "the child follows the condition of its mother," the children of his love were liable to be seized and carried into slavery. Every where, in those humble homes, there was consternation and anguish. But what cared the legislators of the "dominant race" for the blood they were crushing out of trampled hearts?

When my brother William spent his last evening with me, before he went to California, we talked nearly all the time of the distress brought on our oppressed people by the passage of this iniquitous law; and never had I seen him manifest such bitterness of spirit, such stern hostility to our oppressors. He was himself free from the operation of the law; for he did not run from any Slaveholding State, being brought into the Free States by his master. But I was subject to it; and so were hundreds of intelligent and industrious people all around us. I seldom ventured into the streets; and when it was necessary to do an errand for Mrs. Bruce, or any of the family, I went as much as possible through back streets and by-ways. What a disgrace to a city calling itself free, that inhabitants, guiltless of offence, and seeking to perform their duties conscientiously, should be condemned to live in such incessant fear, and have nowhere to turn for protection! This state of things, of course, gave rise to many impromptu vigilance committees. Every colored person, and every friend of their persecuted race, kept their eyes wide open. Every evening I examined the newspapers carefully, to see what Southerners had put up at the hotels. I did this for my own sake, thinking my young mistress and her husband might be among the list; I wished also to give information to others, if necessary; for if many were "running to and fro," I resolved that "knowledge should be increased."

This brings up one of my Southern reminiscences, which I will here briefly relate. I was somewhat acquainted with a slave named Luke, who belonged to a wealthy man in our vicinity. His master died, leaving a son and daughter heirs to his large fortune. In the division of the slaves, Luke was included in the son's portion. This young man became a prey to the vices growing out of the "patriarchal institution," and when he went to the north, to complete his education, he carried his vices with him. He was brought home, deprived of the use of his limbs, by excessive dissipation. Luke was appointed to wait upon his bed-ridden master, whose despotic habits were greatly increased by exasperation at his own helplessness. He kept a cowhide beside him, and, for the most trivial occurrence, he would order his attendant to bare his back, and kneel beside the couch, while he whipped him till his strength was exhausted. Some days he was not allowed to wear any thing but his shirt, in order to be in readiness to be flogged. A day seldom passed without his receiving more or less blows. If the slightest resistance was offered, the town constable was sent for to execute the punishment, and Luke learned from experience how much more the constable's strong arm was to be dreaded than the comparatively feeble one of his master. The arm of his tyrant grew weaker, and was finally palsied; and then the constable's services were in constant requisition. The fact that he was entirely dependent on Luke's care, and was obliged to be tended like an infant, instead of inspiring any gratitude or compassion towards his poor slave, seemed only to increase his irritability and cruelty. As he lay there on his bed, a mere degraded wreck of manhood, he took into his head the strangest freaks of despotism; and if Luke hesitated to submit to his orders, the constable was immediately sent for. Some of these freaks were of a nature too filthy to be repeated. When I fled from the house of bondage, I left poor Luke still chained to the bedside of this cruel and disgusting wretch.

One day, when I had been requested to do an errand for Mrs. Bruce, I was hurrying through back streets, as usual, when I saw a young man approaching, whose face was familiar to me. As he came nearer, I recognized Luke. I always rejoiced to see or hear of any one who had escaped from the black pit; but, remembering this poor fellow's extreme hardships, I was peculiarly glad to see him on Northern soil, though I no longer called it *free* soil. I well remembered what a desolate feeling it was to be alone among strangers, and I went up to him and greeted him cordially. At first, he did not know me; but when I mentioned my name, he remembered all about me. I told him of the Fugitive Slave Law, and asked him if he did not know that New York was a city of kidnappers.

He replied, "De risk ain't so bad for me, as 'tis fur you. 'Cause I runned away from de speculator, and you runned away from de massa. Dem speculators vont spen dar money to come here fur a runaway, if dey ain't sartin sure to put dar hans right on him. An I tell you I's tuk good car 'bout dat. I had too hard times down dar, to let 'em ketch dis nigger."

He then told me of the advice he had received, and the plans he had laid. I asked if he had money enough to take him to Canada. "'Pend upon it, I hab," he replied. "I tuk car fur dat. I'd bin workin all my days fur dem cussed whites, an got no pay but kicks and cuffs. So I tought dis nigger had a right to money nuff to bring him to de Free States. Massa Henry he lib till ebery body vish him dead; an ven he did die, I knowed de debbil would hab him, an vouldn't vant him to bring his money 'long too. So I tuk some of his bills, and put 'em in de pocket of his ole trousers. An ven he was buried, dis nigger ask fur dem ole trousers, an dey gub 'em to me." With a low, chuckling laugh, he added, "You see I didn't *steal* it; dey *gub* it to me. I tell you, I had mighty hard time to keep de speculator from findin it; but he didn't git it."

This is a fair specimen of how the moral sense is educated by slavery. When a man has his wages stolen from him, year after year, and the laws sanction and enforce the theft, how can he be expected to have more regard to honesty than has the man who robs him? I have become somewhat enlightened, but I confess that I agree with poor, ignorant, muchabused Luke, in thinking he had a *right* to that money, as a portion of his unpaid wages. He went to Canada forthwith, and I have not since heard from him.

All that winter I lived in a state of anxiety. When I took the children out to breathe the air, I closely observed the countenances of all I met. I dreaded the approach of summer, when snakes and slaveholders make their appearance. I was, in fact, a slave in New York, as subject to slave laws as I had been in a Slave State. Strange incongruity in a State called free!

Spring returned, and I received warning from the south

that Dr. Flint knew of my return to my old place, and was
making preparations to have me caught. I learned afterwards
that my dress, and that of Mrs. Bruce's children, had been described to him by some of the Northern tools, which slaveholders employ for their base purposes, and then indulge in
sneers at their cupidity and mean servility.

I immediately informed Mrs. Bruce of my danger, and she
took prompt measures for my safety. My place as nurse could
not be supplied immediately, and this generous, sympathizing
lady proposed that I should carry her baby away. It was a
comfort to me to have the child with me; for the heart is reluctant to be torn away from every object it loves. But how
few mothers would have consented to have one of their own
babes become a fugitive, for the sake of a poor, hunted nurse,
on whom the legislators of the country had let loose the
bloodhounds! When I spoke of the sacrifice she was making,
in depriving herself of her dear baby, she replied, "It is better
for you to have baby with you, Linda; for if they get on your
track, they will be obliged to bring the child to me; and then,
if there is a possibility of saving you, you shall be saved."

This lady had a very wealthy relative, a benevolent gentleman in many respects, but aristocratic and pro-slavery. He remonstrated with her for harboring a fugitive slave; told her
she was violating the laws of her country; and asked her if she
was aware of the penalty. She replied, "I am very well aware
of it. It is imprisonment and one thousand dollars fine. Shame
on my country that it *is* so! I am ready to incur the penalty. I
will go to the state's prison, rather than have any poor victim
torn from *my* house, to be carried back to slavery."

The noble heart! The brave heart! The tears are in my eyes
while I write of her. May the God of the helpless reward her
for her sympathy with my persecuted people!

I was sent into New England, where I was sheltered by the
wife of a senator, whom I shall always hold in grateful remembrance. This honorable gentleman would not have voted
for the Fugitive Slave Law, as did the senator in "Uncle Tom's
Cabin;" on the contrary, he was strongly opposed to it; but
he was enough under its influence to be afraid of having me
remain in his house many hours. So I was sent into the
country, where I remained a month with the baby. When it

was supposed that Dr. Flint's emissaries had lost track of me, and given up the pursuit for the present, I returned to New York.

XLI.

FREE AT LAST.

MRS. BRUCE, and every member of her family, were exceedingly kind to me. I was thankful for the blessings of my lot, yet I could not always wear a cheerful countenance. I was doing harm to no one; on the contrary, I was doing all the good I could in my small way; yet I could never go out to breathe God's free air without trepidation at my heart. This seemed hard; and I could not think it was a right state of things in any civilized country.

From time to time I received news from my good old grandmother. She could not write; but she employed others to write for her. The following is an extract from one of her last letters:—

"Dear Daughter: I cannot hope to see you again on earth; but I pray to God to unite us above, where pain will no more rack this feeble body of mine; where sorrow and parting from my children will be no more. God has promised these things if we are faithful unto the end. My age and feeble health deprive me of going to church now; but God is with me here at home. Thank your brother for his kindness. Give much love to him, and tell him to remember the Creator in the days of his youth, and strive to meet me in the Father's kingdom. Love to Ellen and Benjamin. Don't neglect him. Tell him for me, to be a good boy. Strive, my child; to train them for God's children. May he protect and provide for you, is the prayer of your loving old mother."

These letters both cheered and saddened me. I was always glad to have tidings from the kind, faithful old friend of my unhappy youth; but her messages of love made my heart yearn to see her before she died, and I mourned over the fact that it was impossible. Some months after I returned from my flight to New England, I received a letter from her, in which she wrote, "Dr. Flint is dead. He has left a distressed family. Poor old man! I hope he made his peace with God."

I remembered how he had defrauded my grandmother of the hard earnings she had loaned; how he had tried to cheat her out of the freedom her mistress had promised her, and how he had persecuted her children; and I thought to myself that she was a better Christian than I was, if she could entirely forgive him. I cannot say, with truth, that the news of my old master's death softened my feelings towards him. There are wrongs which even the grave does not bury. The man was odious to me while he lived, and his memory is odious now.

His departure from this world did not diminish my danger. He had threatened my grandmother that his heirs should hold me in slavery after he was gone; that I never should be free so long as a child of his survived. As for Mrs. Flint, I had seen her in deeper afflictions than I supposed the loss of her husband would be, for she had buried several children; yet I never saw any signs of softening in her heart. The doctor had died in embarrassed circumstances, and had little to will to his heirs, except such property as he was unable to grasp. I was well aware what I had to expect from the family of Flints; and my fears were confirmed by a letter from the south, warning me to be on my guard, because Mrs. Flint openly declared that her daughter could not afford to lose so valuable a slave as I was.

I kept close watch of the newspapers for arrivals; but one Saturday night, being much occupied, I forgot to examine the Evening Express as usual. I went down into the parlor for it, early in the morning, and found the boy about to kindle a fire with it. I took it from him and examined the list of arrivals. Reader, if you have never been a slave, you cannot imagine the acute sensation of suffering at my heart, when I read the names of Mr. and Mrs. Dodge, at a hotel in Courtland Street. It was a third-rate hotel, and that circumstance convinced me of the truth of what I had heard, that they were short of funds and had need of my value, as *they* valued me; and that was by dollars and cents. I hastened with the paper to Mrs. Bruce. Her heart and hand were always open to every one in distress, and she always warmly sympathized with mine. It was impossible to tell how near the enemy was. He might have passed and repassed the house while we were sleeping. He might at that moment be waiting to pounce upon me if I ventured out of doors. I had never seen the husband of my young mistress, and therefore I could not distinguish him from any other stranger. A carriage was hastily ordered; and, closely veiled, I followed Mrs. Bruce, taking the baby again with me into exile. After various turnings and crossings, and returnings, the carriage stopped at the house of one of Mrs. Bruce's friends, where I was kindly received. Mrs. Bruce returned immediately, to instruct the domestics what to say if any one came to inquire for me.

It was lucky for me that the evening paper was not burned up before I had a chance to examine the list of arrivals. It was not long after Mrs. Bruce's return to her house, before several people came to inquire for me. One inquired for me, another asked for my daughter Ellen, and another said he had a letter from my grandmother, which he was requested to deliver in person.

They were told, "She *has* lived here, but she has left."

"How long ago?"

"I don't know, sir."

"Do you know where she went?"

"I do not, sir." And the door was closed.

This Mr. Dodge, who claimed me as his property, was originally a Yankee pedler in the south; then he became a merchant, and finally a slaveholder. He managed to get introduced into what was called the first society, and married Miss Emily Flint. A quarrel arose between him and her brother, and the brother cowhided him. This led to a family feud, and he proposed to remove to Virginia. Dr. Flint left him no property, and his own means had become circumscribed, while a wife and children depended upon him for support. Under these circumstances, it was very natural that he should make an effort to put me into his pocket.

I had a colored friend, a man from my native place, in whom I had the most implicit confidence. I sent for him, and told him that Mr. and Mrs. Dodge had arrived in New York. I proposed that he should call upon them to make inquiries about his friends at the south, with whom Dr. Flint's family were well acquainted. He thought there was no impropriety in his doing so, and he consented. He went to the hotel, and knocked at the door of Mr. Dodge's room, which was opened by the gentleman himself, who gruffly inquired, "What brought you here? How came you to know I was in the city?"

"Your arrival was published in the evening papers, sir; and I called to ask Mrs. Dodge about my friends at home. I didn't suppose it would give any offence."

"Where's that negro girl, that belongs to my wife?"

"What girl, sir?"

"You know well enough. I mean Linda, that ran away from Dr. Flint's plantation, some years ago. I dare say you've seen her, and know where she is."

"Yes, sir, I've seen her, and know where she is. She is out of your reach, sir."

"Tell me where she is, or bring her to me, and I will give her a chance to buy her freedom."

"I don't think it would be of any use, sir. I have heard her say she would go to the ends of the earth, rather than pay any man or woman for her freedom, because she thinks she has a right to it. Besides, she couldn't do it, if she would, for she has spent her earnings to educate her children."

This made Mr. Dodge very angry, and some high words passed between them. My friend was afraid to come where I was; but in the course of the day I received a note from him. I supposed they had not come from the south, in the winter, for a pleasure excursion; and now the nature of their business was very plain.

Mrs. Bruce came to me and entreated me to leave the city the next morning. She said her house was watched, and it was possible that some clew to me might be obtained. I refused to take her advice. She pleaded with an earnest tenderness, that ought to have moved me; but I was in a bitter, disheartened mood. I was weary of flying from pillar to post. I had been chased during half my life, and it seemed as if the chase was never to end. There I sat, in that great city, guiltless of crime, yet not daring to worship God in any of the churches. I heard the bells ringing for afternoon service, and, with contemptuous sarcasm, I said, "Will the preachers take for their text, 'Proclaim liberty to the captive, and the opening of prison doors to them that are bound'? or will they preach from the text, 'Do unto others as ye would they should do unto you'?" Oppressed Poles and Hungarians could find a safe refuge in that city; John Mitchell was free to proclaim in the City Hall his desire for "a plantation well stocked with slaves;" but there I sat, an oppressed American, not daring to show my face. God forgive the black and bitter thoughts I indulged on that Sabbath day! The Scripture says, "Oppression makes even a wise man mad;" and I was not wise.

I had been told that Mr. Dodge said his wife had never signed away her right to my children, and if he could not get me, he would take them. This it was, more than any thing else, that roused such a tempest in my soul. Benjamin was with his uncle William in California, but my innocent young daughter had come to spend a vacation with me. I thought of what I had suffered in slavery at her age, and my heart was like a tiger's when a hunter tries to seize her young.

Dear Mrs. Bruce! I seem to see the expression of her face, as she turned away discouraged by my obstinate mood. Finding her expostulations unavailing, she sent Ellen to entreat me. When ten o'clock in the evening arrived and Ellen had not returned, this watchful and unwearied friend became anxious. She came to us in a carriage, bringing a well-filled trunk for my journey—trusting that by this time I would listen to reason. I yielded to her, as I ought to have done before.

The next day, baby and I set out in a heavy snow storm, bound for New England again. I received letters from the City of Iniquity, addressed to me under an assumed name. In a few days one came from Mrs. Bruce, informing me that my new master was still searching for me, and that she intended to put an end to this persecution by buying my freedom. I felt grateful for the kindness that prompted this offer, but the idea was not so pleasant to me as might have been expected. The more my mind had become enlightened, the more difficult it was for me to consider myself an article of property; and to pay money to those who had so grievously oppressed me seemed like taking from my sufferings the glory of triumph. I wrote to Mrs. Bruce, thanking her, but saying that being sold from one owner to another seemed too much like slavery; that such a great obligation could not be easily cancelled; and that I preferred to go to my brother in California.

Without my knowledge, Mrs. Bruce employed a gentleman in New York to enter into negotiations with Mr. Dodge. He proposed to pay three hundred dollars down, if Mr. Dodge would sell me, and enter into obligations to relinquish all claim to me or my children forever after. He who called himself my master said he scorned so small an offer for such a valuable servant. The gentleman replied, "You can do as you choose, sir. If you reject this offer you will never get any thing; for the woman has friends who will convey her and her children out of the country."

Mr. Dodge concluded that "half a loaf was better than no bread," and he agreed to the proffered terms. By the next mail I received this brief letter from Mrs. Bruce: "I am rejoiced to tell you that the money for your freedom has been paid to Mr. Dodge. Come home to-morrow. I long to see you and my sweet babe."

My brain reeled as I read these lines. A gentleman near me said, "It's true; I have seen the bill of sale." "The bill of sale!" Those words struck me like a blow. So I was *sold* at last! A human being *sold* in the free city of New York! The bill of sale is on record, and future generations will learn from it that women were articles of traffic in New York, late in the nineteenth century of the Christian religion. It may hereafter prove a useful document to antiquaries, who are seeking to measure the progress of civilization in the United States. I well know the value of that bit of paper; but much as I love freedom, I do not like to look upon it. I am deeply grateful to the generous friend who procured it, but I despise the miscreant who demanded payment for what never rightfully belonged to him or his.

I had objected to having my freedom bought, yet I must confess that when it was done I felt as if a heavy load had been lifted from my weary shoulders. When I rode home in the cars I was no longer afraid to unveil my face and look at people as they passed. I should have been glad to have met Daniel Dodge himself; to have had him seen me and known me, that he might have mourned over the untoward circumstances which compelled him to sell me for three hundred dollars.

When I reached home, the arms of my benefactress were

thrown round me, and our tears mingled. As soon as she could speak, she said, "O Linda, I'm *so* glad it's all over! You wrote to me as if you thought you were going to be transferred from one owner to another. But I did not buy you for your services. I should have done just the same, if you had been going to sail for California to-morrow. I should, at least, have the satisfaction of knowing that you left me a free woman."

My heart was exceedingly full. I remembered how my poor father had tried to buy me, when I was a small child, and how he had been disappointed. I hoped his spirit was rejoicing over me now. I remembered how my good old grandmother had laid up her earnings to purchase me in later years, and how often her plans had been frustrated. How that faithful, loving old heart would leap for joy, if she could look on me and my children now that we were free! My relatives had been foiled in all their efforts, but God had raised me up a friend among strangers, who had bestowed on me the precious, long-desired boon. Friend! It is a common word, often lightly used. Like other good and beautiful things, it may be tarnished by careless handling; but when I speak of Mrs. Bruce as my friend, the word is sacred.

My grandmother lived to rejoice in my freedom; but not long after, a letter came with a black seal. She had gone "where the wicked cease from troubling, and the weary are at rest."

Time passed on, and a paper came to me from the south, containing an obituary notice of my uncle Phillip. It was the only case I ever knew of such an honor conferred upon a colored person. It was written by one of his friends, and contained these words: "Now that death has laid him low, they call him a good man and a useful citizen; but what are eulogies to the black man, when the world has faded from his vision? It does not require man's praise to obtain rest in God's kingdom." So they called a colored man a *citizen*! Strange words to be uttered in that region!

Reader, my story ends with freedom; not in the usual way, with marriage. I and my children are now free! We are as free from the power of slaveholders as are the white people of the north; and though that, according to my ideas, is not saying a great deal, it is a vast improvement in *my* condition. The dream of my life is not yet realized. I do not sit with my children in a home of my own. I still long for a hearthstone of my own, however humble. I wish it for my children's sake far more than for my own. But God so orders circumstances as to keep me with my friend Mrs. Bruce. Love, duty, gratitude, also bind me to her side. It is a privilege to serve her who pities my oppressed people, and who has bestowed the inestimable boon of freedom on me and my children.

It has been painful to me, in many ways, to recall the dreary years I passed in bondage. I would gladly forget them if I could. Yet the retrospection is not altogether without solace; for with those gloomy recollections come tender memories of my good old grandmother, like light, fleecy clouds floating over a dark and troubled sea.

APPENDIX.

The following statement is from Amy Post, a member of the Society of Friends in the State of New York, well known and highly respected by friends of the poor and the oppressed. As has been already stated, in the preceding pages, the author of this volume spent some time under her hospitable roof.

L. M. C.

"The author of this book is my highly-esteemed friend. If its readers knew her as I know her, they could not fail to be deeply interested in her story. She was a beloved inmate of our family nearly the whole of the year 1849. She was introduced to us by her affectionate and conscientious brother, who had previously related to us some of the almost incredible events in his sister's life. I immediately became much interested in Linda; for her appearance was prepossessing, and her deportment indicated remarkable delicacy of feeling and purity of thought.

"As we became acquainted, she related to me, from time to time some of the incidents in her bitter experiences as a slave-woman. Though impelled by a natural craving for human sympathy, she passed through a baptism of suffering, even in recounting her trials to me, in private confidential conversations. The burden of these memories lay heavily upon her spirit—naturally virtuous and refined. I repeatedly urged her to consent to the publication of her narrative; for I felt that it would arouse people to a more earnest work for the disinthralment of millions still remaining in that soul-crushing condition, which was so unendurable to her. But her sensitive spirit shrank from publicity. She said, 'You know a woman can whisper her cruel wrongs in the ear of a dear friend much easier than she can record them for the world to read.' Even in talking with me, she wept so much, and seemed to suffer such mental agony, that I felt her story was too sacred to be drawn from her by inquisitive questions, and I left her free to tell as much, or as little, as she chose. Still, I urged upon her the duty of publishing her experience, for the sake of the good it might do; and, at last, she undertook the task.

"Having been a slave so large a portion of her life, she is unlearned; she is obliged to earn her living by her own labor, and she has worked untiringly to procure education for her children; several times she has been obliged to leave her employments, in order to fly from the man-hunters and woman-hunters of our land; but she pressed through all these obstacles and overcame them. After the

946

labors of the day were over, she traced secretly and wearily, by the midnight lamp, a truthful record of her eventful life.

"This Empire State is a shabby place of refuge for the oppressed; but here, through anxiety, turmoil, and despair, the freedom of Linda and her children was finally secured, by the exertions of a generous friend. She was grateful for the boon; but the idea of having been *bought* was always galling to a spirit that could never acknowledge itself to be a chattel. She wrote to us thus, soon after the event: 'I thank you for your kind expressions in regard to my freedom; but the freedom I had before the money was paid was dearer to me. God gave me *that* freedom; but man put God's image in the scales with the paltry sum of three hundred dollars. I served for my liberty as faithfully as Jacob served for Rachel. At the end, he had large possessions; but I was robbed of my victory; I was obliged to resign my crown, to rid myself of a tyrant.'

"Her story, as written by herself, cannot fail to interest the reader. It is a sad illustration of the condition of this country, which boasts of its civilization, while it sanctions laws and customs which make the experiences of the present more strange than any fictions of the past.

AMY POST.

"ROCHESTER, N. Y., Oct. 30th, 1859."

The following testimonial is from a man who is now a highly respectable colored citizen of Boston.

L. M. C.

"This narrative contains some incidents so extraordinary, that, doubtless, many persons, under whose eyes it may chance to fall, will be ready to believe that it is colored highly, to serve a special purpose. But, however it may be regarded by the incredulous, I know that it is full of living truths. I have been well acquainted with the author from my boyhood. The circumstances recounted in her history are perfectly familiar to me. I knew of her treatment from her master; of the imprisonment of her children; of their sale and redemption; of her seven years' concealment; and of her subsequent escape to the North. I am now a resident of Boston, and am a living witness to the truth of this interesting narrative.

GEORGE W. LOWTHER."

NARRATIVE

OF

THE LIFE

OF

J. D. GREEN,

A RUNAWAY SLAVE,

FROM KENTUCKY,

CONTAINING AN

ACCOUNT OF HIS THREE ESCAPES,

In 1839, 1846, and 1848.

———

EIGHTH THOUSAND.

———

HUDDERSFIELD:
PRINTED BY HENRY FIELDING, PACK HORSE YARD.
1864.

TESTIMONIALS.

Jacob Green, a coloured man and an escaped slave, has lectured in my hearing, on American Slavery, in Springfield School-room, and I was much pleased with the propriety with which he was able to express himself, and with the capabilities which he seemed to possess to interest an audience.

GILBERT Mc.CALLUM.
Minister of Springfield
Independent Chapel, Dewsbury.
Sept 2, 1863.

———

Hopton House, Sept. 10, 1863.

I have much pleasure in bearing my testimony in favour of Mr. Jacob Green, as a lecturer on the subject of American Slavery, having been present when he gave an able and efficient lecture here about a month ago. Having himself witnessed and experienced the fearful effects of that accursed "institution," he is well fitted to describe its horrors, and I have no doubt that amongst certain classes, his labours in the anti-slavery cause may be more telling and efficient than those of more highly educated lecturers who do not profess his peculiar advantages. I shall be well pleased to hear of him being employed by any anti-slavery society.

JAMES CAMERON,
Minister of Hopton Chapel.

———

Eccleshill, Sept. 11, 1863.

Mr. Jacob Green gave a lecture on Slavery, in our School-room here, about two months ago, which I considered a very able one; and it was so considered by my people.

JOHN ASTON.

———

I certify that Mr. Jacob Green has delivered two lectures in the Foresters' Hall, Denholm, to a very numerous audience;

and on each occasion has given great satisfaction. The subjects were, first—Slavery,—second, the American War. He lectures remarkably well, and has a powerful voice; and I have
not the least doubt would give satisfaction in lecturing elsewhere. The chair on each occasion was taken—first, by myself
as incumbent—second, by the Rev. T. Roberts, Independent
Minister.

J. F. N. EYRE.
Incumbent of Denholm.

Oct. 18th, 1863.

I can thoroughly endorse the sentiments of the Rev. J. F. N.
Eyre, herein recorded.

T. ROBERTS.

Mr. J. D. Green has lectured four times in our School-
rooms, and each time he has given very great satisfaction to a
large assembly. From what I have seen of him, I believe him
to be worthy of public sympathy and support.

WILLIAM INMAN, Minister.

Ovenden, Nov. 14, 1863.

NARRATIVE, &c.

My father and mother were owned by Judge Charles Earle, of Queen Anne's County, Maryland, and I was born on the 24th of August, 1813.

From eight to eleven years of age I was employed as an errand boy, carrying water principally for domestic purposes, for 113 slaves and the family. As I grew older, in the mornings I was employed looking after the cows, and waiting in the house, and at twelve years I remember being in great danger of losing my life in a singular way. I had seen the relish with which master and friends took drink from a bottle, and seeing a similar bottle in the closet, I thought what was good for them would be good for me, and I laid hold of the bottle and took a good draught of (Oh, horror of horrors) oxalic acid, and the doctor said my safety was occasioned by a habit I had of putting my head in the milk pail and drinking milk, as by doing so the milk caused me to vomit and saved my life. About this time my mother was sold to a trader named Woodfork, and where she was conveyed I have not heard up to the present time. This circumstance caused serious reflections in my mind, as to the situation of slaves, and caused me to contrast the condition of a white boy with mine, which the following occurrence will more vividly pourtray. One morning after my mother was sold, a white boy was stealing corn out of my master's barn, and I said for this act we black boys will be whipped until one of us confesses to have done that we are all innocent of, as such is the case in every instance; and I thought, Oh, that master was here, or the overseer, I would then let them see what becomes of the corn. But, I saw he was off with the corn to the extent of half a bushel, and I will say nothing about it until they miss it, and if I tell them they wont believe me if he denies it, because he is white and I am black. Oh! how dreadful it is to be black! Why was I born black? It would have been better had I not been born at all. Only yesterday, my mother was sold to go to, not one of us knows were, and I am left alone, and I have no hope of seeing her again. At this moment a raven alighted on a tree over my head, and I cried, "Oh, Raven! if I had wings like you, I would soon find my mother and be happy again." Before parting she advised me to be a good boy, and she would pray for me, and I must pray for her, and hoped we might meet again in heaven, and I at once commenced to pray, to the best of my knowledge, "Our Father art in Heaven, be Thy name, kingdom come.—Amen." But, at this time, words of my master obtruded into my mind that God did not care for black folks, as he did not make them, but the d——l did. Then I thought of the old saying amongst us, as stated by our master, that, when God was making man, He made white man out of the best clay, as potters make china, and the d——l was watching, and he immediately took up some black mud and made a black man, and called him a nigger. My master was continually impressing upon me the necessity of being a good boy, and used to say, that if I was good, and behaved as well to him as my mother had done, I should go to Heaven without a question being asked. My mother having often said the same, I determined from that day to be a good boy, and constantly frequented the Meeting-house attended by the blacks where I learned from the minister, Mr. Cobb, how much the Lord had done for the blacks and for their salvation; and he was in the habit of reminding us what advantages he had given us for our benefit, for when we were in our native country, Africa, we were destitute of Bible light, worshipping idols of sticks and stones, and barbarously murdering one another, God put it into the hearts of these good slaveholders to venture across the bosom of the hazardous Atlantic to Africa, and snatch us poor negroes as brands from the eternal burning, and bring us where we might sit under the droppings of his sanctuary, and learn the ways of industry and the way to God. "Oh, niggers! how happy are your eyes which see this heavenly light; many millions of niggers desired it long, but died without the sight. I frequently envy your situations, because God's special blessing seems to be ever over you, as though you were a select people, for how much happier is your position than that of a free man, who, if sick, must pay his doctor's bill; if hungry, must supply his wants by his own exertions; if thirsty, must refresh himself by his own aid. And yet you, oh, niggers! your master has all this care for you. He supplies your daily wants; your meat and your drink he provides; and when you are sick he finds the best skill to bring you to health as soon as possible, for your sickness is his loss, and your health his gain; and, above all when you die (if you are obedient to your masters, and good niggers), your black faces will shine like black jugs around the throne of God." Such was the religious instruction I was in the habit of receiving until I was about seventeen years old; and told that when at any time I happened to be offended, or struck by a white boy I was not to offend or strike in return, unless it was another black, then I might fight as hard as I chose in my own defence. It happened about this time there was a white boy who was continually stealing my tops and marbles, and one morning when doing so I caught him, and we had a battle, and I had him down on the ground when Mr. Burmey came up. He kicked me away from the white boy, saying if I belonged to him he would cut off my hands for *daring* to strike a white boy; this without asking the cause of the quarrel, or of ascertaining who was to blame. The kick was so severe that I was sometime before I forgot it, and created such a feeling of revenge in my bosom that I was determined when I became a man I would pay him back in his own coin. I went out one day, and measured myself by a tree in the wood, and cut a notch in the tree to ascertain how fast I grew. I went at different times for the space of two months and found I was no taller, and I began to fear he would die before I should have grown to man's estate, and I resolved if he did I would make his children suffer by punishing them instead of their father. At this time my master's wife had two lovers, this same Burmey and one Rogers, and they despised each other from feelings of jealousy. Master's wife seemed to favour Burmey most, who was a great smoker, and she provided him with a large pipe with a German silver bowl, which screwed on the top; this pipe she usually kept on the mantel piece, ready filled with tobacco. One morning I was dusting and sweeping out the dining-room, and saw the pipe on the mantel-piece. I took it down, and went to my young master William's powder closet and took out his powder horn, and after taking half of the tobacco out of the pipe filled it nearly full with powder, and covered it over with tobacco to make it appear as usual when filled with tobacco, replaced it, and left. Rogers, came in about eight o'clock in the morning, and remained until eleven, when Mr. Burmey came, and in about an hour I saw a great number running about from all parts of the plantation. I left the barn where I was thrashing buck-wheat, and followed the rest to the house, where I saw Mr. Burmey lying back in the arm chair in a state of insensibility, his mouth bleeding profusely and from particulars given it appeared he took the pipe as usual and lighted it, and had just got it to his mouth when the powder exploded, and the party suspected was Rogers, who had been there immediately preceding; and Burmey's son went to Rogers and they fought about the matter. Law ensued, which cost Rogers 800 dollars, Burmey 600 dollars and his face disfigured; and my master's wife came in for a deal of scandal, which caused further proceedings at law, costing the master 1400 hundred dollars, and I was never once suspected or charged with the deed.

At this time two or three negroes had escaped, and I heard so much about the free States of the north that I was determined to be free. So I began to study what we call the north star, or astronomy, to guide me to the free States. I was in the habit of driving the master; and on one occasion I had to drive him to Baltimore where two of his sons were studying law; and while there, I stole some sweet potatoes to roast when I got home; and how master got to know I had them I never knew; but when I got home he gave me a note to Mr. Cobb, the overseer, and told me to tell Dick, (another slave on the plantation) to come to Baltimore to him on the following evening, and as soon as I took the note in my hand I was certain there was a flogging in it for me, though he said nothing to me. I held the note that night and following day, afraid to give it to Mr. Cobb, so confident was I of what would be the result. Towards evening I began to reason thus— If I give Cobb the note I shall be whipped; if I withhold the note from him I shall be whipped, so a whipping appears plain in either case. Now Dick having arranged to meet his sweetheart this night assumed sickness, so that he could have an excuse for not meeting master at Baltimore, and he wanted me to go instead of him. I agreed to go, providing he would take the note I had to Mr. Cobb, as I had forgot to give it him, to which he consented, and off I went; and I heard that when he delivered the note to Mr. Cobb, he ordered him to go to the whipping-post, and when he asked what he had done he was knocked down, and afterwards put to the post and thirty-nine lashes were administered, and failed seeing his sweetheart as well. When I arrived at Baltimore my master and young master took their seats and I drove away without any question until we had gone three miles, when he asked what I was doing there that night. I very politely said Dick was not well, and I had come in his place. He then asked me if Mr. Cobb got his note, I answered, yes, sir. He then asked me how I felt, and I said first rate, sir. "The d——l you do," said he. I said, yes sir. He said "nigger, did Mr. Cobb flog you?" No sir. I have done nothing wrong. "You never do," he answered; and said no more until he got home. Being a man who could not bear to have any order of his disobeyed or unfulfilled, he immediately called for Mr. Cobb, and was told he was in bed; and when he appeared, the master asked if he got the note sent by the nigger. Mr. Cobb said "Yes." "Then why," said master, "did you not perform my orders in the note?" "I did, sir," replied Cobb; when the master said, "I told you to give that nigger thirty-nine lashes," Mr. Cobb says, "So I did, sir;" when master replied, "He says you never licked him at all." Upon which Cobb said, "He is a liar;" when my master called for me (who had been hearing the whole dialogue at the door), I turned on my toes and went a short distance, and I shouted with a loud voice that I was coming, (to prevent them knowing that I had been listening) and appeared before them and said "here I am master, do you want me?" He said "Yes. Did you not tell me that Mr. Cobb had not flogged you," and I said "yes I did; he has not flogged me to-day, sir." Mr. Cobb answered, "I did not flog him. You did not tell me to flog him. You told me to flog that other nigger." "What other nigger," enquired Master. Cobb said, "Dick." Master then said, "I did not. I told you to flog this nigger here." Cobb then produced the letter, and read it as follows:

"Mr. Cobb will give the bearer 39 lashes on delivery."
                                            R. T. EARLE.

I then left the room and explanations took place. When I was again called in. "How came Dick to have had the letter," and I then said I had forgot to deliver it until Dick wanted me to go to Baltimore in his place, and I agreed providing he would take the letter. Master then said "you lie, you infernal villain," and laid hold of a pair of tongs and said he would dash my brains out if I did not tell him the truth. I then said I thought there was something in the note that boded no good to me, and I did not intend to give it to him. He said, "you black vagabond, stay on this plantation three months longer, and you will be master and I the slave; no wonder you said you felt first rate when I asked you, but I will sell you to go to Georgia the first chance I get." Then laying the tongs down he opened the door and ordered me out. I knew he had on heavy cow-hide boots, and I knew he would try to assist me in my outward progress, and though expecting it and went as quick as I could, I was materially assisted by a heavy kick from my master's foot. This did not end the matter, for when Dick found out I had caused his being flogged, we had continual fightings for several months.

When I was fourteen years old my master gave me a flogging, the marks of which will go with me to my grave, and this was for a crime of which I was completely innocent. My master's son had taken one of his pistols out, and by some accident it burst. When enquiry was made about the damaged pistol William told his father that he had seen me have it; this, of course, I denied, when master tied me up by my thumbs and gave me 60 lashes, and also made me confess the crime before he would release me. From this flogging my back was raw and sore for three months; the shirt that I wore was made of rough tow linen, and when at work in the fields it would so chafe the sores that they would break and run, and the hot sun over me would bake the shirt fast to my back, and for four weeks I wore that shirt, unable to pull it off, and when I did pull it off it brought with it much of my flesh, leaving my back perfectly raw. Some time after this my master found out the truth about the pistol, and when I saw that he did not offer me any apology for the beating he had given me, and the lie he had made me confess, I went to him and said—now, master, you see that you beat me unjustly about that pistol, and made me confess to a lie—but all the consolation I got was—clear out, you black rascal; I never struck a blow amiss in my life, except when I struck at you and happened to miss you; there are plenty of other crimes you have committed and did not let me catch you at them, so that flogging will do for the lot.

Master had an old negro in the family called Uncle Reuben. This good old man and his wife were very good friends of my mother's, and before she was sold they often met and sung and prayed, and talked about religion together. Uncle Reuben fell sick in the middle of the harvest, and his sickness was very severe; but master having a grudge against uncle Reuben, and his old wife aunt Dinah, respecting a complaint that aunt Dinah had made to mistress about his having outraged and violated her youngest daughter, his spite was carried out by Mr. Cobb, the overseer, who forced Uncle Reuben into the field amongst the rest of us, and I was ordered to cradle behind him to make him keep up with the rest of the gang. The poor old man worked until he fell, just ahead of me, upon the cradle. Mr. Cobb came over and told him to get up, and that he was only playing the old soldier, and when the old man did not move to get up Mr. Cobb gave him a few kicks with his heavy boots and told Reuben, sick as he was, that he would cure him. He ordered us to take off his shirt, and the poor old man was stripped, when Mr. Cobb, with his hickory cane, laid on him till his back bled freely; but still the old man seemed to take no notice of what Mr. Cobb was doing. Mr. Cobb then told us to put on his shirt and carry him in, for he appeared convinced that Reuben could not walk. The next morning I went to see him but he did not seem to know anybody. Master came in along with the Doctor, and master swore at Reuben, telling him that as soon as he was well enough he should have a good flogging for having, by his own folly, caught his sickness. The doctor here checked his master's rage by telling him, as he felt at Reuben by the wrist, he could not live many minutes longer; at this master was silent, and a few minutes Reuben was dead. Poor Aunt Dinah came in out of the kitchen and wept fit to break her poor heart. She had four sons and three daughters, and they all joined in mournful lamentation.

When I was sixteen I was very fond of dancing, and was invited privately to a negro shindy or dance, about twelve miles from home, and for this purpose I got Aunt Dinah to starch the collars for my two linen shirts, which were the first standing collars I had ever worn in my life; I had a good pair of trousers, and a jacket, but no necktie, nor no pocket handkerchief, so I stole aunt Dinah's checked apron, and tore it in two—one part for a necktie, the other for a pocket handkerchief. I had twenty-four cents, or pennies which I divided equally with fifty large brass buttons in my right and left pockets. Now, thought I to myself, when I get on the floor and begin to dance—oh! how the niggers will stare to hear the money jingle. I was combing my hair to get the knots out of it: I then went and looked in an old piece of broken looking-glass, and I thought, without joking, that I was the best looking negro that I had ever seen in my life. About ten o'clock I stole out to the stable when all was still; and while I was getting on one of my master's horses I said to myself—Master was in here at six o'clock and saw all these horses clean, so I must look out and be back time enough to have you clean when he gets up in the morning. I thought what a dash I should cut among the pretty yellow and Sambo gals, and I felt quite confident, of course, that I should have my pick among the best looking ones, for my good clothes, and my abundance of money, and my own good looks—in fact, I thought no mean things of my self.

When I arrived at the place where the dance was, it was at an old house in the woods, which had many years before been a negro meeting-house; there was a large crowd there, and about one hundred horses tied round the fence—for some of them were far from home, and, like myself, they were all runaways, and their horses, like mine, had to be home and cleaned before their masters were up in the morning. In getting my horse close up to the fence a nail caught my trousers at the thigh, and split them clean up to the seat; of course my shirt tail fell out behind, like a woman's apron before. This dreadful misfortune almost unmanned me, and curtailed both my pride and pleasure for the night. I cried until I could cry no more. However, I was determined I would not be done out of my sport after being at the expense of coming, so I went round and borrowed some pins, and pinned up my shirt tail as well as I could. I then went into the dance, and told the fiddler to play me a jig. Che, che, che, went the fiddle, when the banjo responded with a thrum, thrum, thrum, with the loud cracking of the bone player. I seized a little Sambo gal, and round and round the room we went, my money and my buttons going jingle, jingle, jingle, seemed to take a lively part with the music, and to my great satisfaction every eye seemed to be upon me, and I could not help thinking about what an impression I should leave behind upon those pretty yellow and Sambo gals, who were gazing at me, thinking I was the richest and handsomest nigger they had ever seen: but unfortunately the pins in my breeches gave way, and to my great confusion my shirt tail fell out; and what made my situation still more disgraceful was the mischievous conduct of my partner, the gal that I was dancing with, who instead of trying to conceal my shame caught my shirt tail behind and held it up. The roar of laughter that came from both men and gals almost deafened me, and I would at this moment have sunk through the floor, so I endeavoured to creep out as slily as I could; but even this I was not permitted to do until I had undergone a hauling around the room by my unfortunate shirt tail: and this part of the programme was performed by the gals, set on by the boys—every nigger who could not stand up and laugh, because laughing made them weak, fell down on the floor and rolled round and round. When the gals saw their own turn they let me go and I hurried outside and stood behind the house, beneath a beautiful bright moon, which saw me that night the most wretched of all negroes in the land of Dixie; and what made me feel, in my own opinion, that my humiliation was just as complete as the triumph of the negroes inside was glorious, was that the gals had turned my pockets out, and found that the hundreds of dollars they had thought my pockets contained, consisted of 24 cents or pennies, and 50 brass buttons. Everything was alive and happy inside the room, but no one knew or cared how miserable I was—the joy and life of the dance that night seemed entirely at my expense, all through my unfortunate shirt tail. The first thing I thought of now was revenge. Take your comfort, niggers now, said I to myself, for sorrow shall be yours in the morning, so I took out my knife and went round the fence and cut every horse loose, and they all ran away. I then got on my horse and set off home. As I rode on I thought to myself—I only wish I could be somewhere close enough to see how those negroes will act when they come out and find all their horses gone. And then I laughed right out when I thought of the sport they had had out of my misfortune, and that some were ten to twelve, and some fifteen miles away from home. Well, thought I, your masters will have to reckon with you to-morrow; you have had glad hearts to-night at my expense, but you will have sore backs to-morrow at your own. Now, when I got home, the stable was in a very bad situation, and I was afraid to bring my horse in until I could strike a light. When this was done, I took the saddle and bridle off outside. No sooner had I done this than my horse reared over the bars and ran away into the meadow. I chased him till daylight, and for my life I could not catch him. My feelings now may be better imagined than described. When the reader remembers that this horse, with all the rest, master had seen clean at six o'clock the night before, and all safe in the stable, and now to see him in the meadow, with all the marks of having been driven somewhere and by somebody, what excuse could I make, or what story could I invent in order to save my poor back from that awful flogging which I knew must be the result of the revelation of the truth. I studied and tried, but could think of no lie that would stand muster. At last I went into the stable and turned all the rest out, and left the stable door open, and creeping into the house, took off my fine clothes and put on those which I had been wearing all the week, and laid myself down on my straw. I had not lain long before I heard master shouting for me, for all those horses, eight in number, were under my care; and although he shouted for me at the top of his voice, I lay still and pretended not to hear him; but soon after I heard a light step coming up stairs, and a rap at my door—then I commenced to snore as loud as possible, still the knocking continued. At last I pretended to awake, and called out, who's there—that you, Lizzy? oh my! what's up, what time is it, and so on. Lizzy said master wanted me immediately; yes, Lizzy, said I, tell master I'm coming. I bothered about the room long enough to give colour to the impression that I had just finished dressing myself; I then came and said, here I am, master, when he demanded of me, what were my horses doing in the meadow? Here I put on an expression of such wonder and surprise—looking first into the meadow and then at the stable door, and to master's satisfaction, I seemed so completely confounded that my deception took upon him the desired effect. Then I affected to roar right out, crying, now master, you saw my horses all clean last night before I went to bed, and now some of those negroes have turned them out so that I should have them to clean over again: well, I declare! it's too bad, and I roared and cried as I went towards the meadow to drive them up; but master believing what I said, called me back and told me to call Mr. Cobb, and when Mr. Cobb came master told him to blow the horn; when the horn was blown, the negroes were to be seen coming from all parts of the plantation, and forming around in front of the balcony. Master then came out and said, now I saw this boy's horses clean last night and in the stable, so now tell me which of you turned them out? Of course they all denied it, then master ordered them all to go down into the meadow and drive up the horses and clean them, me excepted; so they went and drove them up and set to work and cleaned them. On Monday morning we all turned out to work until breakfast, when the horn was blown, and we all repaired to the house. Here master again demanded to know who turned the horses loose, and when they all denied it, he tied them all up and gave them each 39 lashes. Not yet satisfied, but determined to have a confession, as was always his custom on such occasions, he came to me and asked me which one I had reason to suspect. My poor guilty heart already bleeding for the suffering I had caused my fellow slaves, was now almost driven to confession. What must I do, select another victim for further punishment, or confess the truth and bear the consequence? My conscience now rebuked me, like an armed man; but I happened to be one of those boys who, among all even of my mother's children loved myself best, and therefore had no disposition to satisfy my conscience at the expense of a very sore back, so I very soon thought of Dick, a negro who, like Ishmael, had his hand out against every man, and all our hands were out against him; this negro was a lickspittle or tell-tale, as little boys call them—we could not steal a bit of tea or sugar, or any other kind of nourishment for our sick, or do anything else we did not want to be known, but if he got to know it he would run and tell master or mistress, or the overseer, so we all wanted him dead; and now I thought of him—he was just the proper sacrifice for me to lay upon the altar of confession, so I told master I believed that it was Dick: moreover, I told him that I had seen him in and out of the stable on Saturday night, so master tied Dick up and gave him 39 lashes more, and washed his back down with salt and water, and told him that at night if he did not confess, he would give him as much more; so at night, when master went out to Dick again, he asked if he had made up his mind to tell him the truth, Dick said, yes, master;—well, said master, let me hear it. Well master, said Dick, I did turn the horses out; but will never do so again. So master, satisfied with this confession, struck Dick no more, and ordered him to be untied; but Dick had a sore back for many weeks. And now to return to the negroes I had left at the dance, when they discovered that their horses were gone there was the greatest consternation amongst them, the forebodings of the awful consequences if they dared to go home induced many that night to seek salvation in the direction and guidance of the north star. Several who started off on that memorable night I have since shook hands with in Canada. They told me there were sixteen of them went off together, four of them were shot or killed by the bloodhounds, and one was captured while asleep in a barn; the rest of those who were at the dance either went home and took their floggings, or strayed into the woods until starved out, and then surrendered. One of those I saw in Toronto, is Dan Patterson; he has a house of his own, with a fine horse and cart, and he has a beautiful Sambo woman for his wife, and four fine healthy-looking children. But, like myself, he had left a wife and six children in slavery. When I was about seventeen, I was deeply smitten in love with a yellow girl belonging to Doctor Tillotson. This girl's name was Mary, of whose lovliness I dreamt every night. I certainly thought she was the prettiest girl I had ever seen in my life. Her colour was very fair, approaching almost to white; her countenance was frank and open, and very inviting; her voice was as sweet as the dulcimer, her smiles to me were like the May morning sunbeams in the spring, one glance of her large dark eyes broke my heart in pieces, with a stroke like that of an earthquake. O, I thought, this girl would make me a paradise, and to enjoy her love I thought would be heaven. In spite of either patrols or dogs, who stood in my way, every night nearly I was in Mary's company. I learned from her that she had already had a child to her master in Mobile, and that her mistress had sold her down here for revenge; and she told me also of the sufferings that she had undergone from her mistress on account of jealousy—her baby she said her mistress sold out of her arms, only eleven months old, to a lady in Marysville, Kentucky. Having never before felt a passion like this, or of the gentle power, so peculiar to women, that, hard as I worked all day, I could not sleep at night for thinking of this almost angel in human shape. We kept company about six weeks, during which time I was at sometimes as wretched as I was happy at others. Much to my annoyance Mary was adored by every negro in the neighbourhood, and this excited my jealousy and made me miserable. I was almost crazy when I saw another negro talking to her. Again and again I tried my best to get her to give up speaking to them, but she refused to comply. There was one negro who was in the habit of calling on Mary whom I dreaded more than all the rest of them put together, this negro was Dan, he belonged to Rogers; and notwithstanding I believed myself to be the best looking negro to be found anywhere in the neighbourhood, still I was aware that I was not the best of talkers. Dan was a sweet and easy talker, and a good bone and banjo player. I was led to fear that he would displace me in Mary's affections, and in this I was not mistaken. One night I went over to see Mary, and in looking through the window, saw Mary—my sweet and beloved Mary—sitting upon Dan's knee; and here it is impossible to describe the feeling that came over me at this unwelcome sight. My teeth clenched and bit my tongue—my head grew dizzy, and began to swim round and round, and at last I found myself getting up from the ground, having stumbled from the effects of what I had seen. I wandered towards home, and arriving there threw myself on the straw and cried all night. My first determination was to kill Dan; but then I thought they would hang me and the devil would have us both, and some other negro will get Mary, then the thought of killing Dan passed away. Next morning, when the horn blew for breakfast, I continued my work, my appetite having left me; at dinner time it was the same. At sun-down I went to the barn and got a rope and put it under my jacket, and started off to see Mary, whom I found sitting in the kitchen, smoking her pipe, for smoking was as common among the girls as among the men. Mary, said I, I was over here last night and saw you through the window sitting on Dan's knee. Now, Mary, I want you to tell me at once whose you mean to be—mine or Dan's? Dan's, she replied, with an important toss of her head, which went through my very soul, like the shock from a galvanic battery. I rested for a minute or so on an old oak table that stood by. Mary's answer had unstrung every nerve in me, and left me so weak that I could scarcely keep from falling. Now I was not at that time, and dont think I ever shall be one of those fools who would cut off his nose to spite his face, much less kill myself because a girl refused to love me. Life to me was always preferable, under any circumstances; but in this case I played the most dexterous card I had. Mary, said I sternly, if you dont give Dan up and sware to be mine, I will hang myself this night. To this she replied, hang on if you are fool enough, and continued smoking her pipe as though not the least alarmed. I took out the rope from under my jacket, and got upon a three-legged stool, and putting the rope first over the beam in the ceiling, then made a slip-knot, and brought it down round my neck, taking good care to have it short enough that it would not choke me, and in this way I stood upon the stool for some considerable time, groaning and struggling, and making every kind of noise that might make her believe that I was choking or strangling; but still Mary sat deliberately smoking her pipe with the utmost coolness, and seemed to take no notice of me or what I was doing. I thought my situation worse now than if I had not commenced this job at all. My object in pretending to hang myself was to frighten Mary into compliance with my demand, and her conduct turned out to be everything but what I had expected. I had thought that the moment I ascended the stool she would have clung to me and tried to dissuade me from committing suicide, and in this case my plan was to persist in carrying it out, unless she would consent to give Dan up; but instead of this she sat smoking her pipe apparently at ease and unmoved. Now I found I had been mistaken—what was I to do, to hang or kill myself was the last thing I meant to do—in fact I had not the courage to do it for five hundred Marys. But now, after mounting the stool and adjusting the rope round my neck, I was positively ashamed to come down without hanging myself, and then I stood like a fool. At this moment in came the dog carlow, racing after the cat, right across the kitchen floor, and the dog coming in contact with the stool, knocked it right away from under my feet, and brought my neck suddenly to the full length of the rope, which barely allowed my toes to touch the floor. Here I seized the rope with both hands to keep the weight of my whole body off my neck, and in this situation I soon found I must hang, and that dead enough, unless I had some assistance, for the stool had rolled entirely out of the reach of my feet, and the knot I had tied behind the beam I could not reach for my life. My arms began to tremble with holding on to the rope, and still my mortification and pride for some time refused to let me call on Mary for assistance. Such a moment of terror and suspense! heaven forbid that I should ever see or experience again. Thoughts rushed into my mind of every bad deed that I had done in my life; and I thought that old cloven foot, as we called the devil, was waiting to nab me. The stretch upon my arms exhausted me, with holding on by the rope, nothing was left me but despair; my pride and courage gave up the ghost, and I roared out, Mary! for God's sake cut the rope! No, answered Mary, you went up there to hang yourself, so now hang on. Oh! Mary, Mary! I did not mean to hang! I was only doing so to see what you would say. Well, then, said Mary; you hear what I have to say—hang on. Oh, Mary! for heaven's sake cut this rope, or I shall strangle to death!—oh, dear, good Mary, save me this time: and I roared out like a jackass, and must too have fainted, for when I came round Doctor Tillotson and his wife and Mary stood over me as I lay on the floor. How I got upon the floor, or who cut the rope

I never knew. Doctor Tillotson had hold of my wrist, feeling my pulse; while mistress held a camphor bottle in one hand and a bottle of hartshorn in the other. The doctor helped me up from the floor and set me in a chair, when I discovered that I was bleeding very freely from the nose and mouth. He called for a basin and bled me in my left arm, and then sent me over home by two of his men. Next day my neck was dreadfully swollen, and my throat was so sore that it was with difficulty that I could swallow meat for more than a week. At the end of a fortnight, master having learnt all the particulars respecting my sickness, called me to account, and gave me seventy-eight lashes, and this was the end of my crazy love and courtship with Mary.

Shortly after this, Mary was one Sunday down in her master's barn, where she had been sent by her mistress to look for new nests where a number of the hens were supposed to have been laying, as the eggs had not been found elsewhere. While in the barn, Mary was surprised by William Tillotson, her master's son, who ordered her to take her bed among the hay and submit to his lustful passion. This she strenuously refused to do, telling him of the punishment she had already suffered from her former mistress for a similar act of conduct, and reminding him at the same time of his wife, whose vengeance she would have to dread; but William was not to be put off, nor his base passion to go unsatisfied, by any excuse that Mary could make, so he at once resorted to force. Mary screamed at the top of her voice. Now the negro Dan was just in the act of passing the barn at the time, when he heard Mary's voice he rushed into the barn, and demanded in a loud voice what was the matter? when, to his horror, he beheld William upon the barn floor, and Mary struggling but in vain to rise. William, instead of desisting from his brutal purpose, with a dreadful oath ordered Dan to clear out; but the sight of the outrage on her whom, I now firmly believe he loved better than his own soul, made poor Dan completely forget himself—and made him forget too, in that fatal moment what he afterwards wished he had remembered. Dan seized a pitchfork and plunged it into young Tillotson's back; the prongs went in between his shoulders, and one of them had penetrated the left lung. Young Tillotson expired almost immediately, and Dan seeing what he had done, ran off at once to the woods and swamps, and was seen no more for about two months. Mrs. Tillotson, who had heard Mary scream, was on the balcony, and called out to Dan to know the cause, Dan made no reply but took to his heels. Mrs. Tillotson alarmed at this, and suspecting at once that something was wrong, hastened to the barn, followed by William's wife who happened to be there, and when they saw poor William's corpse, and Mary standing by, they both fainted. Poor Mary, frightened to death, turned into the house and informed her young mistress, Susannah, of what had happened. Miss Susannah spread the alarm, and called some of the slaves to her assistance. She went to the barn and found her mother and sister-in-law lying in a state of insensibility, and her brother William dead. With the assistance of old Aunt Hannah and several of the female servants, the two ladies were somewhat restored to consciousness; and William was carried into the house by the servants. The Doctor himself was away from home attending one of his patients, who was very sick. When Mrs. Tillotson had somewhat recovered, she sent for Mary and enquired as to how William came by his death in the barn. Mary told the whole story as previously related in the presence of about sixty or seventy of the neighbours, who had collected together on hearing of the murder. Of course Mary's story met with no credit from her mistress, and poor Mary stood in the eyes of all as an accomplice in the conspiracy to murder young Tillotson. When the doctor arrived it was dark, and after seeing the corpse and hearing from his wife the story that she had made up for him, he called for Mary, but she was nowhere to be found. The house and plantation were searched in all directions, but no Mary was discovered. At last, when they had all given over looking for her, towards midnight, a cart drove up to the door. Doctor, said the driver, I have a dead negro here, and I'm told she belongs to you. The Doctor came out with a lantern, and as I stood by my master's carriage, waiting for him to come out and go home, the Doctor ordered me to mount the cart and look at the corpse; I did so, and looked full in that face by the light of the lantern, and saw and knew, notwithstanding the horrible change that had been effected by the work of death, upon those once beautiful features, it was Mary. Poor Mary, driven to distraction by what had happened, she had sought salvation in the depths of the Chesapeake Bay that night. Next day the neighbourhood was searched throughout, and the country was placarded for Dan; and Doctor Tillotson and Mr. Burmey, young William's father-in-law, offered one thousand dollars for him alive, and five hundred for him dead; and although every blackleg in the neighbourhood was on the alert, it was full two months before he was captured. At length poor Dan was caught and brought by the captors to Mr. Burmey's, where he was tried principally by Burmey's two sons, Peter and John, and that night was kept in irons in Burmey's cellar. The next day Dan was led into the field in the presence of about three thousand of us. A staple was driven into the stump of a tree, with a chain attached to it, and one of his handcuffs was taken off and brought through the chain, and then fastened on his hand again. A pile of pine wood was built around him. At eight o'clock the wood was set on fire, and when the flames blazed round upon the wretched man, he began to scream and struggle in a most awful manner. Many of our women fainted, but not one of us was allowed to leave until the body of poor Dan was consumed. The unearthly sounds that came from the blazing pile, as poor Dan writhed in the agonies of death, it is beyond the power of my pen to describe. After a while all was silent, except the cracking of the pine wood as the fire gradually devoured it with the prize that it contained. Poor Dan had ceased to struggle—he was at rest.

Mr. Burmey's two sons, Peter and John, were the ringleaders in this execution, and the pair of them hardly ever saw a sober day from one month to another; and at the execution of Dan, Peter was so drunk that he came nigh sharing the same fate. It was not a year after the roasting of Dan that the two brothers were thrashing wheat in the barn, which stood about a quarter of a mile from the house, and being in March, and an uncommon windy day, they had taken their demijohn full of brandy in order to keep the cold out of their bones, as it was their belief that a dram or two had that effect; so they were drinking and thrashing and drinking again until they reeled over dead drunk upon the floor. That same night the barn took fire over them. The first thing that excited the alarm of my master's negroes on Tillotson's plantation was a black smoke issuing from the barn. Suddenly there was a rush from all parts of the plantation, but it was all to no purpose, for scarcely had we got half way before we saw the flames bursting out on every side of the barn, still we continued to run as fast as we could. When we arrived we found the barn door shut and fastened inside. This Mr. Peter and Mr. John had done to keep out the wind which was very high. When old Mr. Burmey arrived with his daughter-in-law, Peter's wife, the first thing demanded was, where is your masters?—oh, my children! my children! while Mrs. Peter screamed, my husband! my husband! oh, pa! oh, pa! The strength of the flames inside at length burst open the barn door, when we beheld through the red flames the figures of the two wretched brothers lying side by side dead drunk and helpless upon the floor. The fire rapidly seized upon everything around. At this moment Mrs. Peter Burmey rushed into the flames to save her husband, but just as she attempted to enter, the beam over the door fell in upon her head, and struck her back senseless and suffocated to the ground; but, notwithstanding the most intense hatred to Burmey and his family, we negroes rushed forward to rescue them—but all in vain. After getting miserably scorched we were compelled to retreat and give them over, and with bleeding hearts to behold the fire consume their bodies. The barn was rapidly consigned to ashes, which being speedily swept away by the violence of the wind, left the victims side by side crisped skeletons on the ground. This was the dreadful end of the two chief actors in the roasting of poor Dan.

When I arrived at the age of 20, my master told me I must marry Jane, one of the slaves. We had been about five months married when she gave birth to a child, I then asked who was the father of the child, and she said the master, and I had every reason to believe her, as the child was nearly white, had blue eyes and veins, yet notwithstanding this we lived happily together, and I felt happy and comfortable, and I should never have thought of running away if she had not been sold. We lived together six years and had two children. Shortly after my marriage my master's wife died, and when he fixed upon Tillotson's daughter as his future wife, she made a condition that all female slaves whom he had at any time been intimate with must be sold, and my wife being one was sold with the children as well as any other female slaves. My wife was sold while I was away on an errand at Centreville, and any one situated as I was may imagine my feelings when I say that I left them in the morning all well and happy, in entire ignorance of any evil, and returned to find them all sold and gone away, and from then until now I have never seen any of them. I went to my master and complained to him, when he told me he knew nothing about it, as it was all done by his wife. I then went to her and she said she knew nothing about, as it was all done by my master, and I could obtain no other satisfaction; I then went to my master to beg him to sell me to the same master as he had sold my wife, but he said he could not do that, as she was sold to a trader.

From 18 to 27 I was considered one of the most devout christians among the whole Black population, and under this impression I firmly believed to run away from my master would be to sin against the Holy Ghost—for such we are taught to believe—but from the time of my wife's being sent away, I firmly made up my mind to take the first opportunity to run away. I had learned that if a Black man wished to escape he will have no chance to do so unless he be well supplied with money; to attain this I arranged with a Dutchman to steal small pigs, chickens, and any poultry that was possible to lay my hands on, and thus I proceeded for nine or ten months, when I found my accumulation to be 124 dollars. Among the plantations I visited was Mr. Rogers', and he had three large bloodhounds let loose about nine at night, but I had made them acquainted with me by feeding them at intervals quietly, unknown to him or his people, and this enabled me to carry on my depredations on his plantation quietly and unmolested. Rogers having suspected these depredations, and not being able to find the thief, set a patrol to watch, who, armed with a double-barreled gun, fixed himself under a fence about seven feet high, surrounded with bushes; but this happened to be my usual way of going to his plantation, and as I made my usual spring to go over, I fell right on the top of his head, and he shouted lustily, and I shouted also, neither of us knowing what really had occurred, and our fears imag-

ining the worst and causing him to run one way and me another. After travelling about a quarter of a mile I thought of
my bag, which had been dropped during my fright, and
knowing that my master's initials were on the bag, and the
consequences of the bag being found would be fearful, I determined to return for the bag and recover it, or die in the attempt. I searched for and found a club, then I returned to the
spot and found the bag there, and by the side of it lay the gun
of the patrol, and I picked the bag up and went home, and
this narrow escape caused me to determine to give up my
thieving expeditions for the obtaining of money from that
time. About one week after the occurrence with the patrol, I
took one of my master's horses to go to a negro dance, and
on my return the patrols were so numerous on the road that
I was unable to return home without observation, and it
being past the usual hour for being at home, I was so afraid
that when two of them observed me I left the horse and took
to my feet, and made my way to the woods, where I remained
all day, afraid to go home for fear of the consequences. But at
night I returned to the barn, where my money was hid in the
hay, and having recovered it, I started for Dr. Tillotson's (my
master's father-in-law), and told him my master had sent for
a horse which he had lent him a few weeks before. After enquiring of the overseer if the horse had not gone home, and
finding it had not, he ordered it to be given up to me. I
mounted the horse and rode off for Baltimore, a distance of
37 miles, where I arrived early in the morning, when I abandoned the horse and took to the woods, and remained there
all day. At night I ventured to a farm-house, and having a
club with me, I knocked over two barn fowl, and took them
to my place in the woods; I struck a light with the tinder,
made a fire of brushwood, roasted them before the fire, and
enjoyed a hearty meal without seasoning or bread.

The following night I went to the city, and meeting with
some blacks I entered into conversation with them, and I
asked if they had heard of any runaways at Baltimore, they
said they had heard of one Jake having run from Eastern
shore, and showed me the bill at the corner which had been
put up that evening. I knew it was no other than me, so I bid
them good evening, and left them saying I was going to

church. I took a back road for Milford, in Delaware, and travelled all night; towards morning I met four men, who demanded to know to whom I belonged, my answer was taking to my heels, and the chase was hot on my part for about half-an-hour, when I got into a swamp surrounded by young saplings, where I remained about two hours, and as soon as it was sufficiently dark to venture out, I made my way to a barn where I secreted myself all day, and in the morning I watched the house to prevent a surprise. At night I again commenced travelling, and at one o'clock in the morning arrived at Milford, where finding no means of crossing the bridge into the town, without being seen by the patrol, I was forced to swim across the river. I passed through Milford, and was ten miles on my road to Wilmington before daybreak, where I again made for the woods, and got into a marshy part and was swamped. I was struggling the whole night to liberate myself, but in vain, until the light appeared, when I saw some willows, and by laying hold of them I succeeded in extricating myself about seven o'clock in the morning. I then made my way to a pond of water, and pulled my clothes off, and washed the mud from them, and hung them up to dry; and as soon as they were dry and night arrived, I put them on, and continued my journey that night in the woods, as the moon was so bright; though I did not progress much on my way, it was more safe. Towards morning I saw a farm-house, and being hungry I resolved to venture to ask for something to eat. Waiting my opportunity, I saw three men leave the house, and judging there then only remained women, I went up and asked if they would please to give me something to eat. They invited me in, and gave me some bread and milk, pitying my condition greatly, one of them telling me that her husband was an Abolitionist, and if I would wait until his return he would place me out of the reach of my pursuers. I did not then understand what was an Abolitionist, and said I would rather not stay. She then saw my feet, which were awful from what I had undergone, and asked me if I should not like to have a pair of shoes, and I said I should. They went in search of a pair up the stairs, and I heard one say to the other, "He answers the description of a slave for which 200 dollars are offered." When they returned I was sitting still in the position I was in before they went up stairs. She said to the other, "I will go and see after the cows;" and the other answered, "Dont be long." But my suspicion was confirmed that going after the cows was only a pretence; and when I thought the other had got far enough away, I laid hold of the remaining one and tied her to the bedstead; went into the closet and took a leg of mutton, and other articles, such as bread and butter, and made my way out as quick as possible; and when I got outside I rubbed my feet in some cow dung to prevent the scent of the bloodhounds, and took to the woods, where I found a sand hole, in which I remained all day. The night was dark, with a drizzling rain; being very fit for travelling, I started again on my journey, but being very cautious, I only managed about 24 miles that night. Towards morning I met with a black, who told me that to Chester, in Pennsylvania, was only twenty-six miles. During the day I again remained in the woods, where I met a black man of the name of Geordie, whom I knew, belonging to Rogers, and who had left two months before me, and he said he had been in those woods five weeks. His appearance was shocking, and from his long suffering and hardships he was difficult to know; and, as he was hungry, I divided with him my leg of mutton and bread and butter, and I was telling him how unwise it was to remain so long in one place, when we were suddenly aroused by the well-known sounds of the hounds. In my fear and surprise I was attempting for a tree, but was unable to mount before they were upon me. In this emergency I called out the name of one of the dogs, who was more familiar with me than the others, called Fly, and hit my knee to attract her attention and it had the desired effect. She came fondling towards me, accompanied by another called Jovial. I pulled out my knife and cut the throat of Fly, upon which Jovial made an attempt to lay hold of me and I caught him by the throat, which caused me to lose my knife, but I held him fast by the windpipe, forcing my thumbs with as much force as possible, and anxiously wishing for my knife to be in hands. I made a powerful effort to fling him as far away as possible, and regained my knife; but when I had thrown him there he lay, throttled to death. Not so, Fly, who weltered in blood, and rolled about howling terribly, but not killed. The other two hounds caught Geordie, and killed him. After this terrible escape I went to a barn, and was looking through a hole and saw two men come to where Geordie's body lay, when a knot of people gathered round, and about ten or eleven o'clock he was buried. I shortly went to sleep among the hay, and slept so soundly that it was the morning after before I was awoke by a boy coming to get hay for the horses, and the prong of the fork caught me by the thigh, which caused me to jump up and stare at the boy, and he at me, when he dropped the fork and ran away. As soon as I recovered, I slipped down the hay-rack, and met six men and the boy, who demanded who I was and what I was doing there. Not knowing what to say, I stood speechless for a long time, and thought my hopes of freedom were now at an end. They again repeated their question, but I made no reply. I was then taken before a magistrate, when I was accused of being in the barn for some unlawful purpose; and as I made no answer to any questions put to me, they concluded I was dumb. When I remembered I had not given evidence of speech, I determined to act as if I was dumb; and when the magistrate called to me, I also thought deafness was often united with dumbness, and I made my mind up to act both deaf and dumb, and when he called "Boy, come here," I took no notice, and did not appear to hear, until one of the officers led me from the box nearer to the magistrate, who demanded my name, where from, and to whom I belonged, and what I was doing in the barn, which I still appeared not to hear, and merely looked at him, and at last acted as if I was deaf and dumb, and so effectually that he discharged me, convinced I was a valueless deaf and dumb nigger; and when told by the officer to go, I dared not move for fear of being found out in my acting, and would not move until I was forced out of the door, and for some time (for fear of detection) I acted deaf and dumb in the streets, to the fear of women and children, until it was dark, when I made for the woods, where I remained until eleven o'clock at night, when I again resumed my journey to Chester (Pennsylvania), which I had been told was only twenty-six miles. Shortly after resuming my journey, I saw four horses in the field, and I determined, if possible to possess one of them, and I chased them two hours, but did not succeed in catching one; so I was obliged to go on walking again, but shortly met with a gentleman's horse on the road which I mounted, and rode into Chester, and let the horse go where he liked. In Chester I met with a quaker, named Sharples, who took me to his house, gave me the best accommodation, and called his friends to see me, never seemed weary of asking questions of negro life in the different plantations. I let them see the money I had, which was in notes, and much damaged by my swimming across the river, but they kindly passed it for me, and I got other money for it; and I was presented with two suits of clothes. He sent in a waggon to Philadelphia and recommended me to a gentleman (who being alive, I wish not to reveal), where I remained in his employ about five weeks. This kind friend persuaded me to make for Canada; and it was with much reluctance I at last complied. My reluctance was in consequence of understanding that Canada was a very cold place, and I did not relish the idea of going on that account; and as a gentleman said he could find employment for me at Derby, near Philadelphia, I went and worked there three years, during which time I was a regular attendant at the Methodist Free Church, consisting entirely of colored people; at which place I heard the scriptures expounded in a different way by colored ministers—as I found that God had made colored as well as white people: as He had made of one blood all the families of the earth, and that all men were free and equal in his sight; and that he was no respecter of persons whatever the color: but whoever worked righteousness was accepted of Him. Being satisfied that I had not sinned against the Holy Ghost by obtaining my freedom, I enlisted in the church, and became one of the members thereof.

About this time, Mr. Roberts, for whom I worked, failed in business, and his property was seized for debt and sold, thereby throwing me out of employment. I was arrested and taken back to Maryland, where I was placed in prison, with a collar round my neck for eleven days.

On the twelfth day my master came to see me, and of course I begged of him to take me home and let me go to work. No, nigger, said master—I have no employment for a vagabond of your stamp; but I'm going to order that collar off

your neck, not because I think that you are sufficiently punished, but because there are some gentlemen coming through
the jail to-morrow, and they want to purchase some negroes,
so you had better do your best to get a master amongst
them—and mind you dont tell them that ever you ran away,
for if you do none of them will buy you. Now I will give you
a good character, notwithstanding you have done your best to
injure me, a good master, and you have even tried to rob me
by running away—still I'll do my best to get you a good master, for my bible teaches me to do good for evil. The next day
I was called out with forty other slaves, belonging to different
owners in the County, and we were marched into the doctor's
vestry for examination; here the doctor made us all strip—
men and women together naked, in the presence of each other
while the examination went on. When it was concluded,
thirty-eight of us were pronounced sound, and three unsound; certificates were made out and given to the auctioneer
to that effect. After dressing ourselves we were all driven into
the slave sty directly under the auction block, when the jail
warder came and gave to every slave a number, my number
was twenty. Here, let me explain, for the better information of
the reader, that in the inventory of the slaves to be sold all go
by number—one, two, three, and so on; and if a man and his
family are to be sold in one lot, then one number covers them
all; but if separate, then they have all different numbers. An
old friend of mine, belonging to William Steel, was also with
his wife and six children in the same sty, all to be sold. The
youngest was a babe in arms, the other five were large enough
to walk; his number was twenty-one, but his wife's number
was thirty-three, and notwithstanding the mournful idea of
parting with relations and friends on the plantation, up to this
moment they had indulged a hope of being sold as a family,
together; but the numbers revealed the awful disappointment.
Even in this hoped for consolation, the painful distress into
which this poor woman was thrown, it is beyond my ability to
describe. The anguish of her soul, evinced by the mournful
gaze first at her children and then at her husband, made me
forget for the time being, my own sufferings and sorrows. Her
looks seemed to say to her husband—these are your children,
I am their mother—there is no other being in this world that

I have to look to for love and protection; cant you help me? I am very much mistaken if these were not the thoughts running through that poor broken-hearted mother's mind. Reuben, for that was his name, called his wife and children into one corner of the sty, and repeated a verse of a hymn which may be found in Watts' hymn book:—

> "Ah, whither shall I go,
>   Burthened, or sick, or faint;
> To whom shall I my troubles show,
>   And pour out my complaint."

Not daring to sing it for fear of disturbing the sale, they both knelt down with the children, and Reuben offered up a long and fervent prayer. In the interval of his prayer nineteen of the slaves were sold, and he had not concluded when my number being twenty was called, and my master handed me out under the hammer; when, after a few preliminary remarks on the part of the auctioneer, my master mounted the auction block and recommended me as a good field hand, a good cook, waiter, hostler, a coachman, gentle and willing, and above all, free from the disease of running away. So after a short and spirited bidding I went at 1,025 dollars. Here the sale policeman, whose business it was to take charge of the negroes sold until bills were settled and papers made out, led me from the block outside the crowd, and placing me by a cart, put on a pair of iron handcuffs; but being well acquainted with me as a troublesome tricky negro, he put the handcuff on my right wrist—took the other cuff through the cart wheel and round the spoke, and then locked it on my left hand, so that if I did start to run, I should carry the cart and all with me. Number twenty-one was now called, and out came poor Reuben, and was placed under the hammer; his weight was said to be two hundred pounds, his age thirty two. Poor Sally, his wife, unable any longer to control her feelings, made her way out of the slave pen, with her babe in her arms, followed by her five small children, and she threw one of her arms around Reuben's neck; and now commenced a scene that beggars all description. Her countenance, though mild and beautiful, was by the keenest pain and sorrow distorted and disfigured: her voice soft and gentle, accompanied

with heart rending gestures, appealed to the slave buyer in
tones so very mournful, that I thought it might have even
melted cruelty itself to some pity—coming as it did from a
woman:—Oh! master, master! buy me and my children with
my husband—do, pray; and this was the only crime the poor
woman committed for which she suffered death on the spot.
Her master stepped up from behind her, and with the butt
end of his carriage whip loaded with lead, struck her a blow
on the side of the head or temples, and she fell her full length
to the ground. Poor Reuben stooped to raise her up, but was
prevented by the jail policeman, who seized him by the neck
and led him over close to where I stood: and whilst he was in
the act of selecting a pair of handcuffs for Reuben, voice after
voice was heard in the crowd—she is dead! she is dead! But
what was the effect of these words upon Reuben—one of the
most easy, good-tempered, innocent, inoffensive, and, in his
way, religious slaves that I ever knew—satisfied apparently
that Sally's death was a fact—he tore himself loose from the
policeman and made his way through the crowd to where
poor Sally lay, and exclaimed, Oh! Sally! O Lord! By this time
the policeman, who had followed him, undertook to drag him
back out of the crowd, but Reuben, with one blow of his fist,
stretched the policeman on the ground. Reuben's pain and
sorrow, mingled with his religious hope, seemed now to terminate in despair, and transformed the inoffensive man into a
raging demon. He rushed to a cart which supported a great
number of spectators, just opposite the auction block, and
tore out a heavy cart stave, made of red oak, and before the
panic-stricken crowd could arrest his arm, he struck his master to the ground, and beat his brains literally out. The crowd
then tried to close upon him, but Reuben, mounted with
both feet upon the dead body of his master, and with his back
against the cart wheel—with the cart stave kept the whole
crowd at bay for the space of two or three minutes, when a
gentleman behind the cart climbed upon the outside wheel
and fired the pistol at him, and shot poor Reuben through the
head. He fell dead about six yards from where the dead body
of his beloved Sally lay, and where his children were screaming terribly. An indescribable thrill of horror crept through
my whole soul, as I gazed from the cart wheel to which I was

ironed, upon the dead bodies first of Reuben and then his wife, who but a few moments before I had seen kneeling in solemn prayer, before what they considered the Throne of Grace—and their master, whom I heard that very morning calling on God not only to damn his negroes, but to damn himself, now, in less than thirty minutes, all three standing before the awful Judgment Seat. After witnessing this dreadful scene I was led into Hagerstown jail, where I remained until my new master was ready, when I went with him to Memphis, Tennessee; but the remembrance of this awful tragedy haunted my mind, and even my dreams, for many months.

Reuben was the son of old Uncle Reuben and Aunt Dinah, and had been swopped away when about twelve years old to William Steele, for a pair of horses and a splendid carriage. Like his father and mother he was very religious, and I had often been to his prayer meetings, where poor Reuben would exhort and preach. Mr. Cobb had made him a class-leader long before he died; and, in fact, we all reverenced Reuben after the death of his father as the most moderate and gifted man amongst us. I had always loved Reuben, but never knew how much until that fatal day. After I went to Memphis I composed some verses on the life and death of Reuben, which run as follows:—

> Poor Reuben he fell at his post,
>   He's gone;
> Like Stephen, full of the Holy Ghost,
>   Poor Reuben's gone away.
> He's gone where pleasure never dies,
>   He's gone,
> In the golden chariot to the skies,
>   Poor Reuben's gone away.
>
> For many years he faced the storm,
>   He's gone;
> And the cruel lash he suffered long;
>   Poor Reuben's gone away.
> But now he's left the land of death,
>   He's gone;
> And entered heaven's happiness;
>   Poor Reuben's gone away.

His friends he bid a long adieu,
    He's gone;
When heaven opened to his view,
    Poor Reuben's gone away;
His pain and sorrow of heart are passed,
    He's gone;
He arrived in heaven just safe at last;
    Poor Reuben's gone away.

Poor Sally, his wife, lays by his side,
    He's gone;
For whom poor Reuben so nobly died;
    Poor Reuben's gone away;
A mournful look on her he cast,
    He's gone,
Five minutes before he breathed his last,
    Poor Reuben's gone away.

In Jordan the angel heard him cry,
    He's gone;
Elijah's chariot was passing by,
    Poor Reuben's gone away;
His body lays in the earth quite cold,
    He's gone,
But now he walks in the streets of gold,
    Poor Reuben's gone away.

After working in Tennessee three years and seven months, my master hired me to Mr. Steele. This gentleman was going to New Orleans, and I was to act as his servant, but I contrived to get away from him, and went to the house of a free black, named Gibson, and after working four days on the levy (or wharf) I succeeded in secreting myself in a ship, well supplied by Mr. Gibson and friends with provisions, and in the middle hold under the cotton I remained until the ship arrived at New York; my being there was only known to two persons on board, the steward and the cook, both colored persons. When the vessel was docked in the pier thirty-eight, North river, I managed to make my way through the booby hatch on to the deck, and was not seen by the watchman on board who supposed I was a stranger, or what they call a

"River Thief." I made a jump to escape over the bow and fell into the river; but before he could raise an alarm, I had reached the next dock, got out and made my way off as fast as possible. I wandered about the streets until morning, not knowing where to go, during which time my clothes had dried on my body. About ten o'clock in the forenoon I met with a colored man named Grundy, who took me to his house, and gave me something to eat, and enquired where I came from and where I belonged; I hesitated about telling my true situation, but after considerable conversation with him, I ventured to confide in him, and when I had given him, all the particulars, he took me to the underground Railway office and introduced me to the officials, who having heard my story determined to send me to Canada, forty dollars being raised to find me clothes, and pay my fare to Toronto, but I was only taken to Utica, in the State of New York, where I agreed to stop with Mr. Cleveland and coachman.

In November I was sent to Post-street on an errand, where I saw my master, who laid hold of me, and called to his aid a dozen more, when I was taken before a magistrate, and that night I was placed in prison, and next day brought before a court, and ordered to be given up to my master. I was taken back to prison that afternoon, and irons placed on my ancles, and hand-cuffed; but, previous to leaving, Mr. Cleveland and family came to take a kind leave of me, and gave me religious advice and encouragement, telling me to put my trust in the Lord, and I was much affected at his little girl, who, when I was placed in the waggon screamed and cried as if she would fall into fits, telling her father to have me brought back, for these men intended to murder me. The waggon drove to the railway depot, and I was placed in the cars, and at three o'clock we started for Buffalo, where I was placed on the steam boat "Milwaukie," for Chicago, Illinois, on Lake Erie. The next night I arrived in Cleveland, and was taken from the boat, and placed in prison, until my master was ready to proceed. While in prison a complaint was made that a fugitive slave was placed in irons, contrary to the law of the state of Ohio, and after investigation, my irons were ordered to be taken off. On the Monday following I was taken on board the steam boat "Sultana" bound for Sandusky, Ohio, and on my way there, the Black people, in large numbers, made an attempt to rescue me, and so desperate was the attack, that several officers were wounded, and the attempt failed. I was placed in the cabin, and at dinner time the steam boat started, and had about half a mile to go before she got into the lake, and, on the way, the captain came down to me, and cautiously asked me if I could swim—I answered I could, when he told me to stand close by a window, which he pointed out, and when the paddle wheels ceased I must jump out. I stood ready, and as soon as the wheels ceased I made a spring and jumped into the water, and after going a short distance, I looked up and saw the captain standing on the promenade deck, who, when he saw I was clear of the wheels, waved a signal for the engineer to start the vessel. I had much difficulty in preventing myself from being drawn back by the suction of the wheels, and before I had gone far I saw my master and heard him shout, "Here, here, stop captain; yonder goes my nigger," which was echoed by shouts from the passengers; but the boat continued her course, while I made my way as fast as possible to Cleveland lighthouse, where I arrived in safety, and received by an innumerable company of both blacks and whites. I was then sent to a place called Oberlin, where I remained a week, and from there I went to Zanesville, Ohio, where I stopped for four months, when I was taken up on suspicion of breaking the windows of a store, and while in prison I was seen by a Mr. Donelson, who declared to the keeper that I belonged to him. I knew him well as the father-in-law of Mr. Steel, with whom I travelled to New Orleans. He was also a methodist minister. He had me discharged by paying the damage, and making affidavit that I was his slave, I was placed in prison, and kept in two weeks, when I was brought before the court for trial; and Mr. Donelson procured papers showing that he had purchased me as a runaway. I therefore saw it was of no use prolonging the matter, and I acknowledged myself. I was then taken and put into the stage and taken to Cincinnati, Ohio, where I was placed upon the steam boat, *Pike*, No. 3, to be taken to Louisville, Kentucky, and there placed in prison a week, and on Thursday brought out to auction and sold to Mr. Silas Wheelbanks for 1,050 dollars, with whom I remained about twelve months, and acted as coachman and waiting in the house. Upon a Saturday evening, my master came and told me to make my carriage and horses so that he could see his face in them, and be ready to take my young mistress, Mary, down to Centreville, to see her grandmother. So I prepared my horses and carriage, and on Monday was ready. The lady got in, and when about seven miles I drove into a blind road, distant about two miles from any house, where I made the horses stand still, and I ordered Miss Mary to get out: and when she asked me why, I thundered out at the top of my voice, "Get out, and ask no questions." She commenced crying, and asked if I was going to kill her. I said "No, if she made no noise," I helped her out, and having no rope, I took her shawl and fastened her to a tree by the roadside; and for fear she should untie the knot and spread the alarm, I took off her veil, and with it tied her hands behind her. I then mounted the box, and drove off in the direction of Lexington, and at a place called Elton I stripped the horses of their harness and let them go. I made my way to Louisville and arrived about 7 o'clock in the evening. I walked about the dock until *Pike* No. 3, the same vessel before spoken of, was nearly ready for starting and I got a gentleman's trunk on my shoulder and went on board, and when I had been paid six cents for carrying the trunk I watched a chance, and jumped down the cotton hold and stowed myself away among the cotton bags and the next day was in Cincinnati, Ohio, where I arrived about daylight in the morning. I waited until the passangers had left the boat and saw neither officer nor engineer about when I ventured to go on shore. On starting up the hill I met my master's nephew, who at once seized hold of me, and a sharp struggle ensued. He called for help but I threw him and caught a stone and struck him on the head, which caused him to let go, when I ran away as fast my legs could carry me, pursued by a numerous crowd, crying "stop thief." I mounted a fence in the street, and ran though an alley into an Irishman's yard, and through his house, knocking over the Irishman's wife and child, and the chair on which she sat, the husband at the time sat eating at the table, jumped into a cellar on the opposite side of the street without being seen by any one, I made my way into the back cellar and went up the chimney, where I sat till dark, and at night came down and slept in the cellar. In the morning the servant girl came down into the cellar, and when I saw she was black I thought it would be best to make myself known to her, which I did, and she told me I had better remain where I was and keep quiet, and she would go and tell Mr. Nickins, one of the agents of the underground Railway. She brought me down a bowl of coffee and some bread and meat, which I relished very much, and that night she opened the cellar door gently, and called to me to come out, and introduced me to Mr. Nickins and two others, who took me to a house in Sixth street, where I remained until the next night, when they dressed me in female's clothes, and I was taken to the railway depot in a carriage—was put in the car, and sent to Cleveland, Ohio where I was placed on board a steam boat called the *Indiana*, and carried down Lake Erie to the city of Buffalo, New York, and the next day placed on the car for the Niagara Falls, and received by a gentleman named Jones, who took me in his carriage to a place called Lewiston, where I was placed on board a steamboat called *Chief Justice Robinson*. I was furnished with a ticket and twelve dollars. Three hours after starting I was in Toronto, Upper Canada, where I lived for three years and sang my song of deliverance,—

WHAT THE "TIMES" SAID OF THE SECESSION IN 1861

(From the *Liverpool Daily Post*, Feb. 3, 1863.)

The following article appeared as a "Leader" in the *Times* on the 7th of January, 1861:—

"The State of South Carolina has seceded from the Union by a unanimous vote of her legislature, and it now remains to be seen whether any of the other Southern States will follow her example, and what course the Federal authorities will pursue under the circumstances. While we wait for further information on these points, it may be well to consider once again the cause of quarrel which has thus begun to rend asunder the mightiest confederation which the world has yet beheld. One of the prevalent delusions of the age in which we live is to regard democracy as equivalent to liberty, and the attribution of power to the poorest and worst educated citizens of the State as a certain way to promote the purest liberality of thought and the most beneficial course of action. Let those who hold this opinion examine the quarrel at present raging in the United States, and they will be aware that democracy, like other forms of government, may co-exist with any course of action or any set of principles. Between North and South there is at this moment raging a controversy which goes as deep as any controversy can into the elementary principles of human nature and the sympathies and antipathies which in so many men supply the place of reason and reflection. The North is for freedom, the South is for slavery. The North is for freedom of discussion, the South represses freedom of discussion with the tar-brush and the pine fagot. Yet the North and South are both democracies—nay, possess almost exactly similar institutions, with this enormous divergence in theory and practice. It is not democracy that has made the North the advocate of freedom, or the South the advocate of slavery. Democracy is a quality which appears on both sides, and may therefore be rejected, as having no influence over the result. From the sketch of the history of slavery which was furnished us by our correspondent in New York last week, we learn that at the time of the American Revolution slavery existed in every State in the Union except Massachusetts; but we also learn that the great men who directed that revolution—Washington, Jefferson, Madison, Patrick Henry, and Hamilton—were unanimous in execrating the practice of slavery, and looked forward to the time when it would cease to contaminate the soil of free America. The abolition of the slave trade, which subsequently followed, was regarded by its warmest advocates as not only beneficial in itself, but as a long step towards the extinction of slavery altogether, it was not foreseen that certain free and democratic communities would arise which would apply themselves to the honourable office of breeding slaves, to be consumed on the free and democratic plantations of the South, and of thus replacing the African slave trade by an internal traffic in human flesh, carried on under circumstances of almost equal atrocity through the heart of a free and democratic nation. Democracy has verily a strong digestion, and one not to be interfered with by trifles.

"But the most melancholy part of the matter is, that during the seventy years for which the American confederacy has existed, the whole tone of sentiment with regard to slavery has, in the Southern States at least, undergone a remarkable change. Slavery used to be treated as a thoroughly exceptional institution—as an evil legacy of evil times—as a disgrace to a constitution founded on the natural freedom and independence of mankind. There was hardly a political leader of any note who had not some plan for its abolition. Jefferson himself, the greatest chief of the democracy, had in the early part of this century speculated deeply on the subject; but the United States became possessed of Louisiana and Florida, they have conquered Texas, they have made Arkansas and Missouri into States; and these successive acquisitions have altered entirely the view with which slavery is regarded. Perhaps as much as anything, from the long license enjoyed by the editors of the South of writing what they pleased in favour of slavery, with the absolute certainty that no one would be found bold enough to write anything on the other side, and thus make himself a mark for popular vengeance, the subject has come to be written on in a tone of ferocious and cynical extravagance, which is to an European eye absolutely appalling. The South has become enamoured of her shame. Free labour is denounced as degrading and disgraceful; the honest triumphs of the poor man who works his way to independence are treated with scorn and contempt. It is asserted that what we are in the habit of regarding as the honorable pursuits of industry incapacitate a nation for civilisation and refinement, and that no institutions can be really free and democratic which do not rest, like those of Athens and of Rome, on a broad substratum of slavery. So far from treating slavery as an exceptional institution, it is regarded by these Democratic philosophers as the natural state of a great portion of the human race; and, so far from admitting that America ought to look forward to its extinction, it is contended that the property in human creatures ought to be as universal as the property in land or in tame animals.

"Nor have these principles been merely inert or speculative. For the last ten or twelve years slavery has altered her tactics, and from a defensive she has become an aggressive power. Every compromise which the moderation of former times had erected to stem the course of this monster evil has been swept away, and that not by the encroachments of the North, but by the aggressive ambition of the South. With a majority in Congress and in the Supreme Court of the United States, the advocates of slavery have entered on a career the object of which would seem to be to make their favourite institution conterminous with the limits of the Republic. They have swept away the Missouri compromise, which limited slavery to the tract south of 36 degrees of north latitude. They have forced upon the North, in the Fugitive Slave Bill, a measure which compels them to lend their assistance to the South in the recovery of their bondmen. In the case of Kansas they have sought by force of arms to assert the right of bringing slaves into a free territory, and in the Dred Scott case they obtained an extrajudicial opinion from the Supreme Court, which would have placed all the territories at their disposal. All this while the North has been resisting, feebly and ineffectually, this succession of Southern aggressions. All that was desired was peace, and that peace could not be obtained.

"While these things were done the South continued violently to upbraid the Abolitionists of the North as the cause of all their troubles, and the ladies of South Carolina showered presents and caresses on the brutal assailant of Mr. Sumner. In 1856 the North endeavoured to elect a President who though fully recognising the right of the South to its slave property, was opposed to its extension in the territories. The North were defeated, and submitted almost without a murmur to the result. On the present occasion the South has submitted to the same ordeal, but not with the same success. They have taken their chance of electing a President of their own views, but they have failed. Mr. Lincoln, like Colonel Freemont, fully recognises the right of the South to the institution of slavery, but, like him, he is opposed to its extension. This cannot be endured. With a majority in both houses of Congress and in the Supreme Court of the United States, the South cannot submit to a President who is not their devoted servant. Unless every power in the constitution is to be strained in order to promote the progress of slavery, they will not remain in the Union; they will not wait to see whether they are injured, but resent the first check to their onward progress as an intolerable injury. This, then, is the result of the history of slavery. It began as a tolerated, it has ended as an aggressive institution, and if it now threatens to dissolve the Union, it is not because it has anything to fear for that which it possesses already, but because it has received a check to its hopes of future acquisition."

SECESSION CONDEMNED IN A SOUTHERN CONVENTION.

SPEECH

Of the Hon. A. H. STEPHENS, made at the Georgia State Convention, held January, 1861, for the purpose of determining whether the State of Georgia was to secede. Notwithstanding this remarkable speech of an extraordinary man, the Convention decided on secession. Mr. Stephens was afterwards elected Vice President of the so-called Confederacy. This distinction shows the estimate of his powers, and adds force to the deliverance, the prophetic declarations of which are now being fulfilled to the letter.

This step (of secession) once taken, can never be recalled; and all the baleful and withering consequences that must follow, will rest on the convention for all coming time. When we and our posterity shall see our lovely South desolated by the demon of war, which this act of yours will inevitably invite and call forth; when our green fields of waving harvests shall be trodden down by the murderous soldiery and fiery car of war sweeping over our land; our temples of justice laid in ashes; all the horrors and desolations of war upon us; who, but this Convention will be held responsible for it? and but him who shall have given his vote for this unwise and ill-timed measure, as I honestly think and believe, shall be held to strict account for this suicidal act by the present generation, and probably cursed and execrated by posterity for all coming time, for the wide and desolating ruin that will inevitably follow this act you now propose to perpetrate? Pause, I entreat you, and consider for a moment what reason you can give that will even satisfy yourselves in calmer moments— what reasons you can give to your fellow-sufferers in this calamity that it will bring upon us. What reasons can you give to the nations of the earth to justify it? They will be the calm and deliberate judges in the case? and what cause or one overt act can you name or point, on which to rest the plea of justification? What right has the North assailed? What interest of the South has been invaded? What justice has been denied? and what claim founded in justice and right has been withheld? Can either of you to-day name one governmental act of wrong deliberately and purposely done by the government of Washington, of which the South has a right to complain? I challenge the answer. While, on the other hand, let me show the facts (and believe me, gentlemen, I am not here the advocate of the North; but I am here the friend, the firm friend and lover of the South and her institutions; and for this reason I speak thus plainly and faithfully—for yours, mine, and every other man's interest—the words of truth and soberness), of which I wish you to judge; and I will only state facts which are clear and undeniable, and which now stand as records authentic in the history of our country. When we of the South demanded the slave trade or importation of Africans for the cultivation of our lands, did they not yield the right for twenty years? When we asked a three-fifths representation in congress for our slaves was it not granted? When we asked and demanded the return of any fugitive from justice, or the recovery of those persons owing labor and allegiance, was it not incorporated in the constitution, and again ratified and strengthened in the Fugitive Slave Law of 1850. But do you reply that in many instances they have violated this compact and have not been faithful to their engagements? As individual and local communities they may have done so; but not by the sanction of government for that has always been true to Southern interest. Again, gentleman, look at another fact, when we have asked that more territory should be added, that we might spread the institution of slavery, have they not yielded to our demands in giving us Louisiana, Florida, and Texas out of which four States have been carved and ample territory for four more to be added in due time, if you by this unwise and impolitic act do not destroy this hope and perhaps, by it lose all, and have your last slave wrenched from you by stern military rule, as South America and Mexico were; or by the vindictive decree of a universal emancipation, which may reasonably be expected to follow. But, again, gentlemen, what have we to gain by this proposed change of our relation to the general government? We have always had the control of it, and can yet, if we remain in it and are as united as we have been. We have had a majority of the presidents chosen from the South, as well as the control and management of most of those chosen from the North. We have had sixty years of Southern presidents to their twenty-four, thus controlling the executive department. So of the judges of the Supreme Court, we have had eighteen from the South, and but eleven from the North; although nearly four-fifths of the judicial business has arisen in the Free States, yet a majority of the court has always been from the South. This we have required so as to guard against any interpretation of the constitution unfavourable to us. In like manner we have been equally watchful to guard our interests in the legislative branch of government. In choosing the presiding president (*pro. tem.*) of the Senate, we have had twenty-four to their eleven. Speakers of the house we have had twenty-three, and they twelve. While the majority of the representatives, from their greater population, have always been from the North, yet we have so generally secured the speaker, because he, to a greater extent, shapes and controls the legislation of the country. Nor have we had less control in every other department of the general government. Attorney-Generals we have had fourteen, while the North have had but five. Foreign ministers we have had eighty-six and they but fifty-four. While three-fourths of the business which demands diplomatic agents abroad is clearly from the Free States, from their greater commercial interests, yet we have had the principal embassies, so as to secure the world's markets for our cotton, tobacco, and sugar on the best possible terms. We have had a vast majority of the higher offices of both army and navy, while a larger proportion of the soldiers and sailors were drawn from the North. Equally so of clerks, auditors, and comptrollers filling the executive department, the records show for the last fifty years that of the three thousand thus employed, we have had more than two-thirds of the same, while we have but one-third of the white popu-

lation of the republic. Again, look at another item, and one, be assured, in which we have a great and vital interest; it is that of revenue, or means of supporting government. From official documents
we learn that a fraction over three-fourths of the revenue collected
for the support of government has uniformly been raised from the
North. Pause now while you can, gentlemen, and contemplate carefully and candidly these important items. Leaving out of view, for the
present, the countless millions of dollars you must expend in a war
with the North; with tens of thousands of your sons and brothers
slain in battle, and offered up as sacrifices upon the altar of your ambition—and for what? we ask again. Is it for the overthrow of the
American government, established by our common ancestry, cemented and built up by their sweat and blood, and founded on the
broad principles of right, justice, and humanity? And, as such, I must
declare here, as I have often done before, and which has been repeated by the greatest and wisest of statesmen and patriots in this
and other lands, that it is the best and freest government—the most
equal in its rights, the most just in its decisions, the most lenient in
its measures, and the most inspiring in its principles to elevate the
race of men, that the sun of heaven ever shone upon. Now, for you
to attempt to overthrow such a government as this, under which we
have lived for more than three-quarters of a century—in which we
have gained our wealth, our standing as a nation, our domestic safety
while the elements of peril are around us, with peace and tranquility
accompanied with unbounded prosperity and rights unassailed—is
the height of *madness*, *folly*, and *wickedness*, to which I can neither
lend my sanction nor my vote.

———

THE CONFEDERATE AND THE SCOTTISH
CLERGY ON SLAVERY.

Some three months ago, we published an "Address to Christians
throughout the world," by "the clergy of the Confederate States of
America;" and yesterday we published a reply to that address, signed
by nearly a thousand ministers of the various Churches in Scotland.
The Confederate address begins with a solemn declaration that its
scope is not political but purely religious—that it is sent forth "in the
name of our Holy Christianity," and in the interests of "the cause of
our most Blessed Master." Immediately after making this declaration, however, the Confederate divines commence a long series of arguments designed to prove that the war cannot restore the Union;

that the Southern States had a right to secede; that having seceded, their separation from the North is final; that the proclamation of PRESIDENT LINCOLN, seeking to free the slaves is a most horrible and wicked measure, calling for "solemn protest on the part of the people of GOD throughout the world;" that the war against the Confederacy has made no progress; and there seems no likelihood of the United States accomplishing any good by its continuance. This may be esteemed good gospel teaching in the Confederate States, but in this country it would be thought to have very little connection with "the cause of our most Blessed Master." But the Southern clergymen reserve for the close of their address the defence of the grand dogma of their religion—the doctrine that negro slavery as carried out in the Southern States of America "is not incompatible with our holy Christianity." Stupendous as this proposition may appear to the British mind, it offers no difficulty to these learned and pious men. Nay, they are not only convinced that slavery is "not incompatible" with Christianity, but they boldly affirm that it is a divinely established institution, designed to promote the temporal happiness and eternal salvation of the negro race, and that all efforts to bring about the abolition of slavery are sacrilegious attempts to interfere with the "plans of Divine Providence." "We testify in the sight of GOD," say the clergy of the Confederate States, "that the relation of master and slave among us, however we may deplore abuses in this, as in any other relations of mankind, is not incompatible with our holy Christianity, and that the presence of the Africans in our land is an occasion of gratitude on their behalf before GOD; seeing that thereby Divine Providence has brought them where missionaries of the cross may freely proclaim to them the word of salvation, and the work is not interrupted by agitating fanaticism. * * * We regard Abolitionism as an interference with the plans of Divine Providence. It has not the signs of the Lord's blessing. It is a fanaticism which puts forth no good fruit; instead of blessing, it has brought forth cursing; instead of love, hatred, instead of life, death—bitterness and sorrow, and pain; and infidelity and moral degeneracy follow its labours." There is no shirking of the question here. Slavery is proclaimed to be the GOD-appointed means for the regeneration of the African race, and those who seek to bring about the emancipation of the slaves are branded as apostles of infidelity. Upon these grounds, the confederate clergy appeal to Christians throughout the world to aid them in creating a sentiment against this war—"against persecution for conscience' sake, against the ravaging of the church of GOD by fanatical invasion."

In their reply to this appeal, the Scottish ministers do what the Confederate ministers professed their intention of doing—they avoid every thing in the shape of political discussion. Among those gentlemen there is no doubt considerable difference of opinion respecting the two parties in the civil war; but they say nothing of that, and address themselves exclusively to the question of slavery. Happily, there is no difference of opinion upon that point among men who take upon themselves the high office of preaching God's word in this country. The Scottish Ministers, in powerful and manly language, express the "deep grief, alarm, and indignation" with which they have seen men who profess to be servants of the Lord Jesus Christ defend slavery as a Christian institution, worthy of being perpetuated and extended, not only without regret, but with entire satisfaction and approval. "Against all this," say they, "in the name of that holy faith and that thrice holy name which they venture to invoke on the side of a system which treats immortal and redeemed men as goods and chattels, denies them the rights of marriage and of home, consigns them to ignorance of the first rudiments of education, and exposes them to the outrages of lust and passion—we must earnestly and emphatically protest." We believe that this is the answer of the whole British community to the appeal of the Confederate clergy. However much the public sentiment may have been misled respecting the rights and the wrongs of the two parties in the war, it cannot but be sound at the core on the subject of slavery. There are many thousands of people who have not the slightest sympathy with slavery, and who yet sympathise with the slave-owners because they have a vague impression that the Southerners are brave gentlemen and the Northerners base mechanics. They have managed by some strange process to separate the cause of slavery from the cause of the slaveowner, and while they rejoice at every success which tends towards the establishment of a confederacy which is to have slavery as the "head stone of the corner," they continue to pray as fervently as ever that the fetters of the slaves may be broken. All such people—and they constitute the mass of the Southern sympathisers in this country—must be ready to repudiate with the sternest indignation this attempt to connect the holy religion of Christ with the most horrible oppression which the cruelty and cupidity of man ever created.

But it is not enough that the Confederate defence of slavery should be rejected. It was proper that the Scottish ministers of religion should deal only with the religious aspect of the question, but it is the duty of every man who feels that he has any influence in the world—and there is no man who has not some—to study the political lessons which the address affords. There can be no doubt that the appeal expresses the genuine sentiment of the Southern States, softened down by whatever softening influence there may be in their peculiar kind of Christianity, and shaped to offend as little as possible the prejudices of British readers. And what does it show us? Does it show us that emancipation is more likely to follow from the success of the Southern society which assumes to be at the helm of all schemes of religion and philanthropy, not only has no desire to put an end to slavery, but regards it in such a light that it will be its duty *to extend it as much as possible.* The Southern clergy say that the relation of master and slave is "not incompatible with our holy Christianity;" why, therefore, should they seek to get rid of it? From a thousand pulpits this language will be sent forth week after week, and it is clear that the religion of the Confederate States will be employed only to convince the slaveowner that he is doing perfectly right in perpetuating a system which enables him to buy men and women as chattels, and to obtain command of human bodies and minds at the prices current of the market. Then, the Southern clergy think it a cause for gratitude to GOD on behalf of the negroes "that He has brought them where missionaries of the Cross might freely proclaim to them the word of salvation." Will it not, therefore, be the duty of the Southern clergy to extend those blessings to new millions of Africans, and thus carry out the "plans of Divine Providence?" Is the whole tendency of this argument not to elevate the horrible trade of the slave-catcher to the same high level with the noble office of the missionary? Proclaiming as they do that the capture of Africans and their removal into slavery in the Southern States is GOD's own missionary plan, the Confederate clergy and people will consider it as much their duty to equip slave-ships with cargoes of manacles and send them forth accompanied by the prayers of the churches, as it is now our duty to send forth missionary-ships laden with Bibles and preachers of the gospel. Then the heathen world will know what missionary Christianity really is. Thousand of Africans, caught on the west coast, will be torn from their families and taken chained on board ship; should they survive the horrors of the passage, they will be set to hard work under laws which permit of almost any degree of corporeal punishment and which deprive them of all the rights of men; and they will be told to thank GOD who has brought them into the blessed light of the Gospel! Let not the man who cannot reconcile his sympathies in the American struggle with his convictions on the question of slavery pooh-pooh this as an extravagant fancy picture of something that never can occur. It is exactly the missionary scheme which the Confederate clergy call "the plan of Divine Providence;" and supposing a powerful Southern Confederacy to be established, what is to prevent its being accomplished? Not the religious and philanthropic feelings of the Confederates; for the religious and philanthropic feelings of the confederates are all for a revival of the slave trade. Not treaties concluded with foreign nations; for a people holding such sentiments could never make a treaty shutting themselves out from the most promising field of missionary labour; or if forced by circumstances to conclude it, their religious convictions would urge them to break it at any moment. In fact, were a powerful nationality once established, with interests and religious convictions all pointing in the way of reviving the slave trade, it would be utterly impossible to prevent a resumption of that abominable traffic.

We have dealt with the professed convictions of the Southern ministers as sincere convictions. We should be sorry to accuse any body of men professing to be teachers of the Christian religion of intentional insincerity, and although we can hardly conceive the possibility of men who base their religion upon the same Bible upon which we rest ours, attempting sincerely to justify slavery upon religious grounds, we would rather attribute the extraordinary moral obliquity which the attempt exhibits to the demoralising influence of the slave system than to actual hypocrisy. The spectacle of a crowd of learned and no doubt pious men standing forth as the avowed apologists of a system which deprives their fellow-men of all the rights of humanity is, perhaps, the most distressing evidence of its blighting and blinding influence which has yet been exhibited to the world. It ought to have its effect. As we have said, it is the duty of every man to study the lessons which this address of the Confederate clergy has for him. If his sympathy and influence be given to the Confederates, let him understand the nature of the cause he is aiding. Let him learn from the statement of the Confederates themselves that their cause is the cause of slavery, and that they look forward to the perpetuation and extension of slavery as the prize of success.

SLAVERY AND LIBERTY.

I'm on my way to Canada,
  That dark and dreary land;
Oh! the dread effects of slavery
  I can no longer stand.
My soul is vexed within me so
  To think I am a slave,
Resolved I am to strike the blow,
  For freedom or the grave.

Chorus
Oh, Righteous Father!
  Wilt thou not pity me,
And help me on to Canada,
  Where coloured men are free.

I've served my master all my days,
  Without one dimes' reward,
And now I'm forced to run away,
  To flee the lash and rod.
The hounds are baying on my track,
  And master just behind,
Resolved that he will bring me back
  Before I cross the line.

Old master went to preach one day,
  Next day he looked for me;
I greased my heels and ran away,
  For the land of liberty.
I dreamt I saw the British Queen
  Majestic on the shore;
If e'er I reach old Canada,
  I will come back no more.

I heard that Queen Victoria said,
  If we would all forsake
Our native land of Slavery,
  And come across the lake:
That she was standing on the shore
  With arms extended wide,
To give us all a peaceful home
  Beyond the swelling tide.

I heard old master pray one night,
  That night he prayed for me,
That God would come with all his might,
  From Satan set me free.
So I from Satan would escape
  And flee the wrath to come,
If there's a fiend in human shape,
  Old master must be one,

CHRONOLOGY

BIOGRAPHICAL NOTES

NOTE ON THE TEXTS

NOTES

Chronology

1510   Spanish begin importation of African slaves into the Caribbean.

1619   Dutch traders sell 20 Africans into servitude at the English settlement at Jamestown, Virginia, beginning importation of slaves into the British colonies in North America.

1662   Virginia adopts law making children born to enslaved mothers slaves from birth. (Other colonies adopt similar laws during the late 17th and early 18th centuries as part of legal codes defining the status of slaves.)

1672   Royal African Company chartered by Charles II of England. Success of the company in the slave trade increases the number of slaves in British North American colonies as the number of white indentured servants declines.

1700   First American antislavery tract, *The Selling of Joseph,* published by Massachusetts judge Samuel Sewall.

1712   Eight whites and 25 blacks are killed in slave uprising in New York City.

1739   At least 30 whites and 44 blacks are killed during Stono slave rebellion in South Carolina.

1750   Estimated population of 13 British colonies is 236,000 blacks, almost all of them slaves, and 934,000 whites.

1772   Publication of the *Narrative* of James Albert Ukawsaw Gronniosaw, the first English-language slave narrative.

1775   Beginning of Revolutionary War.

1776   Declaration of Independence adopted after Continental Congress deletes language in draft condemning the slave trade.

1777   Vermont adopts constitution prohibiting slavery.

1780   Pennsylvania adopts law providing for the gradual abolition of slavery.

1781–83   Judges and juries in several Massachusetts court cases find slavery to be incompatible with the state constitution adopted in 1780, which declared that all men "are born free and equal." (No slaves are reported in Massachusetts in 1790 census.)

1783   Revolutionary War ends; at least 15,000 slaves leave the United States with the evacuating British forces.

1784   Connecticut and Rhode Island adopt laws for gradual emancipation of slaves.

1787   Continental Congress passes the Northwest Ordinance, which bans slavery in the territories north of the Ohio River. U.S. Constitution is framed; it counts slaves as three-fifths of free persons in apportioning representation and direct taxes, provides for the return of fugitive slaves, and forbids ending the importation of slaves before 1808.

1793   Congress passes Fugitive Slave Law, allowing slaveholders to use federal courts to regain possession of runaway slaves. Invention of the cotton gin leads to rapid expansion of cotton cultivation in the South.

1799   New York adopts law for the gradual emancipation of slaves.

1800   Gabriel Prosser and 35 followers are executed for plotting slave rebellion in Richmond, Virginia. United States census lists 108,395 free colored people, 893,041 slaves, and 4,304,489 whites.

1804   New Jersey adopts law for gradual emancipation of slaves.

1807   Congress bans importation of slaves into the United States, effective January 1, 1808. Britain abolishes slave trade throughout its empire and begins using its navy to suppress slave trading by other nations. (It is estimated that 10–11 million Africans were brought to the western hemisphere by the slave trade, of whom approximately 600,000 were landed in the British North American colonies and the United States; more than one million Africans died during the Atlantic passage.) Internal slave trade within the United States increases as large numbers of slaves are sent from tobacco-growing states of the upper South to cotton-growing states of the lower South.

1816   American Colonization Society formed to send free black Americans to Africa.

1820   Congress adopts Missouri Compromise, allowing the admission of Missouri as a slave state while prohibiting slavery in the remainder of the Louisiana Purchase north of latitude 36°30′ N.

1822   Denmark Vesey and 35 other blacks are executed in Charleston, South Carolina, for plotting a slave revolt. Founding of colony (later named Liberia) on the West African coast for expatriated Americans of color.

1827   Final abolition of slavery in New York state.

1829   David Walker, a free black man living in Boston, publishes his *Appeal . . . to the Colored Citizens of the World,* a pamphlet in which he calls on blacks to forcibly overthrow slavery and racial oppression.

1831   Slave rebellion led by Nat Turner in Southampton County, Virginia, ends with the deaths of 57 whites and at least 100 blacks; Turner and 19 followers are hanged.

1832   New England Anti-Slavery Society founded by William Lloyd Garrison to advocate the immediate abolition of slavery through nonviolent means and to oppose the colonization of free blacks.

1838   Final abolition of slavery in the British Caribbean.

1840   Liberty Party, first antislavery political party, founded in Albany, New York.

1845–48   Annexation of Texas and the Mexican War renew debate over the expansion of slavery.

1848   Abolition of slavery in the French Caribbean.

1850   Congress adopts series of measures regarding slavery
            ("Compromise of 1850"), including stronger Fugitive
            Slave Law that denies alleged fugitives any legal protec-
            tions; law provokes widespread opposition and resistance
            in the free states. United States census lists 434,495 free
            colored people, 3,204,313 slaves, and 19,553,068 whites.

1852   Antislavery novel *Uncle Tom's Cabin,* written by Harriet
            Beecher Stowe in response to the Fugitive Slave Law, sells
            300,000 copies in its first year of publication.

1854–56   Kansas-Nebraska Act of 1854 repeals Missouri Compro-
            mise and leads to fighting between pro- and antislavery
            factions in Kansas and the formation of Republican Party
            opposed to the further expansion of slavery.

1857   Supreme Court rules in Dred Scott decision that Con-
            gress cannot exclude slavery from the federal territories
            and that African Americans cannot be U.S. citizens, hav-
            ing "no rights which the white man was bound to re-
            spect."

1859   John Brown seizes federal arsenal at Harpers Ferry, Vir-
            ginia, in an unsuccessful attempt to start slave uprising; 15
            people are killed during the raid, and Brown is later
            hanged along with four other men.

1860   Republican candidate Abraham Lincoln is elected presi-
            dent November 6 on a platform opposing the extension
            of slavery. South Carolina secedes on December 20 (ten
            other states secede by May 1861).

1861   Confederates shell Fort Sumter, South Carolina, on April
            12, beginning Civil War.

1862   Congress abolishes slavery in the District of Columbia
            and the federal territories and passes law freeing slaves
            who escape from the Confederacy, April–July. Lincoln is-
            sues preliminary Emancipation Proclamation on Septem-
            ber 22, declaring that all slaves in Confederate-held
            territory will be freed on January 1, 1863.

1863   Emancipation Proclamation is issued on January 1, autho-
              rizing the enlistment of freed slaves; 180,000 black men
              (including free blacks from northern states) eventually
              serve in the Union army.

1865   Thirteenth Amendment to the Constitution, abolishing
              slavery throughout the United States, is proposed to the
              states by Congress on January 31. Confederate armies sur-
              render, April 9–May 26. Lincoln is assassinated on April
              14. Ratification of the Thirteenth Amendment is com-
              pleted December 6.

Biographical Notes

JAMES ALBERT UKAWSAW GRONNIOSAW (c. 1712–1775) Born in Bornu, near Lake Chad, Gronniosaw was sold into slavery while still a boy and taken on a Dutch ship from the Gold Coast (present-day Ghana) to Barbados. In Barbados he was sold to a master who took him to New York, where he worked as a kitchen servant. His second master, Theodorus Frelinghuysen, a minister in the Dutch Reformed Church, instructed him in Christianity, sent him to school, and manumitted him shortly before his own death c. 1748. Gronniosaw remained with Mrs. Frelinghuysen until her death two years later. After serving as a cook on board an American privateer and as a soldier in the British army in Martinique in 1762, he went to England and then to Holland, where he worked as a butler and told his story to a convocation of Calvinist ministers. Returning to England after a year in Holland, Gronniosaw married a weaver and joined a Baptist congregation. He lived with his family in Colchester and Norwich before moving to Kidderminster, where he told his story to an unnamed amanuensis. *A Narrative of the Most Remarkable Particulars in the Life of James Albert Gronniosaw, an African Prince, as Related by Himself* was published in 1772 and reprinted at least 12 times before 1800 in England, Ireland, and North America. Gronniosaw died in England.

OLAUDAH EQUIANO (c. 1745–March 31, 1797) Born in the southeastern region of present-day Nigeria, Equiano grew up among the Ibo people before he was kidnapped as a young boy and sold into slavery. Sent to Barbados and then to Virginia, he was sold to Michael Henry Pascal, a lieutenant in the British navy, who renamed him Gustavus Vassa and took him to England as a servant. Baptized in 1759, Equiano spent most of his youth aboard ships of the Royal Navy. Expecting to be freed after six years of service, he was instead sold to a West Indian trader in 1762 and then to Robert King, a Philadelphia Quaker and merchant. In 1766 Equiano bought his freedom from King and returned to England the following year to work as a hairdresser and later as a sailor. During this time he learned the French horn, studied mathematics, and underwent a profound religious conversion to Methodism. After participating in an Arctic expedition and voyages to Central America and Turkey, Equiano settled in England in 1777. In 1787 he was appointed "commissary of provisions and stores" for a colonization venture in Sierra Leone, but his criticism of the leaders of the venture led to his dismissal before he could return to West Africa. His autobiography *The Interesting Narrative of the Life of Olaudah Equiano, or Gustavus Vassa, the African, Written by Himself* was published in 1789; after its publication, Equiano traveled extensively in England, Scotland, and Ireland promoting the book and arranging for the publication of eight subsequent editions. He married Susanna Cullen, an Englishwoman, in 1792, and they had two daughters. Equiano died in London.

NAT TURNER (October 2, 1800–November 11, 1831) Born in Southampton County, Virginia, on the plantation of Benjamin Turner, the son of an African-born mother and a father who ran away during Turner's childhood and was never retaken. Raised by his mother and his paternal grandmother, Turner learned to read and write before he began working in the cotton and tobacco fields while a teenager. At the age of 21, he ran away for a month, then returned. In 1822 Benjamin Turner died and Turner was sold for $400 to Thomas Moore, a neighboring farmer. During the late 1820s Turner became convinced that he had been given a messianic task. In 1830 he became the slave of Joseph Travis, a wheelwright who had married Moore's widow, Sally. After an eclipse of the sun in February 1831 Turner formed a small band of slaves to carry out a war against slaveholders. Intending to launch "the work of death" on July 4, 1831, Turner delayed the uprising for six weeks until he saw sunspots in mid-August. On the night of August 21, Turner and seven other slaves killed Travis and his family, and during the next 40 hours the insurrectionists killed more than 50 white men, women, and children as they moved from farm to farm, eventually growing to between 60 and 80 in number. Turner sought to capture arms and ammunition in Jerusalem, the county seat, but on the evening of August 23 the insurrectionists were scattered by white militia and Turner went into hiding. By the time of his capture on October 30 more than 100 African Americans, many of whom had no connection with the uprising, had been killed without trial, and another 19 had been tried and hanged. From November 1 to 3, 1831, Turner was interviewed in his cell by Thomas R. Gray, a local attorney, who kept a written record of Turner's words. After entering a plea of not guilty, Turner was convicted, and hanged on November 11, 1831; he was survived by a wife and children. *The Confessions of Nat Turner*, edited by Gray, was published in Baltimore in late November 1831. By the outbreak of the Civil War 50,000 copies of the *Confessions* are estimated to have been printed.

FREDERICK DOUGLASS (February 1818–February 20, 1895) Born
Frederick Bailey in Talbot County on the eastern shore of Maryland,
the son of Harriet Bailey and an unknown white man. In 1826 he was
sent to Baltimore by Thomas Auld, his master's son-in-law, to live
with Auld's brother, Hugh, and his wife, Sophia. He received reading lessons from Sophia Auld until her husband forbade them; he
then secretly taught himself to read and write. In 1833 he was sent
back to Talbot County, where Thomas Auld hired him out as a field
hand. After a failed escape attempt in 1836 he was again sent to live
with Hugh and Sophia Auld in Baltimore, where he learned ship
caulking and met Anna Murray, a free black woman. With her help,
he escaped to Philadelphia on September 3, 1838, traveling by train
and steamboat with protection papers borrowed from a free black
merchant sailor. Anna Murray soon joined him in New York City,
where they were married. They settled in New Bedford, Massachusetts, where he took the name Douglass; in 1839 the first of their five
children was born. In 1841 Douglass became a lecturer for the radical
American Anti-Slavery Society, led by William Lloyd Garrison, and in
1845 he published his *Narrative of the Life of Frederick Douglass, An
American Slave, Written by Himself*, which is estimated to have sold
more than 30,000 copies by 1850. During his successful lecture tour
in Great Britain and Ireland in 1845–47 a group of English supporters purchased his manumission from the Auld family, allowing Douglass to return to the United States without fear of apprehension by
slavecatchers. He launched his own antislavery newspaper, *North
Star*, in Rochester, New York, on December 3, 1847, and in July 1848
attended the woman's rights convention held at Seneca Falls, New
York. By the early 1850s Douglass had broken with Garrison and become an ally of Gerrit Smith, who advocated an antislavery interpretation of the Constitution and participation in electoral politics. He
published his second autobiography, *My Bondage and My Freedom*, in
1855. Douglass argued for emancipation and the enlistment of black
soldiers as essential war measures at the outbreak of the Civil War
and became a supporter of Abraham Lincoln once the president
adopted these policies. After the war he continued his advocacy of
racial equality and woman's rights while becoming a loyal supporter
of the Republican Party, serving as U.S. marshal (1877–81) and
recorder of deeds (1881–86) for the District of Columbia and as minister to Haiti (1889–91) under Republican administrations. His third
autobiography, *Life and Times of Frederick Douglass*, appeared in 1881
and in an expanded edition in 1892. After the death of Anna Murray
Douglass in 1882, Douglass married Helen Pitts, a white woman's
rights activist, in 1884. He died of a heart attack at Cedar Hill, his estate in the Anacostia section of Washington, D.C.

WILLIAM WELLS BROWN (1814–November 6, 1884) Born on a plantation near Lexington, Kentucky, the son of George Higgins, a white
man, and Elizabeth, an African-American woman. In 1816 his master
moved to Missouri, where Brown worked as a house servant, a field
hand, a tavern keeper's assistant, a printer's helper, an assistant in a
medical office, and as a handyman for James Walker, a Missouri
slavetrader who traveled along the Mississippi River between St.
Louis and the New Orleans slave market. After several failed attempts, he escaped on New Year's Day, 1834, traveling by night
across Ohio from Cincinnati to Cleveland. On his way he met Mr.
and Mrs. Wells Brown, a Quaker couple whose kindness he acknowledged by adopting their name when he became a free man. In
the summer of 1834 Brown married Elizabeth Schooner in Cleveland
and began working as a steamboatman on Lake Erie. Moving to Buffalo, New York, in the summer of 1836, Brown helped fugitive slaves
escape into Canada and organized a temperance society. In 1840 he
visited Haiti and Cuba, and in 1843 he became a lecturer for the
Western New York Anti-Slavery Society, a branch of the Garrisonian
American Anti-Slavery Society. Separating from his wife in 1847,
Brown moved to Boston with their two daughters. His *Narrative of
William W. Brown, A Fugitive Slave, Written by Himself* appeared
that year and went through four American and five British printings
by 1850. In the summer of 1849 Brown attended an international
peace conference in Paris and gave antislavery lectures in England.
While in England he wrote *Three Years in Europe; or, Places I Have
Seen and People I Have Met* (1852), the first travel book authored by
an African American, and *Clotel; or, the President's Daughter* (1853),
generally regarded as the first African-American novel. Returning to
the United States in 1854 after English friends purchased his manumission, Brown published *The Escape; or, A Leap for Freedom* (1858),
the first drama by an African American. In 1860 he married Annie
Elizabeth Gray of Cambridgeport, Massachusetts. During the Civil
War he helped recruit black volunteers for the Massachusetts 54th
and 55th Regiments; his book *The Negro in the American Rebellion*
(1867) is the first military history of African Americans in the United
States. After the Civil War, Brown studied medicine and became a
physician in Boston while continuing his involvement with the temperance movement. In 1874 Brown published his most comprehensive work of African-American history, *The Rising Son; or, the
Antecedents and Advancement of the Colored Race*, biographical
sketches of 110 prominent black Americans. His last book, *My Southern Home*, a reminiscence of his life in slavery combined with a critical assessment of the Reconstruction South, appeared in 1880.
Brown died at his home in Chelsea, a suburb of Boston.

HENRY WALTON BIBB (May 10, 1815–August 1, 1854) Born a slave on a plantation in Shelby County, Kentucky, the son of Milldred Jackson and James Bibb, a Kentucky state senator. Bibb was separated from his mother as a small child and began running away from a succession of masters when he was ten years old. At the age of 18, he fell in love with a slave named Malinda, with whom he had a daughter, Mary Frances. Sold to Malinda's owner, William Gatewood of Bedford, Kentucky, Bibb successfully escaped from slavery by boat, traveling to Cincinnati on Christmas Day 1837, and on to Detroit. He used his earnings in freedom to return to Kentucky in May 1838 to attempt the rescue of his family, but was captured in Cincinnati and sent to Louisville, Kentucky, to be sold. Bibb escaped, then returned in 1839 to Kentucky, but was captured and eventually sold to a Louisiana cotton planter. After several failed attempts, Bibb successfully escaped in 1841 from a Cherokee owner and made his way to Detroit. He soon began lecturing against slavery and in 1844 campaigned for the Liberty Party ticket in Michigan and Ohio. In 1845 he made his final journey South to reclaim his enslaved family, but after learning that Malinda had become her master's concubine, Bibb renounced all obligations to her and in June 1848 married Mary E. Miles, a Boston antislavery activist. He published *Narrative of the Life and Adventures of Henry Bibb, an American Slave, Written by Himself* at his own expense in 1849; by 1850 the book was in its third printing. After the Fugitive Slave Law was passed in 1850, Bibb and his wife immigrated to Ontario, where on January 1, 1851, Bibb launched *The Voice of the Fugitive*, the first black newspaper in Canada. With his wife, Bibb also founded a school and a Methodist church and helped other fugitives settle in Ontario. He died in Canada.

SOJOURNER TRUTH (c. 1797–November 26, 1883) Born Isabella in Hurley, Ulster County, New York, the child of Dutch-speaking slaves named James and Elizabeth. She was separated from her parents around the age of nine. In 1810 she was purchased by John Dumont and began working as a field hand and milkmaid on his farm in New Paltz, New York, where she gave birth to at least five children. When Dumont reneged on his promise to free her, she walked away from the farm with her youngest child and went to live with the neighboring Van Wagenen family, whose name she took. After being emancipated on July 4, 1827, by the New York law that ended slavery in the state, she successfully sued to have her son Peter returned from Alabama, where he had been sent after being illegally sold. In 1829 she moved to New York City, where she worked as a domestic. From 1832 to 1834 she was a member of "the Kingdom of Matthias," a utopian religious commune; when the commune collapsed, Gilbert Vale used her testimony in writing his expose *Fanaticism: Its Source and Influence, Illustrated by the Simple Narrative of Isabella* (1835). On June 1, 1843, she renamed herself Sojourner Truth and left New York City to become an itinerant preacher, settling in 1844 in Northampton, Massachusetts, where she met William Lloyd Garrison, Frederick Douglass, and other prominent antislavery and woman's rights activists. *Narrative of Sojourner Truth,* written by Olive Gilbert, a white abolitionist to whom Truth had told her story, was published in 1850 and reprinted in 1853 and 1855. Beginning in 1850, Truth became a widely traveled speaker for antislavery and woman's rights; her remarks at a woman's rights meeting held in Akron, Ohio, in 1851, have become known as her "Ar'n't I a Woman?" speech, though it is likely that Truth did not use the phrase. In 1857 she moved from Northampton to Battle Creek, Michigan. During the Civil War Truth campaigned for President Lincoln's re-election, helped with relief efforts for the freed people, and participated in the desegregation of the streetcars in Washington, D.C. After the war she campaigned for land grants for blacks in the West and supported temperance while continuing to speak for woman's rights. With the aid of Frances Titus, a white friend, Truth reprinted her *Narrative* in 1875, supplementing it with her "Book of Life," which included personal correspondence, newspaper accounts of her activities, and tributes from her friends; this expanded edition of Truth's biography was reprinted in 1878, 1881, and 1884 as *Narrative of Sojourner Truth; a Bondswoman of Olden Time, with a History of Her Labors and Correspondence Drawn from Her "Book of Life."* Truth died at her home in Battle Creek, Michigan.

WILLIAM CRAFT (c. 1824–1900) was born a slave in Macon, Georgia. ELLEN SMITH CRAFT (1826–1891) was born in Clinton, Georgia, the daughter of an enslaved woman and her master, Major James Smith. At the age of 11 Ellen was given as a wedding present to a white half-sister who lived in Macon. There she met William Craft, a cabinet-maker's apprentice. They married in 1846 and escaped from slavery in December 1848, traveling by train, steamboat, and coach from Macon to Philadelphia with Ellen disguised as an invalid white man and William posing as "his" slave valet. The Crafts settled in Boston, where William worked as a cabinetmaker and Ellen as a seamstress, and spoke together at New England meetings of the Garrisonian American Anti-Slavery Society. After the passage of the Fugitive Slave Law in 1850 they became fearful of recapture and fled to England, where they toured with William Wells Brown and drew large audiences to their antislavery lectures. From 1851 to 1854 they attended the Ockham School in Surrey, a trade school that also taught academic subjects. Moving to London, they started an import-export business while continuing to appear at antislavery meetings. *Running a Thousand Miles for Freedom*, an account of their escape written by William, was published in London in 1860. William went to Dahomey in 1863 in an unsuccessful attempt to persuade King Gelele to abolish slavery, and he later established a school there. He remained in Africa until 1867 while Ellen worked with the British and Foreign Freedmen's Aid Society in London and raised their five children. The Crafts returned to Boston in 1869 and then went to Georgia, where they established an industrial school for blacks in 1870. After it was burned down by the Ku Klux Klan, they purchased the Woodville plantation in Bryan County, Georgia, in 1871 and opened a cooperative farm school. William served as a delegate to state and national Republican conventions and lectured widely in the North to raise money for the school, but insufficient funds and the hostility of local whites forced it to close in 1878. Ellen died at Woodville, and William died at his daughter's home in Charleston, South Carolina.

HARRIET ANN JACOBS (1813–March 7, 1897) Born in Edenton, North Carolina, the daughter of Elijah Jacobs, a house carpenter, and Deliah Horniblow, a domestic servant, both slaves. After the death of her mother in 1819 she was raised by her grandmother, Molly Horniblow, and her white mistress, Margaret Horniblow, who taught her to read, write, and sew. Upon the death of Margaret Horniblow in 1825 Jacobs was sent to the household of Dr. James Norcom, an Edenton physician. Subjected to repeated sexual advances from Norcom, Jacobs formed a clandestine liaison with Samuel Tredwell Sawyer, an Edenton attorney, and had two children by him, Joseph (b. 1829) and Louisa Matilda (b. 1833). In June 1835 Jacobs went into hiding, hoping that her disappearance would cause Norcom to sell her children to their father. Sawyer purchased Joseph and Louisa Matilda in the summer of 1835 and sent them to live with Molly Horniblow, who had been emancipated in 1828. Shortly afterwards Jacobs hid herself in a crawl space above a storeroom in the Horniblow house, where she remained for seven years until her escape by ship to Philadelphia. She found work in New York as a nursemaid to Imogen, the infant daughter of Mary Stace Willis and Nathaniel Parker Willis, a journalist, editor, and poet, and was reunited with her children. To avoid recapture by Norcom she moved to Boston in 1843, where she supported herself as a seamstress. In 1849 Jacobs joined her brother John S. Jacobs in Rochester, New York, where he had opened an antislavery reading room and bookstore above the offices of Frederick Douglass's newspaper *North Star*. In Rochester she met and began to confide in Amy Post, a white abolitionist and woman's rights activist who urged Jacobs to write her autobiography. Without Jacobs' permission, Cornelia Grinnell Willis, the second wife of Nathaniel Parker Willis, purchased her manumission in 1852. Jacobs began writing her autobiography in 1853 while working as a nanny for the Willis family in Cornwall, New York, and in 1860 enlisted Lydia Maria Child, an abolitionist writer, to edit the completed manuscript and help find a publisher for it. *Incidents in the Life of a Slave Girl, Written by Herself* was published pseudonymously in Boston in 1861 with Child listed as the book's editor; an English printing of the autobiography, *The Deeper Wrong*, appeared in 1862. From 1862 to 1868 Jacobs engaged in Quaker-sponsored relief work among former slaves in Washington, D.C., Alexandria, Virginia, and Savannah, Georgia. She then lived with her daughter in Cambridge, Massachusetts, and in Washington, D.C, where she died.

JACOB D. GREEN (b. August 24, 1813) was born a slave in Queen Anne's County, Maryland. During his boyhood he worked as a house servant on a large plantation owned by Judge Charles Earle. When he was 12 years old his mother was sold, and he never saw her again. When his wife and children were sold away from him in 1839, Green made his first escape from slavery. He found employment near Philadelphia and lived quietly as a fugitive until 1842, when he was taken back to Maryland. Sold to a new master, Green was sent to Memphis, Tennessee. He made his second escape in 1846 by stowing away aboard a ship to New York, but was recaptured in Utica, New York, and sold to a third master in Louisville, Kentucky, early in 1847. Green made his final escape in 1848, which took him from Kentucky to Toronto, Canada, where he lived until his immigration to England in 1851. While working as an antislavery lecturer, Green published his 43-page *Narrative of the Life of J. D. Green, a Runaway Slave, from Kentucky* in Huddersfield, Yorkshire, in 1864; according to its title page, 8,000 copies of the *Narrative* were printed. No record of Green exists after the publication of his *Narrative*.

Note on the Texts

This volume collects ten narratives published between 1772 and 1864 that describe the experiences of persons held as slaves in the British North American colonies and in the United States: *Narrative of the Most Remarkable Particulars in the Life of James Albert Ukawsaw Gronniosaw, an African Prince, As related by Himself* (1772); *Interesting Narrative of the Life of Olaudah Equiano, or Gustavus Vassa, the African, Written by Himself* (1789); *The Confessions of Nat Turner, the Leader of the Late Insurrection in Southampton, Va., as fully and voluntarily made to Thomas R. Gray*, by Thomas R. Gray (1831); *Narrative of the Life of Frederick Douglass, An American Slave, Written by Himself* (1845); *Narrative of William W. Brown, a Fugitive Slave, Written by Himself* (1847); *Narrative of the Life and Adventures of Henry Bibb, an American Slave, Written by Himself* (1849); *Narrative of Sojourner Truth: A Northern Slave Emancipated from Bodily Servitude by the State of New York, in 1828*, by Olive Gilbert (1850); *Running a Thousand Miles for Freedom; or, the Escape of William and Ellen Craft from Slavery*, by William Craft (1860); *Incidents in the Life of a Slave Girl, Written by Herself*, by Harriet A. Jacobs (1861); and *Narrative of the Life of J. D. Green*, by Jacob D. Green (1864).

James Albert Ukawsaw Gronniosaw related his story to a young Englishwoman, as yet unidentified, who later helped arrange for its publication. *Narrative of the Most Remarkable Particulars* was published in Bath, England, in December 1772, with William Gye as the printer. At least 12 printings of the *Narrative* appeared by 1800, including printings in Dublin, New York City, and Rhode Island. The text presented here is that of the first printing.

Olaudah Equiano first published his *Interesting Narrative* in London in March 1789 in a two-volume edition supported by 321 subscribers. Between 1789 and 1794 he published eight further editions of the *Narrative* in London, Dublin, Edinburgh, and Norwich, while an unauthorized edition was printed in New York in 1791 and translations appeared in Dutch (1790), German (1792), and Russian (1794). Equiano made substantive changes in each of the authorized editions, adding prefatory material and footnotes and altering wording in the main text; these changes sometimes resulted in the adoption of a more formal and genteel diction. Beginning with the fifth edition, published in Edinburgh in 1793, a paragraph was added to chapter XII describing Equiano's activities in 1791 and 1792, and in all editions after the fourth, published in Dublin in 1791, a 63-word passage (from "While we lay . . ." to ". . . was performed," pp. 230.34–231.1 in this volume) was omitted, possibly as the result of an oversight. The text of the first edition has been chosen for inclusion in this volume because it provides the most immediate version of Equiano's narrative; significant material added in later editions is presented in the notes.

Thomas R. Gray, a Virginia attorney, interviewed Nat Turner in prison from November 1 to November 3, 1831. He deposited the title of his pamphlet for copyright in the District of Columbia on November 10, the day before Turner's execution, and published *The Confessions of Nat Turner* in Baltimore in late November 1831, using Lucas & Deaver as the printers. The text printed here is that of the first edition.

Frederick Douglass was described as "now writing out his story" by the abolitionist Wendell Phillips in a letter written on February 24, 1845. *Narrative of the Life of Frederick Douglass* was published in May 1845 "at the Anti-Slavery Office," 25 Cornhill Street, Boston, the address of the Massachusetts Anti-Slavery Society; by September 1845 it had sold 4,500 copies. Although Douglass made no changes in subsequent American printings of the *Narrative,* he was involved in 1845 and 1846 in the Irish publication of the work, whose sales helped finance his extended speaking tour of Great Britain and Ireland from 1845 to 1847; these printings, as well as an English printing published in 1846, omitted the appendix, in which Douglass parodied a Southern hymn, and contained changes in punctuation, spelling, and wording made to conform to British usage. The text printed here is that of the 1845 first American printing.

William Wells Brown completed the manuscript of his narrative in Boston in June 1847. *Narrative of William W. Brown* was published "at the Anti-Slavery Office," the headquarters of the Massachusetts Anti-Slavery Society at 25 Cornhill Street, Boston, in July 1847. In the revised version of the *Narrative* published in Boston in 1848, Brown made alterations in the wording of some passages, added a lengthy quotation from John Pierpont's poem "The Fugitive Slave's Apostrophe to the North Star," and reorganized the text, reducing the number of chapters from 14 to 11. By August 1849 four printings of the *Narrative* had been published in the United States, amounting to a total of 10,000 copies. By then Brown had gone to Great Britain to deliver antislavery lectures, and in 1849 he arranged for the publication in London of a new edition of his book under the title *Narrative of William W. Brown, An American Slave, Written by*

Himself. For this edition, Brown added a new final chapter describing the rescue in 1836 of a family of fugitive slaves from slavecatchers in upstate New York, as well as extensive prefatory and supplemental material written by Brown and others. The main body of the text followed that of the 1848 revised version, though in chapter V a long quotation from Charlotte Elizabeth's poem "The Slave and Her Babe" was replaced by two paragraphs denouncing the slave trade. The text of the 1847 first American printing has been chosen for inclusion in this volume because it provides the most immediate version of Brown's narrative; some of the changes made in later versions are presented in the notes.

Narrative of the Life and Adventures of Henry Bibb was published "by the author" in New York in 1849. Bibb made no changes to the text in subsequent printings. The text presented here is that of the first printing. (Cross-references to page numbers in the text of the *Narrative* have been changed to correspond to the appropriate page numbers in the present volume, but a cross-reference to an illustration not included in this volume has been omitted.)

Sojourner Truth met Olive Gilbert (1801–84), a white abolitionist and friend of William Lloyd Garrison, around 1846, while Truth was living in the Northampton Association of Education and Industry, a utopian community in western Massachusetts. Truth, who was illiterate, used Gilbert as her amanuensis in recording her story for publication. *Narrative of Sojourner Truth* was published "for the author" in Boston and New York in 1850. It was reprinted, with the addition of a short preface by Harriet Beecher Stowe, in 1853 and 1855. Truth obtained the plates for her *Narrative* in 1875 and, with the help of Frances Titus, her friend and neighbor in Battle Creek, Michigan, republished it, adding selections (edited by Titus) from Truth's "Book of Life," a collection of testimonials, letters, and newspaper articles describing her public activities. This expanded version was reprinted in 1878 and 1881, and in 1884, the year after Truth's death, it was republished with a new "Memorial Chapter" compiled by Titus. The text presented here is that of the 1850 first printing.

Running a Thousand Miles for Freedom; or, the Escape of William and Ellen Craft from Slavery was written by William Craft and published in London by William Tweedie in 1860 and reprinted in 1861 (the Crafts had fled to England after the passage of the Fugitive Slave Law in 1850). The text included in this volume is that of the first printing.

Harriet Jacobs began writing her autobiography in 1853 while living in Cornwall, New York, and completed the manuscript in 1858.

After an unsuccessful attempt to arrange for its publication in England, Jacobs sought the help of Lydia Maria Child, an abolitionist writer. Child agreed to serve as her editor and advised Jacobs to expand her description of the aftermath of Nat Turner's rebellion but to omit a final chapter on John Brown (which Jacobs had apparently added to the manuscript after Brown's raid on Harpers Ferry in 1859). In a letter to her friend Lucy Searle, Child described her editorial work on Jacob's manuscript: "I abridged, and struck out superfluous words sometimes; but I don't think I *altered* fifty words in the whole volume." The Boston publishing firm of Thayer and Eldridge agreed in September 1860 to publish the book and arranged for the production of stereotype plates, but the firm went bankrupt before any copies were printed. Jacobs acquired the plates, and *Incidents in the Life of a Slave Girl* was published "for the author" in Boston in January 1861, with a "Preface by the Author" signed "Linda Brent," Jacobs' pseudonym. The work was published in London by William Tweedie in 1862 under the title *The Deeper Wrong; Or, Incidents in the Life of a Slave Girl. Written by Herself.* The text in the present volume is that of the 1861 first printing.

Jacob D. Green wrote and published his autobiography while touring England as an antislavery lecturer. *Narrative of the Life of J. D. Green* was printed by Henry Fielding in Huddersfield, West Yorkshire, in 1864, and was not reprinted until 1999. The text printed here is that of the original printing.

This volume presents the texts of the original printings chosen for inclusion here, but it does not attempt to reproduce features of 18th-century typography such as the long "s" and the use of quotation marks at the beginning of every line of a quoted passage. The texts are printed without other changes, except for the correction of typographical errors. Spelling, punctuation, and capitalization are often expressive features, and they are not altered, even when inconsistent or irregular. The following is a list of typographical errors corrected, cited by page and line number: 69.6, situa-/; 105.11, Fench; 107.28, gentleman; 115.34, to had,; 141.1 litttle; 143.10, an other; 143.38, amonst; 147.26, said in; 159.22, appelation; 164.12, deliverence; 181.32, onc emore; 197.22, day?; 200.7, twelth; 203.18, MICELLA-NEOUS; 207.2, *ou*; 210.6, bronght; 219.11, *1767*; 227.12, my; 233.27, Comssimioners; 431.35, hem; 435.24, ogic; 446.17, stripes;—; 463.3, boys,; 482.10, No; 498.19, and too; 508.8, superanuated; 521.32–33, pursuaded; 526.26, aud; 541.18, followig; 541.28–29, Perrysbugh; 544.4, "DEAR; 544.21, "You; 548.28, boat?; 548.30, Have; 549.4, Sir; 560.25, instiution; 561.31, faithful.; 562.6, heart rending-shrieks; 562.10, begining; 570.29, 'the; 570.30, brave,—; 593.36, cihldren; 595.30, 'Oh!; 596.5, 'would; 596.6, go.'; 596.9, 'yes,'; 604.35, hat he; 609.33, 'Oh; 609.34, God!"; 660.19, felt—; 688.13–14, *whatsoever.*—; 691.36, "My; 691.36, go?"; 692.4, "Yes,; 692.8, SLAVE!"; 693.15, I; 717.30, It's; 718.7, home.; 720.29, master,"; 727.23, ready.; 785.9, "I; 860.3, Philip; 876.11, "where; 876.12, rest."; 910.20, sent of;1017 911.37, heen; 930.10, you; 953.8, employod; 953.19, heared; 953.26, wipped; 954.19, dertermined; 954.40, niggirs; 955.9, ady; 955.11, hrrd; 955.24, ascertrin; 955.34, pide; 955.36, mantel-piete; 955.39, filleh; 956.32, confidant; 956.34–35, withold; 957.5, adminstered; 957.32, mo; 958.40, thnt; 959.33, fiogging; 960.8, othere; 960.10, fiifty; 960.17, whito; 960.19, wes; 960.23, quit; 961.1, borowed; 961.10, an in impression; 961.23, preformed; 961.27, tm; 961.30, may; 965.6, patroles; 971.36, and and; 972.40, occured; 973.4, were no; 973.5, fearfnl; 973.16, tbe; 973.18, were I; 974.4, half; 975.2, cows;; 975.9, out outside; 975.24, when the we; 975.40, The The; 976.40, did succeed; 977.12, Philadephia; 977.29, he Holy; 982.13, her her; 983.10, suitation; 983.32, buffalo; 985.1, aud; 985.29, my my; 988.14, appaling; 988.15, labour in; 988.39, latitute; 989.5, While; 989.20, contitution; 990.36, yeild; 991.24–25, goverment; 991.35, aboard; 993.21, the plans; 993.28, prolaim; 996.5, momemt.

Notes

In the notes below, the reference numbers denote page and line of this volume (the line count includes chapter headings). No note is made for material included in standard desk-reference books such as Webster's *Collegiate*, *Biographical*, and *Geographical* dictionaries. Biblical references are keyed to the King James Version. Quotations from Shakespeare are keyed to *The Riverside Shakespeare*, ed. G. Blakemore Evans (Boston: Houghton Mifflin, 1974). Footnotes and bracketed editorial notes within the text were in the originals. For further biographical background, references to other studies, and more detailed notes, see *Pioneers of the Black Atlantic: Five Slave Narratives from the Enlightenment, 1772–1815*, edited by Henry Louis Gates Jr. and William L. Andrews (Washington, D.C.: Civitas/Counterpoint, 1998); *The Civitas Anthology of African American Slave Narratives*, edited by William L. Andrews and Henry Louis Gates Jr. (Washington, D.C.: Civitas/Counterpoint, 1999); *I Was Born a Slave: An Anthology of Classic Slave Narratives*, edited by Yuval Taylor (2 vols., Chicago: Lawrence Hill Books, 1999); *Olaudah Equiano, The Interesting Narrative and Other Writings*, edited by Vincent Carretta (New York: Penguin Books, 1995); Harriet A. Jacobs, *Incidents in the Life of a Slave Girl*, edited by Jean Fagan Yellin (Cambridge: Harvard University Press, 1987).

A NARRATIVE OF THE MOST REMARKABLE PARTICULARS IN THE LIFE OF JAMES ALBERT UKAWSAW GRONNIOSAW

2.3   *Countess* of HUNTINGDON] Selina Hastings (1707–91), Countess of Huntingdon, a leading English Methodist who helped Phillis Wheatley publish her *Poems on Various Subjects, Religious and Moral* in London in 1773.

3.4   young LADY] Identified as the English writer Hannah More (1745–1833) in *The Black Prince*, a version of Gronniosaw's narrative published in the United States in 1809, though the identification is uncertain.

4.35   W. SHIRLEY] Walter Shirley (1725–86), a Methodist clergyman, writer of hymns, and cousin of the Countess of Huntingdon.

5.5   BOURNOU] Probably a reference to Bornu, a Muslim-dominated state around Lake Chad.

13.14   Mr. Freelandhouse] Theodorus Frelinghuysen (1691–c 1748), a Dutch Reformed minister and a leading revivalist preacher during the "Great Awakening" of the 1740s.

15.30–31   Bunyan . . . holy war] *The Holy War, Made by Shaddai upon Diabolus, for the Reigning of the Metropolis of the World* (1682), by John Bunyan (1628–88).

16.7   Baxter's . . . *unconverted*] *A Call to the Unconverted to Turn and Live* (1658) by Richard Baxter (1615–91).

16.34   "*Behold . . . God.*"] John 1:29.

18.10–13   "*And I . . . from me.*"] Jeremiah 32:40.

19.3–5   "*And ye are . . . power.*"] Cf. Colossians 2:10.

19.7–9   "*Wherefore He . . . for them.*"] Hebrews 7:25.

22.21–23   Pocock's fleet . . . Havannah] The fleet commanded by Admiral George Pocock (1706–92) captured Martinique and Cuba in 1762. Britain returned Martinique to France and Cuba to Spain under the terms of the Treaty of Paris (1763), which ended the Seven Years War.

24.6   Mr. Whitefield's Tabernacle] A building in Moorfields used by the Methodist preacher George Whitefield (1714–70).

24.10–11   Dr. Gifford's Meeting] Andrew Gifford (1700–84) was the minister of a Baptist meeting on Eagle Street.

24.28–29   Mr. Allen's Meeting] John Allen was the pastor of a Baptist meeting on Petticoat Lane in Spitalsfield.

25.29–30   "*Come unto . . . Soul.*"] Cf. Psalm 66:16.

26.1–2   "*I know . . . liveth,*"] Job 19:25.

33.14–16   *Mr. Fawcet . . . everlasting rest*] Benjamin Fawcett (1715–80), a dissenting minister and friend of the Countess of Huntingdon, had republished *The Saint's Everlasting Rest* (1650) by Richard Baxter.

33.17   Manufactory of *Kidderminster*] Kidderminster was a center of carpet manufacture.

THE INTERESTING NARRATIVE OF THE LIFE OF OLAUDAH EQUIANO

37.1   TO THE LORDS] In later editions Equiano added several letters of recommendation and excerpts from reviews to the prefatory section of the *Narrative*; many of these additions were made after two unsigned articles appeared in the British press in 1792 accusing Equiano of being a native of Santa Cruz in the Danish West Indies.

50.20   Eboe] Ibo.

51.39   Benezet's . . . Guinea"] *Some Historical Account of Guinea, its Situation, Produce, and the General Disposition of its Inhabitants* (1771), by

Anthony Benezet (1713–84). Benezet, a Quaker schoolteacher in Philadelphia, wrote extensively against slavery and the slave trade.

52.29   stickado]   Xylophone.

53.18   eadas]   A tuberous plant.

57.39   Benezet's Account of Africa]   *A Short Account of that Part of Africa, Inhabited by the Negroes* (1762) by Anthony Benezet.

61.27   Leut. Matthew's Voyage]   *A Voyage to the River Sierra-Leone, on the Coast of Africa* (1788), by John Matthews, a lieutenant in the Royal Navy.

62.13–14   Dr. Gill . . . Genesis]   John Gill (1697–1771), *An Exposition of the Old Testament, in Which are Recorded the Original of Mankind, of the Several Nations of the World, and of the Jewish Nation in Particular* (6 vols, 1748–63).

62.18–19   Clarke . . . Christian Religion]   Clarke (1682–1757) had translated *The Truth of the Christian Religion* by Hugo Grotius.

63.1–3   Clarkson . . . Species]   *An Essay on the Slavery and Commerce of the Human Species, Particularly the African* (1786), by Thomas Clarkson (1760–1846).

63.7   Dr. Mitchel]   John Mitchel, whose paper "Causes of the Different Colours of Persons in Different Climates" was presented to the Royal Society in 1744 and published in *The Philosophical Transactions* (1756).

64.8–9   whose wisdom . . . his ways."]   Cf. Isaiah 55:8.

69.1–2   "Ev'ry leaf . . . death."]   Cf. *Cooper's Hill* (1642), lines 287–88, by Sir John Denham (1615–69).

73.18   pomkins]   Pumpkins.

81.22   snow]   A two-masted sailing vessel resembling a brig.

82.18   *Gustavus Vasa*]   King of Sweden from 1523 to 1560, leader of a successful revolt against the Danes and founder of the Swedish navy.

83.17   the Archipelago]   The Aegean Sea.

87.9   the Nore]   Anchorage in the Thames estuary that was frequently used by the Royal Navy.

88.37   Admiral Byng]   John Byng (1704–57) was convicted of neglect of duty and shot after failing to defeat a French fleet off Minorca in 1756.

89.25   Duke of ——]   Changed in the eighth and ninth editions (1794) to "Duke of Cumberland." William Augustus (1721–65), Duke of Cumberland, returned to England in 1757 after having been defeated by the French in Hanover.

90.16–17   the flag . . . the blue] Admirals in the Royal Navy flew blue, red, or white flags, depending upon their seniority.

91.36   At last Louisburgh was taken] The fortress surrendered on July 26, 1758, after a 48-day siege.

92.40–93.1   wore ship, and stood after] Changed course and pursued.

93.34   starting our water] Pumping water out of the ship.

94.21   two and three years] Changed in the fifth edition to "three and four years."

95.26–27   Guide . . . Sodor and Man] *An Essay towards an Instruction for the Indians; Explaining the Most Essential Doctrines of Christianity* (1740), by Thomas Wilson (1663–1755).

95.33   rendezvous-house] A house or inn used as the base of operations for a press-gang.

99.14–16   "Oh Jove! . . . day."] Cf. Alexander Pope's translation of *The Iliad*, Book 17, lines 728–32.

101.12   this engagement] The battle of Lagos, fought August 18–19, 1759.

101.33   that time the king died] George II died on October 25, 1760.

102.15   Belle-Isle] An island in the Bay of Biscay off the southern coast of Brittany.

104.28–29   God . . . cannot fall] Cf. Matthew 10:29.

105.36   "Wing'd . . . rage;"] John Milton, *Paradise Lost*, Book 1, line 175.

106.35   carcases] Incendiary shells.

107.3   Basse-road] Basque Road, anchorage between the Ile de Ré and the Ile d'Oleron at the entrance to the port of Rochefort on the Bay of Biscay.

107.11   springs] Ropes used to hold a vessel in firing position.

107.20   Spanish war began] Britain declared war on Spain on January 4, 1762.

107.23   a cartel] A ship used to carry out a prisoner exchange.

115.24–27   "Regions . . . urges."] Cf. *Paradise Lost*, Book 1, lines 65–68.

115.33   "The Dying Negro,"] By Thomas Day (1748–89) and John Bicknell (d. 1787). Equiano's quotation is not exact.

117.39   droggers] Coasting vessels.

119.17   King's Bench] A debtor's prison.

119.18   The last war] The War of the American Revolution.

121.27–28   woman of her species.] Beginning in the second edition (1789), this was followed by a new paragraph:

"One Mr. D—— told me that he had sold 41,000 negroes, and that he once cut off a negro-man's leg for running away.—I asked him, if the man had died in the operation? How he, as a Christian, could answer for the horrid act before God? And he told me, answering was a thing of another world; but what he thought and did were policy. I told him that the Christian doctrine taught us to do unto others as we would that others should do unto us. He then said that his scheme had the desired effect— it cured that man and some others of running away."

In the eighth edition (1794), Equiano changed "Mr. D——" to "Mr. Drummond."

122.24   a treatise] *Instructions for the Treatment of Negroes, inscribed to the Society for propagating the Gospel in foreign Parts* (1786), by Philip Gibbes (1731–1815).

122.30   the sequel] The second volume of *The Interesting Narrative*.

123.37–38   pot boil over.] Beginning in the fifth edition (1792), this was followed by: "It is not uncommon, after a flogging, to make slaves go on their knees, and thank their owners, and pray, or rather say, God bless them. I have often asked many of the men slaves (who used to go several miles to their wives, and late in the night, after having been wearied with a hard day's labour) why they went so far for wives, and why they did not take them of their own master's negro women, and particularly those who lived together as household slaves? Their answers have ever been—'Because when the master or mistress choose to punish the women, they make the husbands flog their own wives, and that they could not bear to do.' "

124.3–5   "With . . . no rest!"] Cf. *Paradise Lost*, Book 2, lines 616–18.

125.19–20   329th Act] The act was passed on August 8, 1688.

125.36   Samaide] Samoyed.

125.40   Mr. James Tobin] Author of the pro-slavery tract *Cursory Remarks upon the Reverend Mr. Ramsay's Essay on the Treatment and Conversion of African Slaves in the Sugar Colonies* (1785).

127.4   Moses . . . Egyptian] In Exodus 2:11–12.

128.17–25   No peace . . . suffering feel."] Cf. *Paradise Lost*, Book 2, lines 332–40.

137.19–24   "With thoughts . . . slave of man."] The author of these lines has not been identified, and may have been Equiano himself.

145.4   1764] Changed to "1765" in the fifth edition.

170.15   catguts] Stringed musical instruments.

174.3   the Grenades] The Grenadines.

176.14   Cherry-Garden stairs] A landing place in London on the south bank of the Thames.

177.35   barter and alligation] Computational methods used to determine values and prices in commerce.

181.3   refused the temptation] Beginning in the second edition, Equiano added at this point: "thinking one was as much as some could manage, and more than others would venture on."

181.25   Standgate creek] A landing place on the south bank of the Thames in London.

187.39   chucks] Chocks.

190.38   Union Stairs] A landing place on the north bank of the Thames in London.

193.20–22   'Before . . . will hear.'] Isaiah 65:24.

195.17–18   O! to . . . to be!] "Come Thou Fount of Every Blessing," a Methodist hymn by Robert Robinson (1735–90).

196.2–3   "The Conversion . . . Indian."] By Lawrence Harlow (1774).

197.30–31   Mr. P——] Identified by Equiano in the eighth edition as the Calvinist Henry Peckwell (1747–87).

198.16   offends . . . of all?'] James 2:10.

199.25–26   Allen's . . . unconverted.] *An Allarme to Unconverted Sinners* (1673), by Joseph Alleine (1634–68).

200.21   'the commandment . . . died,'] Romans 7:9.

200.31–32   The word . . . honeycomb.] Cf. Psalm 19:9–10.

202.20–21   my Ebenezer] See 1 Samuel 7:12.

202.39   Mr. Romaine] William Romaine (1714–95), a leading Calvinist Methodist preacher.

208.5–13   "Christ . . . things up?"] Adapted from the hymn "The Spiritual Victory."

212.5   Fox's Martyrology] *Acts and Monuments of These Later and Perilous Days* (1563) by John Foxe (1517–87), popularly known as *The Book of Martyrs*, which recorded the persecution of English Protestants under Mary I.

216.27   Mexico or Peru] Changed by Equiano in the ninth edition to "Jamaica."

217.10   casades] Cassava.

218.33–35   'What does . . . soul?'']   Matthew 16:26.

225.19–20   "That he . . . ride."]   Cf. *Love's Last Shift* (1696), play by Colley Cibber (1671–1757).

227.25   Governor Macnamara]   Matthias Macnamara was governor of Senegambia, 1775–78.

228.6   Alexander . . . St. Paul]   See 2 Timothy 4:14.

228.13   late Bishop of London]   Robert Lowth (1710–87) was Bishop of London, 1777–87.

231.29   "Go ye . . . likewise?"]   Cf. Luke 10:37.

231.35–37   your book . . . Negroes]   Originally published in Philadelphia in 1766 by the Quaker writer Anthony Benezet, the book was reprinted and circulated to members of Parliament by English Quakers in 1784 and 1785.

232.35   Lombard-Street.]   In the second, third, and fourth editions, published between 1789 and 1791, this was followed by: "—My hand is ever free— if any female Debonair wishes to obtain it, this mode I recommend." Equiano married in 1792, and from the fifth edition onward changed the sentence to simply read: "This mode I highly recommend."

233.36   Mr. Irving]   Beginning with the second edition, Equiano changed this to read "Mr. Joseph Irwin." Irwin became the agent for the Sierra Leone settlement project in 1786, following the death of Henry Steathman, who had first proposed the plan.

235.19   gentleman in the city]   Identified by Equiano in the ninth edition as Samuel Hoare. A banker and a Quaker, Hoare (1751–1825) was chairman of the Committee for the Black Poor.

236.37   See . . . July 14, 1787]   The newspaper published a letter Equiano had written defending his conduct in the Sierra Leone enterprise.

238.3–4   the Queen]   Queen Charlotte, the consort of George III.

240.8–12   'Those that honour . . . wickedness.']   Cf. Proverbs 14:31, 14:34, 10:29, 11:5.

242.5   return for manufactures.]   This was followed in the fifth and subsequent editions by a paragraph in which Equiano described his travels in Great Britain and Ireland in 1791 and 1792 and mentioned his marriage on April 7, 1792, to "Miss Cullen, daughter of James and Ann Cullen, late of Ely." Beginning with the sixth edition (1793), a footnote to the paragraph mentioned Equiano's descents into tunnels and mines in Manchester, Derbyshire, and Newcastle.

242.22–23   'to do justly . . . God?']   Cf. Micah 6:8.

THE CONFESSIONS OF NAT TURNER

251.10–11   "Seek ye . . . unto you."]   Cf. Luke 12:31.

252.9–11   "For he . . . chastened you."]   Cf. Luke 12:47.

253.30–31   the first . . . be first.]   Cf. Matthew 19:30, 20:16; Mark 10:31; Luke 13:30.

NARRATIVE OF THE LIFE OF FREDERICK DOUGLASS

269.28   "gave . . . MAN,"]   Cf. Shakespeare, *Hamlet*, III.iv.62.

270.5   "created . . . angels"]   Cf. Psalm 8:5, Hebrews 2:7.

271.15   JOHN A. COLLINS]   Collins (1810–79) had resigned as general agent of the Society in 1843 to devote himself to the propagation of Fourierism.

271.36–37   "grow . . . God,"]   Cf. 2 Peter 3:18.

272.4   CHARLES LENOX REMOND]   Born to free parents in Massachusetts, Remond (1810–73) became an agent of the Massachusetts Anti-Slavery Society in 1838 and made anti-slavery speeches in New England, Great Britain, and Ireland. During the Civil War he served as a recruiting officer for the 54th Massachusetts Infantry and was later a clerk in the Boston Custom House.

272.27   Loyal National Repeal Association]   Founded in 1840 by Irish Catholic political leader Daniel O'Connell (1775–1847) to agitate for the repeal of the 1800 act uniting Ireland and Great Britain. The Association sought the restoration of a separate Irish parliament under the British crown.

273.16–17   arm . . . save]   Cf. Isaiah 50:2: "Is my hand shortened at all, that it cannot redeem?"

273.18–19   "in slaves . . . men."]   Cf. Revelation 18:13.

274.18–19   Alexandrian library]   The library in Alexandria, Egypt, said to have been founded by Ptolemy I in the early third century B.C. and destroyed in the late third century A.D.; it was reported to have contained between 400,000 and 700,000 volumes.

276.25   cloud of witnesses]   Hebrews 12:1.

277.17–18   1838 . . . West India]   Emancipation of all slaves in the British West Indies was peacefully completed August 1, 1838, under the conditions of the Abolition Act of August 28, 1833. The Act freed all West Indian slaves under six, bound the remainder to work as apprentices for between five and seven (later reduced to two) years before being emancipated, and granted slaveowners £20 million in compensation; it went into effect on August 1, 1834.

279.10   "hide the outcast,"]   Cf. Isaiah 16:3.

290.29–30   "there . . . heart."] Cf. William Cowper, *The Task* (1785),
Book II—"Time Piece," line 8.

305.17   *gip*] Gypsy.

307.32–33   "The Columbian Orator."] Published in 1797 and edited by
Caleb Bingham (1757–1817), the volume collects excerpts from speeches and
plays, dialogues, and poems, extolling patriotism, education, temperance,
freedom, and courage, and denouncing slavery and oppression. It is introduced by a 23-page essay on speaking by Bingham.

307.34–35   dialogue . . . slave.] Written by Caleb Bingham.

308.6–7   Sheridan's . . . emancipation] The oration on Catholic
Emancipation in the *Columbian Orator* was actually an excerpt from a speech
made in the Irish House of Commons in 1795 by Arthur O'Connor
(1763–1852).

314.14–25   "Gone . . . daughters!"] "The Farewell of a Virginia Slave
Mother to Her Daughters Sold into Southern Bondage" (1838), lines 1–12.

318.31   George Cookman] George Grimston Cookman (1800–41) of
England settled in the United States and became a Methodist minister in
Philadelphia in 1825, then was transferred to Maryland in 1833. He was twice
made chaplain to the House of Representatives.

319.17–18   "He . . . stripes."] Luke 12:47

340.16–17   "rather . . . of."] Cf. *Hamlet*, III.i.80–81.

350.17   not to state all the facts] Douglass first revealed the details of his
escape in a lecture given in Philadelphia in 1873. In his third autobiography,
Life and Times of Frederick Douglass (1881, revised 1892), he described obtaining seaman's protection papers from a free black sailor and using them to
travel from Baltimore to New York by train and steamboat.

351.6–7   western . . . *railroad*] The term apparently first came into public use in Illinois in 1842.

356.38   DAVID RUGGLES] Ruggles (1810–49), born free in Connecticut,
was a grocer, author, secretary of the New York Vigilance Committee (organized 1835), and an abolitionist journalist and lecturer.

357.7   *Darg* case] Ruggles was arrested in New York City on September
6, 1839, and charged with harboring Thomas Hughes, a fugitive Arkansas
slave alleged to have stolen $9,000 from his owner, John P. Darg. The case
was never prosecuted, but Ruggles was forced to remain on bail until the
charge was finally dropped in late 1839.

357.23   the Rev. . . . Pennington] Pennington (1807–70), pastor first of
Congregational then Presbyterian churches, teacher, author, and abolitionist
orator, escaped from slavery in Maryland around 1831.

358.40–359.1   "Lady . . . Douglass."]   The unjustly outlawed Lord James of Douglas is a principal character in Walter Scott's poem *The Lady of the Lake* (1810).

360.24–26   "I was . . . in"]   Cf. Matthew 25:35.

362.1   "Liberator."]   Abolitionist weekly (1831–65) founded at Boston by William Lloyd Garrison (1805–79).

363.23–24   "stealing . . . in."]   Cf. the Rev. Robert Pollok, *The Course of Time* (1827), Bk. 8, lines 616–18: "He was a man / Who stole the livery of the court of Heaven / To serve the Devil in."

364.26–365.4   "Just . . . thine?"]   John Greenleaf Whittier, "Clerical Oppressors" (1836), lines 1–16.

365.7–32   "They . . . iniquity."]   Cf. Matthew 23:4–28.

366.29–31   "Shall . . . this?"]   Jeremiah 5:9.

366.32   A PARODY]   A parody of "Heavenly Union," a hymn especially popular in the South.

NARRATIVE OF WILLIAM W. BROWN

369.11   COWPER]   The quotation is actually from *Cato: A Tragedy* (1713) by Joseph Addison (1672–1719); in Addison, the fourth line reads: "Who owes his Greatness to his Country's Ruin?"

371.3–5   I was a . . . clothed me.]   Cf. Matthew 25:35–36.

372.2   EDMUND QUINCY]   Quincy (1808–77) was corresponding secretary of the Massachusetts Anti-Slavery Society and an editor of the *Anti-Slavery Standard* and the *Abolitionist*.

372.20   "move . . . mutiny"]   Cf. *Julius Caesar*, III.ii.229–30.

373.6–7   "Let me . . . laws;"]   Andrew Fletcher (1655–1716), *An Account of a Conversation Concerning the Right to Regulation of Governments* (1703).

374.13–14   "clothed . . . heaven"]   See note 363.23–24 in this volume.

375.4–7   "Have ye . . . land?"]   James Russell Lowell (1819–91), "The Present Crisis."

375.26–27   "For he . . . tyranny."]   James Russell Lowell, "L'Envoi."

376.4–5   "The common . . . foul."]   Robert Blair (1699–1746), *The Grave* (1743).

376.11   J. C. HATHAWAY]   Joseph Comstock Hathaway (1810–73) was president of the Western New York Anti-Slavery Society.

378.22   It was not yet daylight.]   In the revised version of the *Narrative* published in 1848, Brown replaced this sentence with the following:

"Experience has taught me that nothing can be more heart-rending than for one to see a dear and beloved mother or sister tortured, and to hear their cries, and not be able to render them assistance. But such is the position which an American slave occupies."

383.11–12   Lovejoy . . . Times."] Lovejoy (1802–37) edited the St. Louis *Observer* from 1833 until 1836, when he was forced to leave the city because of his antislavery views. Moving to Alton, Illinois, he edited an antislavery newspaper for a year before being murdered by a proslavery mob.

386.22   "sleep . . . eyelids."] Cf. Psalm 132:4, Proverbs 6:4.

394.27–395.12   "O, master . . . go."] Charlotte Elizabeth (1790–1846), "The Slave and Her Babe." In the version of the *Narrative* published in London in 1849, Brown replaced this quotation with two paragraphs attacking the slave trade within the United States.

395.20–396.6   "See these . . . jubilee!"] This song was first printed in 1844 in *The Liberator*, the antislavery newspaper published by William Lloyd Garrison, under the title "The Plantation Song."

399.10   "Slavery as it is."] *American Slavery As It Is: Testimony of a Thousand Witnesses* (1839), by Theodore Dwight Weld (1803–95).

404.2–3   —the NORTH STAR.] At this point in the revised version of the *Narrative* published in 1848, Brown quoted 21 lines from "The Fugitive Slave's Apostrophe to the North Star" by John Pierpont (1785–1866).

408.28–31   the glory . . . my side."] Elizabeth Margaret Chandler (1807–34), "The Bereaved Father."

409.1–2   "Gone . . . dank and lone!"] John Greenleaf Whittier (1807–92), "The Farewell of a Virginia Slave Mother to Her Daughters Sold into Southern Bondage" (1838).

410.29–30   "He that . . . many stripes!"] Cf. Luke 12:47.

411.1–4   "I would . . . despair."] From the anonymous song "I Am Monarch of Nought I Survey."

419.23   "Thompsonian"] A follower of the American herbalist Samuel Thomson (1769–1843).

NARRATIVE OF THE LIFE AND ADVENTURES OF HENRY BIBB

428.32   Liberty men] Supporters of the antislavery Liberty Party of the 1840s.

429.33   DAWN MILLS] An African-American settlement in southeastern Ontario, founded by the fugitive slave Josiah Henson (1789–1883).

436.13   Judge Wilkins] Ross Wilkins (1799–1872) served as a federal district judge in Michigan, 1837–70.

437.31   LUCIUS C. MATLACK]   An antislavery Methodist preacher and author of *The History of American Slavery and Methodism* (1849).

445.27   "pat juber,"]   To beat out a rhythm with the hands.

446.15–17   "Servants . . . stripes;—"]   Cf. Colossians 3:22, Luke 12:47.

451.23   mestinos]   Mestizos; persons of mixed European and American Indian ancestry.

464.21   "Behind . . . smiling face,"]   William Cowper (1731–1800), "Light Shining Out of Darkness."

486.9   Methodist E.]   Methodist Episcopal.

562.26–27   "Inasmuch . . . unto me."]   Cf. Matthew 25:40.

NARRATIVE OF SOJOURNER TRUTH

569.1   PREFACE.]   The unsigned preface was written by William Lloyd Garrison.

571.29–32   'a swift . . . right?']   Cf. Malachi 3:5.

571.34–37   'Judgment . . . prey.']   Isaiah 59:14–15.

572.4–5   'The Lord . . . oppressed.']   Psalm 103:6.

572.6–10   'O give . . . for ever.']   Cf. Psalm 136:1, 10, 15.

572.10–13   'Sing unto . . . waters.']   Cf. Exodus 15:1, 10.

572.14–16   'Who is . . . wonders?']   Exodus 15:11.

572.34–35   'have no . . . them;']   Ephesians 5:11.

581.31   Juan Fernandes]   Spanish navigator who lived for several years in the 1570s on the Juan Fernandez Islands in the South Pacific off the coast of Chile.

583.34–35   'that bourne . . . returns']   *Hamlet*, III.i.78–79.

587.27–28   emancipation . . . 1828]   The emancipation act of 1817 freed all slaves born before July 4, 1799, on July 4, 1827.

602.19   North River]   Hudson River.

623.20   the Tombs]   A New York City jail.

642.8   Lot's wife,']   See Genesis 19:17–26.

646. 29–30   Ethiopia . . . God.]   Cf. Psalm 68:31.

649.13–14   Mr. Miller's]   William Miller (1782–1849), a traveling preacher who predicted that the Second Coming of Christ would occur between March 1843 and March 1844.

650.30–31   "changed . . . an eye."]   Cf. 1 Corinthians 15:52.

650.40–655.1   Shadrach, Meshach, and Abednego!]   See Daniel 3.

653.2   Fruitlands]   A utopian community founded by Bronson Alcott in Harvard, Massachusetts.

653.11   Northampton Association]   The Northampton Association of Education and Industry, a utopian community founded in Northampton, Massachusetts, in 1842 by Samuel L. Hill and George Benson.

654.10–11   "One . . . to flight"]   Cf. Deuteronomy 32:30.

658.37   'perfect love . . . . fear.']   1 John 4:18.

662.2   'Slavery as It Is.']   See note 399.10 in this volume.

664.37   Clarkson's]   Thomas Clarkson (1760–1846), British antislavery writer.

671.37   WILLIAM MORGAN]   Morgan, a resident of Batavia, New York, disappeared in September 1826. Allegations that he had been murdered by Freemasons in order to prevent him from publishing a book revealing the secrets of the Masonic order resulted in the formation of the Anti-Masonic political party in the northeastern United States.

RUNNING A THOUSAND MILES FOR FREEDOM

677.7–9   "Slaves . . . fall."]   William Cowper (1731–1800), The Task (1785).

679.2–3   "God . . . men,"]   Cf. Acts 17:24–26.

681.9   MILTON]   Paradise Lost, Book 12, lines 67–71.

685.1   calybuce]   Calaboose; jailhouse.

691.14–17   "O, deep . . . death."]   Jesse Hutchinson, "The Bereaved Mother" (1844).

691.25–692.12   "Why stands . . . and thee!"]   "The Slave-Auction—A Fact," published anonymously in The Garland of Freedom: A Collection of Poems, Chiefly Anti-Slavery (1853).

692.35–36   "where the . . . at rest."]   Job 3:17.

693.1–4   "Holds . . . light."]   Henry Wadsworth Longfellow (1807–82), "The Spanish Student" (1842).

693.31–38   "His heart . . . land!"]   Longfellow, "The Quadroon Girl" (1842).

700.24   the engraving]   See page 678 in this volume.

703.10–17   United . . . Negro-scars]   "Epigram to the United States of North America."

704.11–16   "The hill . . . woe."]   John Bunyan, "Pilgrim's Progress."

706.28   opodeldoc]   A soap liniment.

719.10   *Royal Charter*]   British passenger steamer that ran aground and broke up during a storm off Liverpool on October 25, 1859; 447 lives were lost.

735.21–22   "to loose . . . go free."]   Isaiah 58:6.

735.34–39   "I venerate . . . weeds."]   William Cowper, "Expostulation."

741.7–10   "Peace . . . in smiles."]   William Cowper, *The Task* (1785).

742.9   JAMES RUSSELL LOWELL]   "Elegy on the Death of Dr. Channing."

INCIDENTS IN THE LIFE OF A SLAVE GIRL

743.10   A WOMAN OF NORTH CAROLINA]   Angelina E. Grimké (1805–79), *Appeal to the Christian Women of the South* (1836).

743.14   L. MARIA CHILD]   Child (1802–80), a novelist and author of popular advice books, had edited the *National Anti-Slavery Standard* from 1841 to 1849; her antislavery works included *An Appeal in Favor of that Class of Americans Called Africans* (1833) and *Correspondence between Lydia Maria Child and Gov. Wise and Mrs. Mason of Virginia* (1860).

745.20   Bishop Paine]   Daniel A. Payne (1811–93), a bishop of the African Methodist Episcopal Church.

746.5   LINDA BRENT]   Pseudonym used by Harriet Jacobs.

751.8   My father]   Elijah Jacobs (died c. 1826).

751.22   William]   John S. Jacobs (1815?–1875), who published his own narrative, "A True Tale of Slavery," in *The Leisure Hour: A Family Journal of Instruction and Recreation*, a London magazine, in 1861.

751.24   maternal grandmother]   Molly Horniblow (c. 1771–1853).

752.18   Benjamin]   Joseph Horniblow.

753.2   my mother]   Deliah Horniblow (1797?–c. 1819).

753.4   My mother's mistress]   Margaret Horniblow (1797–1825).

754.11–12   her sister's daughter]   Mary Matilda Norcom (b. 1822).

754.14–16   "Thou shalt . . . unto them."]   Mark 12:31; Matthew 7:12.

754.34–35   DR. FLINT . . . the sister]   Dr. James Norcom (1778–1850); Mary Matilda Horniblow Norcom (1794–1868).

758.12   Aunt Nancy]   Betty Horniblow (1794?–1841).

763.40   young master Nicholas]   James Norcom Jr. (b. 1811).

771.29   uncle Phillip]   Mark Jacobs (c. 1800–58).

781.31   "full of . . . uncleanness."]   Matthew 23:27.

782.32   "Not my . . . O Lord!"]   Cf. Luke 22:42.

783.4–7   "Where laughter . . . hell."]   Byron, "The Lament of Tasso,"
iv.7–10.

787.29   Young Mr. Flint]   James Norcom Jr.

790.35–36   "made of . . . men!"]   Acts 17:26.

795.35   "like angels' . . . between."]   Thomas Campbell (1777–1844),
"Pleasures of Hope" (1799).

797.31–33   "The poor . . . gone!"]   William Mason (1724–97), *Elfrida*
(1751).

801.19   Mr. Sands]   Samuel Tredwell Sawyer (1800–65), an attorney in
Edenton who served in the North Carolina House of Representatives,
1829–32, and in the United States House of Representatives, 1837–39.

807.13   my babe]   Joseph Jacobs (born c. 1829).

814.34–36   "Servants . . . Christ."]   Ephesians 6:5.

820.37   "South-Side View of Slavery,"]   *A South-Side View of Slavery; or,
Three Months in the South in 1854* (1854), a defense of slavery written by
Boston minister Nehemiah Adams (1806–78).

823.25   new-born . . . girl]   Louisa Matilda Jacobs (1833–1917).

834.23   Miss Fanny]   Hannah Pritchard (d. 1838).

836.16–19   "There . . . master."]   Cf. Job 3:17–19.

838.14   young Mrs. Flint]   Penelope Hoskins Norcom (1812–43), wife of
James Norcom Jr.

844.32–33   "Give me . . . death,"]   Patrick Henry (1736–99), in a speech
in the Virginia Convention, March 23, 1775.

853.34   "Home, sweet home."]   Song (1823) by John Howard Payne
(1791–1852).

859.34   pent]   Sloping.

867.6–11   Senator Brown . . . slave!"]   Albert Gallatin Brown (1813–80)
served as a Democratic senator from Mississippi, 1854–61, and made these remarks on February 24, 1854, during a debate on the Kansas-Nebraska Bill.

867.30   Thompsonian doctor]   See note 419.23 in this volume.

876.11–12   'where the . . . rest.']   Cf. Job 3:17.

880.4   Astor House]   A New York City hotel.

886.13   Emily Flint]   Mary Matilda Norcom (b. 1822).

905.8   `a levy]   Twelve and a half cents.

905.10   Jeremiah Durham]   Durham was a minister of the African Methodist Episcopal Church.

910.21–22   Mrs. Hobbs]   Mary Bonner Blount Tredwell (1808–69), the wife of James Iredell Tredwell (1799–1846), a first cousin of Samuel Tredwell Sawyer ("Mr. Sands").

913.11   Mrs. Bruce]   Mary Stace Willis (c. 1816–45), wife of Nathaniel Parker Willis (1806–67), a poet, journalist, and magazine editor.

913.29   her lovely babe]   Imogen Willis (b. 1842).

924.5–6   Judge Vanderpool and Lawyer Hopper]   Arent Van der Poel (1799–1870), a Superior Court judge and former congressman; John Hopper (1815–64), a Quaker attorney involved in the protection of fugitive slaves.

928.16   Hon. Miss Murray]   Amelia Matilda Murray (1795–1884) favorably described American slavery in *Letters from the United States, Cuba and Canada* (1856).

930.14–15   " 'Come . . . spy.' "]   Mary Howitt (1799–1888), "The Spider and the Fly."

930.34–35   chains . . . justice]   In 1851 and 1854 chains were placed around the court house in Boston to help prevent the rescue of fugitive slaves being held there.

932.27–28   Isaac and Amy Post]   Isaac Post (1798–1872) and Amy Post (1802–89) were friends of Frederick Douglass who frequently sheltered fugitive slaves; Amy Post was also an early activist in the woman's rights movement.

933.17–18   new Mrs. Bruce]   Cornelia Grinnell Willis (1825–1904).

933.32–33   "short . . . poor."]   Thomas Gray (1716–71), "Elegy Written in a Country Church-Yard" (1751).

933.36   Zion's church]   A mass meeting was held at the Zion Chapel Street Church on October 1, 1850, to protest the arrest of James Hamlet under the new Fugitive Slave Law. The meeting raised $800 to buy his freedom, and on October 5 he returned to the city.

937.34   wife of a senator]   Jacobs was probably sheltered in New Bedford, Massachusetts, by Joseph and Sarah Russell Grinnell, the uncle and aunt of Cornelia Grinnell Willis. Joseph Grinnell had been a Whig member of the House of Representatives from 1843 to 1851.

940.24   Mr. Dodge]   Daniel Messmore.

941.39–40   'Proclaim . . . bound']   Isaiah 61:1.

942.3   John Mitchell] An Irish nationalist, Mitchel (1815–75) was convicted of treason in 1848 and sentenced to 14 years transportation. In 1853 he escaped from Van Diemen's Land (Tasmania) and went to New York, where he began publishing *The Citizen*, a proslavery newspaper, in January 1854.

942.7–8   "Oppression . . . mad;"] Ecclesiastes 7:7.

944.25–26   "where . . . rest."] Job 3:17.

NARRATIVE OF THE LIFE OF J. D. GREEN

979.7–10   "Ah, whither . . . complaint."] From a hymn by Charles Wesley (1707–88) included in a later edition of *Hymns and Spiritual Songs*, first published in 1707 by Isaac Watts.

981.26   Stephen . . . Holy Ghost] See Acts 7:55.

986.22–23   song of deliverance,] See pp. 996–97 in this volume.

989.31–32   SPEECH . . . STEPHENS] Although Stephens did speak and vote against secession in the January 1861 Georgia Convention, the speech printed in *Narrative of the Life of J. D. Green* is a forgery that first appeared in *The Rebuke of Secession Doctrines by Southern Statesmen*, published in 1863 by the Union League of Philadelphia.

Library of Congress Cataloging-in-Publication Data

Slave Narratives

   Originally published in hardcover by The Library of
America in 2000.
   Contents: James Albert Ukasaw Gronniosaw — Olaudah
Equiano — Nat Turner — Frederick Douglass — William
Wells Brown — Henry Bibb — Sojourner Truth — William
and Ellen Craft — Harriet Ann Jacobs — Jacob D. Green
   1. Slaves—United States—Biography.   2. Afro-Americans—
Biography.   3. Slaves' writings, American.   I. Title.
II. Series.
E444.S56   2000
305'.5'67'092396073—dc21

                                              99-40360
                                                  CIP

ISBN 1–931082–11–1 (paperback)
ISBN 1–883011–76–0 (hardcover)

ABOUT THE LIBRARY OF AMERICA

THE LIBRARY OF AMERICA is an award-winning, nonprofit publisher dedicated to preserving America's best and most significant writing in handsome, enduring volumes, featuring authoritative texts. Founded in 1979 with initial funding from the National Endowment for the Humanities and the Ford Foundation, the series, which now numbers over a hundred volumes, has been called "the most important book-publishing project in the nation's history."

For the first time, the full range of outstanding American writing will be permanently available in uniform, hardcover volumes, priced to reach a wide audience. Each volume contains up to 1600 pages and includes a number of works by our country's foremost novelists, historians, poets, essayists, journalists, philosophers, and statesmen. Authoritative, unabridged, scrupulously accurate texts are a hallmark of the volumes, which also feature a handsomely designed page, high-quality, acid-free paper bound in a cloth cover and sewn to lie flat when opened, a ribbon marker, and printed endpapers. The series includes acknowledged classics and neglected masterpieces, and new volumes are added each year.

Library of America hardcover volumes are available singly or by subscription. A jacketed edition, available in bookstores, is priced between $30.00 and $45.00. A slipcased edition is available by subscription at $24.95.

Library of America College Editions bring these authoritative and comprehensive editions to teachers and students for the first time in an affordable paperback format.

For more information, a complete list of titles, or to place an order, contact:

The Library of America
14 East 60th Street
New York, New York 10022
Telephone: (212) 308-3360
Fax: (212) 750-8352
E-Mail: info@loa.org
Websites: www.loa.org
www.LOAacademic.org

LIBRARY OF AMERICA COLLEGE EDITIONS

American Poetry: The Nineteenth Century
John Hollander, editor
ISBN 1-883011-36-1 $14.95   1040 pages

Willa Cather • NOVELS AND STORIES 1905–1918
Sharon O'Brien, editor
The Troll Garden, O Pioneers!, The Song of the Lark, My Ántonia
ISBN 1-883011-74-4 $13.95   975 pages

Stephen Crane • PROSE AND POETRY
J. C. Levenson, editor
Maggie: A Girl of the Streets; The Red Badge of Courage; Stories;
Journalism; Poetry
ISBN 1-883011-39-6 $15.95   1379 pages

Frederick Douglass • AUTOBIOGRAPHIES
Henry Louis Gates, Jr., editor
Narrative of the Life; My Bondage and My Freedom; Life and Times
ISBN 1-883011-30-2 $13.95   1126 pages

W.E.B. Du Bois • WRITINGS
Nathan I. Huggins, editor
The Suppression of the African Slave-Trade; The Souls of Black Folk;
Dusk of Dawn; Essays & Articles from The Crisis
ISBN 1-883011-31-0 $15.95   1334 pages

Ralph Waldo Emerson • ESSAYS AND POEMS
Joel Porte, Harold Bloom, and Paul Kane, editors
Nature; Addresses, and Lectures; Essays: First and Second Series;
Representative Men; The Conduct of Life; Poems 1847;
May-Day and Other Poems; Uncollected Poems
ISBN 1-883011-32-9 $15.95   1360 pages

Nathaniel Hawthorne • TALES AND SKETCHES
Roy Harvey Pearce, editor
Twice-told Tales; Mosses from an Old Manse; The Snow Image
ISBN 1-883011-33-7 $13.95   1181 pages

Henry James • MAJOR STORIES AND ESSAYS
ISBN 1-883011-75-2 $11.95   705 pages

Sarah Orne Jewett • NOVELS AND STORIES
Michael Davitt Bell, editor
Deephaven; A Country Doctor; The Country of the Pointed Firs;
Stories and Sketches
ISBN 1-883011-34-5 $11.95   937 pages

Herman Melville • MOBY-DICK, BILLY BUDD, AND OTHER WRITINGS
G. Thomas Tanselle, Harrison Hayford, John Hollander, editors
Moby-Dick, Bartleby, The Scrivener, Benito Cereno, The Encantadas,
Billy Budd, Hawthorne and His Mosses, Selected Poems
ISBN 1-883011-89-2 $13.95   996 pages

Edgar Allan Poe • POETRY, TALES, AND SELECTED ESSAYS
Patrick F. Quinn and G. R. Thompson, editors
ISBN 1-883011-38-8 $16.95   1506 pages

Slave Narratives
William L. Andrews and Henry Louis Gates Jr., editors
ISBN 1-931082-11-1 $14.95   1035 pages

Mark Twain • HUCK FINN; PUDD'NHEAD WILSON; NO. 44, THE
MYSTERIOUS STRANGER; AND OTHER WRITINGS
Guy Cardwell and Louis J. Budd, editors
ISBN 1-883011-88-4 $12.95   808 pages

Edith Wharton • FOUR NOVELS
R.W.B. Lewis and Cynthia Griffin Wolff, editors
The House of Mirth; Ethan Frome; The Custom of the Country;
The Age of Innocence
ISBN 1-883011-37-x $13.95   1156 pages

Walt Whitman • POETRY AND PROSE
Justin Kaplan, editor
Leaves of Grass 1855; Leaves of Grass 1891–92; Supplementary Poems;
Complete Prose
ISBN 1-883011-35-3 $16.95   1407 pages

Bookstore orders: Penguin Putnam Inc., Attn: Order Processing,
405 Murray Hill Parkway, East Rutherford, NJ 07073-2136;
tel: (800) 526-0275; fax: (800) 227-9604

Exam and Desk Copy Information: www.LOAacademic.org